Medical Radiology

Radiation Oncology

Series Editors

Luther W. Brady
Stephanie E. Combs
Jiade J. Lu

Honorary Editors

Hans-Peter Heilmann
Michael Molls

For further volumes:
http://www.springer.com/series/174

Paolo Montemaggi • Mark Trombetta
Luther W. Brady
Editors

Brachytherapy

An International Perspective

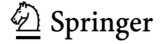 Springer

Editors
Paolo Montemaggi
Department of Radiation Oncology
Allegheny General Hospital
Pittsburgh, PA
USA

Luther W. Brady
Department of Radiation Oncology
College of Medicine, Drexel University
Philadelphia, PA
USA

Mark Trombetta
Division of Radiation Oncology
Allegheny Health Network
Cancer Institute
Drexel University College of Medicine
Pittsburgh, PA
USA

ISSN 0942-5373   ISSN 2197-4187   (electronic)
Medical Radiology
ISBN 978-3-319-26789-0   ISBN 978-3-319-26791-3   (eBook)
DOI 10.1007/978-3-319-26791-3

Library of Congress Control Number: 2016936095

Printed on acid-free paper

This Springer imprint is published by Springer Nature
The registered company is Springer International Publishing AG Switzerland

My professional life has been inspired by two main figures to whom I would like to dedicate this work, Professor Attilio Romanini, my unforgettable mentor and teacher, and Professor Luther W. Brady, who did not only lead me in my professional journey but wanted to honor me also by taking part on this work. Without these two incredible professional figures and outstanding personalities, I couldn't have done the little things I did in my professional life. Along with them I am in debt to the numerous professional figures, students, and residents who helped me to grow up both as a competent and compassionate physician. A special thought to my patients, who, through their courage and suffering taught me the real, essential values of our human life.

Paolo Montemaggi, MD

To God Almighty and Blessed Mother Mary. To the patients whom we have the honor and privilege of assisting in their care and comfort. To our colleagues and trainees with whom collaboration is an absolute and earnest joy. To my family who make life wonderful. Robin, my wife, Stephen, David, and a certain Gunny.

Mark Trombetta, MD

My thanks to all the medical students, residents, faculty, and colleagues who have contributed to the success of radiation therapy in the treatment of cancer. Without their help, the major advances in physics, biology, and clinical treatment would not have been possible. And to the patience of our families who encouraged us.

Luther W. Brady, MD

Acknowledgment

Special thank you: Information Technological assistance
Marc Luick, MS
Division of Radiation Oncology, Department of Oncology
Allegheny Health Network
Pittsburgh, PA, USA

Special thank you: Executive assistance
Lisa Weiss
Division of Radiation Oncology, Department of Oncology
Allegheny Health Network
Pittsburgh, PA, USA

Special thank you: Skin and Sarcoma chapters
Susan King
Department of Radiation Oncology
Botsford Cancer Center
Farmington Hills, MI, USA

Contents

Contributors

Editors

Paolo Montemaggi Department of Radiation Oncology, Allegheny General Hospital, Allegheny Health Network, Pittsburgh, PA, USA

Mark Trombetta Professor, Division of Radiation Oncology, Allegheny Health Network Cancer Institute, Drexel University College of Medicine, Pittsburgh, PA, USA

Luther W. Brady Radiation Oncology, Drexel University College of Medicine, Pittsburgh, PA, USA

Contributors

Douglas W. Arthur Department of Radiation Oncology, Virginia Commonwealth University School of Medicine, Richmond, VA, USA

Dimos Baltas Department of Medical Physics and Engineering, Sana Klinikum, Offenbach, Germany

Sushil Beriwal Department of Radiation Oncology, University of Pittsburgh, Pittsburgh, PA, USA

Maura Campitelli Gemelli ART (Advanced Radiation Therapy), Catholic University of the Sacred Heart, Agostino Gemelli Polyclinic, Rome, Italy

Athanasios Colonias Department of Radiation Oncology, Allegheny General Hospital, Allegheny Health Network, Pittsburgh, PA, USA

Bryan C. Coopey Department of Radiation Oncology, Allegheny Health Network, Pittsburgh, PA, USA

Juanita Crook Department of Radiation Oncology, University of British Columbia, British Columbia Cancer Agency Centre for the Southern Interior, Kelowna, BC, Canada

D. Jeffrey Demanes Professor, Department of Radiation Oncology, Division of Brachytherapy, University of California, Los Angeles, CA, USA

Beth A. Erickson Department of Radiation Oncology, Medical College of Wisconsin, Milwaukee, WI, USA

James Fontanesi Radiation Oncology, Botsford Cancer Center, Oakland University/William Beaumont School of Medicine, Farmington Hills, MI, USA

Rezarta Frakulli Radiation Oncology Center, Department of Experimental, Diagnostic and Specialty Medicine-DIMES, University of Bologna, San Orsola-Malpighi Hospital, Bologna, Italy

Andrea Galuppi Radiation Oncology Center, Department of Experimental, Diagnostic and Specialty Medicine-DIMES, University of Bologna, San Orsola-Malpighi Hospital, Bologna, Italy

Maria Antonietta Gambacorta Gemelli ART (Advanced Radiation Therapy), Catholic University of the Sacred Heart, Agostino Gemelli Polyclinic, Rome, Italy

Alain Gerbaulet Department of Radiotherapy, Institut Gustave-Roussy, Villejuif, France

Patrizia Guerrieri Department of Radiation Oncology, Allegheny Health Network, Temple University of College of Medicine, Pittsburgh, PA, USA

Jean-Michel Hannoun-Levi Radiation Therapy Department, Antoine Lacassagne Cancer Center, Nice, France

Jaroslaw T. Hepel Department of Radiation Oncology, Rhode Island Hospital, Warren Alpert Medical School of Brown University, Providence, RI, USA

Peter Hoskin Consultant in Clinical Oncology, Professor, Mount Vernon Cancer Centre and University College Northwood, London, UK

Thomas B. Julian Department of Surgery, Temple University School of Medicine, Drexel University College of Medicine, Allegheny Health Network, Pittsburgh, PA, USA

Stephen Karlovits Allegheny Health Network Cancer Institute, Allegheny General Hospital, Pittsburgh, PA, USA

Radiation Oncology, Temple University School of Medicine, Pittsburgh, PA, USA

Brian Kopitzki Department of Dermatology, Michigan State College of Osteopathic Medicine, East Lansing, MI, USA

Rodney J. Landreneau Department of Thoracic Surgery, Allegheny General Hospital, Allegheny Health Network, Pittsburgh, PA, USA

Zuofeng Li Department of Radiation Oncology, University of Florida College of Medicine, Gainesville, FL, USA

UF Health Proton Therapy Institute, Jacksonville, FL, USA

Xing Liang Radiation Physics Solution LLC, Garnet Valley, PA, USA

Pei Shuen Lim Specialist Registrar in Clinical Oncology, Mount Vernon Cancer Centre, Northwood, UK

Tibor Major Department of Medical Physics, Center of Radiotherapy, National Institute of Oncology, Budapest, Hungary

Stefania Manfrida Gemelli ART (Advanced Radiation Therapy), Catholic University of the Sacred Heart, Agostino Gemelli Polyclinic, Rome, Italy

Jeffrey Margolis Department of Oncology, Oakland University, William Beaumont Medical School, Rochester, MI, USA

Moyed Miften Department of Radiation Oncology, University of Colorado School of Medicine, Aurora, CO, USA

Konrad Mohnike Department of Radiology and Nuclear Medicine, Otto-von-Guericke-University Magdeburg, Magdeburg, Germany

Gabrielle Monit Oakland Medical Group, Michigan Healthcare Professionals, Oakland, MI, USA

Alessio G. Morganti Department of Experimental Oncology Center, Department of Experimental, Diagnostic and Specialty Medicine-DIMES, University of Bologna, San Orsola-Malpighi Hospital, Bologna, Italy

Michael Mott Orthopedic Oncology, Henry Ford Hospital, Detroit, MI, USA

Jean-Philippe Pignol Radiation Oncology Department, Erasmus Medical Center, Rotterdam, The Netherlands

Csaba Polgár Center of Radiotherapy, National Institute of Oncology, Budapest, Hungary

Cynthia Pope Department of Radiation Oncology, Beth Israel Deaconess Hospital, Plymouth, MA, USA

Paul Renz Department of Oncology, Allegheny General Hospital, Pittsburgh, PA, USA

Jens Ricke Department of Radiology and Nuclear Medicine, Otto-von-Guericke-University Magdeburg, Magdeburg, Germany

Leah K. Schubert Department of Radiation Oncology, University of Colorado School of Medicine, Aurora, CO, USA

Luca Tagliaferri Gemelli ART (Advanced Radiation Therapy), Catholic University of the Sacred Heart, Agostino Gemelli Polyclinic, Rome, Italy

Dorin A. Todor Department of Radiation Oncology, Virginia Commonwealth University Health System, Richmond, VA, USA

Nikolaos Tselis Department of Radiation Oncology and Interdisciplinary Oncology, Sana Klinikum, Offenbach, Germany

Vincenzo Valentini Gemelli ART (Advanced Radiation Therapy), Catholic University of the Sacred Heart, Agostino Gemelli Polyclinic, Rome, Italy

Matthew Van Deusen Department of Thoracic Surgery, Allegheny General Hospital, Allegheny Health Network, Pittsburgh, PA, USA

Erik Van Limbergen Department of Radiotherapy, University of Gasthuisberg, Leuven, Belgium

John A. Vargo Department of Radiation Oncology, University of Pittsburgh, Pittsburgh, PA, USA

Thierry Verstraeten Department of Ophthalmology, Allegheny Ophthalmic and Orbital Associates, Drexel University College of Medicine, Pittsburgh, PA, USA

Frank Vicini Department of Radiation Oncology, St. Joseph Mercy Oakland, Pontiac, MI, USA

Akila N. Viswanathan Department of Radiation Oncology, Brigham and Women's Hospital and Dana-Farber Cancer Institute, Harvard Medical School, Boston, MA, USA

David E. Wazer Departments of Radiation Oncology, Tufts Medical Center, Tufts University School of Medicine, Rhode Island Hospital, Alpert Medical School of Brown University, Boston, MA, USA

Theodore E. Yaeger IV Professor, Department of Radiation Oncology, University of North Carolina, Chapel Hill, NC, USA

Jun Yang Professor, Department of Radiation Oncology, College of Medicine, Drexel University, Philadelphia, PA, USA

Philadelphia Cyberknife Center, Delaware County Memorial Hospital, Havertown, PA, USA

Nikolaos Zamboglou Department of Radiation Oncology and Interdisciplinary Oncology, Sana Klinikum, Offenbach, Germany

Introduction

Theodore E. Yaeger IV , Luther W. Brady,
Mark Trombetta, and Paolo Montemaggi

The second half of the nineteenth century was a time for great discovery. People were introduced to the vacuum cleaner, the light bulb, phonographs, radio, automobiles, and airplanes, among other things. This new beginning was made ever more important because it also ushered in a new era of widespread communication. The new rapid transfer of information was faster, more efficient, and more accurate than ever before.

When William Conrad Roentgen, a professor of physics at Würzburg University, noted the newly developed cathode ray tube produced penetrating "rays," he presented the finding to the Würzburg Society in 1895. For this he shortly thereafter received the very first Nobel Prize in

T.E. Yaeger IV, MD
Professor, Department of Radiation Oncology,
University of North Carolina, Chapel Hill, NC, USA

L.W. Brady, MD (✉)
Radiation Oncology, Drexel University College of
Medicine, Philadelphia, PA, USA
e-mail: luther.brady@drexelmed.edu

M. Trombetta, MD
Professor, Division of Radiation Oncology,
Allegheny Health Network Cancer Institute,
Drexel University College of Medicine,
320 East North Avenue, Pittsburgh, PA, USA
e-mail: mtrombet@wpahs.org

P. Montemaggi, MD
Radiation Oncology (Emeritus), Allegheny Health
Network, Temple University School of Medicine,
Pittsburgh Campus, Pittsburgh, PA, USA
e-mail: montemaggi.p@gmail.com

physics in 1901. It was quickly recognized that very few medical breakthroughs benefitted mankind more than this new "X-ray" and the new communication capabilities rapidly transmitted the discovery. It was (and still is) named "X" because of the unexplained nature of this form of radiation.

Roentgen noted his crudely cardboard-covered "Crookes tube" produced fluorescence from a nearby tube and quickly recognized it must represent a more distant radiation. He thought it indicated something more penetrating that just fluorescence. Thus, on November 8, 1895, the new "X-ray" was discovered. Soon he noted images of his hand bones when it was accidentally exposed onto a barium-plated oxycyanide screen. On December 22, 1895, he produced the now famous image of his wife's left hand, wedding ring obviously visible. This became the first intentionally documented filmed X-ray image. It was immediately reported in Vienna (Die Presse) that the discovery could evaluate bone fractures without the usual painful manipulation. The good news spread like wildfire. Historically it is interesting to note that Professor Goodspeed at the University of Pennsylvania also reported images of common streetcar tokens from radiation exposure onto film but he did not recognize the significance.

Regardless, the news of human images in Europe quickly spread to America within a few days. X-ray images were quickly applied to a variety of medical procedures. Following Roentgen's discovery, clinical and technological

© Springer International Publishing Switzerland 2016
P. Montemaggi et al. (eds.), *Brachytherapy: An International Perspective*, Medical Radiology,
DOI 10.1007/978-3-319-26791-3_1

skills began to accumulate more rapidly than the basic knowledge of the biological effects of radiation. However, the toxicities of radiation exposure began to be reported shortly after the discovery. A British physician, credited with the first clinical X-ray in England, developed skin cancer in his hands while experimenting with X-rays. Thomas Edison noted his assistant developed hair loss and eventually died from metastatic skin cancer. In stark contrast, a patient suffering from advanced breast cancer was exposed to radiation in 1896 by Emil Grubbe. She developed an objective and favorable response. Even given that the treatment technique was crude and exposure time was long, that beneficial response was dramatic.

Because of the growing reports of toxicity, measures were soon adopted to prevent or minimize undesired radiation exposure but the popularity of X-ray continued to grow. Importantly, it was discovered that images of the whole chest could diagnose tuberculosis. This was significant as tuberculosis was the leading cause of death in the last half of the nineteenth century. Besides the new X-ray, radiation was detected from a solid uranium source by Becquerel in 1896. Subsequently Marie and Pierre Curie showed that the Becquerel radiation could be accurately measured using ionization techniques. By December 1898, the Curies were able to produce reliable radiation from a purified source of pitchblende and called it "radium."

The first known patient to have been treated with a combination of external beam radiotherapy and radium was reported at the Memorial Sloan-Kettering Cancer Center for treating a cervix cancer. At the International Congress of Oncology in Paris, about 1922, Coutard and Hautant presented the data in the treatment of advanced laryngeal cancers. They described a technique lasting about 7 weeks. This became the standard by which patients are treated today. Subsequently, and continuing today, there are vast numbers of medical reports identifying the positive and beneficial effects of radiation.

The Curies' radium became a standard source to develop locally applied radiation treatment and eventually evolved into radium needles and the

daughter product radon, captured in glass tubes as a shorter half-life gas for more permanent placements. Both of these devices were often inserted directly into tumors. Edith Quimby demonstrated that a specific pattern of radiation effects could be reproduced using specific implant patterns. Other researchers applied various implant techniques and eventually the "Patterson-Parker" system (also known as the Manchester system) became widely popular and taught as a standard of care beginning circa 1934.

From a historic point of appreciation, the term "brachytherapy" is derived from the Greek word "brachy" meaning close and the more common term "therapy" for treatment. The utilization of this technique was suggested to a physician by Pierre Curie in about 1901 to insert a radium tube directly into a patient's tumor. This was before the advent of megavoltage radiation which would eventually become external beam radiotherapy. So, at least initially, brachytherapy was a significant and integral part of (mostly) palliative but occasionally curative management of cancer patients. It certainly became a standard adjuvant or primary treatment for many cancers such as cervix, breast, head and neck, etc., and is obviously still very much in use today.

It should be noted that both Henri Becquerel and Madame Curie were awarded the Nobel Peace Prize for physics in 1903. After WWI, the Radium Institute was opened in which cancer specialists came from all over the world and converged to study radiation. In 1930 a major center for brachytherapy was opened in England as the Holt Radium Institute where Drs. Patterson, Parker, and Meredith developed a mathematical system of brachytherapy. It was published as the Manchester System in 1934. While other radioactive sources were developed (cobalt-60, cesium-137, iridium-192, etc.), it was not until about 1953 that an afterloader system using plastic tubes and gold-198 seeds was developed. In 1965, Pierquin and Dutreix determined the rules of a new system of dosimetry which was named "the Paris System." Intracavitary application to the cervix and uterine corpus soon followed.

In contemporary practice, many new isotopes have been added to the brachytherapy armamentarium. Many have been developed to improve the safety of using radioactive sources as well as convenience of storage. The original radium-226 has largely been replaced by cesium, iridium, iodine, and palladium and some less commonly used sources. While remote afterloading is not new, the latest iterations employ a small-volume ("rice grain") high-activity source such as a 10 curie iridium-192 source. Remote afterloading has dramatically increased the safety of medical personnel by limiting radiation to the specific patient in a designated radiation-protected (vault) area. This has essentially revolutionized brachytherapy, bringing a revival of the implant treatment modality. Moreover, advances in computer calculation technology have fostered the development of increasingly more sophisticated treatment planning techniques and low-dose afterloading has largely been replaced with high-dose, short-interval implant delivery. Primarily iridium-192-based units with highly sophisticated computer-controlled applicators are most common. It should be noted there is a unique application using a high-dose rate balloon with P-32 for angioplasty to prevent coronary restenosis after dilatation for revascularization and locally applied external beam brachytherapy is developing.

Physicians using various brachytherapy techniques formed the American Radium Society in 1916 intended to allow the exchange of scientific information regarding the utilization of brachytherapy. This society consisted of cancer-interested physicians from various disciplines such as gynecology, surgery, radiologists and now radiation and medical oncologists, and specialist pathologists. The American Radium Society has fostered multiple specialists to better define brachytherapy indications for applications as modern brachytherapy is still defined as the technique of placing treatment sources very close to or within target tumor tissues. Utilizing the concept of rapid dose degradation with distance (inverse square rule), high tumor doses can be safely delivered to localized target regions in a relatively short period of time. This will use implantation techniques of interstitial, intracavitary, or topical molds (plaques) either placed surgically into the tumor or placed clinically depending on the diagnosis and location. The implant can be placed temporarily as in intracavitary cervix cancer or permanently as in a prostate cancer seed implant. Also, there are various types of source loading techniques/technologies. They include preloaded, manually afterloaded, or remotely loaded devices. The dose rate for the first is typically low and can be high or low for the mid and the latter is usually high dose rate. The tumor location typically determines the implantation technique as follows:

Intracavitary brachytherapy is commonly used for the treatment of localized gynecologic, esophageal, or bronchus malignancies. These implants are site-specific equipment which are temporarily left in a patient for a specific period of time to deliver a prescribed dose.

Interstitial brachytherapy uses sources typically placed with needles either individual radioactive seeds or pre-calculated loaded seeds. Older radium or cesium needles are temporary, but radioactive seeds are usually permanent using Pd-103 or I-125. Flexible catheters or ribbons of preloaded I-125 seeds can be temporarily inserted into tumors as seen commonly in oral cancers. Surface-dose applications can be custom molds or pre-constructed plaques which can use either low- or high-dose sources. They are designed to hold the radioactivity onto a surface to allow uniform dose distribution to the intended surface area.

Intraluminal brachytherapy consists of a temporary insertion of a single line source, usually afterloaded using a high dose rate and inserted into a body lumen to treat the surface and proximal and immediately adjacent tumors. Typically this is for palliation of a symptomatic obstruction or bleeding tumor but can be used as part of a curative attempt as a boost to the primary localized tumor site. Until the 1980s, radioactive sources were placed directly into the patient, typically using radium or cesium. Unfortunately this caused radioactive exposure not only to the implanting physician but also to assisting personnel. More recently, remote afterloading has allowed the surgical placement of devices or catheters within the safety of a radiation-protected environment. In the beginning, this concept was done using fairly crude manipulation of the loader. More recently and commonly used today, all loading is automatic and computer controlled for more precise and accurate delivery. After the prescribed treatment is completed, all sources are removed. In this manner, radiation exposure is only given to the desired patient and to the intended target tissues.

The evolution of brachytherapy technologies has progressed consistently. The development of high-dose, afterloading applicators and concomitant delivery technologies has improved significantly during the last decades. Now there is an expectation of precise placement with accurate, reliable delivery and with more appropriate distribution of the desired radiation dose. Beneficially, these newer devices/techniques maximize brachytherapy effectiveness while also maximizing radiation protection to the treating staff. Although low-dose brachytherapy is still applicable to specific diagnoses, almost all modern radiation/brachytherapy treatment programs have the capability for high-dose rate, remote afterloading for the appropriate circumstances.

It is interesting to note that the evolution from low-dose rate, high-personnel exposure implant techniques to the contemporary high dose rate and limited staff exposure has mostly occurred in the absence of repeated and verified randomized controlled clinical trials. However, this paradigm shift is not wholly inconsistent with many other major technological breakthroughs that modern radiotherapy has experienced in recent decades. These would include advanced, precise, accurate,

safe, and computer-controlled radiation delivery techniques and technologies.

The early years of radiation delivery were fueled by the use of the newly discovered X-ray and raw radioactive sources in the diagnosis and crude treatment of cancers. By 1945 nearly 5–6 million people were given diagnostic X-ray chest exams as part of a large-scale public health screening program to diagnose tuberculosis and to assist in surgical interventions. By 1950 the number of radiologic exams had more than doubled to about 15 million per year. Since about 1980 to present, that number has significantly grown to about 80 or 100 million people receiving a diagnostic and 260,000 a therapeutic radiologic procedure with approximately 80,000 patients undergoing some form of brachytherapy annually. Apparently, the treatment efficiency and cost-effectiveness of modern brachytherapy are driving resurgence in this approach to treat cancer. It is now commonplace to see high-dose rate treatment for breast cancer and high- or low-dose rate therapy for prostate and gynecologic cancers. Newer on the scene is the budding technique of low-energy (Kv) electronic brachytherapy for intraoperative or topical applications, including treatment of limited skin cancers.

The intent of this volume is to present contemporary issues in brachytherapy. The authors wish to explore these possibilities to better define the concept and application of brachytherapy, to explore increasing the potential for improved locoregional tumor control, and to diminish any risk increases from various programs, as well as specific therapeutic modalities.

Brachytherapy: A Journey of Hope in the Battle Against Cancer

"Historia Magistra Vitae"

Paolo Montemaggi and Patrizia Guerrieri

When Maria Curie discovered natural radioactivity, she probably did not forecast how much that discovery would impact not only the field of physics but the entire field of medicine. It didn't take long, however, to see how this newly discovered energy could affect living cells and tissues. As early as 1901, we find evidence of radium (^{226}Ra) being used for treating skin conditions of all types, even noncancerous such as lupus erythematosus. And once again, those pioneers did not probably foresee how much ^{226}Ra and its derivatives would change the treatment scenario of cancer treatment. What we know is that as early as 1908 there were already several publications in the literature and that the long journey of radium and radioactive elements in cancer therapy had begun [1–5]. It has been a fascinating journey, not always easy, but always focused on the search for a better, safer, and more effective ways to use this natural energy in the complex and challenging field of cancer therapy.

This book is aimed to help those who are continuing this journey, allowing them to understand where they come from and to move their efforts and research in the right direction, for, as Cicero put it, it

is in our history, in our past, and in its knowledge that we may root to build our future, "historia magistra vitae": history is the teacher of life.

Brachytherapy is a Greek-derived word composed by two words, *brachy*, short, and *therapy*, to cure. The root indicates the use of radioactivity in the treatment of cancer by putting the radioactive sources into a tumor or at short distance from it. In reality, when its history began, the discipline given name was Curietherapy, as a way to honor the work of Maria and Pierre Curie and their contribution to the science of radioactivity. It was only several decades later, when more sophisticated and effective machines for external beam radiotherapy became available, that the discipline was renamed *brachytherapy* to differentiate it from the "teletherapy" (Gr: long or distant) that those machines allowed. Regardless how you want to name it, brachytherapy has been a main focus in the use of radiation as a means to battle cancer. It is in this way that we may view our journey, a continuous and strenuous effort to find a more efficient and effective way to use the new energy to fight the enemy, to ultimately defeat cancer. In this effort we may individuate some major themes:

- The search for dose: the pioneers and the historic systems
- The search for strategy: new isotopes, new systems, new challenges
- The search for the target volume: from clinic to imaging

P. Montemaggi, MD (✉)
Radiation Oncology (Emeritus), Allegheny Health Network, Temple University School of Medicine, Pittsburgh Campus, Pittsburgh, PA, USA
e-mail: montemaggi.p@gmail.com

P. Guerrieri, MD, MS
Radiation Oncology, Allegheny Health Network, Temple University School of Medicine, Pittsburgh Campus, Pittsburgh, PA, USA

© Springer International Publishing Switzerland 2016
P. Montemaggi et al. (eds.), *Brachytherapy: An International Perspective*, Medical Radiology,
DOI 10.1007/978-3-319-26791-3_2

Following these themes, we will review our history up to the present and foresee where we might go and how to continue to pursue our target: our unchanged ultimate scope, the defeat of cancer.

1 The Search for Dose

The earliest attempts to use the newly discovered energy as a possible cancer treatment were, one could say, conducted in tumors arising from easily accessible sites. Among the accessible sites, gynecologic cancers became almost immediately the most important field of application and research. For the early decades of the twentieth century, gynecologic cancers became the fertile field for advancing the knowledge and improving the results that could be obtained through the clinical use of radioactive sources.

When the pioneers of this new methodology began their journey, the preminent method of research was trial and error. The earliest trials consisted of putting a quantity of radioactive material in contact with an accessible lesion and making reference to the time that radioactive source was left in place. In other words, the reference unit milligram-hours (mg/h) was born, a reference that remained unchanged for more than 50 years and that keeps its relevance even to this modern day as a means of comparison of previous and new experiences. It might not seem such a big thing to our now "educated" eyes, but it was a great achievement, allowing the comparison of different experiences and results by a very simple methodology and reference unit [6, 7]. Eventually, however, it became clear that this exclusively quantitative method of evaluation was not enough: that further knowledge and standardization were needed to allow effective comparison and prediction. It was during the first and second decades of the twentieth century that several different systems were designed to allow a rationale planning for the use of radioactive sources. It is beyond the limit of this short review to provide a complete description of those systems, but it is certainly important that we know those systems and learn from what

they were based on. It is not only important that we know those systems; it is also highly educational because, as we will see, the principles on which they were based will remain as cornerstones in the future evolution of the discipline, leading to different ways of thought that still permeate the brachytherapy treatment schedules we use today. In fact, these historic systems will eventually lead the way to the different radiobiological approaches to dose-time relationships and low, high, and pulsed dose rate that presently characterize the discipline. All the diatribes and discussions we have witnessed over the last 40 years root back to those historic systems: to the theoretical principles on which they were based.

Both in Europe and in the United States, the efficacy of ^{226}Ra in gynecologic (GYN) cancer treatment was recognized quite immediately [5, 8, 9] especially for cervical cancer. By the end of 1930s, three major centers had already developed systems to properly and effectively plan how to use radium in the treatment of cervical cancer. They differ in the shape and material of applicators as well as, more importantly, in the quantity and distribution of radioactive sources.

It is also interesting to see, as further endorsement of the continuity referred to earlier, that the different radiobiological considerations and hypotheses underlying low and high dose rate, and continuous and fractionated irradiation, have taken place and originated from the same cultural milieu that introduced and applied similar radiobiological concepts, even if in a preliminary form, in those historic systems for GYN implants:

1. Paris system
2. Manchester system
3. Stockholm system

The main differences between those systems relate to the application length as a function of the radioactive load, basically introducing in clinical practice the fundamentals of what will become eventually the concept of low and high dose rate we deal with today.

The concepts on which those three different systems were based are compared in Table 1.

7

Table 1 Comparison of historic dosimetric systems

Paris [10, 11]	Stockholm [12]	Manchester [13]
Continuous treatment (4–5 days) Uterine tube 30/35 Ra mg Two cylindrical cork vaginal applicators, 10/15 Ra mg	Three insertions every other week Two vaginal silver packers, up to 60/80 Ra mg	Two 72 h insertions over total 10 days' time Three different uterine loadings: 25, 25, and 20 Ra mg for different uterine cavity lengths Large, medium, and small vaginal ovoid, varying in loading from 22.5, to 20, to 17.5 Ra mg

The long journey to find the best way to use the new energy had begun. However, even if those systems helped planning the implants and allowed for comparison of results, still the result was a mere quantitative analysis of the dose.

The first step toward a more sophisticated description of dose distribution came from the Manchester group, through the definition of anatomic reference points [13, 14]. The introduction of those points for the first time defined the dose not just in a generic way, but tried to understand *where* the dose was being delivered; it defined, at the same time, the dose needed both to achieve local control of the disease and to prevent the occurrence of adverse events as much as possible. Points A and B have constituted a cornerstone of GYN brachytherapy everywhere since then, allowing for the comparison of results from different institutions and from different countries. The relevance and significance of those two points were recognized by ICRU 38 which was devoted to the standardization of dose in GYN brachytherapy [15] and still today remain the yardstick to be used when evaluating a brachytherapy implant [16]. However, modern image technology has deeply modified our capacity to see and understand dose distribution, and radiobiology has given us a better way of understanding relationships between dose and fractionation. Even if Manchester points are not any longer decisive in implant evaluation, they remain viv-

idly on the scene, a clear sign that no solid progress can be done if it is not rooted in history and experience.

The definition of points A and B was not the only relevant contribution of the Manchester group in the development of brachytherapy. In a process spanning many years, researchers from Manchester elaborated a system that allowed for the rational planning of a brachytherapy implant according to the surface or volume of the lesion to be treated. The results of this complex elaboration were made available and easy to use through a series of tables, known as Paterson-Parker tables [17]. They were designed with multiple scopes based on the surface and/or volumes to be treated:

1. To predict the amount of radioactive material to be used to deliver 1000 mg/h in the surface/volume
2. To predict the geographic distribution of that material throughout the surface/volume to obtain a "homogeneous" distribution of the dose and to prevent or reduce to the minimum the risk for "cold" or "hot" spot in the implant, through specific mathematic rules determining the relative load at the center and periphery of the implant
3. To be used with different radioactive sources, provided the specific activity of the used isotope is known

The work of the Manchester group provided a great impetus for further spread and implementation of brachytherapy and maintained its value and validity to the present day. Brachytherapy treatment planning systems are still based on the concepts elaborated from that group, and when modern imaging techniques allowed for a more realistic and exact determination of the extent of the lesion, the validity of those concepts was proven again.

Another system, similar to that of Manchester, was elaborated in the United States by Quimby [18], looking at the same goals but simplifying the logistic of the radioactive material. While the Manchester system was based on the availability of radioactive sources of different activity requiring a vast range and number of tubes and/or needles, Quimby proposed the use of sources of homogeneous activity, yet aiming to maintain concepts similar to those of Manchester as far as the geographic distribution of the isotope.

Over the first five decades of the twentieth century, brachytherapy established its role as the main stem of radiotherapy in cancer treatment. It was then that something happened that put a different perspective in the use of its use in cancer treatment.

Following World War II and the research done in the field of nuclear physics, a new generation of machines that allowing more sophisticated external beam radiotherapy was developed and made available for use in clinical practice. In 1953, ^{60}Co machines became available and, a few years later, the in linear accelerators again revolutionized the rapidly developing field of external beam radiotherapy. The natal technology highlighted new possibilities and advantages, in terms of depth dose, dose homogeneity, and radiation safety. At the same time, concerns were growing about the risks connected to the use of ^{226}Ra, both for patients, in connection with integral dose and staff safety due to the high energy and depth penetration of its radiation that required the use of cumbersome and expensive means of surgical tools and radiation protection shields. The balance shifted toward a rapidly declining use of brachytherapy in favor of external beam treatment. Was the end of brachytherapy nigh? No. New isotopes and new systems gave renewed impulse to its practice.

2   The Search for Strategy: New Isotopes, New Systems, New Challenges

It was thanks to French researchers that brachytherapy was "revived" toward the end of the 1950s. The same technological advancements that made possible the linear accelerator were used to improve techniques, clinical indications, and strategies for brachytherapy. The basis of this new impulse was the design of a new family of artificially created isotopes for clinical use, based on a set of differences from the physics and infrastructure requirements typical of ^{226}Ra. New iso-

Table 2 Radium substitute characteristics (ideal)

Characteristic	226 Ra	226 Ra substitutes
Energy	High (average >0.8 Mv)	Low to moderate (29–400 Kv)
Half-life	Long (>1,600 year)	Short (days to months)
Radiation spectrum	Multi energies	Single energy
Source dose rate	Fixed	Variable
Flexibility	No	Yes
Malleability	No	Yes
Miniaturization	No	Yes
Clinical accessibility	Scarce	Ample
Heavy shielding	Yes	No
Afterloading capability	No	Yes
Remote afterloading	No	Yes
Staff protection	Difficult	Yes

topes in development should have specific characteristics devised to ease their application and safety in clinical use. These new isotopes were generally referred to as radium substitutes. Their characteristics in comparison with those of ^{226}Ra are shown in Table 2.

Several ^{226}Ra substitutes were proposed (Table 3) and some of them came to be used in clinical practice for temporary or permanent implants, but one of those became the cornerstone of this new era of brachytherapy: ^{192}iridium. Its success was due not only (nor primarily) to its own physical characteristics but mainly to the system expressly designed by French researchers for its clinical use [19]. This system, which we may refer to as the new Paris system, made ^{192}Ir clinical use simple and reliable, allowing for implant preplanning, image verification, and result comparison. It is not valid for any other isotope, which could ordinarily be a limitation, but its basic concepts can be used more generally to evaluate and optimize the quality of an implant in terms of homogeneity.

The availability of these new isotopes had a great impact on clinical practice of brachytherapy and opened a series of new possibilities and

Table 3 Most used radium substitutes

Element	Isotope	Energy (MeV)	Half-life	Hvl-lead (mm)	Clinical application
Radium	^{226}Ra	0.83 (average)	1,626 years	16	LDR intracavitary – interstitial
Cesium	^{137}Cs	0.662	30 years	3.28	LDR intracavitary
Iridium	^{192}Ir	0.397	73.8 days	6	LDR interstitial, endoluminal, HDR, interstitial, intravascular
Cobalt	^{60}Co	1.25	5.26 years	11	HDR intracavitary
Iodine	^{125}I	0.028	59.5 days	0.025	Permanent interstitial
Palladium	^{103}Pd	0.020	17 days	0.013	Permanent interstitial
Californium	^{252}Cf	2.4 (average) neutron	2.65 years	–	High-LET LDR intracavitary

the development of a new treatment strategy. Many distinguished physicians and physicists contributed to the implementation of the new possibilities using radium substitutes, both in Europe and in the United States. Names such as Pierquin, Chassagne, Pernot, and Dutreix in Europe and others such as Henshcke, Fletcher, Montague, and Anderson in the United States remain and will remain in the history of medicine as eminent researchers who dedicated their entire life to the battle against cancer. It was not just a cultural innovation but opened a completely new world of opportunities for clinical cancer treatment. The last decades of the twentieth century saw the contemporary development of new drugs, new imaging techniques, new surgical procedures, and a new family of isotopes, differently intertwined for a new era of cancer treatment. The fight still rages, but those new perspectives opened the way to new opportunities that completely changed the scenario of the battlefield.

These new strategies developed somewhat differently in Europe and in the United States, but the goals were the same on both sides of the Atlantic Ocean: optimizing the use of radioactive sources in cancer treatment strategies, maximizing clinical results, and minimizing the negative impact of adverse events. New possibilities emerged in terms of dose-time relationship and the integration of brachytherapy in a multidisciplinary approach to cancer treatment. Temporary and permanent implants and low- and

high-dose rate techniques for which specific machines were designed and implemented, along with the development of isotopes specifically designed to fit the requests and needs of these different strategies, have been the backbone of both physics and clinical researchers over the last decades of the twentieth century and the early part of this century.

During these decades, brachytherapy has known a great development but has also been called to face new challenges that emerged from competitors such as stereotactic radiosurgery, stereotactic brain and body radiotherapy, and intensity-modulated radiotherapy which all are able to simulate, even though not always to reproduce, dose distributions and clinical results previously only achievable by a brachytherapy implant. Furthermore, these new technologies do not require additional surgical skills and temporal constraints (as needed with brachytherapy) to add to the heavy burden of knowledge and technical ability already existing on the shoulders of radiation oncologists. All these factors have challenged the clinical practice of brachytherapy, progressively tending to limit its use, and, more importantly, its actual teaching in residency programs. The new generation of radiation oncologists sees less and less of brachytherapy and is more and more focused on the use of images for treatment optimization through external beam radiotherapy. But the battle is not over yet.

3   The Search for Volume: From Clinic to Imaging

As it has been with the advent of new external beam radiotherapy machines, also new medical imagery techniques have determined a series of challenges and opportunities. Clinicians moved from the foggy imagery of traditional bidimensional radiology to the exciting realm of virtually entering the human body to explore and reconstruct in three-dimensional ways the anatomy and the pathological alterations caused by cancer. The concept of cancer volume has been completely modified, as it allowed for a more precise definition of that volume and of its relationship to the adjacent normal structures. This poses new questions and problems regarding the distribution of the dose in the volume. New concepts were proposed to adjust dose distribution to those actual volumes. The contemporary development of more sophisticated and powerful computers made that adjustment possible. All of these did open the way to a more complex and real understanding of the different volumes included in the treated area and to a more detailed description of the dose distribution and dose-effect relationship. Along with new imaging techniques, biological knowledge about the complex biological reality of cancer allowed for a deeper understanding of the impact that different doses and different dose-time relationships would have on the tumor and on the surrounding normal tissues and structures. Lately, imaging techniques moved from solely a morphological representation of the body to describing the functional activity of tissues, organs, and pathological lesions (Table 4). Nowadays a range of morphological and functional imaging techniques give us precise reconstruction of the anatomy and the functionality of normal and pathological structures. This has been reflected in the definition of different volumes of interest both in external beam radiotherapy and in brachytherapy. Several ICRU documents have addressed this new reality, defining and describing these new reference volumes [15, 16].

As a consequence of these new opportunities and deeper knowledge of dose-volume and dose-time relationship, external beam radiotherapy has evolved and has reached a sophisticated level of capacity to focus the dose to small and well-defined areas, mimicking the major advantage of brachytherapy. All these new highly focused external beam radiotherapy techniques have challenged brachytherapists and have promoted a deep reflection to re-imagine the role of brachytherapy in cancer treatment. The first result of that challenge has been a similar process of integrating and using modern images in brachytherapy. Guidelines have been proposed and tested that allow the use, description, and comparison of brachytherapy treatment to image-defined volumes [20–22]. Modern imaging techniques, both morphological and functional, are now taken into account in implant planning, dose prescription, and reporting, as well as in evaluating clinical results both in terms of disease control and adverse event prevention.

We are certainly far from where we started more than 100 years ago. Most of the uncertainties and unknowns we faced then have been clarified and solved. On the other hand, brachytherapy is challenged by highly focused external beam radiotherapy techniques claiming to guarantee the same clinical results and the same normal structure protection against adverse events. Still there are areas in which brachytherapy remains a step ahead and in which it maintains a preemi-

Table 4 Volumes of interest and related imaging techniques

Volume	Definition	CT	MRI	fMRI	PET	Image fusion
GTV	Gross tumor volume as defined clinically and by imaging	Yes	Yes	Yes	No	Yes
CTV	GTV + margins to define the area in which microscopic infiltration of the disease is present	No	No	Yes	Yes	Yes
BTV	Volume that shows a significant variation of biological activity	No	No	Yes	Yes	Yes
PTV	Volume that receives the prescribed dose according to beam or source arrangements	Yes	Yes	Yes	Yes	Yes

nent role and how still important brachytherapy is in clinical practice.

As we have seen earlier in the text, modern radiotherapy is moving more and more toward a sophisticated use of highly focused external beam radiotherapy techniques and we may be tempted to forget about brachytherapy. It is complex, requires skills that are unusual for us, and requires specific training that is not widely available. It seems easier just to sit in front of a computer screen drawing contours and working with physicists and dosimetrists to develop a sophisticated dose plan, all of which is probably true. However, being easier doesn't make it always the right choice.

It is necessary that the principles developed over decades of experience and clinical results of brachytherapy are not forgotten as useless memories. They still can teach us a lot, and must remain a solid knowledge basis in our discipline. This is the purpose of this book. Through a rapid excursion on what brachytherapy has represented in the development of clinical radiotherapy, we want to remind all of us that something good may come from our past and that past lessons must not be forgotten because "historia magistra vitae." Brachytherapy is a fundamental component of our history and we cannot neither forget what it has thought us, nor abandon its path just because it seems easier. It is our duty to carry on this teaching and transmit it to the new generations to build a future solidly rooted in the knowledge and experience that our history has taught.

Bibliography

1. Williams FH (1904) A comparison between the medical uses of the x-rays and the rays from the salts of radium. Boston Med Surg J 150:206–209
2. Williams FH (1908) Early treatment of some superficial cancers, especially epitheliomas, by pure radium bromide than operation or X-rays. JAMA 51:847–849
3. Dallas H (1904) Sur l'action physiologique et therapeutique du radium. Mem Soc Pharmacol 9:65–74
4. Dominici H, Barcat J (1908) L'action therapeutique du radium sur les neoplasies. Arch d'électric méd 16:655–663
5. Wickham L, Degrais P (1910) Radiumtherapy. Cassel and Company, London, Translation of the original French 1909 edition Radiumthérapie
6. Baskerville C (1905) Radium and radio-active substances: their application especially to medicine. Chapter VI. In: The physiological action of radioactive substances and their therapeutic applications. Williams, Brown & Earle, Philadelphia
7. Wickham L, Degrais P (1913) Radium as employed in the treatment of cancer, angiomata, keloids, local tuberculosis and other affectations. Paul B Hebert, New York
8. Pudsey WA, Caldwell EW (1910) The practical application of the Roentgen rays in therapeutics and diagnosis, 2nd edn. Saunders, Philadelphia
9. Abbe R (1914) Die anwedung von Radium bei Karzinom and Sarkom. Strahlentherapie 4:27–35
10. Birkett GE (1931) Radium therapy: principles and practice. Cassel, London
11. Cheval M, Dustin AP (1931) Theorie at pratique de la Telecurietherapie. Masson, Paris
12. Heyman J (1935) The so-called Stockholm method and the results of treatment of uterine cancer at the Radiumhemmet. Acta Radiol 16:129–148
13. Tod M, Meredith WJ (1938) A dosage system for use in the treatment of cancer of the uterine cervix. Br J Radiol 11:809–823
14. Meredith WJ (1967) Dosage for cancer of the cervix uteri. In: Meredith WJ (ed) Radium dosage: the Manchester system, 2nd edn. E&S Livingston, Ltd, Edinburgh
15. ICRU 38: dose and volume specifications for reporting intracavitary treatment in gynecology (1985) International Committee for Radiation Units
16. ICRU 58: dose and volume specification for reporting interstitial brachytherapy (1997) International Committee for Radiation Units
17. Paterson R, Parker HM (1938) A dosage system for interstitial brachytherapy. Br J Radiol 11:313–339
18. Quimby EH (1952) Dosage calculations in radium therapy. In: Glasser O, Quimby EH, Taylor LS (eds) Physical foundations of radiology. Paul Hoecker, New York
19. Dutreix A, Marinello G (1987) The Paris system. In: Pierquin B, Wilson JF, Chassagne D (eds) Modern brachytherapy. Masson, New York, pp 25–42
20. Viswanathan AN, Beriwal S, De Los Santos J et al (2012) The American Brachytherapy Society treatment recommendation for locally advanced carcinoma of the cervix Part II: high dose rate brachytherapy. Brachytherapy 11(1):47–52
21. Nag S, Erickson BA, Parich S et al (for the American Brachytherapy Society) (2000) The American Brachytherapy Society Recommendations for high dose rate brachytherapy for carcinoma of the endometrium. Int J Radiat Oncol Biol Phys 48(3):779–790
22. Viswanathan AN, Erickson BA (2010) Three dimensional imaging in gynecologic brachytherapy: a survey of the American Brachytherapy Society. Int J Radiat Oncol Biol Phys 76:104–109

The Physics of Brachytherapy

Leah K. Schubert and Moyed Miften

Abstract

Just as the right arm of the radiation oncologist is the medical physicist, so the heart of brachytherapy is the science of physics. In this chapter we introduce the basics of brachytherapy physics beginning with the core of the science and culminating with a comprehensive presentation of the known science to date.

1 Introduction

Physics has wide application in brachytherapy. The radioactive sources used for treatment behave according to the laws of nuclear physics. By understanding these principles, one can predict the behavior of radioactive sources and quantify the emitted radiation which ultimately deposits dose into the patient. The development of different sources and constructions has evolved over time, as have various methods of quantifying source strength. The dose deposited in a patient using brachytherapy has unique properties compared with external-beam radiation therapy. Understanding the principles that govern brachytherapy dose distribution provides a foundation that can be applied to decision making in practice. Finally, the quantification of brachytherapy dose distribution has continued to evolve, with most recent developments innovating the way treatments are planned and dose is calculated.

2 Basic Classifications in Brachytherapy

There are various techniques used in brachytherapy, and they can be classified according to different characteristics. In order to gain an overall perspective of the field of brachytherapy physics, it is first useful to understand the terminology used to classify brachytherapy treatment.

2.1 Implant Technique

Brachytherapy is classified according to how the radioactive sources are placed within the patient. This is often governed by the anatomical

L.K. Schubert, PhD (✉) • M. Miften, PhD, DABR, FAAPM
Department of Radiation Oncology, University of Colorado School of Medicine, Aurora, CO, USA
e-mail: Leah.schubert@ucdenver.edu; moyed.miften@ucdenver.edu

© Springer International Publishing Switzerland 2016
P. Montemaggi et al. (eds.), *Brachytherapy: An International Perspective*, Medical Radiology,
DOI 10.1007/978-3-319-26791-3_3

13

treatment site. Interstitial brachytherapy is treatment with sources placed directly in tissue. Brachytherapy treatments for prostate cancer, head and neck cancer, soft tissue sarcomas, and other types of tumors are typically achieved using an interstitial technique. Intracavitary brachytherapy uses sources that are placed in a body cavity, which is near or within the tissue to be treated. Treatments in which radioactive sources are placed within the vagina or uterus for gynecological disease are classified as intracavitary. Intraluminal brachytherapy involves the placement of sources within lumen, such as the esophagus or trachea. Surface mold or plaque brachytherapy uses sources placed on the surface of the tissue, such as the skin or the globe of the eye. Finally, the use of radiation sources placed in blood vessels is classified as intravascular brachytherapy.

2.2 Treatment Duration

Brachytherapy is classified according to how long the radiation remains in the patient. Permanent brachytherapy uses sources that are permanently placed in the patient, never to be removed. Temporary brachytherapy uses sources that are placed for a specified amount of time and are removed at the completion of treatment.

2.3 Dose Rate

Brachytherapy is classified according to dose rate or how quickly dose is delivered to the patient. Low-dose rate (LDR) brachytherapy is defined as the delivery of dose at rates between 0.4 and 2 Gy/h [1]. It may be performed either on an inpatient or outpatient basis. High-dose rate (HDR) brachytherapy is defined as the delivery of dose greater than 12 Gy/h [1]. Using modern HDR delivery equipment, treatment can be delivered at dose rates as high as 7 Gy/min [2]. Due to the short treatment times, HDR treatment can be performed on an outpatient basis. Medium-dose rate (MDR) brachytherapy delivers dose at rates between 2 and 12 Gy/h [1]. Pulsed dose rate

(PDR) involves short pulses of high-intensity radiation that are delivered typically once per hour in order to simulate LDR treatment.

2.4 Source Loading Technique

Brachytherapy is classified according to the technique in which sources are placed within the patient. Different source loading techniques will require variable equipment. Different techniques will also result in varying levels of source placement accuracy and resultant radiation exposure to staff. A vessel is often used to either allow the clinician to place sources without directly touching the source (e.g., a Mick applicator for prostate treatment) or to allow the source to stay in fixed position within the patient during treatment (e.g., a tandem and ovoid applicator for gynecological treatment). That vessel is called an applicator, and applicators have specific designs based on treatment site. Preloaded brachytherapy involves the use of sources that have been loaded into the applicators ahead of time. The applicators with the sources already loaded are then placed into the patient. During manually afterloaded brachytherapy, the applicator is first placed in the patient, after which the clinician manually places sources into the applicator. Remotely afterloaded brachytherapy is different, in that the applicator is first placed in the patient, after which a machine moves the sources into the applicator while the clinician is located remotely (often outside of the room). Remotely afterloaded brachytherapy has the advantage of reducing radiation exposure to staff. Because remotely afterloaded treatments are often carried out using highly technical equipment, the source placement accuracy is high. Uniform loading is the use of all sources either having the same activity or staying within the patient for the same period of time. Nonuniform loading is the use of sources either having different strengths with respect to each other or staying within the patient for variable amounts of time. Uniform and nonuniform loading have different effects on the dose distribution.

In summary, a single brachytherapy treatment can be classified into many different groups. For example, prostate brachytherapy carried out by implanting into the prostate multiple low-strength sources using preloaded needles is classified as interstitial, permanent, LDR, or preloaded brachytherapy. Gynecological brachytherapy carried out by placing into the vagina a high-strength source for a short period of time using a remote afterloading machine is classified as intracavitary, temporary, HDR, or remotely afterloaded brachytherapy. Each classification can have a different impact on the dose distribution, radiobiological effects, treatment delivery accuracy, and staff exposure.

---

3   Principles of Radioactivity

In brachytherapy, the radiation that is used to treat patients is created by radioactive material. Radioactivity involves unstable nuclei. The atom is composed of a nucleus of protons having positive charge and neutrons having no charge, surrounded by orbital electrons having negative charge. The protons within the nucleus are subject to repulsive electrical forces, while nuclear forces hold the nucleus together. Different arrangements of nucleons allow for stable and unstable states of the nucleus. In an unstable state, the nucleus transitions to a lower energy state. This transition results in the release of energy. This emitted energy is the radiation that goes on to the deliver dose to brachytherapy patients.

Radioactivity is the process in which an unstable nucleus transforms into a more stable state, releasing energy as radiation in the process. This transformation to a lower energy state is termed radioactive decay or disintegration.

Radioactive decay is a stochastic process, which means that the disintegration of a nucleus occurs spontaneously. In stochastic processes, one cannot definitively predict when a given nucleus will disintegrate. With a macroscopic sample containing numerous atoms, however, we can quantify the proportion of nuclei that will decay over a given time period based on probability. It is helpful to understand the stochastic nature of radioactive decay by imagining a lottery ball drawing. Many lottery balls are shaken up in a cage. No one knows which specific balls will gain enough energy to jump out of the cage, but we can expect that there will be a ball exiting the cage at a certain rate. Likewise, we can expect that for a group of unstable atoms, a certain proportion of atoms will undergo radioactive decay and emit their excess energy, but we can't know for certain exactly which atom will undergo that transition.

We can predict that the number of atoms disintegrating per unit time (dN/dt) is proportional to the number of radioactive atoms present (N), shown in Eq. 1. This is also known as the decay rate. The constant of proportionality (λ) is called the decay constant. The negative sign in the equation indicates that the number of radioactive atoms remaining in a sample decreases with time because each disintegration corresponds to a decrease in radioactive nuclei present.

$$\frac{dN}{dt} = -\lambda N \qquad (1)$$

The number of remaining radioactive nuclei as a group of atoms undergo radioactive decay can be derived from Eq. 1 and is shown by Eq. 2. This equation determines the number of active nuclei that have not yet decayed. It changes with time, always decreasing at an exponential rate.

$$N(t) = N_0 e^{-\lambda t} \qquad (2)$$

3.1   Half-Life, Mean Life, Effective Half-Life

Another defining characteristic of a radioactive material is the half-life ($T_{1/2}$), which is defined as the time it takes for the number of radioactive atoms to decay to half of its original number. Half-life is calculated by Eq. 3. This is derived by solving for time in Eq. 2 when $N(t)$ is equal to one half of N_0.

$$T_{1/2} = \frac{ln2}{\lambda} \tag{3}$$

After one half-life, the number of radioactive atoms decreases to half of its original amount. After two half-lives, the number decreases to half the original amount and then another half of that remaining amount, i.e., one-fourth of the original amount. After n half-lives, the amount of radioactive material remaining is equal to $(1/2)^n$.

The half-life is a descriptor for how long the material will stay radioactive or alternatively how quickly its radioactivity will decay. For example, Ir-192 has a half-life of 73.83 days. This means that for a given amount of Ir-192, only half of it will remain radioactive after 73.83 days. It is inversely related to the decay constant as shown in Eq. 3. A "long-lived" source stays radioactive for a long period of time, so its half-life is large, while its decay constant is small (since only a small proportion of atoms will decay away).

The average life of a radioactive material is a quantity that describes the average total length of time a material remains radioactive (Eq. 4). The average life is the time required for all radioactive atoms to decay, assuming the rate of decay remains fixed at its initial value. This quantity can be used when calculating the total dose received by a patient receiving permanent brachytherapy, since the radioactive sources will spend their entire lifetime within that patient.

$$T_{avg} = 1.44 T_{1/2} \tag{4}$$

Half-life refers to the lifetime of a material solely due to its physical properties. It describes the time it takes to reduce the amount of radioactivity by the physical radioactive properties of the material itself. When radioactive material is injected into a patient, for example, in radiopharmaceutical procedures, the material may move through the body, ultimately being eliminated through physiological processes. In this situation, there are two processes working simultaneously to reduce the amount of radioactivity within the patient. The effective half-life (T_{eff}) takes into account the radionuclide's physical half-life ($T_{1/2}$) as well as half-life of the body's elimination of the material (T_{biol}). The

effective half-life takes these processes into account and is defined by Eq. 5:

$$\frac{1}{T_{eff}} = \frac{1}{T_{1/2}} + \frac{1}{T_{biol}} \tag{5}$$

3.2 Definition of Activity

The number of atoms disintegrating per unit time (Eq. 1) is known as the decay rate. The decay rate of an atom is referred to as the activity of a radioactive material. Activity is described by Eq. 6:

$$A = -\frac{dN}{dt} = \lambda N \tag{6}$$

The activity of a material will decrease exponentially at the same rate as the number of active nuclei remaining over time. If the activity is known at a certain time, Eq. 7 is used to calculate the activity at a different time either in the future or in the past. For example, a patient's treatment plan for an HDR treatment is calculated using a known source activity on a specific date. If the patient is treated on a different date, the source activity will be different than the plan, so the plan will be adjusted accordingly.

$$A(t) = A_0 e^{-\lambda t} \tag{7}$$

The percent of activity change over a certain time period can be calculation using Eq. 7 and is a useful value to know for clinically used sources. A simple calculation using this value can identify the activity of sources after different time periods. For example, the activity change of I-125 is 1.2 % per day. If I-125 seeds of a certain activity were planned for prostate seed implantation, but the case was delayed by 1 day, then the activity of the seeds would be 1.2 % lower on that rescheduled date. This simple calculation is helpful when determining source activity values on different dates. For example, if different dates are used for sources ordered from seed companies when activity measurements are performed and when treatment actually occurs, this calculation is an easy way to identify the accurate activity on any given day.

Specific activity is another characteristic of a radioactive material. It is defined as the activity per unit mass of radioactive material. The higher the specific activity, the higher the activity for a given mass of material. Alternatively, the higher the specific activity, the smaller the mass of material for a given amount of activity. High specific activity sources are ideal for HDR treatments. They are high in activity in order to produce enough radiation to deliver high dose rates. They are also low in mass such that they are small enough to fit in body cavities for treatment.

4 Source Strength Specification

There are multiple methods to define the strength of a source. Many of these definitions have been used historically and are now obsolete, while many are still used interchangeably in various practices. The definitions of source strength can be grouped into two main perspectives. The first perspective quantifies source strength in terms of amount of material present (standardized as mass of radium and activity). The second perspective is from the point of view of the output of emitted radiation (exposure rate and air-kerma strength).

4.1 Mass of Radium

The oldest quantity of source strength is the mass of radium (Ra-226) contained within a source. Ra-226 was the first radioisotope used for brachytherapy treatment. Since Ra-226 was the only source used at the time, it was straightforward to quantify the amount of radiation emitted. It was simply related to the physical amount of radium, or the mass of radium (in units of mg of radium). In this situation, for a given mass of radium, the amount and type of emitted radiation and the impact of the source construction were always consistent. When new sources were introduced, the mass of those sources did not produce the same effects as the same mass of radium, since the emitted radiation and source construction were not the same. Equivalent masses to Ra-226 were used for the newly introduced sources. The equivalent mass of radium is defined as that mass of radium encapsulated in 0.5 mm Pt that produces the same exposure rate at the calibration distance as the source of interest. Mass of radium and equivalent mass of radium, while now considered obsolete quantities to define source strength, continue to be used in Cs-137 brachytherapy treatment.

4.2 Activity

Activity is defined as the number of nuclei undergoing radioactive decay per unit time. Standard international (SI) units of activity are becquerel (Bq) [3]. One Bq is equivalent to the activity of a quantity of radioactive material in which one nucleus decays per second (1 dps). Another unit of activity is a curie (Ci). Although Ci is not the SI unit of activity, it is still used in clinical practice. The typical activity of the Ir-192 source used in HDR is 5–10 Ci. The Ci is related to the Bq by Eq. 8:

$$1\,Ci = 3.7 \times 10^{10}\,Bq \qquad (8)$$

Modern sealed radioactive sources are constructed such that they are encapsulated within a strong metal lining. This lining will absorb some of the radiation emitted by the radioactive source within, thereby diminishing the radiation reaching the patient. Apparent activity is defined as the activity of a hypothetic unfiltered point source that has the same exposure rate at the calibration distance as the source of interest. It is considered an obsolete quantity [1, 4] although still in use for specifying source strength in permanent brachytherapy treatments.

4.3 Exposure Rate

Exposure rate is a source strength quantity that is defined in terms of the emitted radiation from the radioactive material. Exposure rate refers to the rate at which air is ionized by indirectly ionizing radiation [5]. In the context of brachytherapy, gamma rays emitted during radioactive decay ionize the air. Specifically, exposure rate is the charge rate produced in air by indirectly ionizing radiation, per unit mass of air (C/kg-h). The SI unit of exposure rate is C/kg-h, but a commonly used unit is roentgen per hour (R/h). The two units are related to each as

$$1\frac{R}{hr} = 2.58 \times 10^{-4} \frac{C}{kg\, hr} \qquad (9)$$

The strength of a gamma-emitting radioactive source is specified in terms of exposure rate normally at a calibration distance of 1 m. The exposure rate is inversely related to the square of the distance away from the source. For example, if one were to move twice as far away from the source, the exposure rate will decrease by a factor of four. Therefore, in order to compare quantities of radiation based on the properties of the sources themselves, the exposure rate is specified at a constant, known distance.

Exposure rate at a specific distance ($\dot{X}(r)$) is related to activity (A) by the exposure rate constant (Γ) (Eq. 10). The exposure rate constant describes rate at which air is ionized by photons emitted by radioactive decay. Using the exposure rate constant, one can calculate the exposure rate for a given source activity and at a given distance away from the source. For example, the exposure rate constant of Ra-226 is 8.25 R-cm^2/mg-h. This means that for 1 mg of radium, the exposure rate is 8.25 R/h at 1 cm away.

$$\Gamma = \frac{\dot{X}(r)}{A} r^2 \qquad (10)$$

4.4 Air-Kerma Strength

Air-kerma strength is the quantity endorsed by the American Association of Physicists in Medicine (AAPM) to specify source strength for gamma-emitting brachytherapy sources [4, 6–8]. Kerma quantifies the energy that is transferred to charged particles per unit mass in a volume of medium [5]. Air-kerma strength is a measure of the energy transferred to air. S_k is defined as the product of the air-kerma rate, measured at a specific distance from the source center along the transverse axis of the source, multiplied by the square of the measurement distance (Eq. 11). The air-kerma rate measurement is performed in free air geometry at a large distance from the source, typically 1 m. The units of air-kerma strength are in U, which is equivalent to cGy-cm^2/h or μGy-m^2/h.

$$S_k = \dot{K}(d) \times d^2 \qquad (11)$$

4.5 Relationships Between Different Source Strength Quantities

The various quantities and units used for source strength can be converted between each other. Treatment planning programs often allow for different source strength quantities to be used for treatment planning. When ordering radioactive sources from vendors, one can define the source strength using various quantities. Activity calibration can also be performed by independent companies or via in-house measurements, and different source strength quantities may be used. In all of these steps, it is critical to know which quantity is being used and, when differing quantities are used, how to convert between them. Source strength quantities have been mistakenly switched in practice in the past, resulting in dose errors as high as 30 % dose difference [9].

5 Radioactive Sources Used in Brachytherapy

A variety of radioactive sources have been used for different brachytherapy procedures. There are historical, physical, or practical reasons why different sources are used. There are several desirable properties that make an ideal source for treatment. The first property is the type and energy of radiation emitted by the source. These impact the dose delivered to the patient and the radiation exposure to the staff involved in the procedure. The energy should be low enough to provide a desired sharp dose falloff, yet high enough to treat in depth with acceptable dose heterogeneity. Higher energy gammas that can penetrate through the patient will result in higher staff exposure. The source's specific activity should be an optimal value to allow for the delivery of desired dose rates while sufficiently small to be placed within the body. Finally, the source's half-life should be optimal to support the working life of the source such that it can deliver sufficient doses over the desired treatment duration.

Sources for brachytherapy treatment are uniquely constructed with various sizes and shapes. The radioactive portion of the source is surrounded by an encapsulating material. The encapsulation prevents radioactive material from leaking out. The encapsulation also absorbs non-penetrating radiation emitted from the source, including low-energy gammas, betas, and alphas, which would otherwise increase the surface dose with minimal contribution to the treatment therapeutic goal. Different sources are constructed with various thicknesses and types of encapsulating materials. The construction of the radioactive material within the encapsulation will also vary. Some may be in the form of small pellets or rods all held within the encapsulation.

Table 1 summarizes the properties of common radioactive sources used historically and currently.

6   Brachytherapy Dose Distributions

6.1   Characteristics and Clinical Impact

Brachytherapy dose distributions have unique characteristics compared with external-beam dose distributions. It is important understand these characteristics, as they can impact various practices in brachytherapy.

Brachytherapy dose distributions exhibit a high dose gradient, which allows for a rapid dose falloff from the radioactive source. This is due to the low energy of radiation emitted. The energy of the emitted radiation is in the keV range as opposed to the MeV range. The main advantage of this dose gradient is to allow for sparing of nearby normal tissue. On the other hand, there are consequences for this high dose gradient. The first consequence is that the more rapid the dose fall-off, the more difficult it can be to provide dose coverage for targets farther away from the source. In order to cover tissue that extends farther away from the source, the tissue closest to the source will receive a higher dose. Brachytherapy treatments are thus characterized by heterogeneous dose distributions. For example, in vaginal cylinder treatments, when prescribing to a depth of 0.5 cm from the surface of the applicator, the vaginal mucosa on the surface of the cylinder can receive a dose up to twice as high as the prescription dose. In order to mitigate hotspots, the largest possible applicator that can be comfortably fitted is used. This practice especially applies when selecting vaginal applicator sizes (particularly cylinders and ovoids). The reason for this practice is that dose gradient is sharper closer to the source than farther away. Therefore, the largest applicator moves the tissue as far away from the source as possible in order take advantage of the lower dose gradient. Finally, high-dose heterogeneity is the reason for pretreatment quality assurance evaluation in balloon-based brachytherapy. The balloon integrity must be confirmed prior to delivering every treatment fraction. If the balloon were to inadvertently deflate during the course of treatment, the tissue surface would move close to the source and could receive up to ten times higher dose (Fig. 1).

Another consequence of the sharp dose falloff is the need for delivery of radiation with high accuracy. The higher the dose gradient, the more stringent the delivery accuracy need. Brachytherapy using remote afterloading technology requires millimeter accuracy of the source position relative to the applicator position [4]. While a discrepancy of several millimeters in positioning may be not a cause for concern in external-beam radiotherapy (RT), it may be critical for brachytherapy treatments using remote afterloading technology.

Table 1 Physical properties of radioactive sources commonly used in brachytherapy

Isotope	Common clinical applications	Common treatment sites	Form	Clinical emission particle	Average particle energy (keV)	HVL (mm lead)	Half-life	% activity change
Ra-226	LDR intracavitary and interstitial	Historically used	Tubes, needles	Gamma	830	12	1600 years	0.04 % per year
Cs-137	LDR intracavitary and interstitial	Cervix, uterus	Tubes, needles	Gamma	662	5.5	30 years	2.3 % per year
Co-60	LDR intracavitary and interstitial, HDR intracavitary	Multiple sites	Wire	Gamma	1250	11	5.26 years	12.3 % per year
Au-198	LDR interstitial	Prostate	Seeds	Gamma	412	2.5	2.7 days	22.6 % per day
Ir-192	HDR intracavitary, interstitial, and surface; LDR interstitial	Cervix, uterus, sarcoma, head and neck, prostate, breast	Seeds, wires, ribbons	Gamma	380	2.5	73.8 days	0.9 % per day
I-125	LDR interstitial and surface	Prostate, eye	Seeds	Gamma	28	0.025	59.4 days	1.2 % per day
Pd-103	LDR interstitial	Prostate	Seeds	Gamma	21	0.008	17 days	4.0 % per day
Cs-131	LDR interstitial	Prostate	Seeds	Gamma	29	0.025	9.7 days	6.9 % per day
Sr-90	HDR surface	Eye	Applicator	Beta	224 (max)	N/A	28.8 years	2.4 % per year

Abbreviations: HVL half-value layer, HDR high dose rate, LDR low dose rate, keV kilo-electron volt, R roentgen, cm centimeter, mCi millicurie, hr hour, mm millimeter

The Physics of Brachytherapy

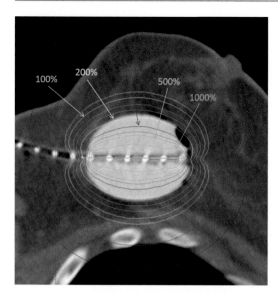

Fig. 1 Dose distribution for a MammoSite® breast treatment. The 100 % line refers to the prescription dose at 1.0 cm depth from the balloon surface. In this figure, the dose to the balloon surface is twice as high as the prescription. If the balloon were to completely deflate, breast tissue could receive dose up to ten times higher than the prescription dose

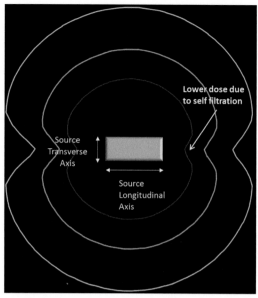

Fig. 2 Dose distribution in water for a realistic Ir-192 source, visualized by the *gray rectangle*. The *red*, *green*, and *blue lines* show select isodose volumes. The reduction of dose along the source longitudinal axis is due to an increase of self-filtration of radiation as it passes through more source material

6.2 Factors That Influence the Shape of Brachytherapy Dose Distributions

In the simplest scenario, a single radioactive source, three main factors impact the shape of brachytherapy dose distributions. The first factor is distance from the source. For external-beam RT, the radiation intensity as a function of distance is described by the inverse-square law, which states that radiation intensity decreases by the square of the distance from the source. In brachytherapy, this law is an adequate approximation at large distances from the source. Large distance generally means a distance that is at least twice the size of the source [8]. When closer to the source, however, the inverse-square law starts to break down.

The second factor is the impact of the source itself and its encapsulation on the emitted radiation. Emitted radiation is absorbed or scattered as it exits the source, prior to reaching the surrounding tissue. In reality, sources are constructed with a finite shape and size. The impact of the source on the dose distribution depends on the specific source construction, namely, the source and encapsulation dimensions and material. Typical sources are cylindrical in shape, so there will be more attenuation along the longitudinal axis as opposed to the transverse axis of the source. This is because the emitted radiation needs to penetrate more material along the longitudinal axis before reaching the surrounding tissue and is therefore more attenuated. The resulting dose is lower along the longitudinal axis of the source as opposed to the transverse axis (Fig. 2).

Finally, the material surrounding the source will impact the emitted radiation. The surrounding material will cause photons to attenuate as they move deeper. In addition to attenuation, the surrounding material will also cause photons to scatter.

7 Dose Calculation Methods

7.1 Cumulative Dose Calculations

Cumulative dose calculations determine the total dose delivered over the duration of treatment (t). The dose rate ($\dot{D}(t)$) at a particular time (t) is proportional to activity. The dose rate changes over time because the source activity changes over time. Therefore, the dose rate is calculated as

$$\dot{D}(t) = \dot{D}_0 e^{-\lambda t} \qquad (12)$$

where $\dot{D}_0$ is the dose rate at the start of treatment and λ is the source decay constant. The total delivered dose over a specific period of time is determined by taking the integral of Eq. 12, which results in Eq. 13. Depending on the relationship between the treatment duration and the source half-life, this equation can be simplified in the following ways:

$$D(t) = \dot{D}_0 \times T_{\frac{1}{2}} \times 1.44 \times \left(1 - e^{-\lambda t}\right) \qquad (13)$$

For permanent brachytherapy using short-lived sources, the treatment duration is much longer than the source half-life. Dose is delivered over the lifetime of the source. Therefore, the total delivered dose is proportional to the average lifetime of the source and is calculated in Eq. 14. An example treatment of this type is LDR prostate seed implants.

$$D = \dot{D}_0 \times T_{\frac{1}{2}} \times 1.44 = \dot{D}_0 \times T_{avg} \qquad (14)$$

For temporary brachytherapy when the treatment duration is very short compared to the half-life of the source, the source strength, and therefore the initial dose rate, changes only minimally throughout treatment. The total delivered dose can be approximated using Eq. 15 [2]. An example treatment of this type is HDR treatments using Ir-192 or LDR treatments using Cs-137.

$$D = \dot{D}_0 T \qquad (15)$$

For brachytherapy in which the treatment duration is similar to the source half-life (more than 5 % of the half-life), the source strength changes throughout the treatment. Thus, the changing dose rate must be taken into account when calculating the total delivered dose (Eq. 13).

7.2 Integral and Interpolation Methods

Dose distributions around linear brachytherapy sources, such as sources in the form of tube or needles, were historically calculated using either an integral method (Sievert integral) or using an interpolation method [10, 11]. The Sievert integral method subdivides a linear source into several equal segments, where each segment is small enough to be considered a point source. For a given location with respect to the source, corrections for distance, oblique filtration, attenuation and scatter are separately applied and contributions summed. Interpolation methods use a set of data points that has been determined either using experimental methods or theoretical calculations. Along-and-away tables have been used for Cs-137 treatments, and tabulated data are also used in Paterson-Parker [11] and Quimby systems [12].

7.3 AAPM TG-43: Modular Formulism

The dose calculation formulism by the AAPM Task Group 43 (TG-43) is the current standard dose calculation method [7, 13]. It can be used for 1D and 2D dose calculations, and it accounts for differences in the construction of clinically used sources. Current treatment planning systems commonly use TG-43 calculations. The formulism assumes a cylindrically symmetric source. It is a homogeneous dose calculation, assuming that all surrounding media is water. When performing a CT-based plan, the material of the applicator and surrounding tissue are not taken into account during dose calculation.

The TG-43 formulism is a modular formulism, breaking up the various factors that impact the dose distribution into individual parameters. Each parameter is specific to individual sources in clinical use. This approach uses measured experimental data and Monte Carlo-generated data for known sources. The values of the parameters are dependent on the position of the dose calculation point with respect to the source. The position of the dose calculation point is in the polar coordinate system, where the position is described as a radial distance from the source, r, and an angular position from the source's longitudinal axis, θ (Fig. 3).

The TG-43 formulism to calculate dose as a function of position is shown in Eq. 16, where S_k is the source strength (defined as air-kerma strength), Λ is the dose rate constant, $G(r, \theta)$ is the geometry function, $g(r)$ is the radial dose function, and $F(r, \theta)$ is the anisotropy function. The standard reference position (r_0, θ_0), is at a radial distance of 1 cm along the transverse axis ($\theta = 90°$). This form of the equation is a 2D calculation, which takes into account realistic line, cylindrically symmetric sources.

$$\dot{D}(r,\theta) = S_k \Lambda \frac{G(r,\theta)}{G(r_0,\theta_0)} g(r) F(r,\theta) \quad (16)$$

The dose rate constant, Λ, is defined as the dose rate to water per unit air-kerma strength at the reference position. Its units are in cGy/U-h.

The geometry function, $G(r, \theta)$, accounts for the variation of relative dose due to the spatial distribution of activity within the source. It does not account for scatter and attenuation, but rather provides an effective inverse-square law, which is based on an approximate model of the distribution of radioactivity within the source. It is dependent on both radial distance and angular position and its units are in cm^{-2}. For a point source, the geometry function is equal to $1/r^2$. For a cylindrical line source, the geometry function takes the following form (Eq. 17), where L is the active source length and $\Delta\beta$ is the angle subtended by the source with respect to the calculation point:

$$G(r,\theta) = \begin{cases} \dfrac{\beta}{Lr\sin\theta} & for\ \ \theta \neq 0° \\[2ex] \left(r^2 - \dfrac{L^2}{4}\right)^{-1} & for\ \ \theta = 0° \end{cases} \quad (17)$$

The radial dose function, $g(r)$, is a dimensionless quantity that accounts for the dose falloff along

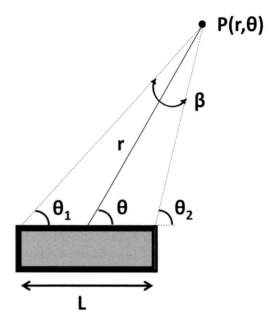

Fig. 3 Coordinate system describing the position of the calculation point ($P((r, \theta)$) with respect to the brachytherapy source. The source is visualized by the rectangle, where the active length (L) indicates the length of the radioactive material shown in *gray*. The source transverse axis is shown in the vertical direction and the longitudinal axis is in the horizontal direction. The angle θ is the angle that the calculation point makes between the longitudinal source axis and the source center. The angles θ_1 and θ_2 are the angles from each source end, while β is the angle subtended by the source, with respect to the calculation point. The distance (r) is the radial distance between the calculation point and the source center

the transverse plane due to scatter and attenuation in the surrounding material. At the reference distance of r_0 the quantity becomes unity. It is defined along the transverse axis of the source and therefore is only dependent on the radial distance.

The anisotropy function, $F(r, \theta)$, accounts for the anisotropic shape of the dose distribution around the source due to source self-filtration and oblique transmission through the source encapsulation. It describes the variation in dose away from the transverse plane (i.e., when θ is not equal to θ_0). When the angle θ is equal to the reference angle θ_0 (i.e., along the transverse plane), the quantity F becomes unity.

The line-source calculation given in Eq. 17 takes into account the anisotropic shape of radiation emitted from realistic sources. One can simplify this equation by assuming the source is a point, thus ignoring the anisotropic shape of the emitted radiation and instead assuming an isotropic distribution. This simplification is known as a point-source approximation (Eq. 18). Because the dose distribution is isotropic, the angular position of the dose calculation point is no longer a variable, and the dose is solely dependent on radial distance away from the source. In the point-source approximation, the anisotropy function, $F(r, \theta)$ is replaced by the 1D anisotropy factor, $\Phi(r)$. The anisotropy factor is found by averaging the dose rate at each distance with respect to the solid angle.

$$\dot{D}(r) = S_k \Lambda \left(\frac{r_0}{r} \right)^2 g(r) \Phi(r) \qquad (18)$$

The point-source approximation ignores realistic source geometry and its dosimetric impact and is less accurate. This approximation is an adequate approximation if either of the following two conditions apply: (1) if the distance from the source is greater than twice the source active length, such that the calculation point is far enough so that the distribution of radioactivity does not largely impact the calculated dose, and (2) if sources are distributed with random orientations, such that the dose anisotropy effects are averaged out [8]. LDR prostate treatments often use point-source approximations because of the random orientation of the sources placed within the tissue. Alternatively, HDR treatments commonly use line-source calculations in order to determine a more accurate dose distribution; because the source travels within applicators of known, rigid geometry, the source orientation in the patient can be accurately predicted.

7.4 Image-Based Dose Calculation

Traditional brachytherapy planning has been based on applicators, where optimized dose distributions were determined from applicator positions, source loading schema, and standard rules. Dose is usually prescribed and tracked to a few defined points. Three-dimensional (3D) imaging now allows for patient-specific anatomy to be explicitly taken into account [13–19]. Computed tomography [18, 20, 21] and ultrasound [22–25] are primarily used for anatomy-based planning, with magnetic resonance imaging [18, 26–29] and functional imaging such as positron emission tomography [30–32] starting to be adopted. Similar to planning practices for external-beam RT, the planning target volumes (PTVs) and organs at risk (OAR) are contoured on the 3D images. The brachytherapy applicators are defined on the image to identify the source positions. The source dwell times (for HDR) or treatment duration or source activity (for LDR) may then be adjusted in order to provide an optimal dose distribution for target coverage and OAR avoidance. Three-dimensional isodose distributions and dose-volume histograms (DVHs) are used to evaluate plan quality. Forward and inverse planning [8, 33–38] may be used to achieve the desired dose distribution.

Image-based brachytherapy planning can use the standard TG-43 formulism, which is a homogeneous dose calculation that assumes that the applicators and patient anatomy are water density. Model-based algorithms are alternative dose calculation algorithms which take into account the surrounding material. These algorithms either simulate the coupled photon-electron radiation transport in the material or they use multiple dimensional scatter integration techniques to take into account the material's impact on scatter dose. Three current methods are collapsed cone convolution-superposition (CS) [39], grid-based Boltzmann solvers (BSs) [40–43], and Monte Carlo simulations (MCSs) [44–47]. In CS, dose from primary and scatter radiation is calculated using kernels which map the spatial energy deposition response of radiation in a medium. A CS algorithm is being integrated to the Oncentra® brachytherapy treatment planning system (Elekta, Crawley, UK). BSs use deterministic approaches to directly solve the linear Boltzmann transport equation. A BS algorithm called Acuros® is implemented in the Brachyvision® treatment planning system (Varian Medical Systems, Palo Alto, CA). MC simulations use stochastic approaches to solve the linear Boltzmann transport equation using random sampling. The use of these model-based algorithms is currently an active area of research [48–50]. The current recommendation from the AAPM is to perform TG-43 calculations in parallel with model-based calculations [50].

8   Summary

Physics has advanced the development of brachytherapy treatment. Different radioactive sources and source construction designs continue to be developed for use in various treatment applications. Throughout the history of brachytherapy, the methods with which to quantify source strength have evolved as different sources have been introduced: starting with the mass of radium to the current standard of air-kerma strength. The methods of calculation of dose distributions from brachytherapy treatments have also evolved. These methods include simple calculations of total absolute dose delivered, calculations using tabulated data that take into account the source size and construction, calculations which separate the impact of source construction into modular components, and the most recent developments using three-dimensional images and sophisticated radiation transport algorithms. Brachytherapy physics, while having a long history, continues to innovate and advance the field.

Bibliography

1. Units, I.C.o.R (1991) Measurements: dose and volume specification for reporting intracavitary therapy in gynecology; Repr, vol 38. International commission on radiation units and measurements
2. Halperin EC, Brady LW, Wazer DE et al (2013) Perez & Brady's principles and practice of radiation oncology. Lippincott Williams & Wilkins, Philadelphia
3. NCRP (1985) A handbook of radioactivity measurements procedures. NCRP report 58
4. Nath R, Anderson LL, Meli JA et al (1997) Code of practice for brachytherapy physics: report of the AAPM Radiation Therapy Committee Task Group No. 56. Med Phys 24(10):1557–1598
5. Units, I.C.o.R (1998) Fundamental quantities and units for ionizing radiation, vol 58. International commission on radiation
6. Nath R (1987) Specification of Brachytherapy Source Strength: Report of AAPM Task Group 32
7. Rivard MJ, Coursey BM, DeWerd LA et al (2004) Update of AAPM Task Group No. 43 Report: A revised AAPM protocol for brachytherapy dose calculations. Med Phys 31(3):633–674
8. Thomadsen B, Rivard MJ, Butler WM, Medicine, A.A.o.P.i (2005) Brachytherapy physics. American association of physicists in medicine
9. Richardson S (2012) A 2-year review of recent Nuclear Regulatory Commission events: what errors occur in the modern brachytherapy era? Pract Radiat Oncol 2(3):157–163
10. Krishnaswamy V (1972) Dose distributions about 137Cs sources in tissue 1. Radiology 105(1):181–184
11. Paterson JRK, Meredith WJ (1967) Radium dosage: the Manchester system. E. & S. Livingstone, Edinburgh
12. Glasser O, Quimby H, Taylor LS et al (1961) Physical foundations of radiology. Hoeber, New York, p 581
13. Rivard MJ, Butler WM, DeWerd LA et al (2007) Supplement to the 2004 update of the AAPM Task Group No. 43 Report. Med Phys 34(6):2187–2205
14. Fellner C, Pötter R, Knocke TH et al (2001) Comparison of radiography-and computed tomography-based treatment planning in cervix cancer in brachytherapy with specific attention to some quality assurance aspects. Radiother Oncol 58(1):53–62
15. Gebara WJ, Weeks KJ, Hahn CA et al (1998) Computed axial tomography tandem and ovoids (CATTO) dosimetry: three-dimensional assessment of bladder and rectal doses. Radiat Oncol Investig 6(6):268–275
16. Mizoe J (1990) Analysis of the dose-volume histogram in uterine cervical cancer by diagnostic CT. Strahlentherapie und Onkologie: Organ der Deutschen Rontgengesellschaft[et al] 166(4):279–284
17. Schoeppel SL, Lavigne ML, Martel MK et al (1994) Three-dimensional treatment planning of intracavitary gynecologic implants: analysis of ten cases and implications for dose specification. Int J Radiat Oncol Biol Phys 28(1):277–283
18. Haie-Meder C, Pötter R, Van Limbergen E et al (2005) Recommendations from Gynaecological (GYN) GEC-ESTRO Working Group☆(I): concepts and terms in 3D image based 3D treatment planning in cervix cancer brachytherapy with emphasis on MRI assessment of GTV and CTV. Radiother Oncol 74(3):235–245
19. Viswanathan AN, Erickson BA (2010) Three-dimensional imaging in gynecologic brachytherapy: a survey of the American Brachytherapy Society. Int J Radiat Oncol Biol Phys 76(1):104–109
20. Willins J, Wallner K (1997) CT-based dosimetry for transperineal I-125 prostate brachytherapy. Int J Radiat Oncol Biol Phys 39(2):347–353

21. Pötter R, Haie-Meder C, Van Limbergen E et al (2006) Recommendations from gynaecological (GYN) GEC ESTRO working group (II): concepts and terms in 3D image-based treatment planning in cervix cancer brachytherapy—3D dose volume parameters and aspects of 3D image-based anatomy, radiation physics, radiobiology. Radiother Oncol 78(1):67–77

22. Blasko J, Ragde H, Schumacher D (1987) Transperineal percutaneous iodine-125 implantation for prostatic carcinoma using transrectal ultrasound and template guidance. Endocuriether Hypertherm Oncol 3:131–139

23. Edmundson GK, Yan D, Martinez AA (1995) Intraoperative optimization of needle placement and dwell times for conformal prostate brachytherapy. Int J Radiat Oncol Biol Phys 33(5):1257–1263

24. Holm H, Juul N, Pedersen J et al (2002) Transperineal 125 iodine seed implantation in prostatic cancer guided by transrectal ultrasonography. J Urol 167(2):985–988

25. Vicini FA, Jaffray DA, Horwitz EM et al (1998) Implementation of 3D-virtual brachytherapy in the management of breast cancer: a description of a new method of interstitial brachytherapy. Int J Radiat Oncol Biol Phys 40(3):629–635

26. Nag S, Cardenes H, Chang S et al (2004) Proposed guidelines for image-based intracavitary brachytherapy for cervical carcinoma: report from Image-Guided Brachytherapy Working Group. Int J Radiat Oncol Biol Phys 60(4):1160–1172

27. Ménard C, Susil RC, Choyke P et al (2004) MRI-guided HDR prostate brachytherapy in standard 1.5 T scanner. Int J Radiat Oncol Biol Phys 59(5):1414–1423

28. Pouliot J, Kim Y, Lessard E et al (2004) Inverse planning for HDR prostate brachytherapy used to boost dominant intraprostatic lesions defined by magnetic resonance spectroscopy imaging. Int J Radiat Oncol Biol Phys 59(4):1196–1207

29. Viswanathan AN, Dimopoulos J, Kirisits C et al (2007) Computed tomography versus magnetic resonance imaging-based contouring in cervical cancer brachytherapy: results of a prospective trial and preliminary guidelines for standardized contours. Int J Radiat Oncol Biol Phys 68(2):491–498

30. Malyapa RS, Mutic S, Low DA et al (2002) Physiologic FDG-PET three-dimensional brachytherapy treatment planning for cervical cancer. Int J Radiat Oncol Biol Phys 54(4):1140–1146

31. Lin LL, Mutic S, Low DA et al (2007) Adaptive brachytherapy treatment planning for cervical cancer using FDG-PET. Int J Radiat Oncol Biol Phys 67(1):91–96

32. Mutic S, Grigsby PW, Low DA et al (2002) PET-guided three-dimensional treatment planning of intracavitary gynecologic implants. Int J Radiat Oncol Biol Phys 52(4):1104–1110

33. Lessard E, Pouliot J (2001) Inverse planning anatomy-based dose optimization for HDR-brachytherapy of the prostate using fast simulated annealing algorithm and dedicated objective function. Med Phys 28(5):773–779

34. Lee EK, Gallagher RJ, Silvern D et al (1999) Treatment planning for brachytherapy: an integer programming model, two computational approaches and experiments with permanent prostate implant planning. Phys Med Biol 44(1):145

35. Lachance B, Béliveau Nadeau D, Lessard É et al (2002) Early clinical experience with anatomy-based inverse planning dose optimization for high-dose-rate boost of the prostate. Int J Radiat Oncol Biol Phys 54(1):86–100

36. Lahanas M, Baltas D, Giannouli S (2003) Global convergence analysis of fast multiobjective gradient-based dose optimization algorithms for high-dose-rate brachytherapy. Phys Med Biol 48(5):599

37. Milickovic N, Lahanas M, Papagiannopoulou M et al (2002) Multiobjective anatomy-based dose optimization for HDR-brachytherapy with constraint free deterministic algorithms. Phys Med Biol 47(13):2263

38. Pouliot J, Tremblay D, Roy J et al (1996) Optimization of permanent 125 I prostate implants using fast simulated annealing. Int J Radiat Oncol Biol Phys 36(3):711–720

39. Tedgren ÅC, Ahnesjö A (2008) Optimization of the computational efficiency of a 3D, collapsed cone dose calculation algorithm for brachytherapy. Med Phys 35(4):1611–1618

40. Zourari K, Pantelis E, Moutsatsos A et al (2010) Dosimetric accuracy of a deterministic radiation transport based I192r brachytherapy treatment planning system. Part I: single sources and bounded homogeneous geometries. Med Phys 37(2):649–661

41. Petrokokkinos L, Zourari K, Pantelis E et al (2011) Dosimetric accuracy of a deterministic radiation transport based I192r brachytherapy treatment planning system. Part II: Monte Carlo and experimental verification of a multiple source dwell position plan employing a shielded applicator. Med Phys 38(4):1981–1992

42. Zourari K, Pantelis E, Moutsatsos A et al (2013) Dosimetric accuracy of a deterministic radiation transport based 192Ir brachytherapy treatment planning system. Part III. Comparison to Monte Carlo simulation in voxelized anatomical computational models. Med Phys 40(1):011712

43. Mikell JK, Klopp AH, Price M et al (2013) Commissioning of a grid-based Boltzmann solver for cervical cancer brachytherapy treatment planning with shielded colpostats. Brachytherapy 12(6):645–653

44. Thomson R, Taylor T, Rogers D (2008) Monte Carlo dosimetry for I125 and Pd103 eye plaque brachytherapy. Med Phys 35(12):5530–5543

45. Carrier JF, D'Amours M, Verhaegen F et al (2007) Postimplant dosimetry using a Monte Carlo dose calculation engine: a new clinical standard. Int J Radiat Oncol Biol Phys 68(4):1190–1198

46. Poon E, Williamson JF, Vuong T et al (2008) Patient-specific Monte Carlo dose calculations for high-dose-rate endorectal brachytherapy with shielded intracavitary applicator. Int J Radiat Oncol Biol Phys 72(4):1259–1266

47. Poon E, Le Y, Williamson JF et al (2008) BrachyGUI: an adjunct to an accelerated Monte Carlo photon transport code for patient-specific brachytherapy dose calculations and analysis. J Phys Conference Series 102:012018, IOP Publishing

48. Papagiannis P, Pantelis E, Karaiskos P (2014) Current state of the art brachytherapy treatment planning dosimetry algorithms. Br J Radiol 87(1041):20140163

49. Rivard MJ, Venselaar JL, Beaulieu L (2009) The evolution of brachytherapy treatment planning. Med Phys 36(6):2136–2153

50. Beaulieu L, Tedgren ÅC, Carrier JF et al (2012) Report of the Task Group 186 on model-based dose calculation methods in brachytherapy beyond the TG-43 formalism: current status and recommendations for clinical implementation. Med Phys 39(10):6208–6236

Physics: Low-Energy Brachytherapy Physics

Jun Yang, Xing Liang, Cynthia Pope, and Zuofeng Li

Abstract

Low-energy brachytherapy has been a standard for more than one century of clinical cancer application. We present the isotopes used, the characteristics of these elements, and the physics of use.

1   Introduction

Low-energy brachytherapy sources, with mean energy ≤50 keV [1, 2], are widely used in the radiotherapy treatment of several tumors, including the permanent implant treatment of prostate

J. Yang, PhD (✉)
Professor , Department Of Radiation Oncology,
College Of Medicine, Drexel University,
Philadelphia, PA 10102, USA

Philadelphia Cyberknife Center, Delaware County
Memorial Hospital, 2010 Westchester Pike,
Havertown, PA 10102, USA
e-mail: junbme@yahoo.com

X. Liang, PhD
Radiation Physics Solution LLC,
Garnet Valley, PA, USA

C. Pope, MS
Department of Radiation Oncology, Beth Israel
Deaconess Hospital, Plymouth, MA, USA

Z. Li, DSc, FAAPM
Department of Radiation Oncology, University of
Florida College of Medicine, Gainesville, MA, USA

UF Health Proton Therapy Institute,
Jacksonville, FL, USA

cancer [3] and the plaque treatment of ocular melanoma [4]. Commonly used low-energy brachytherapy sources include a large number of iodine-125 seed sources of various designs, palladium-103, and cesium-131 sources. Their lower energies make them clinically attractive, and radiation safety concerns for patients implanted with these sources can easily be addressed either by patient tissue attenuation for permanent implants or with minimal lead shielding for temporary implants such as the eye plaques. However, dosimetry of these lower-energy sources, due to their lower mean energies, is highly perturbed by the source design and construction, in-tissue attenuation and scattering, and tissue inhomogeneity.

Clinical applications of low-energy brachytherapy sources have seen significant increases due to their successful use in the transrectal ultrasound (TRUS)-guided permanent implant treatment of prostate cancer following the reports of pioneers of this technique [5, 6]. Other clinical applications, albeit more limited, include treatment of intraocular melanomas [4] and early-stage lung cancer [7].

This chapter discusses currently or historically used low-energy brachytherapy isotopes,

© Springer International Publishing Switzerland 2016
P. Montemaggi et al. (eds.), *Brachytherapy: An International Perspective*, Medical Radiology,
DOI 10.1007/978-3-319-26791-3_4

how seed construction and design can alter delivered, dose distributions by these sources, currently recommended dosimetry calculation formalism for these sources, and current clinical applications of low-dose brachytherapy.

2 Isotopes

Radiation therapy for curing disease began as brachytherapy following the discovery of X-rays by Röntgen in 1895. The first reported brachytherapy treatment was performed in 1903 using radium needles [8]. In these early days, not many sources of radiation were known. In modern radiotherapy, isotope choice for a particular therapy includes weighing many physical properties, such as half-life, type of radiation, energy, radiation protection concerns, specific activity (amount of activity per unit mass), and production cost.

The following radiation sources have been or are currently being used for brachytherapy [9], listed in order of active half-life. They are also conveniently grouped into high-energy photon-emitting sources, low-energy photon-emitting sources, and beta-emitting sources.

2.1 High-Energy Sources

^{226}**Ra**: γ-ray, 1,600 year half-life, 0.83 MeV avg energy

Radium was the first source used for radiotherapy/brachytherapy shortly after the discovery of radioactivity and the potential of such therapy to cure cancer. Radium was used by early cancer physicians as brachytherapy techniques were developed and improved. Because of the early experience with radium, there is a large body of clinical experience using radium needles. Successful prescriptions were developed using milligrams of radium required for a desired effect. As new sources were developed, the activity prescribed was often based on the equivalent milligrams of radium.

The energy emitted by radium, averaging 0.83 MeV, makes it useful in many interstitial clinical situations. Unfortunately, other physical properties are less desirable. Radium produces a harmful daughter product, radon-222, as well as helium gas, which leads to a buildup of pressure inside sealed sources. Eventually the sources may crack due to the pressure and release the harmful daughter products.

^{137}**Cs**: γ-ray, 30 year half-life, 0.662 MeV energy

Cesium sources were developed as an alternative for radium. Cesium's 0.662 MeV energy allows it to penetrate tissue to a similar degree as radium. Due to the 30-year half-life of cesium sources, calibration and treatment times must be adjusted as the sources age. Eventually the higher-activity sources must be replaced to keep the treatment times clinically acceptable. Cesium sources were widely used in low-dose gynecological implants such as cylinder, tandem, and ovoid implants. Cs-137 sources are used in low-dose afterloading devices [10].

^{60}**Co**: γ-ray, 5.26 year half-life; 1.17 MeV and 1.33 MeV

Cobalt-60 has a high specific activity, which allows for a very small source size. It has been used as a replacement for radium, but due to the short half-life, cesium is used more often. Cobalt's short half-life means more replacement sources will be required. Co-60 is also used as a source for external beam therapy machines.

^{192}**Ir**: γ-ray, 73.8 day half-life, 0.38 MeV avg energy

Iridium-192 was chosen as a source because its 0.38 avg MeV energy is less penetrating than that of cesium or radium but is strong enough for use in similar interstitial implants. It also has a high specific activity, so small sources may still contain a large amount of activity. Sources may be seeds spaced in a pattern on ribbons or wires. Iridium is also used in high-dose afterloading devices.

^{198}**Au**: γ-ray, 2.7 day half-life, 0.412 MeV energy

Gold-198 is used in seed form for permanent interstitial implants. It has advantages over radium because of lower energy and short half-life. Gold seeds became less favored after the introduction and popularity of I-125.

2.2 Low-Energy Sources

¹²⁵I: X-ray, 59.4 day half-life, 0.028 MeV avg energy

Iodine-125 is a low-energy source often used in small seeds. In more recent years, it is mostly commonly used in permanent prostate seed implants. It has also been used in eye plaques and brain implants. I-125 is a low-energy photon source that has a very steep dose falloff in tissue. Shielding needs for radiation protection purposes are very minimal. The low energy also means that the dosimetry of the source is more complex and strongly dependent on source design.

¹⁰³Pd: X-ray, 17 day half-life, 0.021 MeV avg energy

Palladium-103 is an alternative to I-125, with a similar energy but a shorter half-life. The shorter half-life may be a biological advantage as the dose is given over a shorter period of time. Pd-103 is used in permanent prostate brachytherapy and eye plaques.

¹³¹Cs: γ-ray, 9.7 day half-life, 0.03 MeV avg energy

Cesium-131 is another alternative to I-125, with a shorter half-life and similar energy.

It should be noted that the isotopes of ¹³⁷Cs, ⁶⁰Co, ¹⁹²Ir, and ¹⁹⁸Au are considered to be "radium equivalent," in that their energy spectra are dominated by high-energy photons that are minimally perturbed by source construction and tissue attenuation [11]. This results in the definition of "milligram radium equivalence" as a specification of source strength and the much simplified dose calculation methods that apply only to this class of high-energy sources. In contrast, dose distributions of low-energy sources of ¹²⁵I, ¹⁰³Pd, and ¹³¹Cs are significantly modified by the attenuation and scattering of low-energy photons, both in the

source construction components and in tissue. The source strength calibration standard and patient dose calculation formalism must be appropriately modified to account for these differences, as described in the following sections of this chapter.

2.3 Beta Sources

³²P: β-rays, 14.3 day half-life, 0.695 MeV avg energy, 1.71 MeV max energy

P-32 is a pure beta emitter. It is used in a disk or plaque form for skin lesions, as well as in a wire for interventional vascular brachytherapy for cardiac artery in-stent restenosis.

⁹⁰Sr: β-rays, 28.9 year half-life, 0.196 MeV avg energy, 0.546 MeV max energy

⁹⁰Y: β-rays, 64.1 h half-life 0.933 MeV avg energy, 2.28 MeV max energy

Strontium-90 has a daughter product, yttrium-90, that is a pure beta emitter. Sr-90 and Y-90 are used for eye plaques and other cancers where depth of penetration is an issue. Y-90 has been used in microspheres for treatment of hepatic malignancies. Microsphere brachytherapy uses glass or resin microspheres embedded with the nuclide [12].

3 Seed Design and Construction

In the United States, national source strength calibration standards of low-energy brachytherapy sources were first established using the Ritz free-air chamber for model 6702 and 6711 I-125 seeds [13]. The calibration, however, included effects of the 4.5 keV K-edge characteristic X-rays produced in the seed's titanium encapsulation, leading to an exaggerated estimate of the source strength. Loftus and Kubo et al. analyzed the dosimetric effect of this overestimate, leading NIST to develop the wide-angle free-air chamber (WAFAC) system as the source strength calibration standard for low-energy brachytherapy sources [14–16]. Multiple analyses have subsequently been published by relevant American Association of Physicists in Medicine (AAPM) committees on the impact of this standard change on the clinical dosimetry of prostate implants [17–19].

In 1995, the AAPM Task Group 43 published its recommendations on dosimetry of interstitial brachytherapy sources [20], unveiling the now well-accepted TG43 dose calculation formalism for the only seed sources available at the time: the Nycomed-Amersham 6702 and 6711 I-125 seeds, the Theragenics TP-200 Pd-103 seed, and the Ir-192 seeds from Best Medical and Alpha-Omega. This report was subsequently updated to correct for inconsistencies in the original report and to include later AAPM recommendations on low-energy brachytherapy sources, recommended dosimetry data sets for newly available I-125 and Pd-103 seeds, and guidelines for determination of dosimetric parameters of low-energy brachytherapy sources [21]. This updated TG43U1 report remains, to this day, the standard for clinical dose calculation, as well as reference dosimetry data determination of such sources.

Low-energy brachytherapy seed sources have traditionally been designed to geometrically conform to the precedent set by the Amersham model 6702 and 6711 I-125 seeds, with external dimensions of 4.5 mm in length and 0.8 mm in diameter. While no official explanations on these dimensions may be identified, it is likely that the diameter is determined by the intention of needle gauge size to be used for interstitial implants (a seed of 0.08 cm diameter would fit into an 18 gauge implant needle), while the length is dictated by the US Department of Transportation regulations relevant to special-form radioactive materials (with lower limit of 0.5 cm or 0.2 inches in length) for packaging and shipping purposes. Figure 1, from the TG43U1 report [21], shows the construction diagrams of some I-125 and Pd-103 sources, illustrating several common construction characteristics of low-energy brachytherapy sources:

1. A titanium capsule that serves as source encapsulation, typically a thin titanium tube manufactured through an extrusion process

2. End enclosures in the form of end welds, cups, or other mechanisms to seal the titanium tubes after internal components are inserted into the tube

3. Active source carriers, in the shape of spheres or cylinders

4. Active source materials containing the radioactive isotope, impregnated in or absorbed onto the source carriers

An ideal low-energy brachytherapy source would be expected to have uniform dose distribution around the source, as well as intersource dose distribution reproducibility.

Source design, construction, and manufacturing processes can impact dosimetric characteristics:

1. The titanium encapsulation should have uniform thickness. This is usually achievable via state-of-the-art manufacturing processes.

2. The end enclosure design should be thin and uniform and have minimal interseed variations. Thicker end enclosures, such as end welds or cups, may increase the anisotropy of dose distribution near the ends of the seed sources, thereby reducing accuracy of point-source-based dose calculation for these sources. Variations in end-weld thicknesses among seeds cause actual dose distributions to deviate from calculated ones, especially in anisotropic aspects (Fig. 2). These variations, although likely clinically insignificant, have the potential to significantly increase the uncertainties of calculated source anisotropy function values, due to uncertainties in the thickness of the average end-weld thickness used in the calculations. They also increase the uncertainties of measured anisotropy function values.

3. The geometry and material compositions of active source carriers may affect the dosimetric characteristics:

(a) Use of silver as an active source carrier, with its 25.51 keV K-edge X-rays, will effectively soften the photon energy spectrum of the encapsulated source, as noted by Daskalov et al. [22]. Dosimetrically, this results in lower dose rate constants

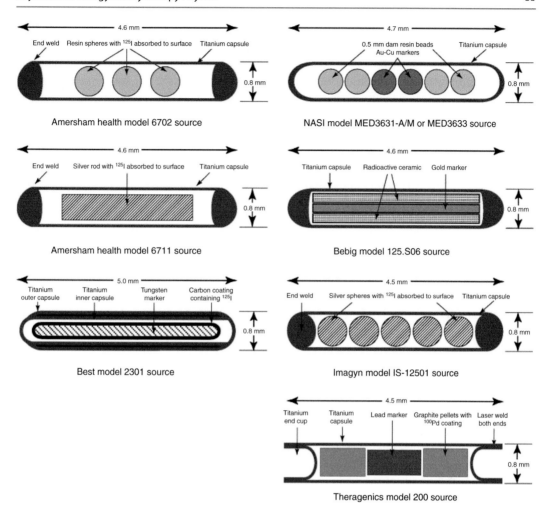

Fig. 1 Low-energy brachytherapy sources examined in the AAPM TG43U1 report [22]

Fig. 2 A radiograph of Amersham 6711 seed sources. Note the interseed variations of end-weld thicknesses and silver source carrier locations within the encapsulations

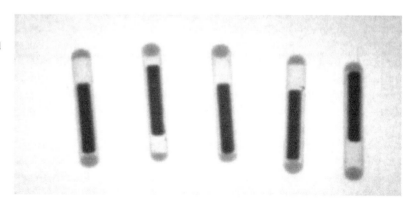

(DRC) of silver-based I-125 seed sources than of those using other source carriers. For example, the average DRC value of silver-based I-125 seeds (Amersham 6711 and Imagyn IS-12501) in the TG43U1 report is 0.953 cGy h^{-1} U^{-1}, while the average DRC value of the other seeds (Amersham 6702, Best 2301, NASI

MED3631-A/M, and Bebig/Theragenics I25.S06) is 1.026 cGy h^{-1} U^{-1}, a difference of 7.6 % (see [22]).

(b) Lack of positional reproducibility of source carriers within the titanium encapsulation can negatively impact accuracy of measured dose distribution around the source, in a manner similar to the interseed thickness variations of end enclosures, as shown in Fig. 2 for the Amersham 6711 seeds.

(c) Lack of interseed reproducibility of geometry of source carriers may increase the anisotropy values for calculated and measured source dose distribution, similar to variations in end-weld thicknesses. Figure 3 shows electron micrographs of the ends of two silver rods. The different degrees of beveling shown in the photos lead to differences in the calculated and measured source anisotropy function values.

4. Lack of uniformity of radioactive source material deposition on the source carriers can increase calculated and measured source dose distribution anisotropy (and even radial dose function). This can also be seen in Fig. 3, where one of the ends of the silver rods had little if any active source deposited.

In many clinical applications, the dose distribution uncertainties introduced by source construction and manufacturing variations are mostly mitigated by the number of sources used for patient treatments, as well as the fact that dosimetric uncertainties due to these variations are mostly limited to short distances away from each source, where the magnitude of such uncertainties is overshadowed by uncertainties in source position determination. It is therefore reasonable to state that point-source-based patient dose calculations may allow adequate accuracy of prescription dose calculation.

The sensitivity of low-energy source dose distribution to source design and construction also mandates that manufacturers should take into consideration potential dosimetry impacts of any changes in their source designs and manufacturing processes. Even more importantly, any such changes should be communicated in a timely manner to the users, such that potential changes in the sources' TG43 parameters may be identified. Chen et al. performed spectrometric and phantom measurements of DRC of the model CS-1 Cs-131 sources before and after production revisions and found the DRC changed by 0.7 % ± 0.5 % due to a significant decrease of fluorescent X-rays produced by the niobium used as the new source carrier [23].

Newer designs of low-energy brachytherapy sources continue to be developed. Frank et al. reported on their development and dosimetric evaluation of an MRI marker for prostate brachytherapy [24]. By placing cobalt chloride complex contrast agent markers adjacent to an I-125 seed, they were able to verify the improved visibility of the I-125 seeds on MR images. Phantom measurements of such modified seeds confirmed that the presence of markers does not alter the original source's anisotropy function values. Gautam et al. reported on their dosimetric analysis of an I-125 seed modified for thermotherapy by replacing the original tungsten source carrier with a ferromagnetic alloy material [25]. An 8 % change of the DRC of the source was determined by Monte Carlo calculations, while only small relative dose distribution parameters were identified. Rivard et al. calculated the TG43 parameters using the Monte Carlo method for a new Pd-103 source design, with the source available in lengths from 1.0 cm up to 6.0 cm, at 1.0 cm steps [26]. They found minimal variations of the normalized source strength as a function of source lengths. The dose rate constants, however, showed significant dependence on active source lengths, with percent reductions ranging between 18 and 8 % as active source length increases.

4 Dosimetry

Low-energy radionuclide sources in clinical use have different strengths, which historically have been described as apparent activity. This quantity was usually derived from exposure rate at a distance, which is a calibrated quantity

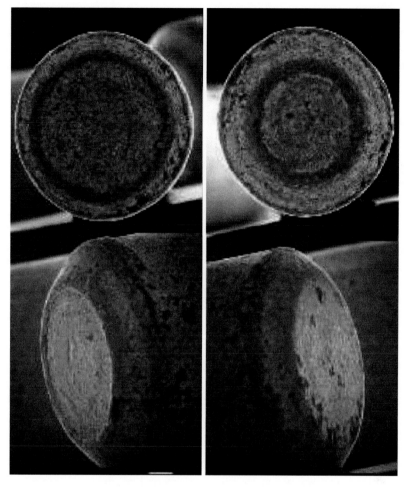

Fig. 3 Variations of active source deposition on source carriers. Note that the ends of the silver rods have different amounts of beveling and of active source depositions due to manufacturing deviations

directly traceable to National Institute of Standards and Technology (NIST) laboratories or American Association of Physicists in Medicine (AAPM) accredited dosimetry calibration laboratories (ADCL). Two-dimensional dose distribution was calculated based on these quantities. Currently, air kerma strength (S_K) is the standard brachytherapy source strength quantity, which can be converted to exposure rate ($\dot{X}$) at 1 m as

$$S_K = \dot{X}\left(\mathrm{Rh}^{-1}\right)(0.876\ \mathrm{cGy/R})(1\mathrm{m})^2, \quad (1)$$

where $\dot{X}$ is exposure rate measure in Rh^{-1}. Air kerma strength is defined as the product of air kerma rate due to photons of energy ($\dot{K}$) greater than a cutoff energy (δ) at a distance (d) and the square of the distance:

$$S_K = \dot{K}_\delta\left(d\right)d^2. \quad (2)$$

The cutoff energy, δ, is 5 keV for low-energy brachytherapy sources according to the update of AAPM Task Group No. 43 [21].

The air kerma strength of a clinical source should be calibrated by direct comparison with a NIST- or ADCL-calibrated source of the same kind. At NIST, air kerma strength of a source is calibrated by the wide-angle free-air chamber (WAFAC) with a precision of 0.01 ..Gy m^2 h^{-1}. An aluminum filter in the WAFAC is used to exclude low-energy contamination photons, which reflects the cutoff energy in the air kerma strength definition, to minimize the measurement uncertainty.

Using the calibrated air kerma strength, the 2D dose rate can be calculated as

$$\dot{D}(r,\theta) = S_K \cdot \Lambda \cdot \frac{G(r,\theta)}{G(r_0,\theta_0)} \cdot g(r) \cdot F(r,\theta), \quad (3)$$

where Λ is the dose rate constant (DRC), $G(r,\theta)$ is the geometry function, $g(r)$ is the radial dose function, and $F(r,\theta)$ is the 2D anisotropy function. The DRC is the ratio of dose rate at the reference point in water and air kerma strength. This quantity reflects the fundamental difference between the current dose calculation and the traditional. The calculation is done in water/water equivalence, which makes it more proper for dosing in patients. The geometry function reflects inverse square law falloff based on the source geometry. For instance, the geometry function for point source is $G_p(r,\theta) = r^{-2}$. Falloff due to scattering and attenuation is not part of the geometry function; rather, these factors are incorporated in the radial dose function, which is given in a lookup table in the update of AAPM Task Group No. 43 [21] and its supplement [27]. Since most of the sources are in linear form, the 2-D anisotropy function describes the dose variation as a polar angle relative to the transverse plane. For point sources, the dose distribution can be written in one dimension as

$$\dot{D}(r) = S_K \cdot \Lambda \cdot \left(\frac{r_0}{r}\right)^2 \cdot g_P(r) \cdot \phi_{an}(r), \quad (4)$$

where $\phi_{an}(r)$ is the anisotropy factor. Similarly for linear sources, the dose distribution can be written as

$$\dot{D}(r) = S_K \cdot \Lambda \cdot \frac{G_L(r,\theta_0)}{G_L(r_0,\theta_0)} \cdot g_L(r) \cdot \phi_{an}(r). \quad (5)$$

Consensus data sets of dose calculation quantities are given by the update of the AAPM Task Group No. 43 [21] and its supplement [27] for clinical implementation of low-energy I-125 and Pd-103 source models by different manufacturers. These data sets were derived from published Monte Carlo simulations or experimentally derived parameters. Consensus data sets of most low-energy brachytherapy sources available on the market as of 2005 can be found in the reports.

Once the dose rate at the time of the procedure is known, dose rate after a certain amount of time t can be written as

$$\dot{D}(t) = \dot{D}(0)e^{-\frac{0.693t}{T_{1/2}}}, \quad (6)$$

where $T_{1/2}$ is the half-life of the isotope and $\dot{D}(0)$ is the initial dose rate. The cumulated dose at this time then can be written as

$$D(t) = \dot{D}(0)(1.44T_{1/2})\left(1 - e^{-\frac{0.693t}{T_{1/2}}}\right). \quad (7)$$

Total dose after complete decay becomes

$$D_{total} = 1.44\dot{D}(0)T_{1/2}. \quad (8)$$

Below an example of treatment planning for prostate implant is introduced as an example of low-energy brachytherapy dosimetry implementation. Intraoperative planning is a popular option currently for prostate implants, in which TRUS images are acquired in the operating room and transferred to the treatment planning system. Target volume, rectum, and urethra are contoured on TRUS images, from which a treatment plan is generated. Point source assumption is usually used for the treatment planning algorithm. Linear source models may be used, given the assumption that sources are parallel to the needle. However, this assumption may cause calculation inaccuracies. On the other hand, source orientation may be more accurately determined on CT images during post-implant dose evaluation by using more advanced automatic segmentation methods. Dose distribution can then be calculated as a sum of the dose from each seed.

4.1 Example

Amersham 6702 I-125 seeds are used for a prostate implant case. The air kerma strength is

0.5 U. One seed is 3 cm from the anterior rectal wall. What is the dose rate from this seed to the closest point on the rectum? How much dose will this point get from this source after 1 month? After complete decay?

We explore these questions based on the point source model. The dosimetric quantities can be found in the update of AAPM Task Group No. 43 [21] as

$$S_k = 0.5\,\mathrm{U}; \Lambda = 1.036\ \mathrm{cGy\,h^{-1}\,U^{-1}};$$
$$g_P(r) = 0.702; \phi_{an}(r) = 0.951;$$

$$T_{1/2}12 = 59.4\ \mathrm{days} = 1425.6\ \mathrm{h}.$$

Therefore, the dose rate at the point is

$$\dot{D}(r) = S_K \cdot \Lambda \cdot \left(\frac{r_0}{r}\right)^2 \cdot g_P(r) \cdot \phi_{an}(r)$$
$$= 0.5 \cdot 1.036 \cdot \left(\frac{1}{3}\right)^2 \cdot 0.702 \cdot 0.951$$
$$= 0.0384\ \mathrm{cGy\,h^{-1}}.$$

After 1 month, the cumulated dose at this point is

$$D(t) = \dot{D}(0)(1.44T_{1/2})\left(1 - e^{-\frac{0.693t}{T_{1/2}}}\right)$$
$$= 0.0384 \cdot 1.44 \cdot 1425.6 \cdot \left(1 - e^{-0.693\cdot\frac{30}{59.4}}\right)$$
$$= 23.28\ \mathrm{cGy}.$$

The total dose is

$$D_{total} = 1.44\dot{D}(0)T_{1/2} = 0.0384 \cdot 1.44 \cdot 1425.6$$
$$= 78.83\ \mathrm{cGy}.$$

Note the above-calculated doses are from one source only. The total dose to this point should be summed from dose from all seeds.

5 Clinical Applications of Low-Dose Brachytherapy

Compared with higher-energy X-rays, low-energy X-rays have a higher linear energy transfer (LET), which associates with higher relative biological effectiveness (RBE), an advantage in terms of tumoricidal effect [28]. Typical energies of the low-energy brachytherapy discussed in this

chapter are below 50 keV, with effective energies similar to low-energy X-rays between 30 and 150 keV. Specifically, with reference to Co-60, I-125, the most commonly used low-energy brachytherapy source, has an RBE in the range of 1.1–2.0. Pd-103 has a lower energy and slightly larger LET compared with iodine-125, and its RBE values are generally accepted to be about 10 % higher [29–32].

The RBE also depends on the prescription dose and the dose rate. The dose and dose rate will be determined primarily by the nature and duration of implant. Temporary implants deliver a typical dose of 60–90 Gy in a few days, with a dose rate ranging from 0.5 to 0.8 Gy h⁻¹ using high-activity seeds. The typical permanent implant dose rate is less than 0.2 Gy h⁻¹ using low-activity seeds. For I-125, RBE values of 1.15–1.20 are observed for temporary implants, and higher RBE values (up to 2) are observed in permanent implants.

The dose D and biologically effective dose (BED) of temporary implants can be calculated as

$$D(t) = \frac{1}{\lambda}\dot{D}(0)(1 - e^{-\lambda t}), \quad (9)$$

$$\mathrm{BED} = \frac{1}{\lambda}\dot{D}(0)(1 - e^{-\lambda t})$$
$$\left\{1 + \frac{2\dot{D}(0)\lambda}{(\mu-\lambda)(\alpha/\beta)(1-e^{-\lambda t})}\right.$$
$$\left.\left[\frac{1}{2\lambda}(1-e^{-\lambda t}) - \frac{1}{(\mu+\lambda)}(1-e^{-(\mu+\lambda)t})\right]\right\} \quad (10)$$

[33, 34]. The total dose and BED of permanent implants can be calculated as

$$D = \frac{1}{\lambda}\dot{D}(0),$$

$$\mathrm{BED} = \frac{1}{\lambda}\dot{D}(0)\left(1 + \frac{\dot{D}(0)}{(\mu+\lambda)\alpha/\beta}\right), \quad (11)$$

where $\dot{D}(0)$ is the initial dose rate, $\lambda = 0.693/T_{1/2}$ is the decay constant, and μ is the recovery constant for sublethal damage.

While brachytherapy has a long history of treating many tumors, such as cancers of the cervix, oral cavity, lip, and penis, low-energy brachytherapy did not start until new radioactive sources became available. Because of its lower γ-ray energy, radiation protection issues are relatively easy to manage. The patient usually is allowed visitors, and medical staff can care for the patient with limited exposure to radiation. Patients often can be treated as outpatients and released shortly after the procedure.

The half-life is also important in the choice of isotope for practical purposes. The half-life should be long enough to allow sufficient time for shipping, assays, and the clinical procedure. On the other hand, the half-life used in permanent implantations should be fairly short to minimize time of exposure for relatives of the patient and members of the public.

Since the dose rate falls off as the inverse square of distance from the seeds and penetrating power is lower, a highly heterogeneous tumoricidal dose is delivered within the target, and the dose to the tissue outside the implanted volume falls off rapidly. This is an obvious advantage of brachytherapy compared with external beam radiation and often allows a high prescription dose to be delivered with fewer radiation complications. However, the seeds have to be placed directly inside or very close to the target, which generally requires an invasive procedure. Compared with higher-energy brachytherapy isotopes (Cs-137, Co-60, Ir-192, etc.), each low-energy seeds irradiate a relatively smaller target volume, and many seeds are commonly used for a large treatment volume. The most prominent application of low-energy brachytherapy is permanent seed implant of prostate adenocarcinoma using I-125 or Pd-103 encapsulated sources (seeds), with the choice determined by the physician or patient. The typical prescribed minimal peripheral doses are 145 Gy for monotherapy with 110 Gy boost for I-125 seeds and 110–130 Gy monotherapy with 100 Gy boost for PD-103 seeds. The patient is usually placed in an extended lithotomy position under anesthesia to allow transperineal needle insertion under the image guidance of TRUS. Based on the patient-specific treatment plan, from 60 to 120 seeds are injected into the prostate gland using 10 to 20 needles. The procedure and clinical aspects are discussed in another chapter of this book.

Temporary implants using eye plaques treating choroidal melanoma is another well-established clinical application. The pre-assayed seeds are placed inside a gold or lead plaque, which shields the extraocular tissues behind. The plaque is sewn on the outside of the eyeball to irradiate the intraocular target for a few days. After comparing various isotopes (Ra-226, Au-198, Co-60, Ir-192, and I-125, as well as tantalum-182 and ruthenium-10), the Collaborative Ocular Melanoma Study chose I-125 ophthalmic plaque radiation therapy to treat medium-sized choroidal melanomas. In the study, 85 Gy was prescribed at the apex of tumor for 3–7 days at a dose rate of 0.42–1.05 Gy h^{-1} [35, 36]. Some researchers chose to deliver the apical dose of 73.3 Gy over 5–7 days using Pd-103 and reported a favorable outcome [37–39]. The procedure and clinical aspects are discussed in another chapter of this book.

References

1. Li Z, Das RK, DeWard AL et al (2007) Dosimetric prerequisites for routine clinical use of proton emitting brachytherapy sources with average energy higher than 50 kev. Med Phys 34(1):37–40
2. Butler WM, Bice WS, DeWerd LA et al (2008) Third-party brachytherapy source calibrations and physicist responsibilities: report of the AAPM Low Energy Brachytherapy Source Calibration Working Group. Med Phys 35(9):3860–3865
3. Nath R, Bice WS, Butler WM et al (2009) AAPM recommendations on dose prescription and reporting methods for permanent interstitial brachytherapy for prostate cancer: report of Task Group 137. Med Phys 36(11):5310–5322
4. Chiu-Tsao ST, Astrahan MA, Finger PT (2012) Dosimetry of (125)I and (103)Pd COMS eye plaques for intraocular tumors: report of Task Group 129 by the AAPM and ABS. Med Phys 39(10):6161–6184
5. Blasko JC, Grimm PD, Ragde H (1993) Brachytherapy and organ preservation in the management of carcinoma of the prostate. Semin Radiat Oncol 3:230–239
6. Holm HH, Juul N, Pedersen H et al (1983) Transperineal 125Iodine seed implantation in prostate cancer guided by transrectal ultrasonography. J Urol 130:283–286
7. Smith RP, Schuchert M, Komanduri K et al (2007) Dosimetric evaluation of radiation exposure during I-125 vicryl mesh implants: implications for ACOSOG z4032. Ann Surg Oncol 14(12):3610–3613

8. Lemoigne Y, Caner A (eds) (2009) Radiotherapy and brachytherapy. Springer, Dordrecht
9. Venselaar J, Baltas D, Meigooni AS et al (eds) (2012) Comprehensive brachytherapy: physical and clinical aspects. CRC Press, Boca Raton, FL
10. Sina S, Faghihi R, Meigooni AS et al (2011) Impact of the vaginal applicator and dummy pellets on the dosimetry parameters of Cs-137 brachytherapy source. J Appl Clin Med Phys 12:3480
11. Williamson JF, Brenner DJ (2008) Physics and biology of brachytherapy. In: Halperin CE, Perez CA, Brady LW (eds) Perez and Brady's principles and practice of radiation oncology. Lippincott Williams & Wilkins, Philadelphia, pp 423–475
12. TG144.http://www.aapm.org/pubs/reports/RPT_144.pdf
13. Loftus TP (1984) Exposure standardization of 125I seeds used for brachytherapy. J Res Nat Bur Stand 89:295–303
14. Kubo H (1985) Exposure contribution from Ti K x rays produced in the titanium capsule of the clinical 125I seed. Med Phys 12:215–220
15. Seltzer S, Lamperti P, Loevinger R et al (1998) New NIST Air-kerma strength standards for I-125 and Pd-103 brachytherapy seeds. Med Phys 25:A170
16. Williamson J (1988) Monte Carlo evaluation of specific dose constants in water for 125I seeds. Med Phys 15:686–694
17. Kubo HD, Coursey BM, Hanson WF et al (1998) Report of the ad hoc committee of the AAPM radiation therapy committee on 125I sealed source dosimetry. Int J Radiat Oncol Biol Phys 40(3):697–702
18. Williamson JF, Butler W, DeWerd LA et al (2005) Recommendations of the American Association of Physicists in Medicine regarding the impact of implementiong the 2004 Task Group 43 report on Dose Specification for Pd-103 and I-125 interstitial brachytherapy. Med Phys 32:1424–1439
19. Willliamson JF, Coursey BM, DeWerd LA et al (1999) Guidance to users of Nycomed Amersham and North American Scientific, Inc., I-125 interstitial sources: dosimetry and calibration changes: recommendations of the AAPM RTC ad hoc committee on low-energy seed dosimetry. Med Phys 26(4):570–573
20. Nath R, Anderson LL, Luxton G et al (1995) Dosimetry of interstitial brachytherapy sources: report of the AAPM Radiation Therapy Committee Task Group 43. Med Phys 22(2):209–234
21. Rivard MJ, Coursey BM, DeWerd LA et al (2004) Update of AAPM Task Group no. 43 report: a revised AAPM protocol for brachytherapy dose calculations. Med Phys 31(3):633–674
22. Daskalov GM, Kirov AS, Williamson JF (1998) Analytical approach to heterogeneity correction factor calculation for brachytherapy. Med Phys 25(5):722–735
23. Chen Z, Bongiorni P, Nath R (2010) Impact of source-production revision on the dose-rate constant of 131Cs interstitial brachytherapy source. Med Phys 37(7):3607–3610
24. Frank SJ, Tailor RC, Kudchadker R et al (2011) Anisotropy characterization of I-125 seed with attached encapsulated cobalt chloride complex contrast agent markers for MRI-based prostate brachytherapy. Med Dosim 36(2):200–205
25. Gautam B, Parsai EI, Shvydk D et al (2012) Dosimetric and thermal properties of a newly developed thermobrachytherapy seed with ferromagnetic core for treatment of solid tumors. Med Phys 39(4):1980–1989
26. Rivard MJ, Reed JL, DeWerd LA (2014) 103Pd strings: Monte Carlo assessment of a new approach to brachytherapy source design. Med Phys 41(1):011716
27. Rivard JM, Butler WM, DeWerd LA et al (2007) Supplement to the 2004 update of the AAPM Task Group No. 43 Report. Med Phys 34(6):2187–2205
28. Eckerman MB (2013) Relative biological effectiveness of low-energy electrons and photons, letter report. U.S. Environmental Protection Agency October
29. Ling CC, Li WX, Anderson LL (1995) The relative biological effectiveness of I-125 and Pd-103. Int J Radiat Oncol Biol Phys 32:373–378
30. Scalliet P, Wambersie A (1988) Which RBE for iodine 125 in clinical applications? Radiother Oncol 9:221–230
31. Wuu CS, Zaider M (1998) A calculation of the relative biological effectiveness of 125I and 103Pd brachytherapy sources using the concept of proximity function. Med Phys 25:2186–2189
32. Wuu CS, Kliauga P, Zaider M et al (1996) Microdosimetric evaluation of relative biological effectiveness for palladium-103, iodine-125, americium 241 and iridium 192 brachytherapy sources. Int J Radiat Oncol Biol Phys 36:689–697
33. Dale RG (1985) The application of the linear quadratic dose-effect equation to fractionated and protracted radiotherapy. Br J Radiol 58:515–528
34. Gagne NL (2012) Radiobiology for eye plaque brachytherapy and evaluation of implant duration and radionuclide choice using an objective function. Med Phys 39:3332–3342
35. Earle JD (1987) Selection of iodine 125 for the collaborative ocular melanoma study. Arch Ophthalmol 100:763–764
36. Melia BM, Abramson DH, Albert DM et al (2001) Collaborative ocular melanoma study (COMS) randomized trial of I-125 brachytherapy for medium choroidal melanoma. visual acuity after 3 years COMS report no. 16 Collaborative Ocular Melanoma Study Group. Ophthalmology 108:348–366
37. Dolan J, Li Z, Williamson JF (2006) Monte Carlo and experimental dosimetry of an I-125 brachytherapy seed. Med Phys 33(12):4675–4684
38. Finger PT, Berson A, Ng T et al (2002) Palladium-103 plaque radiotherapy for choroidal melanoma: an 11-year study. Int J Radiat Oncol Biol Phys 54:1438–1445
39. Finger PT, Chin KJ, Duvall BS et al (2009) Palladium-103 ophthalmic plaque radiation therapy for choroidal melanoma: 400 treated patients. Ophthalmology 116:790–796

Balloon Brachytherapy Physics

Dorin A. Todor

Abstract

Brachytherapy utilizing intracavitary balloon and strut devices is a recent therapeutic offering. As such, the specifics of the physics of what might appear superficially to be simple devices can be quite challenging. We present this chapter to explain the balloon device and its physical properties, including the nuances that may arise in planning and quality assurance.

1   Introduction

Accelerated partial breast irradiation (APBI) treatments can be delivered using external beam or brachytherapy techniques. Interstitial brachytherapy using low-dose-rate (LDR) Ir-192 seeds was historically the first modality used for APBI and consequently has the longest follow-up. More recently, external beam treatment has been used, either as photon beams or highly collimated electron beams, the latest being more often associated with intraoperative techniques relatively popular in Europe. New brachytherapy sources have been developed, one example being the miniature low-energy (~50 kV) source known as electronic brachytherapy, but existent sources (e.g., Pd-103) commonly associated with treatment of prostate cancer are also used as permanent seed implant for permanent breast seed implant (PBSI) [1–3]. However, most commonly (at least in the USA), APBI is associated with high-dose-rate (HDR) treatment using Ir-192. The relatively high-energy source (~380 keV) at the tip of a thin wire is placed, using a computer-controlled afterloader device, in precisely specified positions for time intervals determined in the planning phase. Given the fact that the treatment is delivered quickly compared with the average half-life of cellular repair processes, one can establish an equivalence between multiple sources loaded simultaneously (LDR) and one source – which is the case for the HDR paradigm, being placed in specified positions called dwell positions, along applicators, and kept for well-specified amounts of time called dwell times. Thus, for a well-determined target and a specified applicator typically inserted close to the site to be treated and a given strength of an Ir-192 source,

D.A. Todor, PhD
Department of Radiation Oncology, Virginia
Commonwealth University Health System,
Richmond, VA, USA
e-mail: dorin.todor@vcuhealth.org

© Springer International Publishing Switzerland 2016
P. Montemaggi et al. (eds.), *Brachytherapy: An International Perspective*, Medical Radiology,
DOI 10.1007/978-3-319-26791-3_5

an HDR treatment plan consists of specifying dwell positions and their associated dwell times. Since the radioactive source is placed in the body but cannot come in contact with tissues, one has to use an "applicator" to both contain and to guide the source in the desired positions. The simplest applicator is a plastic catheter inserted in the tissue, and a multitude [15–24] of such well-spaced catheters is called an interstitial implant. Each catheter is connected to a channel in the afterloader using a transfer (or guide) tube.

The first technique developed for APBI was the multi-catheter interstitial brachytherapy [4]. With this approach, the treatment time is reduced from the traditional 5–7 weeks to 5–8 days or less. The technique was initially used to deliver a tumor bed boost after whole breast irradiation, and it has been one of the most used methods for APBI in North America and Europe. Catheters are placed through the breast tissue surrounding the lumpectomy cavity typically at 1–1.5 cm intervals. The number of catheters is determined by the size and shape of the target, and the configuration of the catheters is guided by the understanding of brachytherapy dosimetry. Initially, the target volume was defined as the lumpectomy cavity plus a 2 cm margin, except where these target dimensions were limited by the extent of breast tissue (i.e., chest wall and skin). One has to remember though that initially the catheter placement was guided by fluoroscopy (with surgical clips placed to mark the lumpectomy cavity), while the planning was based on orthogonal radiographs, so no true planning target volume (PTV) was actually defined.

Even though from a technical perspective, the interstitial implant is the most flexible technique, it does require specialized training and considerable experience. In an effort to make APBI more accessible, a number of devices were created with the goal of reducing the level of invasiveness, making the technique simpler and more reproducible [4, 5]. Essentially, there are two categories of devices: balloon-based devices (MammoSite®, Contura MLB®, and MammoSite ML®) and strut-based devices (SAVI®, ClearPath®). MammoSite®, historically the first balloon device for breast brachytherapy, was in fact following in the footsteps of another balloon device for brain brachytherapy: GliaSite RTS® – a balloon filled with liquid I-125 [6].

1.1 Description of Devices Available

MammoSite® is a silicone balloon that can be placed in a lumpectomy cavity and then inflated with water to a diameter of 4–5 cm. It has a 15 cm long central shaft and a 0.6 cm diameter that contains a larger "treatment" channel for placement of the high-dose-rate source and a smaller channel used for inflation (Fig. 1). Given the central placement of the lumen, the dose distribution created by one or multiple dwell positions is always cylindrically symmetrical. The lack of symmetry of the central lumen relative to the balloon or the asymmetry of the PTV (due to closeness to skin or chest wall) could only be dealt with by the MammoSite®

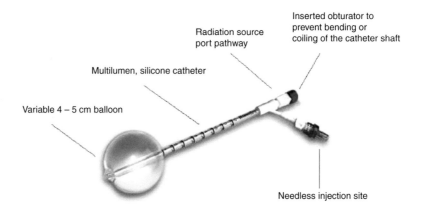

Fig. 1 MammoSite® balloon

RTS by compromising target coverage or dose to the critical normal structures (skin and chest wall). Given that the prescription dose is always at 1 cm from the surface of the balloon, the radius of the balloon will influence dose to the surface of the balloon and consequently the dose gradient in the target. For a medium-sized balloon (diameter of about 4.5 cm), the dose to the surface of the balloon is approximately 200 % of the prescription dose, with slightly smaller values for a larger diameter balloon and slightly larger values for a smaller diameter balloon. A slight anisotropy of dose along the direction of the wire (picture an apple vs. an orange at the north and south "pole") can be reduced by the use of multiple dwell times [7]. The theoretical advantage of using the largest possible balloon diameter is that it allows one to create a more homogeneous dose distribution. However, some centers have noticed higher rates of seroma formation and fat necrosis with higher balloon fill volumes.

Because treatment planning is performed under the conditions of an inflated balloon, it is critical that the integrity of the balloon is verified prior to each fraction to avoid delivery of higher than intended doses directly to the surrounding breast tissue. Typically such verification is done using ultrasound, fluoroscopic, or CT images.

For the central lumen balloon, there is a tight coupling between dose coverage of the target and dose to organs at risk (OARs). An attempt to decrease the dose to an organ at risk when using only central lumen balloons will unavoidably decrease the dose to the target. The lack of flexibility in planning with the central lumen only balloon device leads to the creation of the multi-lumen devices: Contura MLB® and MammoSite ML®. Both devices preserved the central lumen but added offset treatment lumens. The Contura MLB® also has two vacuum ports at the distal and proximal aspects that can be used for removal of air and fluid thus increasing conformity of the tissue to the surface of the balloon (Fig. 2a, b). The major advantage of the multi-lumen devices is that they decouple the dose coverage of the target from minimizing the dose to critical structures.

A treatment plan for an asymmetric target can now simultaneously maximize the prescription dose coverage while minimizing dose to skin and chest wall. The "penalty" comes in the form of creating an asymmetric dose distribution (which conforms very well to the asymmetric target) outside a symmetric balloon, thus increasing the volume of tissue in the target receiving a larger than prescription dose (e.g., V200, the volume of the target that receives 200 % of prescribed dose).

Even though initially developed by different companies, all three balloon devices commercially available are now offered by the same company (Hologic Inc., Bedford, MA): MammoSite® single-lumen balloon catheter (in two sizes, 4.0–5.0 cm and 5.0–6.0 cm), MammoSite® multi-lumen (ML) balloon catheter (3.5–5.0 cm), and Contura® multi-lumen balloon (MLB) (also in two sizes, 4.0–5.0 cm and 4.5–6.0 cm). For each device, a balloon device is offered for cavity size evaluation, the Cavity Evaluation Device® (CED) which is placed at the time of the lumpectomy and replaced with a treatment balloon at the time of treatment. The MammoSite® device consists of a silicone balloon connected to a catheter (Fig. 1). The balloon is inflated with saline solution and a small amount of radiographic contrast to aid visualization. The designs of the multi-lumen balloon applicators are different. The Contura MLB® has five lumens, one central lumen and four equally spaced peripheral lumens which are 0.5 cm away (at their largest separation) from the central lumen (Fig. 2b). The MammoSite ML® has four lumens: one central lumen and three equally spaced peripheral lumens, parallel with and at 0.3 cm from the central lumen (Fig. 3a, b). Another balloon applicator, with just a central lumen, was developed in conjunction with the 50 kV electronic brachytherapy source Axxent EBT® system (Xoft, Inc., Sunnyvale, CA) (Fig. 4). Other than the size of the central lumen designed to accommodate the much larger X-ray source and its cooling housing, there is nothing else that would distinguish the Axxent® from the MammoSite® balloon.

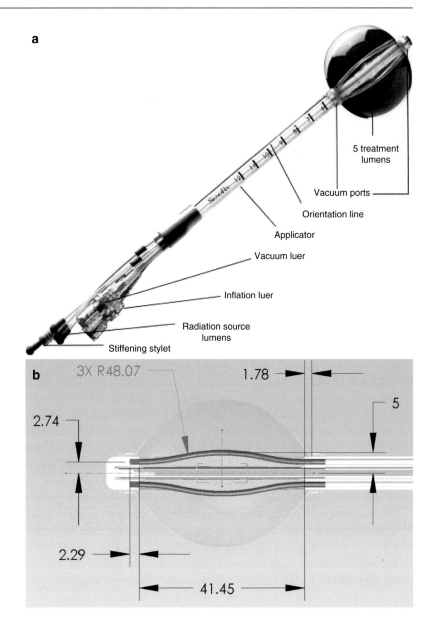

Fig. 2 (**a**, **b**) Contura MLB®

1.2 Radiation Sources for Breast HDR

[192]Iridium has long been the workhorse of brachytherapy. The history starts with iridium in seed form having been used in brachytherapy in 1958 by Ulrich Henschke and then, from the early 1960s, mainly as wires [8]. Andrassy, in a debate on the best HDR isotope, sets up the history, pointing out the fact, sometimes forgotten that

there was a time when most afterloaders used cobalt-60: "In the 1950-60s, when the production of isotopes by neutron activation became feasible, Co-60 complemented Cs-137 as the standard nuclide in radiation therapy. Its application has been studied in many countries all over the world, and broad clinical experience in teletherapy, as well as in brachytherapy has been gained. All in all, several hundred HDR afterloader units equipped with Co-60-sources have been utilized

Fig. 3 (**a**, **b**) MammoSite
ML®

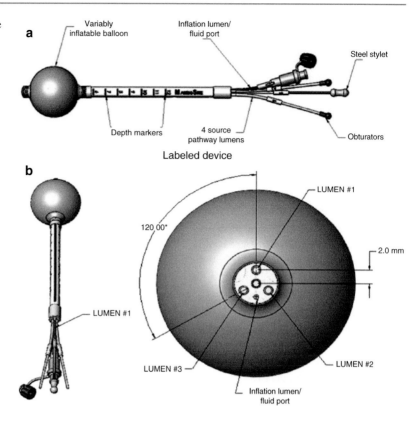

a

Variably
inflatable balloon

Inflation lumen/
fluid port

Steel stylet

Depth markers

4 source
pathway lumens

Obturators

Labeled device

b

LUMEN #1

120.00°

2.0 mm

LUMEN #1

LUMEN #3

LUMEN #2

Inflation lumen/
fluid port

Fig. 4 Axxent®
applicator

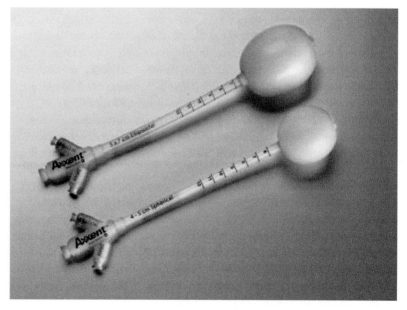

in clinics ever since, the majority of them for gynecological applications. The technical development of sources with higher specific activity was the starting point for HDR remote afterloading. Clinical data and dose delivery concepts to achieve equivalent outcomes in Low Dose Rate (LDR) and HDR-applications had been worked out using Co-60 sources. In the

1970s, the manufacture of miniaturized ^{192}Ir sources shifted market preference to this nuclide. Smaller size and source diameter allowed new application modalities, e.g. interstitial therapy, as well as dose optimization due to stepping source technology. At the same time, the extrapolation of experience obtained from traditional brachytherapy nuclides to Ir-192 was based on the similarity of physical dose distributions" [9]. ^{192}Iridium has a reasonably long half-life (73.81 days) so a typical source exchange occurs approximately every 2 months. Two other technical advantages are a relatively low average energy (~.38 Mev, with a range from 0.136 to 1.062 MeV) and a half value layer of ~0.3 cm Pb so it is relatively easily shielded. Nevertheless, the lead shielding for a room designated solely for brachytherapy can be expensive. The other advantage is its high specific activity (450 Ci/g) allowing the construction of high activity sources (10 Ci) of small diameter (0.06–0.11 cm). ^{192}Ir is produced from enriched ^{191}Ir targets (37 % natural abundance) in a reactor by the (n, γ) reaction, creating HDR ^{192}Ir sources (typically 0.1 cm diameter by 0.35 cm length cylinders) with activities exceeding 4.4 TBq. High-dose-rate ^{192}Ir sources are encapsulated in a thin titanium or stainless steel capsule and laser welded to the end of a flexible wire. Electrons from β-decay are absorbed by the core and the capsule.

Instead of using HDR ^{192}Ir, the Xoft Axxent source is an electronic microminiature X-ray tube [1]. Despite a small diameter of the X-ray tube – 0.225 cm – the need for a flexible cooling catheter makes the HV catheter 0.54 cm large enough to make its use impossible in most, if not all, applicators designed for ^{192}Ir. The electronic source generates a 50-kV photon spectrum in a roughly spherical distribution. The depth dose characteristics of this source were designed to roughly mimic HDR ^{192}Ir; however, there are important differences. The lower photon energy of this source results in greater attenuation. Unlike HDR ^{192}Ir, electronic brachytherapy (EBB) does not require a shielded vault. This reduces costs and allows for portability of the system, which can lead to greater access for patients particularly in more remote locations or non-shielded operating and treatment rooms. There are also dosimetric implications of a lower-energy spectrum that results in more rapid dose falloff with depth in tissue. With a standard dose prescription at 1 cm from the balloon surface, the dose to structures proximal to this point is higher, and the dose to structures beyond this point is lower with EBB. Dickler et al. evaluated the dosimetric differences between Xoft® and MammoSite® [10]. They showed that the dose to lung and heart was significantly lower with EBB. The lung V30 was 1.1 % vs. 3.7 % and heart V5 of 9.4 % vs. 59.2 % for EBB and intracavitary breast brachytherapy (IBB), respectively. The dose to nontarget breast was also lower; breast V50 was 13 % vs. 19.8 %, respectively. However, the volume of dose hotspots was significantly higher with EBB. The V150, V200, and V300 were 59.4 % vs. 41.8 %, 32 % vs. 11.3 %, and 6.7 % vs. 0.4 %, respectively. Another consideration for EBB is that the relative biological effectiveness (RBE) for low-energy photons is higher on the order of 1.2–2, depending on energy and depth. This has currently not been taken into account in the prescribed dose for EBB, which uses the same prescription of 34.0 Gy in 10 fractions as used with IBB using HDR ^{192}Ir. Electronic sources do not fall under existent regulatory scrutiny of radioactive sources. The American Society for Radiation Oncology (ASTRO) Emerging Technology Committee issued a report on electronic brachytherapy providing a descriptive overview of the technologies' current and future projected applications, comparison of competing technologies, potential impact, and potential safety issues [11].

^{169}Ytterbium has been mentioned for a long time as a possible alternate HDR source and the advantages of Yb-169 compared with Ir-192 for a balloon device have been described [12]. ^{169}Ytterbium emits photons with energies ranging from 50 to 308 keV (average energy 93 keV) and decays with a half-life of 32 days. While the shorter half-life is a disadvantage, the lower average energy clearly would require significantly less shielding than iridium. In the balloon study, the plans using ^{169}Ytterbium source results in less volume receiving doses of 150 and 200 % of the prescription, a greater dose homogeneity index (DHI), and lower maximum dose [12]. The X-ray source performed worse in all categories.

1.3 Process Description

Once a patient has been identified as an appropriate candidate for APBI, one has to assess the appropriateness of balloon brachytherapy. The patient typically undergoes a CT or ultrasound of the involved breast, and the options are discussed in a multidisciplinary team involving a surgeon, radiation oncologist, and physicist. A balloon is deemed a suitable choice if the lumpectomy cavity is situated in a region of the breast where there is enough surrounding tissue to allow the inflation of a balloon (the typical diameter is between 4 and 6 cm). After placement under ultrasound (US) guidance, other conditions are necessary or desirable: a balloon-to-skin distance 0.3 cm or more (preferably $\geq$0.7 cm), good conformance of the balloon's surface to the walls of the lumpectomy cavity, and, for a single-lumen device, (MammoSite®) balloon symmetry around the catheter's center shaft. Patients are excluded if the cavity is excessively large, if there is poor conformance of the balloon to the cavity walls or inadequate balloon-to-skin distance.

Zannis et al. identified three different techniques for insertion of a breast brachytherapy balloon catheter [13]: (1) at the time of lumpectomy into an open cavity, (2) after surgery with ultrasound guidance through a separate small lateral incision into a closed cavity, or (3) after surgery by entering directly through the lumpectomy wound (the scar entry technique). Analyzing clinical outcomes after each of the insertion methods, they concluded "There was a statistically significant increased incidence of premature catheter removals for pathologically related reasons with the open-cavity technique compared with the 2 postoperative methods secondary to final histology reports disqualifying the patient" after placement. Thus, postoperative placement, after the final pathology report is issued, decreases the incidence of premature removal of the catheter because of disqualifying pathology.

The ultrasound-guided placement technique takes place after surgery and uses ultrasound visualization of the lumpectomy cavity. After skin and subcutaneous tissue infiltration with lidocaine solution, a sharp metal trocar provided by the manufacturer is inserted with ultrasound guidance into the lumpectomy cavity through a small skin incision made in the lateral breast. The cavity seroma decompresses through the trocar lumen, the trocar is removed, and then the deflated balloon catheter is inserted into the cavity through the trocar tract or using a split sheath. Using a syringe with a saline and contrast solution, the balloon is progressively inflated. Another CT or ultrasound is taken to ensure the conformity of the balloon to the lumpectomy cavity, to estimate the balloon-to-skin distance, and to make sure that the balloon catheter is in an optimal position. A photograph is taken at the CT time and used to verify catheter position before each fraction. A reference mark is placed on the breast commensurate with the index mark on multi-lumen balloons to verify correct positioning in the event of rotation of the device. A planning CT is used for treatment planning and dose optimization. The plan is verified, applicator treatment lengths are measured, and treatment is administered in the planned number of fractions (typically 10 fractions of 3.4 Gy) using a ^{192}Ir computer-controlled remote afterloader. Prior to each fraction, the integrity of the balloon (its size/ diameter) is verified using ultrasound, fluoroscopy, CT, or CBCT, along with the rotational position. After the last treatment is delivered, the balloon is deflated and the balloon catheter removed and incision closed. Rotation of the balloon in the breast prior to explantation breaks adhesions and facilitates the removal.

1.4 Target Delineation in Balloon Brachytherapy

The vast majority of authors describing early experience with interstitial implants report a clinical target volume (CTV) defined as lumpectomy cavity + 2 cm [4, 14, 15]. It is not clear when the accepted interstitial margin became 1.5 cm, but most likely it is related to the CT-based planning, when careful, systematic, reproducible, and true three-dimensional volumes were created. It is also likely that it occurred at the time of the National Surgical Adjuvant Breast and Bowel Project (NSABP) protocol B-39 [16] writing. The 1.5 cm was chosen as a compromise between the 2 cm margin for interstitial implants and the 1 cm margin for the "new" balloon applicator that was to be included in the brachytherapy arm of the trial.

When the balloon brachytherapy method using MammoSite® was introduced, Edmundson et al. made a point in demonstrating, using the concept of "effective thickness," that the target irradiated by the MammoSite® was in fact "nearly 2 cm" [17]. This demonstrates that at the time (2002) the 2 cm margin was still the accepted margin for interstitial implants. Dickler et al. also calculated the effective thickness for 13 patients and produced a mean result of 1.6 cm [18]. These results were consistent with the CTV margins used for multi-catheter interstitial brachytherapy, supporting the hypothesis that the two APBI modalities treat effectively similar target volumes. Dickler's paper was published in 2004, therefore sometime between 2002 and 2004 the margin for interstitial implants was transformed from 2 cm to 1.5 cm.

A more recent paper, acknowledging the fact that the effective thickness might not be uniform due to the fact that the tissue adjacent to the balloon may compress or stretch, used deformable registration to propagate contours from one CT set to another [19]. Their conclusion was that "The effective CTV treated by the MammoSite® was on average $7\% \pm 10\%$ larger and $38\% \pm 4\%$ smaller than three-dimensional conformal radiotherapy (3D–CRT) CTVs created using uniform expansions of 1 and 1.5 cm, respectively. The average effective CTV margin was 1.0 cm, the same as the actual MammoSite® CTV margin.

However, the effective CTV margin was non-uniform and could range from 0.5 to 1.5 cm in any given direction."

Contouring of CTV is known to be associated with low interobserver concordance, due to a number of factors: dense breast parenchyma, benign calcifications in the breast, and tissue stranding from the surgical cavity. Surgically placed clips after lumpectomy as radiographic surrogates of the cavity have been shown to help with the delineation of the lumpectomy cavity. In balloon-based methods, the uncertainty of delineating the lumpectomy cavity is removed and replaced by the much more reliable delineation of the balloon surface. Of course the implicit assumption is that the balloon is correctly placed in the center of lumpectomy cavity and that the inflated balloon stretches the tissue isotropically. For increased visibility on CT images and automatic delineation, a small quantity of iodine-based contrast is used in the water. A planning target volume for evaluation (PTV_EVAL) is created using a 1.0 cm expansion from the balloon surface of the CTV but limited by the first 0.5 cm from the skin surface and abutting the chest wall. A 1 cm expansion is used in the case of balloon-based brachytherapy devices due to stretching of the tissue surrounding the lumpectomy cavity. A majority of the seroma will be expelled during the placement of the brachytherapy applicator. Some additional fluid may be present at the time of simulation and may be removed using the device's vacuum port, if available. Time will also almost always allow for resorption or dissolution of fluid and air. Waiting 1–2 days before treatment usually remedies the issue. If air or fluid is retained within the lumpectomy cavity after inflation of the applicator's balloon, the displacement of the tissue away from the applicator's surface must be accounted for. The air/fluid trapped should be contoured separately on each CT slice and a total volume should be calculated to determine the percentage of the PTV_EVAL that is displaced. This percent displacement must be limited so that:

$$\left(\% \, PTV\_EVAL \, coverage\right) - \left[\left(vol. \, trapped \, air \, / \, vol \, PTV\_EVAL\right) \times 100\right] = \geq 90\%$$

The PTV_EVAL originated as a structure used to *evaluate* an existent plan for APBI under the NSABP B-39 clinical trial (also known as the Radiation therapy Oncology Group (RTOG) trial 0413). The simple idea was that since the external beam (EB) dose calculation algorithms were unreliable close to interfaces (i.e., skin) and since the trial was supposed to compare brachytherapy and external beam treatments, creating a structure that would remove the 0.5 cm of skin seemed almost normal. The pectoralis muscle, chest wall, and ribs were deemed "nontarget" tissues and also removed from the PTV.

While the PTV, as a 1 cm margin from the balloon surface, would almost always be symmetrical (unless the balloon would be less than 1 cm away from the skin), the PTV_EVAL, by being limited by the 5 mm skin structure and the chest wall and pectoralis, would be, in many cases, asymmetric. In the MammoSite® era, there was nothing one could do to customize the coverage for an asymmetric PTV_EVAL. Whether the PTV would be "whole" – as in the case of a balloon placed deep in the breast – or "chopped" (Fig. 5), the dose distribution created was invariably a radially symmetrical blob. So even though there were no two explicit structures, one for planning and one for evaluation (as that was the case, e.g., in EBRT), there was in fact an implicit planning structure simply because the device could only create a radially symmetrical dose distribution. With the advent of multiple treatment lumens, which have the potential to create a dose distribution truly conformal to the PTV_EVAL, the question whether PTV_EVAL is in fact a planning structure, an evaluation structure, or both should be revisited. The answer is far from being of just academic interest and more likely has important implications for how the new devices are being used.

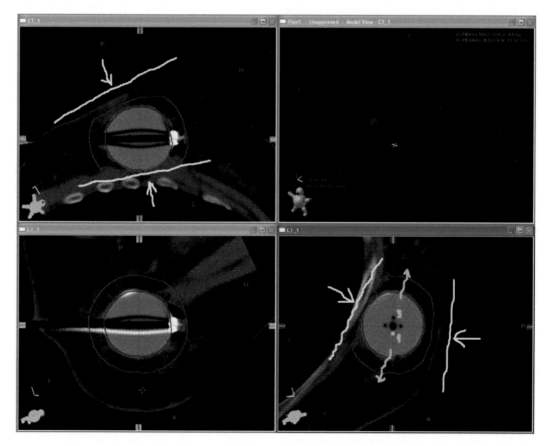

Fig. 5 Orthogonal views of a Contura Multi-lumen® plan. In *yellow* are the "bounding" planes of the PTV_EVAL

A planning exercise using Contura® balloons attempted to elucidate the implications of removing the 0.5 cm of skin from the PTV on dosimetric parameters currently reported (Todor D, 2007, personal communication).

A "classic" PTV_EVAL is shown in Fig. 6. The uniform 1 cm expansion of the balloon is limited by both the pectoralis muscle and 0.5 cm of the skin layer. The "novel" PTV_EVAL is shown for the same anatomy as above (Fig. 7). One can see (in bright red contours) that in its anterior aspect, the "novel" PTV_EVAL is now limited by the skin surface.

Two plans were created per patient, each optimizing the "coverage" for its intended structure. The coverage of each intended target for the two

plans was similar (within 1 %), so meaningful conclusions can be drawn for all other parameters. Dose–volume histogram (DVH)-based optimization with constraining pseudo-structures was employed in all cases. By including the 0.5 cm of skin in the PTV_EVAL, the volume of this structure increased by up to 20 %. Despite an increase in target volume, when the dose is correctly optimized, the dose received by breast tissue is very similar with a slight increase (1–4 %) for the larger PTV_EVAL. So, even though one outlined and optimized on a different structure, the volume of breast tissue receiving prescription dose was virtually the same. The one parameter clearly different was the maximum dose to the skin: for the NSABP B-39 PTV_EVAL, the max dose to skin was between 11 and 17 % lower than for the larger PTV_EVAL, even though in all cases it was kept under 125 % of prescription.

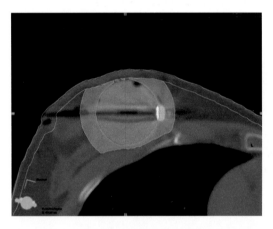

Fig. 6 A "classic" (NSABP-B49/RTOG 0413) PTV_EVAL

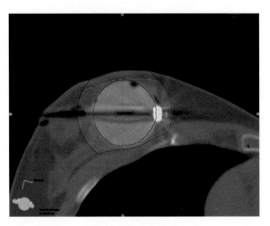

Fig. 7 A "novel" PTV_EVAL containing the 0.5 cm of skin normally removed

1.5   Fundamentals of Physics

The physics of balloon brachytherapy is in no way different from the physics of brachytherapy in general. In fact, while essential to our understanding of dose delivered to target tissues, physics is one component in a long list of "ingredients" necessary for a successful brachytherapy treatment. Without the claim that this is an exhaustive one, here is a comprehensive list of such ingredients:

1. One or more radiation sources with calibration traceable to a standard laboratory
2. Good understanding of the radiation emitted by the sources and the effects of encapsulation, wires, etc.
3. Good dosimetric system/model for the computation of dose distribution and treatment time
4. Good understanding and good geometrical and material description of applicators
5. Accurate positioning of sources
6. Accurate timing of source placement
7. Accurate description of tissues (composition and mass energy absorption coefficients)
8. Accurate description of radiation biological effects in the targeted tissues as well as "normal" tissues

In August 2012, a report of the High Energy Brachytherapy Source Dosimetry (HEBD) Working Group published its "Recommendations of the American Association of Physicists in Medicine (AAPM) and the European Society for Radiotherapy and Oncology (ESTRO) on dose calculations for high-energy (average energy higher than 50 keV) photon-emitting brachytherapy sources" was presented, including the physical characteristics of specific ^{192}Ir, ^{137}Cs, and ^{60}Co source models as well as consensus datasets for commercially available high-energy photon sources [11]. Without getting in the details of the dose computation formalism and radiation source descriptions within this formalism, all of which are well described in literature, we will address physics issues directly related to balloon brachytherapy. In general, four factors influence the single-source dose distribution for photon-emitting sources:

- Distance (inverse-square law)
- Absorption and scattering in the source core and encapsulation
- Photon attenuation
- Scattering in the surrounding medium

The inverse-square law is the best known and strictly geometric consequence of any isotropic source emitting photons in a 3D space. It assumes no attenuation or scattering of photons by the medium. Of the four factors influencing the dose distribution, the inverse-square law is by far the most important. For a pure isotropic point source, the dose will decrease by a factor of 100 between the distances of 0.5 and 5 cm. The influence of the remaining factors over the same distance range rarely exceeds a factor of 2 or 3. The tissue surrounding the source affects the dose distribution in two competing ways: dose is reduced by the attenuation of primary photons and at the same time is increased by the scattered photons. Photons are being emitted in all directions from the source and are interacting with the tissue by means of Compton scattering and photoelectric absorption. Thus, each volume element of tissue is effectively radiating scattered photons in all directions, many of which contribute to the dose at the point of interest.

One can see that up to distances of about 5 cm, the attenuation of primary photons and the buildup of dose from scattered photons are compensating each other, leading to an almost "pure" inverse-square distance law (Fig. 8). At larger distances, seldom of interest for clinical purposes, attenuation wins and the falloff is faster. Compton scattering, which dominates photon absorption and scattering above 100 keV, depends mainly on electron density (electrons/g) of the medium, which is nearly constant for all biologic materials. Thus, for ^{192}Ir HDR brachytherapy, tissue composition is largely irrelevant, and water as a medium is a very good approximation, validating the use of TG-43 formalism in most clinical applications. The only limitation of TG-43 is assuming that medium is infinite and thus scatter contribution is always in full. In the "evolution of brachytherapy treatment planning," the authors examined the sensitivity of common treatment sites to dosimetric limitations of the current dose computation formalism (TG-43) [20]. They concluded that for breast HDR, significant differences between planned and delivered dose are likely to occur due to one factor only: scatter. In the breast, relatively close to the radiation source and applicators are two interfaces: one between the breast and air and the other between breast tissue and the lung. As a

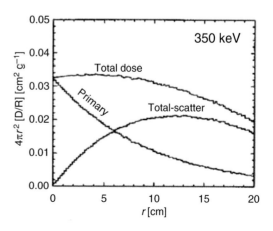

Fig. 8 Contributions of primary and scattered photons to total absorbed dose at the photon energies of 350 keV. The dose distributions are multiplied by the distance squared and normalized to the primary photon energy (From Carlsson and Ahnesjö [43])

result, a part of the contribution from scatter will be lost, and likely the planned dose will be an overestimation of the dose actually delivered. It is interesting to note that this is also applicator dependent. In interstitial implants, the source is in the immediate proximity of the tissue, thus dose is delivered largely by primary photons and thus the missing scatter will impact very little the difference between planned and delivered dose (typically 2–3 %). In balloon brachytherapy, the tissue is a few cm away (as much as 3–4 cm) from the source, making the scatter a more important component of dose. Thus, the missing scatter due to the breast tissue–air interface can bring the difference between planned and delivered dose to 10–15 %.

1.6   Prescription Dose and Fractionation Schedules

The whole breast treatment of standard breast conservation therapy typically lasts 5–7 weeks with daily treatments delivering a dose of 45–50 Gy to the whole breast, sometimes followed by a boost of 10–16 Gy to the tumor bed volume. Multi-catheter interstitial brachytherapy is the APBI technique with the longest follow-up and most mature data supporting APBI. It was initially developed as a technique to deliver the boost part of the treatment after whole breast irradiation (WBI). A clinical trial, RTOG 95–17, evaluated interstitial brachytherapy as a sole modality after lumpectomy. This was based on the pioneering work at the Ochsner Clinic (New Orleans, LA, USA) and the William Beaumont Hospital (Royal Oak, MI, USA). Patients were treated with LDR ^{192}Ir at a dose of 45Gy over 4.5 days or HDR, with 34 Gy in 10 fractions over 5 days. In the era of interstitial implants, alternative fractionation schemes were 4 Gy×8 fractions [21] and 4.33 Gy×7 fractions or 5.2 Gy×7 fractions [22]. There are a number of MammoSite® APBI series describing long-term outcomes with a number of fractionation schemes: 3.4 Gy×10 fractions [23–25] and 7 Gy×4 fractions [26]. Ultrashort-course APBI using the Contura® device, with conservative

dosimetric parameters, is actively being investigated in a phase II multi-institutional trial. Early data using a fractionation regimen of 7 Gy in four fractions (delivered twice daily) shows tolerable rates of acute toxicities comparable to typical APBI fractionation schemes [27]. Based on the linear-quadratic model and acknowledging its limitations, three "ultrashort" fractionation regimens were developed using a multi-lumen balloon device: 7 Gy×4 fractions, 8.25 Gy×3 fractions, and 10.5 Gy×2 fractions. A minimum of 6 h was required between fractions, irrespective of the fractionation schedule and very conservative dosimetric criteria were defined. Four-year results were presented using balloon brachytherapy (MammoSite®) delivered with a 2-day fractionation schedule [26]. In a recent dosimetric study comparing HDR using ^{192}Ir vs. 50 kV X-rays for breast intraoperative radiation therapy the authors proposed using a multi-lumen balloon to deliver 1 fraction of 12.5 Gy [28]. An ongoing prospective clinical trial will evaluate the safety and feasibility of this technique.

1.7   CT Planning and Dose Optimization

Before discussing dose optimization, one needs to stress the importance of optimal placement of the device (s). While there are many constraints in how a device (in this case a balloon) is being implanted, many of them relate to patient anatomy and convenience, lumpectomy position within the breast, and the position of OARs relative to lumpectomy. Optimal placement takes into account the particularities of the device and the way dose distribution is created. An example is given in Fig. 4 for the Contura MLB®. One can see that the asymmetry of the PTV_EVAL can be bounded by two lines (in yellow) in two of the orthogonal views. Ideally, the central lumen would be oriented along the bisector (upper panel left) and catheters 1 and 3 would also be positioned along the bisector (lower panel right). While the position of the shaft can be dictated (as in this case) by the length of the tissue that needs to be traversed to reach the cavity, there is no reason not to rotate the balloon, once inserted, in such a way to place it in an optimal position. If catheters 1–3 are along the bisector and catheters 2–4 are oriented along the shorter "axis" of PTV_EVAL, the planning system optimizer would very likely weigh heavily on 1–3 in order to create an elongated dose distribution, and it would use very little catheters of 2 and 4. In a less than optimal position, the optimizer would likely distribute dwell times in all catheters, thus leading to a more spherical, less conformal dose distribution.

A preliminary CT scan can be used for rotating the balloon in the optimal position. For the final treatment planning of CT, the patient should be in a supine position, and that position should be reproduced in each of the treatments. Every particular aspect (arm, wedges used to rotate the patient, etc.) should be recorded and reproduced in each of the treatment positions. The CT should start at or above the mandible and extend several cm below the inframammary fold (including the entire lung) if one wants to develop comprehensive DVH parameters. A CT scan thickness of ≤0.5 cm (preferably 0.2–0.3 cm) should be employed. The following structures would be contoured: the balloon surface, the clinical target volume (CTV), the planning target volume (PTV), PTV_EVAL, trapped air and/or fluid in the cavity, and the ipsilateral breast. The chin, shoulders, and entire ipsilateral breast would be included in the scan. The target and normal tissue structures must be outlined on all CT slices. Immediately after the scan (or immediately before), a photo should record the position and orientation of the shaft relative to the incision. Sometimes a small dot on the skin helps reproduce the orientation prior to each treatment. Some devices have built-in markers to help the planner identify the catheter number. Contura®, for example, has a wire underneath catheter No. 1 (showing bright in Fig. 4). Radiopaque plugs at the tip of each catheter help identify the most distal point for the applicator. MammoSite ML® does not have any of these features, so the use of at least a wire marker is absolutely necessary to identify a reference offset catheter. Knowledge of the device orientation and indexing of the offset catheters can then help identify the other

catheters. Once a CT scan is obtained, the planning phase includes delineation of anatomical and planning structures, delineation of applicators, establishment of "allowed" positions for the radioactive source within applicators (dwell positions), and dose optimization.

The balloon can be outlined (segmented) automatically based on an increased CT number compared with adjacent tissue (Fig. 9). This can be easily achieved using a few milliliters of an iodine-based dilute in the water or saline used to inflate the balloon. The contour of the balloon becomes a surrogate definition of the lumpectomy cavity (gross target volume or GTV). The PTV_EVAL is created by uniformly expanding the balloon surface by 1 cm. The structure is limited to 0.5 cm from the skin surface and limited to exclude the chest wall and pectoralis muscles.

Very important for the planning for these types of devices is an arbitrarily constructed avoidance structure. The pseudo-structure is obtained by expanding the PTV_EVAL by 0.3–0.4 cm then subtracting the PTV_EVAL itself, resulting in a thin rim surrounding the PTV_EVAL (Fig. 6). Additional constraints can be imposed on this structure, together with the ones already described for the PTV_EVAL.

The next step is defining the geometry of the applicators. For the balloon-based devices, the rigid relative geometry of the treatment lumens (e.g., Contura MLB®, MammoSite ML®) allows the importing of an archived applicator from a

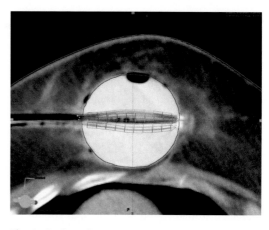

Fig. 9 Outline of a multi-lumen balloon after automatic segmentation. Also shown are the applicators

template library, dramatically reducing the time needed to outline the applicators and at the same time insuring a perfect and reproducible definition of the applicators even on less than optimal quality images. Once applicators are delineated, one defines the dwell positions by specifying, for each catheter, the lumen or strut a starting dwell position and a dwell increment (typically 0.5 cm but it can be any value greater than 0.1 cm).

While there are many ways of creating a dose distribution, among them, manual and geometrical optimization, the only "true" optimization is the so-called volume or DVH-based optimization. Each of the structures that will be subjected to dose–volume constraints is sampled in a number of points, typically hundreds to thousands, depending on the volume. The reason for doing this is that in order to speed up the optimization process, one can choose to calculate dose in a much smaller number of points than the total number of dose voxels that the structure inherently has, based on the resolution of the dose matrix. While upper and lower constraints are placed on the dose–volume histogram for the target PTV_EVAL, the avoidance structure placed outside the target is the one limiting higher than prescription dose "spilling" into the normal tissue, thus driving the dose conformance. Good structures and good constraints will produce optimal plans. If one needs to manually "tweak" an already optimized plan, it is very likely that either the optimizer is not performing adequately (might be too sensitive and easily "captured" by local minima), or the set of constraints does not adequately or completely reflect the goals for the plan.

During "volume optimization," dose–volume constraints are placed on the histograms for PTV_EVAL and the avoidance structure (an example with typical constraints is shown in Fig. 7). Depending on the shape of the PTV_EVAL, one can limit the volume of the avoidance structure receiving prescription dose to a small percentage (1–10 %), thus increasing the conformality of the dose to the PTV_EVAL. The volume of the PTV_EVAL receiving 150 % PD is, for a balloon-based device, depending on its diameter, around 25–30 % of the total volume.

Optimization of dose for a multi-catheter balloon device is clearly the best way to produce a dose distribution conformal to an asymmetric PTV_EVAL. Conformity implicitly means lowest dose to the adjacent OARs. The cost for the best dose coverage of the target and the best sparing of OARs is an increase in V200. If one would attempt to minimize V200, the best way to achieve that would be to create a dose distribution for which the 200 % isodose line falls either on the surface of the balloon (thus conforming) or inside the balloon, which is meaningless clinically. The latter is only possible for large diameter balloons where the distance between the prescription dose (PD) isodose line and the 200 % PD isodose line is slightly more than 1 cm, given the simple fact that being farther away from the source places the target in a region of gentler gradient. One cannot simultaneously meet these two conflicting requirements: a 200 % PD isodose conforming to a symmetrical shape (the balloon) and a 100 % PD isodose conforming to an asymmetric target (PTV_EVAL). As a consequence, V200 will be slightly increased but well under the 10 cm^3 limit.

1.8 Dosimetry in Balloon Brachytherapy: Outcome Measures and Toxicity Analysis

Since the balloon devices are relatively new, the short follow-up after balloon brachytherapy and the constant evolution of the devices and accepted dosimetry does not yet permit a definite judgment concerning the long-term effectiveness of balloon-based APBI. NSABP B-39/RTOG 0413 "A Randomized Phase III Study of Conventional Whole Breast Irradiation (WBI) Versus Partial Breast Irradiation (PBI) for Women with Stage 0, I, or II Breast Cancer" is the key to answering the question, "Is partial breast irradiation (PBI) safe and as effective as whole breast irradiation (WBI) for these patients?" Mature phase III data documenting the long-term efficacy of PBI and the group of patients most suitable for its application are not yet available. However, toxicities and side effects tend to develop in a shorter time frame, and as a result, a significant number of papers have been published on this subject. Data about toxicity and dosimetric limits associated with various side effects originated after studying interstitial implants, historically the first APBI modality. A well-known paper by Wazer et al. analyzed variables associated with late toxicity such as long-term cosmetic outcome after high-dose-rate interstitial brachytherapy [29]. They found that suboptimal cosmetic outcome was significantly associated with the number of source dwell positions, V150 and V200, and inversely associated with DHI (0.77 vs. 0.73; $p=0.05$). The risk of grade 1/2 skin toxicity was significantly associated with V150 and V200 and inversely associated with DHI (0.77 vs. 0.71; $p=0.009$). The risk of grade 0/1 vs. grade 2–4 subcutaneous toxicity was significantly associated only with a lower value of DHI (0.77 vs. 0.73; $p=0.02$). To further explore factors that might contribute to the risk of fat necrosis (symptomatic or asymptomatic), a separate analysis showed that only dose hotspots as reflected in V150 and V200 were significantly associated with elevated risk. It is interesting that while DHI proved to be a very strong indicator of late skin toxicity and late subcutaneous toxicity, its use in balloon brachytherapy completely disappeared. A reason is probably the fact that most balloons can only achieve a DHI of about 0.7, and the type of dose inhomogeneity in the target tissue around a balloon is very different from the one found in an interstitial implant. Below are listed (for comparison) the NSABP B-39/RTOG 04–13 guidelines for target and normal tissue constraints [16]:

Treatment technique	Determination factors	Dose constraints
Interstitial brachytherapy	Dose homogeneity	DHI ≥ 0.75
		$DHI = (1 - V150\ \%/V100\ \%)$
		V150 % ≤ 70 cm^3
		V200 % ≤ 20 cm^3
	Skin	Skin Dmax <100 %
	Ipsilateral breast	V50 % ≤ 60 %
	Target	>90 % of the prescription dose covers >90 % of the PTV_EVAL

Treatment technique	Determination factors	Dose constraints
MammoSite	Tissue-balloon conformance air/PTV_EVAL	Volume of trapped <10 %
	Balloon symmetry	Deviation of <2 mm from expected dimensions
	Minimum balloon surface–skin distance	Ideal: ≤ 7 mm
		Acceptable: 5–7 mm if Dmax to skin <145 %
	Ipsilateral breast	V150 % ≤ 50 cm^3
		V200 % ≤ 10 cm^3
		V50 % <60 %
	Target	>90 % of the prescription dose covers >90 % of the PTV_EVAL (after accounting for volume of trapped air)

In later trials (e.g., the multi-institutional phase IV Contura® registry trial), the coverage was increased to V95 $\geq$95 %, while the max skin dose was decreased to 125 % PD, and the max dose to the proximal rib, previously unconstrained, was set to no more than 145 %. In a comparison between multi-catheter implants, Contura® multi-lumen balloon, and MammoSite® single lumen [30], the multi-catheter implants were found to have the lowest skin and chest wall dose, but between the two balloons, Contura® was found to have the lowest skin and rib dose: 82 % PD and 82 %, respectively, vs. 94 % PD and 105 % for MammoSite®. A recent study of patterns of failure, patient selection, and dosimetric correlates for late toxicity after APBI using MammoSite® balloon brachytherapy [31] established an even lower limit for max skin dose, skin dose >100 % significantly predicted for the development of telangiectasia (50 % vs. 14 %, $p < .0001$), rediscovering the initial constraint set for multi-catheter implants. Despite reports on late chest wall toxicity after MammoSite® breast brachytherapy [31] describing "fractures occurred in ribs with V37 and V44

Gy, no clear thresholds were detected". In the first analysis of the American Society of Breast Surgeons MammoSite® breast brachytherapy registry trial [32], excellent results were noted which compared favorably with other forms of APBI with similar follow-up. The toxicity rates with single-lumen brachytherapy-based APBI were low with fewer than 10 % of patients developing infections, 13 % symptomatic seromas, and 2.5 % fat necrosis. These numbers are comparable with WBI outcomes.

One interesting issue is the dose estimation for OARs, most notably, skin and chest wall/ ribs. It is the current practice to measure the maximum dose to the surface of the skin and the maximum dose to the proximal rib. The obvious question is whether this is the best thing to do and whether it is reproducible and/or accurate.

In a study of the pathogenesis of late radiation-related fibrosis, the issue how to most meaningfully estimate skin dose was raised:

Although subcutaneous radiation induced fibrosis is probably the most common manifestation of radiation injury, the exact depth in the skin most responsible for the fibrotic process is unclear. Bentzen et al proposed range of 3.3–5.5 mm as acceptable reference points for subcutaneous fibrosis in the breast, with the best estimate at a depth of 4.1 mm. … Unless consistency in describing dose and measuring outcome is used, we will remain at a disadvantage in predicting the true incidence and dose response of RIF. [33]

How is this relevant for balloon brachytherapy and why do we estimate the surface dose as opposed to dose at a depth? The choice of depth itself is only an issue if the dose to surface is not correlated (uniquely determined) by dose to some arbitrary depth (say 0.4 or 0.5 cm). In the case of a balloon like MammoSite®, where the source can only be placed along the central lumen, dose to the surface is likely in a fixed relationship (in a first approximation, not taking into account the lack of scatter that TG-43 does not take into account) with dose to depth. Therefore, whether reporting dose to surface (as we do now) or dose to a "meaningful depth" (say, 0.41 cm) would likely not change any clinical correlation between dose to skin and toxicity. In the case of an interstitial implant or even a multi-lumen balloon,

the number of dwell positions and their variable position would make it such that the dose to the surface would not be in a unique relationship with dose at depth but would be case dependent. Clinical correlations with dose will likely be perturbed depending on the choice of depth for reporting dose to skin.

Dose limits to these structures have evolved in time, similar with definitions of PTV. In the interstitial implants, as Edmundson describes "… the skin dose is typically less than half the prescribed dose, and no skin response is usually seen. High local skin doses may result in small areas of moist desquamation and perhaps an excess of telangiectasia" [17]. In NSABP B-39 the skin dose for interstitial implants is established to ≤100 % PD [16]. For the MammoSite® device, however, the maximum dose to skin is coupled to the distance from the balloon to skin surface. As the prescription is ideally delivered at 1 cm from the balloon surface, the constraint that worked for interstitial implants would have been met every time the balloon-to-skin surface distance would have been 1 cm or more. Since usage of the balloon was also envisioned for shorter distances, a higher limit for skin dose was placed, namely, 145 % PD. This is approximately the equivalent of a 4 cm diameter balloon placed 0.5 cm from the skin surface. A larger balloon would slightly improve things (e.g., a 5 cm diameter balloon at 5 mm from skin would only produce 136 % PD on the skin surface). There are multiple publications reporting on dose limits for OAR based on clinical outcome, and these publications emphasize the initial knowledge that a skin dose of 100 % or less is safe. While initially no dose constraint for ribs was declared in the NSABP-B39, studies on rib fractures and chest wall pain lead to the conclusion that there is a safe limit and it is likely around 125 % PD. Brashears et al. hypothesized volumes receiving 37 and 44 Gy might be important, but they concluded that given the possibility of a history of osteoporosis or exposure to adjuvant chemotherapy "As long-term toxicity data accrue from APBI series, the traditional models for estimating the biologic equivalent dose may benefit from refinements that specifically address the unique radiobiologic and physical properties intrinsic to high-dose-rate brachytherapy for breast conservation therapy" [31].

1.9 Dose Calculation Formalism: Effects of Contrast and Air

In 1995, the American Association of Physicists in Medicine (AAPM) Task Group No. 43 published a clinical protocol on dosimetry for interstitial brachytherapy sources, known as the "TG-43 formalism," and provided reference dosimetry datasets for commercially available ^{192}Ir, ^{125}I, and ^{103}Pd sources.

While AAPM has reviewed and published reference-quality dosimetry datasets for low-energy brachytherapy sources in a number of reports (TG-43, TG-43 U1, and TG-43 U1S1), no similar effort has been attempted by AAPM or the European Society for Radiotherapy and Oncology (ESTRO) for high-energy sources. To fill this void, the AAPM Brachytherapy Subcommittee (BTSC) formed the High Energy Brachytherapy Source Dosimetry (HEBD) working group to focus on photon-emitting brachytherapy sources with average energy higher than 50 keV. The report [34] reviewed published dosimetry for commonly used high-energy ^{192}Ir, ^{137}Cs, and ^{60}Co sources, critically reviewed the TG-43 U1 formalism, and developed a complete consensus dataset to support clinical planning for each source model.

New advances of dose calculation algorithms using sophisticated model-based dose calculations (MBDC) have been recently introduced for brachytherapy treatment planning systems (TPS). While TG-43 models a single source in an effectively infinite water phantom, MBDC models sources, applicators, patient heterogeneities, interfaces, and boundaries.

The two commercially available systems are the BrachyVision Acuros (BV-Acuros) (Varian, Palo Alto, CA) and the Oncentra Advanced Collapsed Cone Engine (ACE) (Elekta, Netherlands) MBDCs. BV-Acuros is a grid-based Boltzmann solver (GBBS) that deterministically solves the linear Boltzmann transport equation.

Oncentra ACE is a collapsed cone convolution (CCC) algorithm which has been developed specifically for performing dose calculations for brachytherapy.

AAPM issued a report of a Task Group 186 [35] on the topic of model-based calculation formalism beyond TG-43. In conclusion, it was stated that "…it is important to acknowledge that the bulk of clinical brachytherapy dosimetry experience is with radiation transport and energy deposition in water, with dose to water reported (as calculated under the TG-43 approach). Hence, for the time being the recommendation that TG-43 calculations be performed in parallel with model-based dose calculations is crucial. Only in this way will the radiation therapy community become familiar with dose differences, including the impact on prescription dose and doses to points, organs and regions of interest."

For breast irradiation with ^{192}Ir, the most important factor impacting TG-43 dose calculation is the lack of complete scatter around the implant, leading to an overestimate of the skin dose (and to a smaller extent, target coverage). The magnitude of this overestimation was addressed by a number of investigators [36, 37] using multiple methods (TLD measurements, Monte Carlo simulations, etc.). The effects were found to be dependent on the balloon diameter, with up to 9.8 % for a 4 cm balloon and 13.2 % for a 6 cm balloon with no tissue beyond the prescription distance at the breast–skin interface. Smaller magnitude effects were noted on the breast–lung interface, with 6.7–9.6 % differences for the small and large balloon diameters, respectively.

Also studied intensively were the effects of contrast in the balloons and that of air pockets. While mixing radiopaque iodine-based contrast with water or saline helps visualizing the balloon contour, an increased absorption and attenuation can lead to a dose reduction if only a TG-43 calculation is performed (as opposed to a heterogeneity corrected calculation). In a study [37], concentrations ranging from 5 to 25 % by volume of iodine-based radiopaque solution were simulated in balloons with diameters between 4 and 6 cm. The dose rate reduction at the typical prescription line of 1 cm from the balloon surface ranged from –0.8 % for the smallest balloon diameter and contrast concentration to a maximum of –5.7 % for the largest balloon diameter and contrast concentration, relative to a water-filled balloon. Limiting the contrast concentration to 10 % would insure less than 3 % reduction in the prescription dose, regardless of balloon diameter. In terms of air pockets effects, the dose near the balloon surface may be increased by 0.5 %/cm^3 of air [38]. Monte Carlo simulation suggests that the interface effect (enhanced dose near surface) is primarily due to Compton electrons of short range (<0.05 cm).

Some of the issues regarding inhomogeneity and boundaries are exacerbated by the use of low-energy source like Xoft Axxent®. In a study comparing TG-186-based calculations with TG-43 for balloon applicators [39], based on a prescription dose of 34 Gy, the average D90 to PTV was reduced by between ~4 % and ~40 %, depending on the scoring method (dose to water ($D_{w, m}$) and dose to medium ($D_{m, m}$)), compared to the TG-43 result. Max skin dose was also reduced by 10–15 % due to the absence of backscatter not accounted for in TG-43. The final conclusion of the study was that "Tissue heterogeneities, applicator, and patient geometries demonstrate the need for a more robust dose calculation method for low energy brachytherapy sources."

1.10 Uncertainties in Planning and Delivery

All balloons, independent on whether they use one lumen or multi-lumens, have the theoretical possibility to rotate once implanted in a patient. Of course, rotation of a balloon with a perfectly central lumen would not produce any changes in dose, as dose distributions with cylindrical symmetry are invariant to rotation around the central axis. It is interesting to note that while the balloon rotation became a real issue with the development of the multi-lumen balloon, NSABP B-39 acknowledged the fact that the single-lumen MammoSite® balloon can be asymmetrical and placed a limit (≤0.2 cm) to the asymmetry but

without acknowledging the potential effect of an asymmetrical balloon rotating during treatment (between fractions). The Contura® multi-lumen balloon has a black line, an orientation line, on the shaft of the applicator to identify the position of Lumen #1. If at the time of the CT the patient had a skin mark drawn to align with the orientation line, a photo is taken and subsequently verified before each fraction, this should ensure an accurate non-rotational position of the balloon. In a study of sixteen patients in which the patients underwent CT scans before each fraction, a method was validated to accurately confirm the orientation of the Contura® multi-lumen balloon catheter before each fraction, and they determined if any residual device rotation remains after adjustment [40]. Using the external alignment of a skin mark with the orientation line was deemed an accurate and reliable method to align the balloon before treatment and no significant internal device rotation (<0.02 cm) occurred.

Dosimetric impact due to MLB rotation has been recently studied by Kim et al. [41]. For a plan with both of skin and rib distance less than 0.7 cm, the maximum degradation on D95 of the PTV_EVAL was about 6.5 % when there was a 120° rotation error. They found that in a clinical situation, which had a rotation error smaller than 10°, the degradation on D95 and D90 of the PTV_EVAL were less than 1 % and the deviation of the skin and rib dose were less than 2.5 % of the prescription dose.

In the process of planning and delivery, there are sources of error and uncertainty. Among them are the size and shape of balloon, the seroma volume, the delineation and the length measurement of the applicators, the positional accuracy of planned vs. delivered dwell positions, etc. Some of these were examined in a study on 42 CT images scanned from seven patients [42]. The original plans (as group A) had a mean value of 96.8 % on V95 of the PTV_EVAL. Another group (B) was created in which that the mean value of the V95 was relaxed to 90.4 %. A geometrical uncertainty with a mean deviation of 0.27 cm per root of sum of square caused the degradations of V90 and V95 by mean values of 1.0 % and 1.2 %, respectively. A systematic error of 0.3 and 0.4 cm would degrade both of V90 and V95 by 4 % and 6 %, respectively. The degradations on target coverage of the plans in group A were statistically the same as those in group B, concluding that "Overall, APBI treatments with MLB based brachytherapy are precise from day to day."

Conclusions

Accelerated partial breast irradiation is a new technology that provides faster, more convenient treatment after breast conservation surgery. Of all the APBI modalities, balloon brachytherapy is probably the technique at the confluence of an important number of desirable features. Given the single entry catheter as opposed to multiple catheters in interstitial implants, it is probably the easiest for patients to tolerate. Relying on a balloon surface as a GTV surrogate instead of the delineation of an uncertain lumpectomy cavity, together with the use of library plans, makes planning an easy task. While our dose computation formalisms are evolving, we do have a reasonable good understanding of the dosimetric factors which play a role in good outcomes of the treatment. Long-term follow-up and guidelines like those outlined in RTOG 0413/NSABP B-39 national phase III trial will hopefully demonstrate the long-term effectiveness and safety of this method for selected patients with early breast cancer.

References

1. Rivard MJ et al (2006) Calculated and measured brachytherapy dosimetry parameters in water for the Xoft Axxent X-ray source: an electronic brachytherapy source. Med Phys 33:4020–4032
2. Rivard MJ, Venselaar JL, Beaulieu L (2009) The evolution of brachytherapy treatment planning. Med Phys 36(6):2136–2153
3. Pignol JP, Keller B, Rakovitch E et al (2006) First report of a permanent breast 103Pd seed implant as adjuvant radiation treatment for early-stage breast cancer. Int J Radiat Oncol Biol Phys 64(1):176–181
4. Arthur DW, Koo D, Zwicker RD et al (2003) Partial breast brachytherapy after lumpectomy: low-dose-rate and high-dose-rate experience. Int J Radiat Oncol Biol Phys 56:681–689
5. Cuttino LW, Todor D, Arthur DW (2005) CT-guided multi-catheter insertion technique for partial breast brachytherapy: reliable target coverage and dose homogeneity. Brachytherapy 4(1):10–17
6. Monroe JI, Dempsey JF, Dorton JA et al (2001) Experimental validation of dose calculation algorithms for the GliaSite RTS®; a novel 125I liquid-filled balloon brachytherapy applicator. Med Phys 28(1):73–85
7. Astrahan MA, Jozsef G, Streeter OE (2004) Optimization of MammoSite® therapy. Int J Radiat Oncol Biol Phys 58(1):220–232
8. Baltas D, Sakelliou L, Zamboglou N (2007) The physics of modern brachytherapy for oncology. New York, Taylor & Francis
9. Andrassy M, Niatetsky Y, Perez-Calatayud J (2012) Controversies. Co-60 versus Ir-192 in HDR brachytherapy: scientific and technological comparison. Rev Fis Med 13(2):125–130
10. Dickler A, Kirk MC, Coon A et al (2008) A dosimetric comparison of Xoft Axxent® Electronic Brachytherapy and iridium-192 high-dose-rate brachytherapy in the treatment of endometrial cancer. Brachytherapy 7(4):351–354
11. Park CC, Yom SS, Podgorsak MB et al (2010) Electronic Brachytherapy Working Group. American Society for Therapeutic Radiology and Oncology (ASTRO) emerging technology committee report on electronic brachytherapy. Int J Radiat Oncol Biol Phys 76(4):963–972
12. Munro J, Medich D (2007) Dosimetric comparison of three radiation sources used in balloon-based breast brachytherapy. Brachytherapy 6:77–118
13. Zannis V, Beitsch P, Vicini F et al (2005) Descriptions and outcomes of insertion techniques of a breast brachytherapy balloon catheter in 1403 patients enrolled in the American Society of Breast Surgeons MammoSite® breast brachytherapy registry trial. Am J Surg 190(4):530–538
14. Kuske RR, Bolton JS, Hanson W (1998) RTOG 95–17: a phase I/II trial to evaluate brachytherapy as the sole method of radiation therapy for stage I and II breast carcinoma. Radiation Therapy oncology Group, Philadelphia, pp 1–34
15. Nag S, Kuske RR, Vicini FA et al (2001) Brachytherapy in the treatment of breast cancer. Oncology 15(2):195–202
16. NSABP (2006) B-39, RTOG 0413: A randomized phase III study of conventional whole breast irradiation versus partial breast irradiation for women with stage 0, I, or II breast cancer. Clin Adv Hematol Oncol 4:719–721
17. Edmundson GK, Vicini FA, Chen PY et al (2002) Dosimetric characteristics of the MammoSite RTS®, a new breast brachytherapy applicator. Int J Radiat Oncol Biol Phys 52(4):1132–1139
18. Dickler A, Kirk M, Choo J et al (2004) Treatment volume and dose optimization of MammoSite® breast brachytherapy applicator. Int J Radiat Oncol Biol Phys 59(2):469–474

19. Shaitelman SF, Vicini FA, Grills IS et al (2012) Differences in effective target volume between various techniques of accelerated partial breast irradiation. Int J Radiat Oncol Biol Phys 82(1):30–36

20. Rivard MJ, Davis SD, DeWerd LA et al (2006) Calculated and measured brachytherapy dosimetry parameters in water for the Xoft Axxent® x-ray source: an electronic brachytherapy source. Med Phys 33:4020–4032

21. Ott OJ, Hilderbrand G, Potter R et al (2007) Accelerated partial breast irradiation with multi-catheter brachytherapy: local control, side effects and cosmetic outcome for 274 patients; results of the German-Austrian multi-centre trial. Radiother Oncol 82:281–286

22. Polgár C, Major T, Fodor J et al (2010) Accelerated partial-breast irradiation using high dose rate interstitial brachytherapy: 12-year update of a prospective clinical study. Radiother Oncol 94:274–279

23. Khan AJ, Vicini FJ, Beitsch P et al (2012) Local control, toxicity, and cosmesis in women >70 years enrolled in the American Society of Breast Surgeons accelerated partial breast irradiation registry trial. Int J Radiat Oncol Biol Phys 84:323–330

24. Cuttino LW, Keisch M, Jenrette J et al (2008) Multi-institutional experience using the MammoSite® radiation therapy system in the treatment of early-stage breast cancer: 2 year results. Int J Radiat Oncol Biol Phys 71:107–114

25. Benitez MR, Keisch M, Vicini FJ et al (2007) Five-year results: the initial clinical trial of MammoSite® balloon brachytherapy for partial breast irradiation in early-stage breast cancer. Am J Surg 194:456–462

26. Wilkinson JB, Martinez A, Chen P et al (2012) Four-year results using balloon-based brachytherapy to deliver accelerated partial breast irradiation with a 2 day dose fractionation schedule. Brachytherapy 11:97–104

27. Khan AJ, Vicini FJ, Brown S et al (2013) Dosimetric feasibility and acute toxicity in a prospective trial of ultrashort-course accelerated partial breast irradiation (APBI) using a multi-lumen balloon brachytherapy device. Ann Surg Oncol 20:1295–1301

28. Jones R, Libby B, Showalter SL et al (2014) Dosimetric comparison of 192Ir high-dose-rate brachytherapy vs. 50 kV x-rays as techniques for breast intraoperative radiation therapy: conceptual development of image-guided intraoperative brachytherapy using a multilumen balloon applicator and in-room CT imaging. Brachytherapy 13(5):502–507

29. Wazer DE, Kaufman S, Cuttino L et al (2006) Accelerated partial breast irradiation: an analysis of variables associated with late toxicity and long-term cosmetic outcome after high-dose-rate interstitial brachytherapy. Int J Radiat Oncol Biol Phys 64(2):489–495

30. Cuttino L, Todor D, Rosu M et al (2011) A comparison of skin and chest wall dose delivered with multi-catheter, Contura multilumen balloon, and MammoSite® breast brachytherapy. Int J Radiat Oncol Biol Phys 79(1):34–38

31. Vargo JA, Verma V, Kim H et al (2014) Extended (5-year) outcomes of accelerated partial breast irradiation using MammoSite® balloon brachytherapy: patterns of failure, patient selection, and dosimetric correlates for late toxicity. Int J Radiat Oncol Biol Phys 88(2):285–291

32. Shah C, Badiyan S, Wilkinson J et al (2013) Treatment efficacy with accelerated partial breast irradiation (APBI): final analysis of the American Society of Breast Surgeons MammoSite® breast brachytherapy registry trial. Ann Surg Oncol 20(10):3279–3285

33. O'Sullivan LB, Levin W (2003) Late radiation-related fibrosis: pathogenesis, manifestations, and current management. Sem Radiat Oncol 13(3):274–289

34. Perez-Calatayud J, Ballester F, Das R et al (2012) Dose calculation for photon-emitting brachytherapy sources with average energy higher than 50 keV: report of the AAPM and ESTRO. Med Phys 39(5):2904–2929

35. Beaulieu L, Tedgren A, Carrier JF et al (2012) Report of the Task Group 186 on model-based dose calculation methods in brachytherapy beyond the TG-43 formalism: current status and recommendations for clinical implementation. Med Phys 39(10):6208–6236

36. Raffi JA, Davis SD, Hammer CG et al (2010) Determination of exit skin dose for 192Ir intracavitary accelerated partial breast irradiation with thermoluminescent dosimeters. Med Phys 37(6):2693–2702

37. Kassas B, Mourtada F, Horton JL et al (2004) Contrast effects on dosimetry of a partial breast irradiation system. Med Phys 31(7):1976–1979

38. Cheng CW, Mitra R, Li XA, Das IJ (2005) Dose perturbations due to contrast medium and air in MammoSite® treatment: an experimental and Monte Carlo study. Med Phys 32(7):2279–2287

39. White SA, Landry G, Fonseca GP et al (2014) Comparison of TG-43 and TG-186 in breast irradiation using a low energy electronic brachytherapy source. Med Phys 41(6):061701

40. Ouhib Z, Benda R, Kasper M et al (2011) Accurate verification of balloon rotation correction for the Contura® multilumen device for accelerated partial breast irradiation. Brachytherapy 10(4):325–330

41. Kim Y, Trombetta MG (2014) Dosimetric evaluation of multilumen intracavitary balloon applicator rotation in high-dose-rate brachytherapy for breast cancer. J Appl Clin Med Phys 15(1):4429

42. Kuo HC, Mehta KJ, Hong L et al (2014) Day to day treatment variations of accelerated partial breast brachytherapy using a multi-lumen balloon. J Contemp Brachytherapy 6(1):68–75

43. Carlsson AK, Ahnesjö A (2000) The collapsed cone superposition algorithm applied to scatter dose calculations in brachytherapy. Med Phys 27(10):2320–2332

Part I

Disease Site Specific Topics

Ocular Brachytherapy

Stephen Karlovits and Thierry Verstraeten

Abstract

Episcleral plaque brachytherapy (EPB) has been utilized since the first half of the last century to treat intraocular tumors [1]. The two most common indications for EPB are ocular/choroidal melanoma (CM) and retinoblastoma. Although the techniques are similar, the focus of this chapter will be on the treatment of CM.

1 Introduction

CM is the most common primary malignancy of the globe but its incidence is only 4.3 cases/million in the USA [2]. Local control is paramount as failure to achieve this goal results in both local (vision loss, pain) and systemic (liver, lung, bone metastasis) consequences including death. In the 1960s enucleation with subsequent histopathology demonstrated close to 20 % of erroneous diagnosis, and as the observational skills of ophthalmologists improved, that rate fell to less than 5 % by the mid-1970s [3]. Prior to the 1980s, the treatment of choice was enucleation (eye removal) with the associated major downside of ipsilateral vision loss. Along with improving skills, the introduction of fine needle aspiration biopsy in the mid-1980s improved the accuracy of diagnosis [4].

Historically EPB was first introduced by Stallard in England in the 1950s using cobalt 60 [5]. This technique could offer the possibility of both organ and resultant vision preservation while controlling or eradicating the tumor. Subsequently, different isotopes were tried, including iridium 192, ruthenium 106, iodine 125, and later palladium 103 [6]. Episcleral brachytherapy using various radionuclides has been performed in the treatment of CM at numerous institutions across the globe for years. However, the only randomized study reflecting class 1 evidence for effectiveness compared to enucleation is the Medium Tumor Collaborative Ocular Melanoma Study (COMS) [7, 8]. This multi-institutional trial enrolled more than 1300 patients with medium-sized CM, and patients

S. Karlovits, MD (✉)
Allegheny Health Network Cancer Institute,
Allegheny General Hospital, Pittsburgh, PA, USA

Radiation Oncology, Temple University
School of Medicine, Pittsburgh, PA, USA
e-mail: SKARLOVI@wpahs.org

T. Verstraeten, MD
Department of Ophthalmology, Allegheny
Ophthalmic and Orbital Associates, Drexel University
College of Medicine, Pittsburgh, PA, USA

© Springer International Publishing Switzerland 2016
P. Montemaggi et al. (eds.), *Brachytherapy: An International Perspective*, Medical Radiology,
DOI 10.1007/978-3-319-26791-3_6

were randomized to either enucleation or ^{125}I EPB. At 12 years' mean follow-up, there was no survival difference including death from histopathologically confirmed melanoma metastases [8]. Eighty-seven percent of patients treated with EPB retained their eye at 5 years with 43 % of the treated eyes demonstrating visual acuity of 20/200 or worse at 3 years [9, 10].

Prior to 2002, the main standardized clinical guidelines were those as set forth in the COMS study, but these were based on [125]I. However, many other sources in addition to ^{125}I have been used and are in use with EPB globally including ^{60}Co, [106]Ru (Europe), [103]Pd, ^{90}Sr, and [131]Cs [5, 11–20]. The American Brachytherapy Society (ABS) therefore convened an EPB consensus conference in 2002 focusing on CM and then again in 2013 focusing on both CM and retinoblastoma and published guidelines [21, 22]. In addition, the American Association of Physicists in Medicine (AAPM) Task Group (TG) 129 medical physics guidelines were published in two reports 2011 and 2012 [23, 24]. The first compared the dosimetry of the two most common radionuclides in use in North America ([103]Pd and ^{125}I). The second focused on ideal dose calculation, radiation safety, and quality assurance [22].

1.1   Workup and Staging

Since 2002, the ABS has recommended that EPB be performed only in specialized medical centers as both the complexity of the workup and ultimate treatment require an experienced multidisciplinary team [21]. Recommended initial ABS workup includes full ophthalmic exam including intraocular pressure and visual acuity as well as ophthalmoscopy, fundus photography, and ultrasound [25, 26]. Clinical diagnosis is adequate for treatment and histopathologic confirmation is optional [22]. Increasing benefits of obtaining tissue prior or during the application of EPB include the ability to identify the molecular genetics of the tumor with prognostic value and quantification of metastasis risk [27]. In the mid-1990s, the discovery of a chromosome

3 monosomy mutation in enucleated globes led to the observation of a 50 % risk of metastasis by 3 years compared to eyes not affected by the mutation [28]. Once the diagnosis is established, a metastatic workup should be performed including complete physical exam, liver function studies, and chest X-ray. Computed axial tomography (CT) of the chest and abdomen is performed if indicated [21]. The ABS Ophthalmic Oncology Task Force (ABS-OOTF) [22] has adopted the seventh edition American Joint Committee on Cancer (AJCC) eye cancer staging system for uveal melanoma [22, 29].

1.2   Case Selection

As stated in their 2013 report, the ABS exclusion criteria for EPB have become more limited, basically now including only gross extraocular extension (T4e or >5 cm), basal diameters that exceed brachytherapy limits, blind painful eye, and no light perception [22]. Patients with tumors near the fovea or optic nerve need to be counseled on potential brachytherapy morbidity such as blindness [30–32]. Visual outcomes generally improve as the distance increases, between the plaque and macula or optic nerve, and as the tumor volume decreases [33]. Recent advances include intravitreal injection of triamcinolone and anti-vascular endothelial growth factor (anti-VEGF) agents to limit the incidence of radiation retinopathy and optic neuropathy [34, 35].

1.3   Treatment Planning

Required information from the ophthalmologist includes eye laterality, tumor AJCC stage, tumor size (basal diameter and height) confirmed by ultrasound, and a detailed fundus diagram [29, 36]. The fundus diagram should include tumor location, tumor measurements, as well as the distances from the tumor to the fovea, optic nerve, lens, and opposite eye [22]. Ideally, this information is then transferred from the fundus diagram to a computerized treatment planning program per AAPM/ABS TG 129 [23, 24]. The radionuclide of choice dosimetric information is inputted, and then tumor dosing as well as dose to critical structures at risk such as the macula, optic disk, and lacrimal gland can then be calculated per COMS and TG 129 [23, 24].

Tumor diameters must not be greater than the planning target volumes or the diameter of the plaque to avoid a geographic miss [22]. In accordance with COMS, the ABS-OOTF recommends the tumor apex (point of maximal thickness) as the prescription point. Also, the prescription isodose line should encompass the entire tumor volume to maximize local control. Depending upon the radionuclide chosen, the total dose to the apex may vary between 70 and 100 Gy. Additionally, the dose rate should not be less than the equivalent COMS standard of 0.60 Gy/h for [125]I [22] At our institution, we follow the COMS guidelines and use ^{125}I plaques with a 0.2 cm margin around the basal diameter of the tumor and prescribe 85 Gy to the tumor apex with a mandated minimum of 85 Gy to 5 intraocular millimeter thickness.

1.4   Surgery

First and foremost the ABS-OOTF recommends that these procedures be performed by a team comprised of ophthalmic oncologists, radiation oncologists, and medical physicists in experienced subspecialty centers. Actual placement of the eye plaque is done under local and/or general anesthesia. The tumor first needs to be localized by the surgeon. In most cases, the scleral shadow of the tumor base is identified by trans-pupillary or transocular illumination and marked. Measurements are then taken to confirm that the fabricated eye plaque is adequate to cover the tumor base and planning margin. Sutures are placed into the sclera with or without the aid of a "dummy" plaque and the eye plaque is affixed (Fig. 1). If an ocular muscle encroaches on the site, thereby preventing proper EPB placement, it is temporarily relocated. Insertion time is recorded into the radiation record and a lead eye patch is placed over the affected eye. The EPB

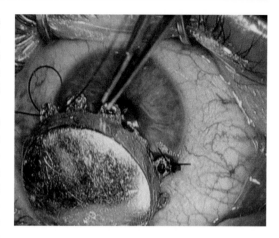

Fig. 1 External photograph of gold COMS plaque sewn to the sclera after localization

then remains in place for the preplanned duration calculated to deliver the appropriate dose at depth and then removed under local and/or general anesthesia and any relocated muscles are reattached. The removal time, seed count, and radiation survey (patient, operating room, and if applicable patient's hospital room) are then recorded in the radiation record [21, 22].

1.5   Follow-Up

In general, most patients are then followed every 3–6 months with a complete physical and ophthalmic exam to assess for tumor response/recurrence, radiation-related morbidity, and metastatic disease. The ABS-OOTF recommends (with level I consensus) that periodic hepatic imaging be performed to detect subsequent metastases to allow for more prompt systemic management [22]. At our institution, the patient is discharged after the initial 4-day hospital stay and is followed on an outpatient basis at 1 week, 1 month, 3 months, and then every 6 months for 5 years. Serial fundus photography (Figs. 2, 3, and 4) and ultrasound A and B scans are performed to monitor the treatment response. Longer follow-up is recommended as we have seen liver metastasis occur at 7 years post brachytherapy with local ocular tumor control.

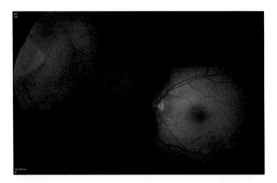

Fig. 2 Fundus color photograph (montage) of the left eye in a 67-year-old white female showing a sessile tumor of the nasal periphery measuring 12 mm diameter and 6 mm elevation. Vision is 20/25

Fig. 4 Same eye 30 months after treatment. Note disappearance of vascular changes and excellent tumor control (measurements: 10 mm diameter and 3 mm elevation)

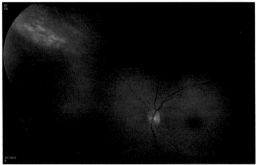

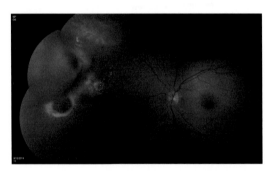

Fig. 3 Same eye 18 months after I125 brachytherapy. Note radiation retinopathy over tumor surface with hemorrhaging and exudation. No additional treatment performed. Vision is 20/25

1.6   Clinical Outcomes

Clinical outcomes are difficult to quantify due to the variability of technique, skill level, treatment planning, isotopes used, and tumor-related characteristics (mainly location and size) between institutions and continents. The only class I evidence pertains to medium-sized CM treated with ^{125}I EPB versus enucleation with results published in multiple outcome-specific reports by the COMS. As published in COMS Report No. 16, baseline visual acuity in the affected eye was 20/32 (median) with 70 % at least 20/40 and 10 % at best, 20/200. Three-year visual acuity results were 20/125 (median), 34 % and 45 %, respectively. Visual decline was progressive post implant with those with baseline affected eye visual acuity greater than

20/200 worsening to (at best) 20/200 at a rate of 17 % by year 1 and 43 % by year 3. Other than baseline visual acuity, the factors most strongly associated with a posttreatment visual acuity of 20/200 or worse were greater initial apical tumor height and shorter distance between the tumor and foveal avascular zone (FAZ) [10]. In those patients randomized to eye preservation, the 5-year risk of tumor recurrence was 10.3 % and the 5-year need for salvage enucleation was 12.5 % per COMS Report No 19. The most common reason for enucleation within the first 3 years was tumor recurrence. After 3 years, pain was the most common reason. Mirroring the risk factors for visual decline, common risk factors for both recurrence and enucleation were greater tumor thickness and shorter distance between the tumor and FAZ [9]. Overall 12-year mortality rates and prognostic factors were published in COMS Report No. 28. Cumulative all-cause 5-year mortality was 19 % overall, and the 12-year mortality in the brachytherapy arm versus enucleation arms was 43 % versus 41 %, respectively. Five- and 12-year risk of death with histopathologically confirmed melanoma metastasis was 10 % versus 11 % and 21 % versus 17 %, respectively [8]. COMS Report No. 26 included both the medium and large CM COMS trials and showed the majority of metastatic disease occurred with the first 5 years of follow-up, with the liver being the most common location (89 %). The overall 5- and 10-year metastatic rates were 25 % and 35 %, respectively. The death rate after diagnosis of metastatic disease was 80 % at 1 year with few long-term survivors [37].

1.7 Complications

Both acute and late complications are related to treatment and tumor-related factors such as total dose, dose rate, treatment volume, and location [38, 39]. Late complications predominate, and the incidence increases over time with the most common being radiation retinopathy [21, 22]. The onset of retinopathy is rare in the first year but increases between 12 and 18 months following brachytherapy. The proximity of the tumor to the macula or posterior pole increases the risk. Peripheral retinal vascular leakage with exudation and hemorrhage is often seen over and around the perimeter of larger or thicker tumors (Fig. 3). Often these complications can be controlled by the administration of intravitreal steroids, anti-VEGF agents, and the applications of laser photocoagulation. The development of a cataract is often expected for tumor located anterior to the equator of the globe and in the ciliary body. Overall the incidence of cataract formation was 68 % within the first 5 years in COMS Report No. 27 [40]. It is preferable to delay the performance of cataract surgery or other penetrating surgeries like glaucoma surgery or vitrectomy surgery until tumor regression is observed (1–2 years post procedure). This is advisable to lower the risk of extraocular dissemination of malignant cells. COMS Report No. 30 showed a 5-year risk of optic neuropathy of 27.4 % with ^{125}I EPB with major risk factors being diabetes and proximity to the optic nerve, FAZ, and fovea [41]. A late complication seen in about 5 % of the eyes is the development of scleral necrosis with the appearance of progressive extraocular dark pigmentation (Fig. 5). It has been our experience and that of others (Shields personal communication) that these can often be managed by conservative monitoring as these visible cells are no longer malignant. Rarely though, a scleral patch graft or possibly enucleation may have to be performed.

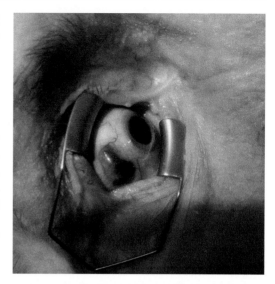

Fig. 5 External photograph of the right eye in an 88-year-old white female 5 years after brachytherapy. The initial tumor measured 14 mm diameter and 8 mm elevation in the temporal equatorial region. Note dark pigmentation with 2 mm elevation and the absence of sclera. This is not representing extrascleral tumor growth. Internally the tumor is regressed and measures 2 mm elevation. The vision is 20/80 and the patient is comfortable

Conclusions

This chapter represents our multidisciplinary approach to EPB for choroidal melanomas, and the reader is encouraged to refer to the ABS-OOTF and AAPM/ABS TG 43 and TG 129 guidelines for expanded information on specific clinical scenarios, technical issues, and quality assurance.

References

1. Moore R (1930) Choroidal sarcoma treated by the intraocular insertion of radon seeds. Br J Ophthalmol 14:145–156
2. Singh AD, Bergman L, Seregard S (2005) Uveal melanoma: epidemiologic aspects. Ophthalmol Clin North Am 18:75–84
3. Shields JA (1878) Accuracy and limitations of the 32P test in the diagnosis of ocular tumors: an analysis of 500 cases. Ophthalmology 85:950–966
4. Augusburger JJ, Shields JA (1984) Fine needle aspiration biopsy of solid intraocular tumors: indications, instrumentation and techniques. Ophthalmic Surg 15:34–40

5. Stallard HR (1966) Radiotherapy for malignant melanoma of the choroid. Br J Ophthalmol 50:147–155
6. Finger PT, Bufa A, Mishra S et al (1994) Palladium 103 plaque radiotherapy for uveal melanoma: clinical experience. Ophthalmology 101:256–263
7. Collaborative Ocular Melanoma Study Group (1995) Ch 12: Radiation therapy. In: National technical information service (NTIS). COMS manual of procedures, Springfield, pp PB95–PB179693
8. Collaborative Ocular Melanoma Study Group (2006) The COMS randomized trial of iodine 125 brachytherapy for choroidal melanoma: V. Twelve-year mortality rates and prognostic factors: COMS report No. 28. Arch Ophthalmol 124:1684–1693
9. Collaborative Ocular Melanoma Study Group (2002) The COMS randomized trial of iodine 125 brachytherapy for choroidal melanoma: IV. Local treatment failure and enucleation in the first 5 years after brachytherapy: COMS report No. 19. Ophthalmology 109:2197–2206
10. Collaborative Ocular Melanoma Study Group (2001) The COMS randomized trial of iodine 125 brachytherapy for choroidal melanoma: I. Visual acuity after 3 years: COMS Report No. 16. Ophthalmology 108:348–366
11. Lommatzsch PK (1987) Results after beta-irradiation (106Ru/106Rh) of choroidal melanomas. Twenty years' experience. Am J Clin Oncol 10:146–151
12. Packer S, Rotman M (1980) Radiotherapy of choroidal melanoma with iodine-125. Ophthalmology 87:582–590
13. Sealy R, le Roux PL, Rapley F et al (1976) The treatment of ophthalmic tumors with low-energy sources. Br J Radiol 49:551–554
14. Finger PT, Chin KJ, Duvall G et al (2009) Palladium-103 ophthalmic plaque radiation therapy for choroidal melanoma: 400 treated patients. Ophthalmology 116:790–796
15. Rivard MJ, Melhus CS, Sioshansi S et al (2008) The impact of prescription depth, dose rate, plaque size, and source loading on the central axis using 103Pd, 125I and 131Cs. Brachytherapy 7:327–335
16. Finger PT (1997) Radiation therapy for choroidal melanoma. Surg Ophthalmol 42:215–232
17. Leonard KL, Gagne NL, Mignano JE et al (2011) A 17 year retrospective study of institutional result or eye plaque brachytherapy of uveal melanoma using (125)I, (103)Pd., and (131)Cs and historical perspective. Brachytherapy 10:331–339
18. Vakulenko MP, Dedenkov AN, Brovkina AF et al (1980) Results of beta-therapy of choroidal melanoma. Med Radiol (Mosk) 25:73–74
19. Brovkina AF, Zarubei GD, Val'skii VV (1997) Criteria for assessing the efficacy of brachytherapy of uveal melanomas, complications of therapy and there prevention. Vestn Ofalmol 113:14–16
20. Murakami N, Suzuki S, Ito Y et al (2012) Ruthenium plaque therapy (RPT) for retinoblastoma. Int J Radiat Oncol Biol Phys 84:59–65
21. Nag S, Quivey JM, Earle JD et al (2003) The American Brachytherapy Society recommendations for brachytherapy of uveal melanomas. Int J Radiat Oncol Biol Phys 56(2):544–555
22. American Brachytherapy Society – Opthalmic Oncology Task Force (2014) The American Brachytherapy Society consensus guidelines for plaque brachytherapy of uveal melanoma and retinoblastoma. Brachytherapy 13(1):1–14
23. Rivard MJ, Chiu-Tsao ST, Finger PT et al (2011) Comparison of dose calculation methods for brachytherapy of intraocular tumors. Med Phys 38:306–316
24. Chiu-Tsao S, Astrahan MA, Finger PT et al (2012) Dosimetry of 125I and 103Pd COMS eye plague for intraocular tumor: report of Task Group 129 by the AAPM and ABS. Med Phys 2396:6161–6184
25. Ferry AP (1964) Lesions mistaken for malignant melanoma of the posterior uvea: a clinical pathologic analysis of 100 cases with ophthalmoscopically visible lesions. Arch Ophthalmol 72:463–469
26. Albert DM, Marcus DM (1990) Accuracy of diagnosis of choroidal melanomas in the Collaborative Ocular Melanoma Study. COMS Report No. 1. Arch Ophthalmol 108:1268–1273
27. Harbour JW (2009) Molecular prognostic testing and individualized patient care in uveal melanoma. Am J Ophthalmol 148:823–829
28. Prescher G, Bornfeld N, Hirsche H et al (1996) Prognostic implications of monosomy 3 in uveal melanoma. Lancet 347:1222–1225
29. Uveal melanoma (2009) In: Edge SE, Byrd DR, Compton CC et al (eds) The AJCC cancer staging manual. 7th ed. New York: London, Springer, pp 547–559
30. Finger PT (2000) Tumor location affects the incidence of cataract and retinopathy after ophthalmic plaque radiation therapy. Br J Ophthalmol 84:1068–1070
31. Finger PT, Chin KJ, Yu GP (2010) Risk factors for radiation maculopathy after ophthalmic plaque radiation for choroidal melanoma. Am J Ophthalmol 149:608–615
32. Finger PT, Chin KJ, Yu GP et al (2010) Risk factors for cataract after palladium-103. Ophthalmic plaque radiation therapy. Int J Radiat Oncol Biol Phys 80:800–806
33. Quivey JM, Char DH, Phillips TL et al (1993) High intensity 125-iodine (125I) plaque treatment of uveal melanoma. Int J Radiat Oncol Biol Phys 26:613–618
34. Shields CL, Demirci H, Dai V et al (2005) Intravitreal triamcinolone acetonide for radiation maculopathy after plaque radiotherapy for choroidal melanoma. Retina 25:868–874
35. Shah SU, Shields CL, Bianciotto CG et al (2014) Intravitreal bevacizumab injection at 4 month intervals for prevention of macular edema following plaque radiotherapy of uveal melanoma. Ophthalmology 121:269–275

36. Evans MDC, Astrahan MA, Bate R (1993) Tumor localization using fundus view photograph for episcleral plaque therapy. Med Phys 20:769–775

37. Diener-West M, Reynolds SM, Agugliano DJ et al (2005) Development of metastatic disease after enrollment in the COMS trials for treatment of choroidal melanoma: Collaborative Ocular Melanoma Study Group Report No. 26. Arch Ophthalmol 123(12):1639–1643

38. Robertson DM, Earle J, Anderson JA (1983) Preliminary observations regarding the use of iodine-125 in the management of choroidal melanoma. Trans Ophthalmol Soc U K 103(pt2):155–160

39. Houdek PV, Schwade JG, Medina AJ et al (1989) MR technique for localization and verification procedures in episcleral brachytherapy. Int J Radiat Oncol Biol Phys 17:1111–1114

40. Collaborative Ocular Melanoma Study Group (2007) Incidence of cataract and outcomes after cataract surgery in the first 5 years after iodine 125 brachytherapy in the Collaborative Ocular Melanoma Study: COM Report No 27. Ophthalmology 114(7):1363–1371

41. Collaborative Ocular Melanoma Study Group (2009) I-125 brachytherapy for choroidal melanoma: photographic & angiographic abnormalities. Collaborative Ocular Melanoma Study: COMS Report No 30. Ophthalmology 116(1):106–115

Head and Neck Brachytherapy: A Description of Methods and a Summary of Results

D. Jeffrey Demanes

Abstract

Brachytherapy applications for head and neck are diverse and sometimes complicated. Knowledge of anatomy and the ability to perform complex procedures are basic prerequisites. This chapter addresses most head and neck brachytherapy other than radionuclide treatment of thyroid cancer and eye plaques for melanoma. The literature is comprehensively reviewed, but it is not exhaustive. It is recommended that the reader also consult *Modern Brachytherapy* [1], *GEC-ESTRO Handbook of Brachytherapy* [2], *Head and Neck Cancer* [3], and *Brachytherapy: Applications and Techniques* [4].

1 Introduction

1.1 History of Technical Developments

Head and neck brachytherapy began with radium-226 applications to the skin and lip. Radiation dose was described as the amount of radium and the duration of the application (milligram-hours). Treatment of deeper head and neck lesions required development, mostly by surgeons, of interstitial techniques. As the specialty evolved, radiologists became more adept and proficient at interstitial insertion of permanent radon seeds or temporary radium needles. Such applications were, by necessity, done quickly to limit radiation exposure to medical personnel.

In the 1950–1960s, with the advent of cyclotrons, scientists such as William G Meyer developed man-made radioactive sources, which could be delivered through small needles and catheters. Ulrich Henschke in the United States and Bernard Pierquin in France pioneered their clinical use. As a result, permanent gold-198 and iodine-125 seeds replaced radon seeds, and iridium-192 seeds replaced radium-226 needles for head and neck brachytherapy [5].

Permanent seeds have sufficiently low energy to allow safe handling in the operating room and tissue attenuation such that patients can be safely discharged home after the procedure. The radia-

D.J. Demanes, MD, FACRO, FACR, FASTRO
Professor, Division of Brachytherapy, Department of Radiation Oncology, , University of California Los Angeles (UCLA), Los Angeles, CA, USA
e-mail: jdemanes@mednet.ucla.edu;
jeffreydemanes@gmail.com

© Springer International Publishing Switzerland 2016
P. Montemaggi et al. (eds.), *Brachytherapy: An International Perspective*, Medical Radiology,
DOI 10.1007/978-3-319-26791-3_7

tion dose is dependent upon the source activity and the geometry of the implant. The duration of treatment varies according to the radionuclide half-life: iodine-125 (59 days), palladium-103 (17 days), and cesium-131 (9.7 days) as the sources decay to become essentially inert. Permanent seeds are convenient because they are inserted in a single procedure, but their distribution is often difficult to control, especially at mucosal surfaces or in mobile soft tissue. Once inserted, seeds cannot be purposefully moved or adjusted.

Iridium-192 became the source of choice for temporary interstitial implants. It emits a high-energy photon, so treatment must be delivered in controlled areas for radiation safety. The interstitial implants are performed by the insertion of a scaffolding of hollow applicator tubes without hurry or concern of radiation exposure. The iridium-192 is later temporarily inserted into catheters for treatment delivery (i.e., afterloaded). The sources may be inserted by hand or by a robotic delivery device. Once the sources have been removed, there is no residual radiation exposure. Iridium-192 is supplied for manual loading as low-activity seeds embedded at 0.5 cm intervals along the length of nylon "ribbons" (which looks like a monofilament fishing line) or as a component of a continuous wire. More commonly now, it is inserted robotically as a single very high-intensity radiation source attached to the end of a fine cable (remote afterloading).

Temporary brachytherapy is classified by the rate at which the dose is delivered. Low dose rate (LDR) is defined as <2 Gy/h. It involves the insertion of low-intensity iridium-192 seeds in ribbons, by hand, into the afterloading catheters. The dose is determined by multiplying the "dose rate" by the duration of treatment (typically 1–3 days). The problems with manual source loading are radiation exposure to medical personnel, patient isolation, and restrictions on nursing care.

High dose rate (HDR) is defined as >12 Gy/h (medium dose rate is 2–12 Gy/h). It uses remote afterloading devices, which are the necessary and logical solution to the problem of radiation exposure to medical personnel. Engineers, all over the world, began to develop reliable robotic afterloading devices in the 1980s. The number and size of the doses given per day classify the application as HDR or pulsed dose rate (PDR). High dose rate typically gives 3–6 Gy (up to about 20 Gy) per session. The dose is often given twice (occasionally three times) per day with 4–6 h intervals between treatments. There are significant radiobiological implications to these large doses "per fraction" in that the biological effect increases exponentially with dose. PDR mimics the radiobiology of continuous LDR by giving small doses of radiation hourly on either 12 or 24 hour schedule. A detailed history of afterloading brachytherapy has been published [6].

Interstitial implants are the primary method used for head and neck brachytherapy. Dosimetry is as important as total dose and dose rate. As brachytherapy became more widely used in the middle of the twentieth century, various systems of dosimetry evolved. In the 1930–1940s, Quimby (New York) developed a uniform loading system for brachytherapy sources which resulted in high doses in the center of the implant where less sensitive hypoxic cells are located [7–9]. Patterson-Parker (Manchester), on the other hand, preferred a more uniform distribution based upon geometric arrangements of sources in planes or volumes [10–12]. In France in the 1970s, Pierquin et al. developed rules for interstitial dosimetry to describe mean doses at locations between planes of sources and the minimal peripheral dose concepts (i.e., the minimum dose that encompasses the target) [13]. All of these systems have given way to computer-based treatment planning and dosimetry [14].

Dosimetry was initially based upon two-dimensional imaging that gave isodose depictions and point doses without precise anatomic correlations. However, the advancement of 3D imaging by the third quarter of the twentieth century provided anatomic data in which tumor volumes and critical structures (organs at risk (OAR) such as the eye, spinal cord, and mandible) could be accurately incorporated into dosimetry calculations. Dose volume histograms (DVH) provided virtual image reconstructions, standard target volume isodose descriptions (V100, V150, V200), and doses to specified target volumes (D90 or D100). Similarly, normal tissue doses were reported in terms of doses to specified volumes of normal tissue such as 0.1 cc (surrogate for maximum dose), 1 cc, and 2 cc (D0.1 cc, D1cc, and D2cc). Finally, "inverse treatment planning" became available in brachytherapy where target dose specifications and normal tissue dose constraints could be entered and calculated through an iterative process to find optimal dosimetry solutions [15].

2 Indications and Uses of Brachytherapy for Head and Neck Cancer

2.1 Pretreatment Workup of Head and Neck Cancer

The staging and workup of head and neck cancer depends upon the primary site and type of cancer. A complete general patient evaluation and a careful head and neck examination are the first steps. In an office, fiberoptic nasopharyngoscopy or direct laryngoscopy under anesthesia is typically needed for complete examination of the mucosa and to assess the airway. Pathologic confirmation of disease is a prerequisite to radiation therapy. Biopsy of the mucosal lesion confirms the primary, and a fine-needle aspiration or neck dissection is usually diagnostic of regional spread. Imaging often includes a high-quality MRI (assuming no contraindications to the study) to determine the soft tissue and bone marrow components of disease, a CT with contrast to assess cortical bone invasion, and a PET-CT to identify local functional activity and distant metastasis. Dental evaluation and psychosocial assessments are also basic components of the workup.

2.2 General Considerations

Radiation therapy is an effective treatment for head and neck cancer, but it has acute and chronic side effects. Mucositis, salivary dysfunction, and taste impairment are expected, and there is a potential for deeper injuries to mucosa, glandular

tissue, muscle, neurovascular structures, and bone. The long-term clinical consequences may include impairments of speech and swallowing, tooth decay, soft tissue or bone necrosis, neuropathy, and vascular disease. Radiation therapy also negatively affects surgical wound healing and exacerbates postoperative fibrosis. There is a small risk of radiation-induced second malignancy (typically sarcoma), although such cancer is rare compared to recurrent cancer and second mucosal primaries. All of these radiation effects are radiation dose and dose distribution dependent.

Brachytherapy delivers a high radiation dose to a localized target without having to traverse normal tissue to reach the target. It thus has a dosimetric advantage for accessible and sufficiently well-defined targets. Brachytherapy requires anesthesia and thus carries some procedural risks. However, there are no major wounds to heal, and the anatomy, function, and appearance of the implanted structures are typically preserved. The outcomes with brachytherapy are dependent on implant quality and proper case management.

Brachytherapy may be used in virtually any head and neck cancer, primary or recurrent, where hollow catheters can be safely inserted. The relative risks and benefits of surgery, external radiation with or without chemotherapy, and brachytherapy should be considered for all patients with head and neck cancer. Brachytherapy may be an alternative or complementary to surgery. As an alternative, it avoids the morbidity associated with tissue removal and reconstruction. Most experts agree that there are significant advantages to surgery when disease invades bone and it is preferred in certain tumors like salivary gland cancers that are less responsive to radiation than squamous cell carcinoma. Surgery also provides important pathological information about the local and regional (when a neck dissection is performed) extent of disease. Brachytherapy can be complementary to surgery by extending treatment for close or positive pathological margins. It can be done simultaneously with the surgery where intraoperative exposure is useful, or it can be done after surgery to allow wound healing and full evaluation of surgical pathology. Postoperative brachytherapy might be selected instead of EBRT for an oral cavity lesion, for example, to reduce postoperative radiation side effects when the treatment target is believed to be localized and where lymph node irradiation is not indicated.

Because of its physical characteristics, brachytherapy delivers relatively higher tumor doses and lower doses to adjacent normal anatomy than EBRT. As a result, it usually does not cause long-term symptomatic injury to salivary glands, taste buds, pharyngeal musculature, or the carotid arteries. The decision to use brachytherapy alone or in combination with EBRT primarily depends upon the likelihood of regional spread of disease. When used with EBRT, brachytherapy offers precise delivery of the high doses needed to control gross disease (at the primary site or in bulky lymph nodes) while EBRT delivers more uniform doses needed for control of microscopic lymphatic or perineural disease. Therefore, brachytherapy offers the opportunity, with or without EBRT, to optimize the radiation distribution for organ preservation and to maximize local disease control. Cosmetic results with brachytherapy are typically good.

The connection of human papillomavirus (HPV) to squamous cell carcinoma of the oropharynx has altered our understanding of the disease, and it has been found to have a better prognosis than tumors associated with alcohol and tobacco. This discovery has led to new treatment strategies of radiation dose de-intensification [16]. It appears that the cure rates may not be adversely affected by less treatment, and therefore the side effects could be diminished [17]. The reductions may be in dose, volume, or the need for sensitizing chemotherapy. Since the brachytherapy is intrinsically target volume and dose specific, it should be considered as a form of treatment with de-intensification to normal tissue without sacrificing tumor dose for local control.

The chance for disease control, the functional outcome, and the likelihood of major complications in head and neck cancer depend upon many factors, including the kind of cancer, stage of disease, and comorbidity status. Treatment must be offered in the context of the patient's overall health,

smoking and alcohol history, human papillomavirus association (HPV/P16), and psychosocial circumstances. The relative risks and benefits of surgery, radiation, or chemoradiation are often debated, and it is not always possible to recommend one specific best treatment. Since there are few direct comparative studies and even fewer controlled trials that incorporate brachytherapy, the benefits of brachytherapy may not be fully recognized or made available to the patient. Ultimately, the individual patient must decide which of the various treatment alternatives to accept.

3   Brachytherapy Without External Beam

3.1   Early Cancers of the Lip, Buccal Mucosa, Nasal Vestibule Oral Cavity

Brachytherapy can be administered as a sole treatment (monotherapy) or in conjunction with EBRT. Used alone, brachytherapy is typically done as a single interstitial implant followed by several days to a week of therapy [18]. Monotherapy causes little in the way of long-term xerostomia or decrease in taste function. By way of intent, it is the radiotherapeutic equivalent of a wide local excision without lymph node dissection. The use of brachytherapy alone reduces the volume of normal tissue irradiated, and it allows subsequent irradiation or surgery, if needed. If successful, it provides disease control with preservation of structure and function of the affected site.

Treatment to the primary site alone is predicated upon the disease being localized (i.e., no nodal metastasis); therefore, the indications relate to lesion size, location, and histology. Stage T1 or small T2, anterior (lip, nasal vestibule, and oral cavity), and well-differentiated lesions without perineural (PNI) or lymphovascular invasion (LVI) are prime indications because they are more likely to be localized than large, posterior (pharyngeal), or poorly differentiated cancers. To achieve success, the curative brachytherapy dose should fully encompass the primary disease with a 1–1.5 cm margin in all dimensions.

Properly selected lesions of the localized type can be effectively managed with either wide local excision or brachytherapy or by a combination of excision and postoperative brachytherapy. There is no consensus and few comparative studies to determine whether surgery or brachytherapy is more effective for early lesions or if they are equivalent. The use of brachytherapy instead of EBRT reduces the side effects (dry mouth and taste impairment) and reduces the dose to surrounding soft tissue and the mandible. The decision to use surgery versus radiation may be influenced by the lesion characteristics. For example, exophytic growth patterns are well oxygenated and more responsive to radiation. Endophytic or infiltrating lesions, which may be ulcerated or necrotic, might be resected and treated with postoperative brachytherapy or external beam or both. The indications for postoperative brachytherapy include pathological assessment of surgical margins, the pathological extent of disease, the presence of LVI or PNI, and any concerns by the surgeon that surgery alone is insufficient.

Surgery is generally preferable to radiation therapy for lesions involving bone because the needed tumor doses are likely to exceed normal tissue tolerance, and the combination of surgery and radiation yields better outcomes. Once the relatively thin gingival mucosa has given way, the exposed bone is more prone to infection and osteonecrosis, especially the mandible (body more than ramus) with its limited blood supply. Edentulous patients and those with healthy gums are at less risk of mandibular necrosis than patients with teeth or gingivitis. Brachytherapy helps avoid injury to the mandible, if properly administered, because lower doses are delivered to the bone and salivary function is relatively preserved. Bone and teeth are impediments to the placement of brachytherapy catheters. However, in some cases when need arises, they can be successfully managed by wrapping around or attaching brachytherapy catheters to the surface of the bone to treat lesions that are not too deep or extensively erosive.

Neck dissection and elective nodal irradiation are not necessarily routine measures for early cancer of the lip or oral cavity cancer, but patients with clinical or surgical-pathological evidence of lymph node involvement are prime candidates for neck irradiation. Selected cases with limited adenopathy after neck dissection may not need postoperative radiation therapy [19, 20]. Without neck surgery, the decision to administer elective nodal irradiation would depend upon the nature and extent of the primary or imaging evidence such as PET-CT to suggest the neck is involved. Recurrence in the untreated neck can (often) be successfully salvaged with a neck dissection and postoperative EBRT, but salvage treatment is typically more complicated and morbid than initial treatment [21, 22].

3.2 Cancer of the Oropharynx

Regional metastases are common in cancers of the oropharynx. Consequently, management of these tumors usually involves treatment of at-risk lymph nodes with EBRT. As our ability to identify microscopic spread improves, local treatment only and the benefits of reduced morbidity may become feasible. In the meantime, highly selected patients with T1N0, whose PET scans are negative, might be treated with brachytherapy alone (monotherapy). Tonsil and soft palate lesions are probably more suitable candidates for monotherapy than base of tongue primaries where it can be difficult to determine the extent of the primary lesion. Patients with oropharynx cancer who decline surgery and external beam may be offered brachytherapy.

3.3 Brachytherapy with External Beam

EBRT is fundamental to comprehensive therapy in diseases with a high rate of lymph node involvement. Intensity-modulated radiation therapy (IMRT) with or without concomitant or neoadjuvant chemotherapy, when used without brachytherapy, is usually given to about 70 Gy.

Randomized clinical trials of EBRT alone versus EBRT with chemotherapy favor combined therapy [23]. The morbidity of IMRT with chemotherapy, however, is greater than when radiation is used alone. The acute side effects of chemoradiation commonly result in treatment breaks and hospitalization. Reduction of late toxicity by "dose de-escalation" can be achieved in HPV (P16)-positive cases where there is a better prognosis [17]. Decreases in both acute and late toxicity can also be effectively achieved with brachytherapy. When brachytherapy is used with IMRT, the rationale is to take advantage of both technologies to optimally deposit the dose in the primary and nodal targets to limit the dose as much as possible to pharyngeal muscles, salivary tissue, and major blood vessels. There have been no clinical trials to compare IMRT (or chemoradiation) versus IMRT with brachytherapy. It would be valuable to study to what extent brachytherapy would enhance local tumor control or reduce morbidity.

Chemotherapy should be discontinued before brachytherapy to avoid metabolic perturbations and blood count depressions that will complicate the procedure. The primary benefit of chemotherapy is to enhance the effect of radiation on local and regional disease. However, this goal might as well be achieved with brachytherapy without chemotherapy. Although it is not widely recognized, brachytherapy can be used to boost gross adenopathy as well as the primary, and it simplifies the integration of EBRT and brachytherapy. Lesions suitable for combined brachytherapy and IMRT are large oral cavity lesions, cancers of the pharynx, poorly differentiated cancers, and adenoid cystic carcinoma.

3.4 Locally Advanced Oral Cavity Not Suitable for Brachytherapy Alone

Brachytherapy is used as a boost to EBRT for locally advanced or regionally disseminated cancers of the lip and oral cavity that are not suitable for brachytherapy alone [18, 24]. These larger lesions, particularly those with endophytic growth, are more difficult to control, and there is a greater likelihood of regional spread. Under these circumstances, brachytherapy offers the advantage over EBRT alone of localized dose escalation with the potential for enhanced tumor control and less dose to the mandible, salivary glands, and taste buds. Surgical resection of the lesion followed by brachytherapy and EBRT is a common strategy for locally advanced disease that may improve local control rates, but it is also associated with more functional impairment of the tongue. Indications for postoperative brachytherapy are LVI, PNI, positive or close margins, or lymph node involvement [25]. There must be a suitable interval and careful assessment for wound healing to avoid disruption of free-flap grafts. Chemotherapy may have a role in cases of locally or regionally advanced cancers of the oral cavity [26].

3.5 Oropharynx (Base of Tongue, Tonsil, Soft Palate, and Pharyngeal Wall)

Oropharynx cancer usually presents as adenopathy or as a locally advanced primary. The distinction between various subsites is more anatomical and clinical than biological, but base of tongue cancers are more difficult to detect. Oropharynx cancers may be treated with comparable disease control with surgery (usually with postoperative radiation therapy) or chemoradiation therapy. The use of brachytherapy with EBRT results in excellent functional outcomes and good quality of life preservation [27]. The same appears to be true for tonsillar cancer. A comparison study of surgery and brachytherapy with EBRT revealed equally high local control but more trismus with surgery and more (transient) soft tissue necrosis with brachytherapy [28–30]. Traditional surgery may be replaced by transoral robotic surgery (TORS) for some cases of oropharynx cancer; it eliminates the need for tracheostomy and reduces the complexity of surgical access [31]. There are no randomized prospective trials to compare IMRT with or without brachytherapy to standard surgery or TORS for these cancers.

The main role of brachytherapy in oropharynx is as a boost to EBRT. Base of tongue, tonsil, and soft palate cancers are all accessible and amenable to brachytherapy. Tracheostomy is often, but not always, performed to protect the airway during brachytherapy or the oropharynx. Combined EBRT and brachytherapy for soft palate cancers has the advantage of leaving the soft palate intact and usually avoids the need for a prosthetic device. The use of brachytherapy in pharyngeal wall cancer minimizes injury and removal of the pharyngeal constrictors.

3.6 Nasopharynx

Chemoradiation is treatment of choice for locally advanced or regionally metastatic nasopharynx cancer [32]. Brachytherapy boost of early (T1 or T2) disease with little or no bone erosion and no intracranial extension is performed by outpatient placement of an intracavitary applicator under local anesthesia. In more advanced disease, the use of brachytherapy is less likely to impact the outcome because the base of the skull or the intracranial extension precludes disease encompassing anatomic access [33, 34].

3.7 Hypopharynx, Larynx, and Trachea

Lesions of the hypopharynx and larynx are technically challenging for brachytherapy due to the relatively inaccessible location, laryngeal cartilage concerns, and vascular anatomy. For the most part, these cancers are treated with either surgery or radiation therapy or some combination. Brachytherapy is used in selected cases as salvage or for palliation. Outpatient intraluminal brachytherapy is applicable to tracheal stomal recurrences and for lesions in the trachea. Stomal recurrences are usually palliative whereas early lesions of the trachea can be treated with brachytherapy or EBRT and brachytherapy with curative intent. Extensive peristomal disease may require the use of complex interstitial implants.

3.7.1 Head and Neck Brachytherapy Used for Salvage of Previously Irradiated Patients

Local recurrence of disease and new primaries in previously irradiated patients are common. Normal tissue tolerance places limits on additional radiation therapy, so brachytherapy has been used when the disease is amenable and the patient's general condition allows a procedure to be performed. The surgical option should always be considered and the condition of the previously irradiated tissues assessed before proceeding with salvage brachytherapy. Doses to the spinal cord need to be reviewed, so that total spinal cord can be kept within tissue tolerance. Salvage interstitial implant are often complicated and challenging procedures [35–45].

4 Techniques of Head and Neck Brachytherapy

4.1 Overview

The techniques for brachytherapy are as varied as the modality itself. The GEC-ESTRO handbook is an excellent reference and overview of head and neck brachytherapy [2].

4.2 Dental Evaluation and Prosthodontics

Dental evaluation before radiation therapy is an essential part of treatment planning. The teeth should be cleaned, caries filled, and extractions performed as needed. Dental trays are prepared for long-term fluoride treatment to prevent tooth decay. Management of gingivitis is essential for prevention of bone necrosis (BN). Custom-fitted mandible trays with or without shielding for displacing normal tissues from the radiation sources are valuable and necessary devices prepared for the reduction of dose and radiation injury of the mandible and other normal tissues. The proper use of these devices reduces the likelihood of mandible necrosis [46–49] (Fig. 1).

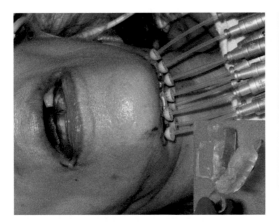

Fig. 1 Oral tongue implant with mandible spacer (insert) shown in treatment position

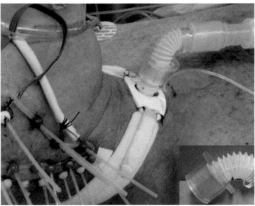

Fig. 2 Base of tongue implant with tracheostomy and Omni flexible connector to facilitate access for needle placement

Management of tissue reactions after radiation affects the extent and severity of long-term complications. Extractions after radiation therapy should be avoided unless there are strong indications to do them. Only dentists or maxillary facial surgeons experienced in the care of radiation therapy patients should do these procedures. Hyperbaric oxygen therapy before and after the extractions may be indicated to reduce complications of the procedure and improve wound healing [50]. Hyperbaric oxygen has also been used to treat soft tissue and bone necrosis after treatment of head and neck cancer [51, 52].

4.3 Tracheostomy and Airway Management

Brachytherapy involves the placement of hardware that can impair the airway. Interstitial catheters may be associated with edema, bleeding, and obstructing secretions, which can accumulate around the devices and obstruct the airway. Urgent intubation with a brachytherapy device in place can be difficult so the airway must be assessed before and during the performance of the brachytherapy procedure. The patient should be consented for a tracheostomy, and there must be an anesthesia plan on how to best secure the airway (direct, fiberoptic, transoral, or transnasal intubation). The patient should not be paralyzed until the airway is clearly manageable.

The lesion size and location, prior to surgery or radiation, the dental status, the presence of trismus, and the general condition of the patient all affect decisions about airway management and whether to do a prophylactic tracheostomy. In general, smaller anterior lesions pose less airway risk. Trismus, thick secretions, a full set of teeth, and medical infirmity are detrimental. Standard direct or video-assisted transoral intubation is done for easier airway control. Oral intubation impedes the brachytherapy procedure, so if there is no tracheostomy planned, nasal intubation using a right-angle endotracheal (RAE) tube which curves superiorly over the forehead out of the operative field is preferable. When in doubt about the airway, a tracheostomy should be performed. In patients with a prior tracheostomy or a tracheal stoma, a cuffed "Armor" tube can be used. Another very useful device is an "Omni" tracheostomy connector device. It has a short flexible tube with a low profile that allows the airway control device to be out of the way and fixed on the patient's chest so that it does not interfere with access to the submental region during the implant (Fig. 2).

If intubation is not feasible, then an "awake" tracheostomy can be done under local anesthesia with the patient sedated. On occasion, the implant turns out to be more extensive than expected, in which case a tracheostomy can be performed after completion of the implant. A size 6–8 cuffed (fenestrated) tracheostomy tube is most suitable.

The fenestration is helpful for alleviating later airway obstruction related to the tracheostomy cuff, which can become encrusted with secretions over the course of several days. The fenestration also facilitates decannulation. Most patients who need to return to the operating room for implant removal should probably have a tracheostomy and vice versa. The tracheostomy is typically removed the day after the implant catheters are taken out, and in most cases, the tracheostomy is removed prior to hospital discharge.

5 Intracavitary and Intraluminal Applications

5.1 Intracavitary Custom Applications

The head and neck region has complex anatomy with natural cavities and potential spaces created by surgery that affect placement of radiation sources; they include the nasal cavity, nasopharynx, trachea, oral cavity, external auditory canal, sinuses, and orbits. The nasopharynx presents a small, somewhat irregular accessible site for intracavitary brachytherapy. The nasal cavity is more accessible, but more irregular and less amenable to standard shaped brachytherapy applicators. The external auditory canal is another cylindrical site occasionally treated with intracavitary brachytherapy. Various custom applicators can be designed and constructed by maxillofacial prosthodontics to fit in and around accessible lesions such as the lip or hard palate, which serve to position the applicator and displace normal tissues [53–56].

5.2 Nasopharynx

Intracavitary brachytherapy can be used as a boost for EBRT in NPC without major base of skull bone or intracranial involvement. One technique is to place symmetrical balloon-type applicators directly through the nose and into the nasopharynx. Such applicators, however, are not customized to fit the nasopharynx, and they give undesirably large dose to the soft palate. The Rotterdam dual-channel applicator is a more suitable device; it is slightly more complicated to insert, but the dosimetry is far better than the symmetrical balloon [34]. The patient may require some sedation, and the mucous membranes should be topically anesthetized before insertion. Small (10–12-French) feeding tubes are inserted through the nose until they present in the oropharynx. They are retrieved through the mouth and threaded into the two channels of the Rotterdam applicator. The assembly is pulled upside down and backward through the mouth so that it seats correctly into the nasopharynx with channels presenting out each nostril. This two-channel applicator has a tissue spacer to displace the soft palate away from the sources while the dorsal part of the applicator is pressed snugly onto the nasopharyngeal mucosa. There are two versions; one with parallel channels and the other with somewhat lateralized channels to improve dosimetry. The applications are given on an outpatient basis (Fig. 3).

5.3 Supraglottic Larynx

Custom applicators have been invented based upon laryngeal mask anesthesia (LMA) devices. This applicator can be used for a variety of indications. It requires anesthesia to apply. It is a relatively simple applicator to insert, and it permits custom source positioning [57].

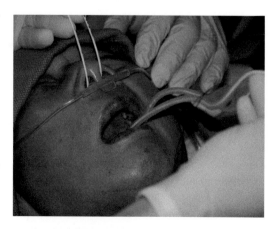

Fig. 3 Double feeding tubes are inserted in the nose and exit the oral cavity for placement of the Rotterdam nasopharynx applicator

5.4 Trachea and Tracheal Stoma

Primary or metastatic cancer in the trachea is amenable to intraluminal brachytherapy. The patient is sedated and prepared for bronchoscopy. One or more closed-ended 5–6-French "endo-bronchial" brachytherapy catheters are inserted into the anesthetized trachea through biopsy port of the bronchoscope. As the scope is withdrawn, the brachytherapy catheter is simultaneously advanced (using a wire) until the bronchoscope is removed, leaving the brachytherapy catheter in the desired location. Inability to control the position of endobronchial catheters within the relatively large trachea lumen is a dosimetry limitation, which can be somewhat mitigated by the use of multiple catheters. A larger "centering" catheter (Fritz adjustable intraluminal catheter) has been designed to improve the dosimetry, but its size prevents it from fitting through a broncho-scope and poses some challenges for use in the intact airway. It can be inserted into a tracheal stoma. Other solutions for patients with intralumi-nal tracheal stoma recurrence have been designed. One such device was fashioned from a tracheal stent, an endobronchial catheter, and a tissue spacer to allow custom dosimetry and delivery of radiation to the involved side of the tracheal stoma with sparing of the opposite wall [58]. A typical course of intraluminal HDR brachytherapy is 3–5 sessions with or without EBRT.

5.5 Postoperative Mold Brachytherapy (Sinuses, Nasal Cavity, or Orbit)

Cancers of the sinuses or orbit are most commonly treated with surgery. In some cases, the pathological margins are close or positive or there may even be gross residual disease. Depending upon the circumstances, brachytherapy alone or in combination with EBRT may be applied to enhance local tumor control. Custom-shaped applicators or molds with multiple embedded channels are made in conjunction with the maxillofacial and prosthetics department. The catheters located within the custom form-

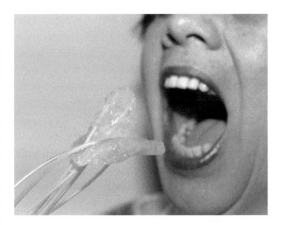

Fig. 4 Custom prosthodontic device with catheters embedded for postoperative intracavitary application

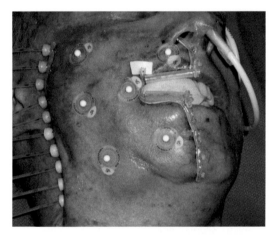

Fig. 5 Complex interstitial brachytherapy with tissue displacement device for T4N0 buccal cancer treated in combination with external beam

fitting device can then be applied directly to the target (Fig. 4). Treatment is given as an outpatient series, usually without sedation or anesthesia. These special applicators may also be designed for a combination of intracavitary and interstitial brachytherapy (Fig. 5).

5.6 Complex Interstitial Brachytherapy

Head and neck brachytherapy is mostly performed as an interstitial implant. Virtually, any soft tissue can be implanted. The complexity and risk of the procedure are related to the lesion size, its anatomic location, and the relationship of the implant to bone and vascular structures. The implant design, catheter distribution, and dosimetry are always customized to accommodate the highly variable clinical circumstance. The implant process can be described as minimally invasive (i.e., no incision), but it is complex, spatially challenging and often time-consuming to perform. Edema can occur as the implant proceeds, which can affect the process of catheter insertion and subsequently impact the dosimetry and clinical management. In general, the salivary glands can be ignored as organs at risk, but bone, especially the mandible, and blood vessels cannot.

5.7 Clinical Management of the Head and Neck Brachytherapy Patient

The clinical management during the brachytherapy procedure should be standardized. There is no literature consensus about some of the recommendations presented here; they are the policies of the author. Please see appendices A and B for template order sets, which are presented as example ideas rather than patient-specific recommendations.

Perioperative measures:

1. Routine preoperative orders (Appendix A).
2. Patient comfort: patient-controlled analgesia (PCA) usually hydromorphone, if patient is able to manage it.
3. Prophylactic antibiotics: intraoperative antibiotics typically cefoxitin (or levofloxacin and clindamycin if penicillin allergic). The author prefers continuation of antibiotics during the entire time the applicator is in place. This policy has led to low infection rates of approximately 1–2 %.
4. Dexamethasone 8–10 mg given just before the procedure and may be given daily until the implant is removed. It is not needed for all cases (such as smaller or more superficial implants) and must be used with caution in diabetic patients.

5. Antacid medications to prevent stress peptic ulceration as needed.
6. Nasogastric feeding tube placement (usually a wire-guided 12 French) unless the patient already has a percutaneous endoscopic gastrostomy (PEG).
7. Intensive care unit (ICU) or similar level of care monitoring is recommended for patients with fresh tracheostomies, questionably stable patients, patient with implants anywhere near the major blood vessels, or those where there are concerns about secretion production or mental status.
8. Routine postoperative orders (Appendix B).

5.8 Implant Timing and Target Volume

The implant may be done before or after EBRT for combined treatment indications. The advantage of performing brachytherapy first is that the lesion is most apparent for implantation. The advantage of administering EBRT or chemoradiation first is to shrink the lesion and make it less friable and easier to implant. It may be debated whether to implant the original extent of disease or just the residual gross disease volume. These concepts have been addressed by GEC-ESTRO using the terms (1) gross tumor volume (GTV) for scan or clinically apparent residual disease at the time of brachytherapy, (2) high-risk clinical tumor volume (HR-CTV) for some margin around the GTV, (3) intermediate risk (IR-CTV) for the original extent of gross disease, and (4) low risk (LR-CTV) for regions that may have harbored undetectable microscopic disease.

The challenge with making a rule is that tumor regression is variable and there are no compelling studies for guidance of implant volume in the head and neck. The author prefers to implant a volume closer to the original extent of disease or at least give a generous margin to residual palpable disease. One can always elect not to use certain catheters or to treat a smaller volume than implanted or to shrink the dosimetry volume during the course of brachytherapy. If in doubt, it is better to place more rather than fewer catheters.

In addition, if the physician is knowledgeable and sufficiently experienced, gross adenopathy can be implanted with these same concepts in mind. A clear strategy for distributing and integrating the internal and external radiation therapy components is best developed before starting radiation therapy.

5.9   The Implant Procedure: Needle Insertion

Needle insertion is the first of a two-step process, and brachytherapy catheter insertion is the second step. The level of difficulty of inserting open ended interstitial needles (usually 17 gauge) depends upon the tissue location and its degree of fibrosis associated with disease or prior surgery or radiation therapy. At 15 cm long, they are relatively easy to use and usually sufficient for the head and neck region. It is best to use 30° bevel metal needles because they pass through tissue with reasonable facility. They are sharp enough to penetrate the skin and cervical fascia, yet their tips can be safely palpated and advanced through tissue (never do both simultaneously). Once inserted beneath the skin, the needles can be carefully advanced (not stabbed) through the tissue so they can be moved past rather than through the vessels. Sharper needles (14° bevel open ended) are rarely necessary and not recommended, except in cases of extreme fibrosis, because they are more likely to enter vessels, and it is more dangerous for the physician to palpate the sharper needle tips during insertion (Fig. 6).

5.10   Direct Catheter Insertion (Exchanging the Needle for the Brachytherapy Catheter)

The second step of the process is to replace the needle with an implant catheter (Fig. 7). It is safest to insert needles and replace them with catheters one needle at a time. Brachytherapy catheters come with an internal stent, which

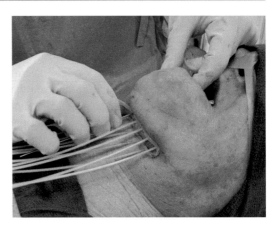

Fig. 6 Bimanual technique of needle insertion during tube and button interstitial tongue brachytherapy procedure

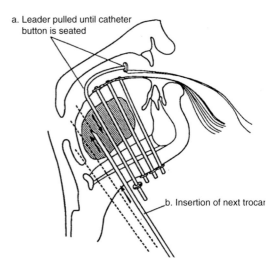

Fig. 7 Catheter insertion method for interstitial tubes and buttons with silk ties during a tongue implant (Reprinted from Demanes et al. [59])

helps prevent the catheters from stretching and thinning as they are pulled through the tissue. It must be removed with wire strippers to make the catheter hollow and ready for source insertion. For "direct" catheter insertion, the beveled open end of the trocar presents visibly at the mucosal surface. A brachytherapy catheter, with a narrow hollow proximal leader and a larger diameter distal closed-ended functional portion, is prepared by adding a small button on the end to fix the catheter at the mucosal surface. Prior to catheter insertion, a 30 in. #1 needless silk suture is tied, with ends of equal length, to one of the two side holes of the button. The leader end of the assembly is threaded with medium smooth pickups into the (face-up) needle bevel until it presents at the proximal end of the needle, which exits the skin. The needle is then removed and the leader is pulled to seat the hollow catheter and button snugly, but not too tightly, on the (distal) mucosal surface.

A colored-coded external fixing button is threaded over the leader and pushed to the skin surface to make both ends of the catheter stable. Internal buttons are usually flat and preferably countersunk, so the tip of the catheter does not project above the level of the button. The end of the silk ties, attached to the mucosal buttons, is left outside of the mouth to aid later in retrieval of the tube and button during the removal procedure. The silk ties are gathered, twisted into a bundle, tied together, and covered with a ¼ inch Penrose drain. The ties are fixed externally to one of the entry site fixing the buttons, so they cannot be swallowed (Figs. 8, 9, and 10). Notice the metal buttons in Fig. 10, which are used to hold LDR source ribbons in place. They can also be used to close one end of a double leader catheter when they are used for loops or arches by leaving some portion of the inner leader within the catheter.

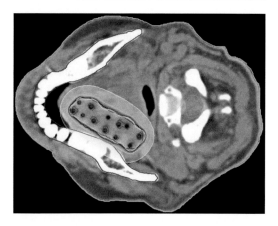

Fig. 9 Axial CT of tongue implant dosimetry with color wash isodose display

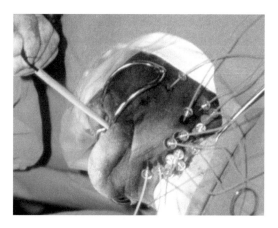

Fig. 10 Base of tongue implant with silk ties gathered and covered with ¼-inch Penrose drain, which will be fixed to one of the external fixing buttons to prevent the patient from swallowing it

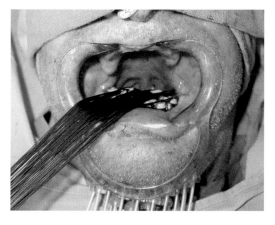

Fig. 8 Interstitial tube and button with silk ties (used later for catheter removal) during implantation of a T4N0 oral tongue cancer

5.11 Wire-in-Leader Catheter Insertion

When the bevel end of the trocar is not visible, the brachytherapy catheter can still be inserted by a method called the "leader-in-wire" technique [59]. A 27-gauge wire is inserted into the skin entry (proximal) end of the trocar and advanced until it is palpable at the internal beveled end. The wire is carefully directed with the palpating double-gloved finger superiorly without kinking it by applying continuous gentle pressure on the external end of the wire rather than pulling it from the inside. Once the wire is visible in the oral cavity, it is retrieved from the mouth. A small clamp is placed on the external (proximal) end to prevent the external part of the wire from slipping into the needle. The thin hollow leader of the catheter (with the tip squared off with scissors) is threaded over the part of the wire presenting from the mouth for 4–6 in. (at minimum the thickness of the tissue being implanted). The wire and leader are fixed together by placing a tonsil clamp on the leader outside the mouth near the end of the wire. The end of the wire, projecting from the skin side of the needle, is then grasped and pulled to "seat" the leader into the bevel of the needle, so it won't fray as it is being pulled through the tissue. As the external catheter and wire are pulled out through the skin, the tonsil clamp advances into the mouth until the needle finally exits the skin and the leader becomes visible. The leader is grasped, the tonsil clamp is released, and then the wire is pulled out and discarded. The needle is set aside for reuse. The catheter is then pulled into position with the button on the mucosal surface as usual (Fig. 11).

5.12   Avoidance of Vascular Injury

Vascular structures are to be avoided during interstitial implants. Thin-walled veins are more likely to be penetrated than thicker-walled arter-

ies, where consequences are more serious. The technique to avoid implanting vascular structures is somewhat difficult to describe because there is some "feel" to it. The common and internal carotid arteries are of particular interest in head and neck brachytherapy because of the potential for bleeding and neurovascular injury about which the patient should be apprised in advance of the procedure. The course and anatomy of the large blood vessels must be known, and the relationships to the target volume must be understood by the physician doing the implant. Smaller arteries are usually not at great risk of injury because they are more difficult to penetrate with brachytherapy needles and the consequences are clinically less significant. Placement of a brachytherapy catheter into the carotid artery or jugular vein, although undesirable, is not necessarily associated with a morbid clinical outcome. With proper technique, the risk of major bleeding or stroke in the unoperated neck is low. Risks are increased, sometimes significantly, in patients with prior radical neck dissection, ulcerated or necrotic lesions, and preexisting vascular disease. Major bleeding during the brachytherapy insertion is unusual because the brachytherapy catheters tamponade penetrated vessels. The greatest risk for bleeding is during implant removal when the catheter is taken out of an inadvertently penetrated vessel (Fig. 12).

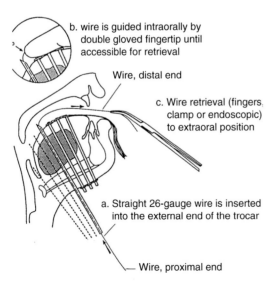

b. wire is guided intraorally by double gloved fingertip until accessible for retrieval

Wire, distal end

c. Wire retrieval (fingers, clamp or endoscopic) to extraoral position

a. Straight 26-gauge wire is inserted into the external end of the trocar

Wire, proximal end

Fig. 11 Wire-in-leader technique for loading catheters, which are not directly visible for catheter loading (see text description) (Reprinted from Demanes et al. [59])

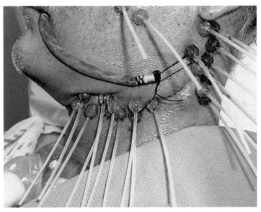

Fig. 12 Complex interstitial implantation of T3N2 oropharynx cancer (base tongue, tonsil, and soft palate) including implantation of adenopathy

5.13 Bone Issues

The mandible, maxilla, hard palate, pterygoid plates, base of skull, and hyoid bone may be obstacles to the placement of brachytherapy catheters. When significantly involved, they are challenges to good dosimetry. Surgery and external beam radiotherapy should be considered for any resectable lesion with significant bony involvement. The body of the mandible is at greatest risk for necrosis, so attempts should always be made to displace the brachytherapy catheters from resting directly upon the gingiva. Spacers, with or without shielding, should be used when feasible. Disease with limited bone involvement can be managed by wrapping catheters around the bone. A strongly curved catheter, however, can kink and prevent passage of the radiation source (especially with HDR afterloading), so catheters with a tightly curved radius must be checked to be sure they are not obstructed.

5.14 Double Leader Arches

When lesions involve midline structures, such as the soft palate, posterior pharyngeal wall, or nasopharynx, double leader catheters without buttons are preferred. They permit creation of an arch, which crosses from one side of the site to another. A pair of beveled implant needles is inserted symmetrically on either side of the neck or face. Then each needle is advanced into tissue, so it exits the mucosa at or near the midline. Each end of a double leader catheter is inserted through the mouth into the matching pair of needles, and they are advanced until the leader projects from the proximal (skin) end of the needles. The needles are then withdrawn leaving the leaders protruding from the skin on opposite sides. The leaders are pulled until the functional portion of the arch exits the skin on each side. The catheter lumen can be stopped from one side (at any point along the arch) by leaving a segment of the inner leader inside the arch and fixing it at one end with a metal crimping button (again as seen in Fig. 10). The treatment plan and virtual image of a palatal arch are shown in Fig. 13 [38, 43, 60, 61].

5.15 Dual Catheters and Internally Connected Buttons to Avoid Catheter Kinking

Catheters that wrap around bone in an acute angle have the potential to kink to make the double leader arch dysfunctional. A better solution is the use of two independent single leader catheters, which meet internally. Needles are inserted on either side of the bone to meet at a common internal mucosal site. Catheters are prepared by connecting their button tip ends together with silk ties. The two catheters are then inserted like a double leader catheter to wrap around bone such as the mandible [62].

5.16 Jackson-Pratt Drain Scaffolding, Catheter Spacing and Stabilization

The placement of tubes and buttons is typically done freehand. The spacing relationships and stability of the catheters, therefore, is subject to variability. A method has been developed using commercially available Jackson-Pratt drains to stabilize brachytherapy catheters [63]. It has holes at 0.5 cm intervals that can be used to space the catheter entry and exit points and connect them together as a unit. For the head and neck regions, 10-French round drains are typically used on the skin (Fig. 14). The drains are threaded over the needles or the catheter leaders typically at 1–1.5 cm intervals to create stable catheter groupings. Planes of catheters can be connected with crossing connections to create stable scaffolding. Stabilization and internal mucosal spacing can be improved by tying selected buttons together with silk.

5.17 French Hairpin (Guide Gutter) Technique

A technique was developed and used primarily in Europe and Asia to facilitate the placement of sources in the tongue [2, 24, 64]. It consists of the transoral placement of a doubly pointed needle connected on the ends by a bar, which stabilizes

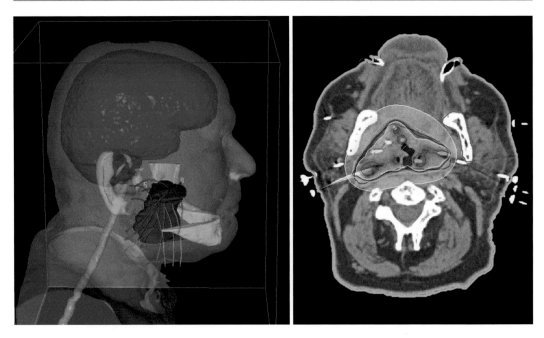

Fig. 13 3D virtual image of the implant catheters and axial color wash isodose of a T3N0 soft palate primary with extension to tonsil and base of tongue in a previously irradiated patient

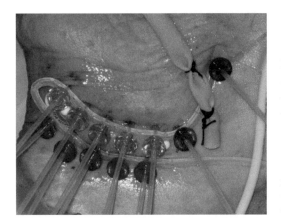

Fig. 14 Base of tongue implant demonstrating the use of size 10 round Jackson-Pratt drains to space and stabilize implant catheters

the needles and defines the interval between the two arms. A series of these devices can be placed at approximately 1 cm intervals to make a two-plane implant. The procedure may be done under general or local anesthesia. The guide gutters are afterloaded with iridium-192 wires for LDR brachytherapy. This method, to the author's knowledge, has not been adapted for HDR brachytherapy.

5.18 Entry Site Design and Catheter and Spacing

Each implant design is unique. Selection of entry sites can be challenging because of the variability of the target anatomy, the bony obstructions, and the need to avoid vascular structures. Catheter spacing must consider both external and internal anatomy. In some cases, the catheters converge (lower base of tongue and vallecula), and in others, it may fan out (larger oral tongue lesions). Access to the deep tongue base is limited by the hyoid bone, and access to the oral tongue is limited by the mandible. The tentative catheter entry sites and spacing should be marked on the skin with a sterile marker before proceeding with the implant. Integration of implantation of the primary mucosal lesions with implantation of gross cervical adenopathy, if any, must be planned in advance. It has been noted that spacing the catheters more widely at the skin entry and having them converge to the desired location within the target help reduce the dose to the mandible, and it is thus believed to lower complication rates [18]. This is good advice for LDR brachytherapy with uniform loading. HDR dwell time optimization can be used to similar ends, particularly if the catheter entry sites are somewhat too close together.

5.19 Fully Encompassing the Lesion

Optimal dosimetry is achieved when the target volume is fully encompassed by relatively uniformly spaced peripheral catheters. Failure to do so results in markedly higher than desired doses (inhomogeneity and possible tissue necrosis) to the tissues within the implant volume in the attempt to deliver the full dose to the periphery of the tumor (i.e., poor dose uniformity). Similarly, poorly spaced peripheral catheters can lead to scalloping of the dose margin, which may result in inadequate target coverage. Uniform spacing is more important for smaller than larger implants. Catheter spacing for larger implants can be increased from 1 to 1.5 cm because of the beneficial effect of the additional source positions on dosimetry. Correct catheter spacing impacts complication rates [65].

5.20 Implant Quality

One of the problems with head and neck brachytherapy is that the spacing of catheters and planes is not known with certainty until the patient has a post-implant CT scan. When inserting catheters, there is a tendency (especially in the oral tongue) to have the planes converge at depth even though they appear to be properly spaced at the entrance and exit sites. It is therefore important to place the medial plane needles sufficiently deep (medial) in the tissue to achieve proper spacing between the catheter planes along their entire length. Therefore, placement of additional catheters medial to the target is preferable to having an implant of insufficient thickness or volume. Too many catheters too close together can be easily managed with HDR brachytherapy where the moving source can compensate by adjusting dwell times. Additional needle insertions are less harmful to the patient than inadequate dosimetry (poor target coverage or excessive hot spots).

5.21 Tissue Displacement and Mandible Shielding

The physics (inverse square law) and methods of brachytherapy provide intrinsically localized radiation. Advantage may be taken of these principles by tissue displacement devices and shielding. These devices may be as simple as several tongue blades wrapped together and inserted between the tongue implant and the mandible or (preferably) a custom prosthodontic device that fits snugly on the teeth and gingiva to displace the implant from normal tissue. Embedded lead shields further improve the protection. They are most applicable to lip and oral cavity, but they may be applied to any site.

5.22 Implant Removal

Implant removal may be simple or complex depending upon the location and extent of the implant. Catheter removal is relatively painless, but the physician must be prepared to manage secretions, hemorrhage, and the patient's well-being. Oral cavity, lip, buccal, and neck catheters can generally be removed in the clinic or at the bedside. Deeper pharyngeal lesions are best removed in the operating room under anesthesia to control bleeding, evaluate the airway, do wound debridement, and optimize patient comfort. A cuffed tracheostomy tube allows anesthesia to be introduced without a second intubation, and the fenestration makes it easier for the patient with a cuffed tube to breathe and to be decannulated. The patient should be paralyzed for removal to allow optimal internal access. The procedure should start with a standard head drape without a sterile preparation and then pharynx should be thoroughly suctioned and rinsed to eliminate debris and secretions. The physician will do the sterile preparation of the brachytherapy catheter sites during removal.

The most accessible (anterior) and least likely to bleed catheters are removed first. The Penrose drain is removed, and the silk ties are separated to clarify their connections to the catheter buttons. Tugging on individual ties helps identify the connection. Once the individual assembly has been identified, the external portion of the catheter is gently retracted from the skin and generously cleaned with sterilization solution (usually povidone-iodine unless the patient is allergic). The surface is depressed to expose the portion of the catheter beneath the button just deep to the skin, so it can be cut to minimize introduction of contaminated material. The remaining portion of the catheter and the internal button attached to the silk tie are then pulled from the tissue using the index finger on the silk tie. The assembly is delivered through the mouth and discarded. Catheters are removed sequentially to manage bleeding one catheter at a time. Deep catheters or those thought to be located near larger blood vessels are best removed last. The palpating finger can often locate the mucosal site of the button that marks where internal pressure should be applied. Tamponade performed using a single fingertip to occlude the catheter exit site is preferable to general packing. A catheter count should be performed after implant removal to assure all the catheters have been removed. At the end of the procedure, the oral cavity, pharynx, nasal cavity, and trachea should be suctioned clear and debrided of secretions and necrotic material. A terminal direct laryngoscopy should be performed to confirm hemostasis and assess the tissue condition and the airway for the potential for uncomplicated decannulation. Antibiotic ointment should be applied to external catheter exit sites and the tracheostomy site, and a clean tracheostomy collar applied. If there is a nasogastric feeding tube, it can be removed in the operating room or later when swallowing status has been determined. As soon as the patient's vital signs and blood pressure are stable, the head of the bed can be raised to facilitate secretion management, to decrease head and neck venous pressure, and to unweight the diaphragm for improved breathing and recovery.

5.23 Site-Specific Commentary

Lip The lip is an accessible site amenable to brachytherapy. Tube and button techniques and steel needles in a template have been used. Plastic tube catheters are generally easier for the patient to manage.

Oral Commissure This area is problematic in that the tissues are thin and mucositis is exacerbated by motion during eating, speaking, and facial expression. The superficial aspect of the tumor must not be underdosed, so it may be necessary to place catheters outside the lesion on the surface. Superficial lesions are potentially amenable to a wrap technique where the catheters are positioned transversely in a U-shape across the lip on the mucosa, vermillion region, and skin around the lip to sandwich the lesion without an interstitial component. Implant displacement away from the gingiva and bone by custom-fitted dental prosthetic devices reduces the dose and injury to normal structures [2, 54, 66–69].

Buccal Mucosa The buccal mucosa extends from the anterior commissure to the intermaxillary fissure and from the mandible to the maxilla with attachment at the gingival buccal sulci. Implants are similar to lip except posteriorly where the structures end medially near the retromolar trigone and the intermaxillary fissure. Posterior lesions must be implanted in such a way to fully encompass the posterior extent of the lesion with either a looping catheter or a perpendicularly crossed end near the posterior border of the masseter muscle. Displacement of the soft tissue with a dental device is indicated, keeping in mind that lesions in the sulcus or which are otherwise adjacent to bone must be encompassed. Although it is difficult to distinguish during the procedure, implantation of the parotid (Stensen's) duct is, in principle, to be avoided [2, 70–73] (Fig. 5).

Oral Tongue Cancer of the oral tongue occurs most commonly on the lateral undersurface. The approach for brachytherapy catheters placement is to utilize the relatively narrow region between the body of the mandible and the hyoid bone. From there, the tongue fans out from the tip to the base and in the normal state rests with a deformable mushroomlike dorsal surface projecting from the floor of mouth. Implantation must take into consideration the anatomic access and the extent and location of the lesion. There are three implant methods: (1) plastic tube loop, (2) guide gutter–hairpin, and (3) the single leader plastic tube and button. The latter is most suitable for HDR because the single leader method avoids the tight curves that are troublesome for the HDR afterloader. The plastic tube loop and hairpin techniques are well described in brachytherapy literature [2, 18, 24, 56, 64, 74] (Figs. 6, 7, and 8).

The single leader catheter with button technique should begin with the lateral plane and start with the most anterior position, especially if the lesion is near the tip. The needle is inserted into the submental skin and passed through soft tissue into the tongue musculature. A finger in the floor of mouth is used to guide the needle along the undersurface of the tongue to exit at the junction with the dorsum (where the mucosa changes from smooth to rough by taste buds). Care must be taken not to accidentally impale the guiding finger, so advancement of the needle and palpation are not done simultaneously. The needle is replaced with the single leader catheter with button and silk tie by inserting the leader of the catheter into the beveled tip and advancing it until it exits the other end of the needle. The needle is then removed leaving the leader exposed. The catheter can then be pulled to bring the functional hollow catheter into the tissue with the button coming to rest on the dorsal mucosal surface. Subsequent needles are inserted in a parallel fashion between 1 and 1.5 cm apart. The cutaneous entry sites generally follow the body of the mandible somewhat diagonally, from anterior medial to posterior lateral, approximately 0.5 cm medial to the bone. Lateral entry, if is located too close to the mandible, will impede needle placement and potentially cause overdose to the bone. If entry is too medial, there will not be enough space for the medial planes. In the author's opinion, a second more medial plane is usually required to generate a volume implant for proper dose uniformity and complete target coverage. The second plane should be at least 1–1.5 cm deep and parallel to (i.e., medial) the first plane. Button to button touching on the tongue surface

is a good guide to catheter spacing. It is advisable for the needles of the second plane to enter the skin and be directed more medial than might be expected before heading superiorly to the exit in the dorsum in order to avoid catheter convergence deep in the tongue upon tongue relaxation when the retraction is eased. A third plane may be needed if the lesion is bulky or if there is any doubt about catheter spacing. The additional catheters will be valuable for dosimetry in cases where unintended catheter convergence has occurred. Generally, fewer catheters are required for more medial than for lateral planes [61, 75, 76].

Floor of Mouth Floor of mouth implants must be directed into a relatively limited horseshoe-shaped space between the gingiva and tongue. These lesions are challenging because of the thinness of the mucosa and their relationship to the mandible. In the relatively narrow confines of the floor of mouth, the catheters may need to converge somewhat from the skin to the mucosal surface to improve dose uniformity [18]. It is more relevant to LDR brachytherapy than HDR where dwell time modulation can help achieve the desired uniformity. Tumor extension to the tongue is easily implanted with a plane of catheters similar to the lateral plane of a tongue implant, but gingival extension is more problematic. When possible, lesions involving the gingiva should be managed surgically. When surgery is not an option, brachytherapy catheters should be placed approximately 0.5 cm from the gingival surface of the lesion. It is necessary to understand the sloping anatomy of the mandible in order to maintain a suitable (>0.5 cm) distance from the mandible during the implant. Submental needle entry into the skin must not be too close to the edge of the mandible because it will cause the needle to exit the mucosa too close to the attachment of the tongue. There are two possible solutions to how to bring the treatment sufficiently superior to the floor of mouth to encompass the gingival extension. One solution, used for LDR, is to wrap the brachytherapy catheter over the mandible with submental and lower lip entry sites [77]. Teeth impede but do not necessarily preclude such an approach. The other solution, more suitable to patients with teeth and when using HDR, is to place multiple buttons on the ends of the catheters in the floor of mouth, so the source projects above the mucosa far enough to provide dose to the medial gingiva [62].

Base of Tongue These implants pose a greater airway risk, and tracheostomy is advisable. The base of tongue converges from a broad upper portion to a relatively more narrow termination in the vallecula. The implant design, therefore, must account for the radial anatomy spacing of catheters by inserting them approximately 1.5–2 cm apart on the skin and allowing them to converge to 1 cm spacing where they enter the mucosa. Five converging catheters are sufficient for the most inferior or deepest row even for a bilateral vallecular lesion with extension to the lateral pharyngeal wall. As the implant proceeds superiorly, a somewhat more parallel needle path can be used. It is generally advisable to insert the deepest and medial catheters first because reaching this location with the palpating finger becomes increasingly difficult and the lesion progressively harder to appreciate as catheters and buttons are added. Gentle on-and-off countertraction can be applied to the initial catheters to help guide subsequent needle trajectories. The hyoid bone, anchors and protects the base of the tongue. Therefore, for deep lesions, the needle path may need to pass inferior to the hyoid bone, or the needles may be superior to it for lesions that spare the vallecula. The paired lingual arteries are unlikely to be pierced, but they are occasionally a source of bleeding during these procedures. The "wire-in-leader technique" is often used for base of tongue implants because the internal needle tips are often not visibly for direct loading [78–80].

Figure 10 shows an LDR base of tongue implant, and Fig. 11 is one drawing of the wire-in-leader technique.

Tonsil Like the base of the tongue, the tonsil is amenable to brachytherapy, except that the ramus of the mandible impedes access. This barrier can be circumvented by the use of looping catheters or a dual catheter technique as described previously. The anterior loop is limited superiorly by the zygoma and maxilla and inferiorly by the body of the mandible. The posterior loop is more broad and open to the lateral pharynx. Spread of the lesion to the base of tongue or pharyngeal wall can be implanted with the single leader catheters with buttons and silk ties. The risk of vascular injury and bleeding is somewhat greater for tonsil implants, which are lateral and more posterior in the neck and, therefore, closer to the carotid artery and jugular vein [28, 29, 33] (Fig. 12).

Hard and Soft Palate The soft palate is implanted with a double leader arch technique [38, 43, 51, 60] (Fig. 13). Three, or sometimes four, catheters are used. The first catheter entry site is 1 cm below and slightly posterior to the angle of the mandible. The examining finger must be inserted into the oral cavity and placed behind the soft palate to appreciate the correct trajectory through the lateral pharyngeal fold (posterior tonsillar pillar) then up and along the free border of the soft palate so that it exits the mucosa near the midline. A contralateral catheter is similarly inserted so that the beveled tips meet at or near the midline. A double leader catheter is inserted, as previously described, to create an arch. The second catheter is inserted 1 cm superior and slightly forward of the first catheter just behind the angle of the mandible. It runs through the anterior tonsillar pillar into the soft palate about 1 cm anterior to the first catheter. If there is room, a third catheter can be inserted behind the mandible. The most anterior catheter is inserted in front of the angle of the mandible at the junction of the ramus and the body. It passes posterior to the maxillary tubercle and through the tissue at the junction of the soft and hard palate. If disease extends to the hard palate, then more anterior catheters can be inserted that pass over the gums or between the teeth. They are sutured to the surface of the hard palate and spaced and stabilized by the Jackson-Pratt drain technique. Alternatively, a prosthodontic surface applicator device can be created as previously described and referenced [53]. Cancer of the hard palate is more often treated with surgery than radiation therapy.

Nasopharynx and Posterior Pharynx Early nasopharyngeal cancers may be managed with an intracavitary brachytherapy boost; however, more extensive disease (primary or recurrent) may require a complex interstitial implant. Deep invasion into the skull base or through the foramina is beyond the dosimetric range of curative transcutaneous brachytherapy. The complex interstitial implants are technically challenging and may be done independently or in conjunction with intracavitary applications. Two approaches have been described. One is through the lateral face and neck, and the other is endoscopic guided through the nose. Both approaches are facilitated by CT or fluoroscopic image guidance. CT is preferable, but it is not widely available in most operating rooms where the lateral procedure should be performed.

In the *lateral approach*, implant needles (15 cm) are inserted on either side of the face to meet in the midline in an arch technique, or alternatively, a single long needle (20 cm) can be passed entirely across the pharynx to exit the contralateral face like the pencil in *Grant's Atlas of Anatomy*. The entry site for the first catheter is below the zygoma through the mandibular notch. It traverses the superior nasopharynx above the torus tubarius. The leader-in-wire and arch techniques can be used if paired needles enter the nasopharynx as extracting the wire from the nasopharynx is technically challenging. On the other hand, traversing the entire skull from mandibular notch to mandibular notch with one long needle may require image guidance, but it is easier to load the plastic catheter. A second needle is inserted just behind the head of the mandible posterior and slightly inferior to the first needle. Forward thrust of the jaw facilitates needle insertion and exit. This second catheter traverses at the level of the junction of the roof and posterior wall of the nasopharynx. One to three additional catheters can be placed at 1–1.5 cm intervals in the posterior pharyngeal wall going fully across from side to side anterior to the carotid arteries. As one proceeds inferiorly, the tissue volume expands, and there may be need to place an additional row of single leader catheters with buttons which terminate in the lateral pharyngeal wall just anterior

to the traversing plane. More inferiorly, the large vessels may be within the needle trajectory (possibly tortuous or displaced by disease or prior treatment). Preoperative CT or MRI of vascular anatomy is advisable before proceeding with these kinds of implants [81] (Figs. 15, 16, and 17).

The *endoscopic approach* consists of direct visualization of the lesion with a rigid scope and the guided placement of specially formatted curved catheters. The extent of the lesion and its relationship to the carotid artery and jugular vein is determined by CT or MRI image guidance before or during the procedure. The lateral extent of the implant by this method is limited by the anatomic constraints of access through the nose and the nature of the catheters, but it is probably easier to perform and might be more widely applicable than the lateral method [82, 83]. Nasal packs with hollow tubular centers may also be used.

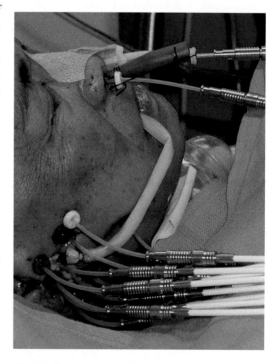

Fig. 15 Complex interstitial and intracavitary implant of a recurrent nasopharynx cancer (previously irradiated) with HDR transfer tubes connected to brachytherapy catheters

Nasal Vestibule The nasal cavity has a complex internal structure. It was already addressed as a potential site for intracavitary brachytherapy mostly in the postoperative setting. Lesions of the nasal vestibule (columella, nasal alae, and distal nasal cavity) may be treated with interstitial techniques. The implant may consist of tubes and buttons, or it can be done with closed-ended catheters with obturators implanted through a template or stabilized with Jackson-Pratt drains or done free-hand. Transverse or axial trajectories have been used. The principles of catheter spacing are the same as for other mucosal sites just described. The presence of cartilage and bone affects the execution of interstitial brachytherapy of this region [84–86].

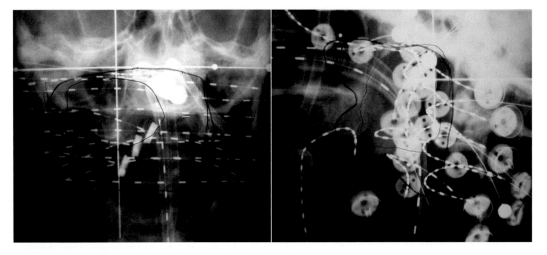

Fig. 16 Anterior-posterior and lateral plane film views of an extensive recurrent posterior pharyngeal wall cancer in a previously irradiated patient

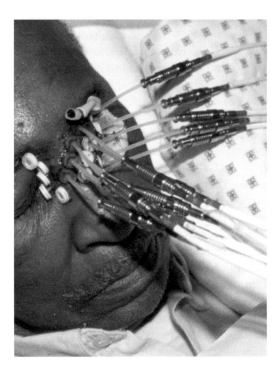

Fig. 17 Interstitial implant of the ethmoid sinus, medial orbit, and bridge of the nose in a patient who had recurrent sinus cancer, after maxillectomy, orbital exenteration, and postoperative external beam radiation therapy

Paranasal Sinuses The challenges for paranasal sinus brachytherapy are that access is limited by bony anatomy and the clinical presentation is often of advanced disease with bone involvement. Surgery is the treatment of choice in most cases. Surgical margins may be close or positive, and preservation of normal structures, such as the eye, can be difficult. The use of brachytherapy may enhance the therapeutic index by extending the surgical margin and reducing radiation morbidity associated with external beam. Brachytherapy may be intraoperative or postoperative. After the lesion is resected, brachytherapy catheters or devices can be fashioned. It is also possible to drill or remove bone and fashion a stable applicator from plastic catheters and other materials. If a shielded operating room is available, treatment can be delivered in a single intraoperative fraction. Alternatively, afterloading catheters can be inserted at the time of the procedure, and treatment can be delivered through the usual process of simulation, computerized dosimetry, and source loading (LDR, PDR, or HDR) [87, 88] (Fig. 18).

Peristomal Recurrences Recurrent cancer involving the tracheostomy stoma can result in necrosis, pain, bleeding, and airway stenosis or obstruction. These lesions, often present in previously irradiated field, are potentially clinically morbid and usually difficult to resect. Brachytherapy catheters can be inserted directly into these lesions with the tube and button technique with proper attention to maintenance of airway patency [89] (Fig. 18).

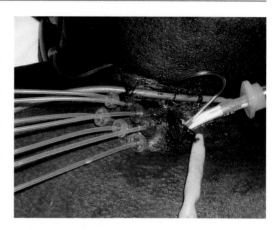

Fig. 18 Interstitial brachytherapy of a deeply invasive peristomal recurrence of larynx cancer

5.24 Brachytherapy of Cervical Adenopathy

Lower Neck Adenopathy in the lower neck can be implanted with a tangential (to the vertical axis of the spine) skin-to-skin catheter placement. In the lower neck, the great vessels are anteriorly situated, and they may traverse the intended implant target volume. In the nonoperated neck, it is possible to place catheters both deep (between the vessels and the vertebrae) and

superficial to the carotid to fully encompass adenopathy involving the carotid space. Ultrasound and CT image guidance are helpful, but equally important is the technique of gently advancing the 30° bevel needle through the tissue (rather than stabbing), so they do not penetrate the artery. Typically more than one plane is required to create a volume around adenopathy. In patients who have undergone a prior neck dissection, and especially in previously irradiated cases, the vessels will have lost supporting soft tissue, and they are not as pliable or mobile. These unprotected, partially fixed vessels are more prone to penetrating injury. In these cases, proceed with neck implantation with caution and preferably with image guidance. Another even more challenging situation is when the lesions ulcerate through the skin or are associated with a fistula. These circumstances are relative contraindications to neck brachytherapy [39–44, 79] (Figs. 19 and 20).

Upper Neck Upper cervical adenopathy is not generally amenable to implantation by a tangential approach. The lower border of the mandible generally demarcates where the tangential technique is no longer applicable. The upper neck is best implanted with a "trans-pharyngeal" approach. A prophylactic temporary tracheostomy is advisable. The carotid artery curves posterior in the upper neck. At the base of the skull, it is posterior to the vertebral body and behind the plane of implantation. Image guidance may be helpful, but the mandible usually interferes with ultrasound. Needles are inserted perpendicular to the skin and directed into the neck toward the pharynx. Single leader tube and button catheters with silk ties are either loaded directly or with the wire-in-leader technique. Two or more planes may be needed. These upper neck implants should be removed in the operating room [90] (Fig. 10).

5.25 Intraoperative Brachytherapy

Brachytherapy can be done with head and neck surgery, as just described, where disease is excised, radiation targets are identified, and brachytherapy catheters are inserted safely around important normal structures. The catheter spacing and stabilization technique described earlier is often helpful [63]. A 10-French flat drain is placed in the wound perpendicular to the plane of the catheters to maintain internal catheter spacing. This drain should not be pulled or adjusted prior to implant removal since it is attached to brachytherapy catheters. Wound closure must be planned and tested during the catheter insertion to be sure the catheters don't become distorted in the process. It is advisable to allow several days for wound healing before starting radiation treatment. Timing depends upon the extent of surgery, blood supply, nature of the lesion, prior radiation, and the relationship of dose to the tissues that need time to heal. This approach, which involves afterloading of the radiation source, takes full advantage of 3D simulation, computerized dosimetry, and normal tissue sparing fractionation of the dose.

Brachytherapy doses can be delivered in the operating room as intraoperative radiation therapy (IORT). It has the advantage of displacement of normal structures and wound closure margins from the radiation dose but lacks the imaged-based precision dosimetry, time for wound healing, and benefits of dose fractionation associated with postoperatively source loading. It requires either an HDR-shielded operating room or a lower-energy source such as generated with low-energy electronic devices [91–93]. Electronic radiation sources are currently larger and more cumbersome than radionuclides. Applicators for

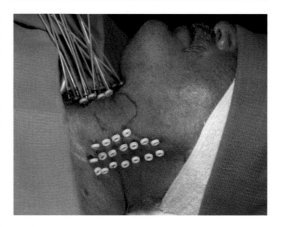

Fig. 19 Complex interstitial transcutaneous brachytherapy of low cervical adenopathy in a patient with recurrent hypopharynx cancer

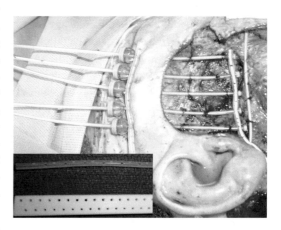

Fig. 20 Intraoperative placement of brachytherapy catheters and the use of Jackson-Pratt-type drains to position and stabilize the catheters within the wound. (Larger 10 flat are preferred in wounds in most operative cases because they are less likely to break off in the wound during implant removal)

these devices, suitable for IORT in the head and neck, are yet to be fully developed (Fig. 21).

5.26 Permanent Seed Brachytherapy

Permanent seeds may be used in the head and neck region when the lesion volume accommodates the sources or there is a surface onto which a seed-embedded mesh can be applied. Individual permanent seeds or seeds in needles with absorbable spacers may be injected into gross tumor.

Insertion of seeds into primary mucosal cancer can be technically challenging because good source distributions are difficult to achieve in deformable soft tissue and at mucosal surfaces. Tissue necrosis at mucosal surfaces may result in seed loss, degradation of dosimetry, and possible seed aspiration. Permanent seed implants are most commonly used to treat recurrent disease presenting in a definable soft tissue volume. Permanent seed sources can be individually injected, inserted as strands on absorbable suture or embedded in a mesh and sutured onto an exposed wound surface. Since irradiation begins immediately upon application, the relationship of the sources to the tissues may affect wound healing. Three technical challenges with permanent seeds are as follows: (1) source distributions are unknown until after the procedure has been completed; (2) once inserted, the sources cannot be modified; and (3) there is no HDR-like dwell time dose optimization. Medical personnel are exposed to radiation and the patient must follow radiation safety precautions. The advantage of permanent seeds is their simplicity and efficiency of source delivery [5, 37, 39, 56, 94–100].

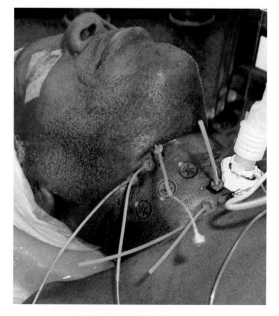

Fig. 21 Complex interstitial implant of recurrent larynx cancer (which, parenthetically, requires direct laryngoscopy for catheter insertion)

5.27 Salvage Brachytherapy

Brachytherapy may be used for recurrent cancer at almost any site in the head and neck region. It can be applied to recurrent disease at the primary site, lymph nodes, or other soft tissue locations. Surgery should always be considered an option, especially in previously irradiated patients (Fig. 22).

6 Guidelines for Head and Neck Brachytherapy

The Groupe European de Curietherapie and European Society for Therapeutic Radiology and Oncology (GEC-ESTRO) for Head and Neck Cancer have defined standards for head and neck brachytherapy. These standards have been adopted by the American Brachytherapy Society (ABS) as well [101].

The stated aims of head and neck brachytherapy are to control cancer, preserve structure and function, and achieve a good cosmetic outcome. High doses are delivered to the target relative to normal tissue without target motion problems associated with EBRT [102]. The use of shields and spacers to protect the mandible and other structures enhances the therapeutic index. The current data indicate that, for early oral cavity cancer (T1–T2 N0), brachytherapy is comparable to surgery, and it is preferable to EBRT or EBRT with brachytherapy [2]. Doses of 65–70 Gy LDR (or HDR equivalent) at dose rates between 0.3 and 0.6 Gy/h are recommended. For more advanced lesions, brachytherapy is used as a boost combined with EBRT to the primary and lymph nodes. Surgery may be used for any of these lesions. For larger T2, T3, and T4N0 tumors, post-elective neck dissection radiation therapy may be indicated. Planned surgery and postoperative radiation therapy are indicated for N+ disease. Surgery is preferred for lesions within 0.5 cm of the mandible or that involve bone. For oropharyngeal cancer, EBRT and brachytherapy appears to result in better functional and quality of life outcomes compared to surgery and postoperative radiation therapy [28–30]. The relative efficacy of brachytherapy and EBRT to EBRT alone (with or without chemo-

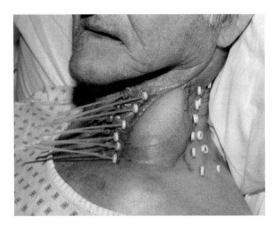

Fig. 22 Transcutaneous implantation of recurrent neck disease in a previously operated patient who had had a deltopectoral wound closure

therapy) has not been systematically studied for cancer of the oropharynx. The management of neck in oropharynx cancer usually involves EBRT, surgery with EBRT, or brachytherapy for gross adenopathy. The impact and significance of HPV-associated head and neck cancer were not available in 2009 when the GEC-ESTRO guidelines were written.

The brachytherapy clinical target volume (CTV) is the gross tumor volume (GTV) plus a 0.5–1.0 cm margin. The planning target volume equals the clinical target volume (CTV = PTV). Concomitant chemotherapy with brachytherapy is not recommended except perhaps in the salvage setting [103, 104]. Completion of the radiation within 8 weeks is advised by GEC-ESTRO, but after chemoradiation, it often takes more than 2 weeks for recovery of mucous membranes. In the author's experience, a 9–10-week time frame is a more realistic goal. It has been suggested that there be two brachytherapy competent persons present in the operating room for implant procedures; however, this may be impractical. Brachytherapy catheters should be placed parallel with spacing of 1–1.5 cm (up to 2 cm with large implants). The author agrees with this recommendation but would add that implant orientation can be complex and variable in head and neck cancer, so not all catheters will necessarily be inserted in uniformly parallel rows. The basic concept is that the lesion should be fully encom-

passed in all dimensions. Image guidance (ultrasound, fluoroscopy, or 3D scanning) is encouraged where technically feasible. Management of tight curves with HDR afterloading requires methods such as dual catheter and button technique [62].

Simulation and dosimetry have evolved from older 2D systems (New York, Quimby as modified by Henschke and Hilaris et al.; Manchester, Paterson-Parker; and Paris, Pierquin-Chassagne) to 3D simulation and computerized dosimetry [7, 8, 10, 13]. Three-dimensional dose volume histogram (DVH) analysis allows in-depth analysis of tumor and normal tissue dosimetry. The specific dose optimization method should be specified in the treatment planning documentation. The GEC-ESTRO brachytherapy quality parameters are dose nonuniformity ratio (DNR), homogeneity index (HI), and uniformity index (UI). The reporting recommendations (ICRU 58) are to describe the implant technique, source specifications (air kerma rate and total dose), and time-dose patterns [105]. Brachytherapy physics descriptors, such as the mean central dose, minimum target dose, and various other doses and volumes, are described in the report. Any of three valid source loading and dose rate methods (LDR, PDR, or HDR) may be employed [106]. The recommended LDR dose rate was between 0.3 and 0.5 Gy/h [107]. The averaged 24 h PDR dose rate was similarly 0.3–0.7 Gy/h with consideration given to daytime-only treatment schedules [108, 109]. Recommendations for HDR fraction size were 3–4 Gy including twice-daily treatment [110]. The much used dose schedules with 6 Gy fractions used in Japan were not addressed [111].

The patient's clinical condition and the stability of the applicator must be regularly monitored. According to GEC-ESTRO, brachytherapy catheter removal should be done in the OR, although the nature and location of the implant may allow nonoperative removal. A follow-up program was recommended to monitor disease control and to identify and manage complications. Patient education should include information on expected inflammatory reactions, which usually peak at 1 week and resolve in 3–6 weeks. Preparations should be made for home oral care, for tracheostomy and catheter entry site wound care, and for nutritional support (Fig. 23).

6.1 Site-Specific Issues

Lip and Buccal Brachytherapy was preferred over surgery for lip cancer, except in small superficial lesions (<0.5 cm), where surgery alone may be curative with a good cosmetic and functional result [2, 66, 79, 177]. A rigid set of needles is recommended for lip cancer, but tube and button techniques were also considered acceptable. Buccal cancer is similar to lip cancer, but brachytherapy is suboptimal if the lesion extends to deep into the buccal alveolar sulcus adjacent to bone.

Technically, 1–2 planes of catheters are used with a mandatory posterior loop in medial and posterior tumors to encompass disease in the intermaxillary commissure. The excellent outcomes for lip are somewhat better than for buccal mucosa.

Tongue and Floor of Mouth For tongue and floor of mouth cancer, the plastic tube and button technique is the most commonly employed technique [2, 18, 110, 116, 224]. The guide gutter LDR technique can be used for small tongue or floor of mouth tumors, especially for older or infirm patients who are anesthesia risks, because it can be done under local anesthesia [64]. Tissue expanders or lead shielding should be used to protect the mandible.

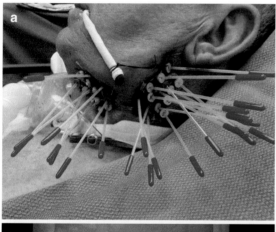

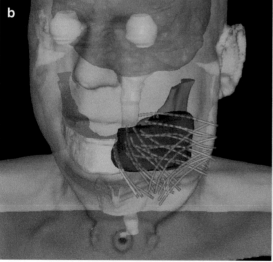
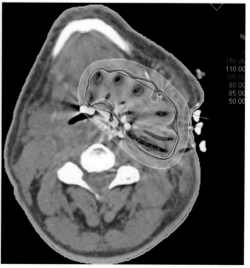

Fig. 23 (**a, b**) Dosimetry of a complex interstitial implant of tongue and upper neck adenopathy

Brachytherapy alone is the treatment of choice for T1–2 N0 tongue cancer and T1–2 N0 floor of mouth cancer if lesions are <3 cm and >0.5 cm from the mandible. The relative risk of normal tissue injury is greater in the floor of mouth. Since surgery is commonly utilized for tongue cancer, there is a role for postoperative brachytherapy when pathology margins are close or positive. Surgery is the treatment of choice for floor of mouth cancer that is <0.5 cm from bone. To decrease risk of bone injury, the brachytherapy catheters should run parallel to the contour of the mandible at some distance (0.5 cm) and thereby avoid excessive doses to the mandible.

In T3–T4 or N+ lesions, surgery and postoperative EBRT with or without brachytherapy or combined EBRT and brachytherapy may be used. Relative contraindications to brachytherapy are T4 tumors involving bone or the inability to encompass the lesion with catheters. Postoperative brachytherapy should be considered for close or positive margins. External beam would be used for positive lymph nodes or in cases with extensive bone involvement. Patients with extensive floor of mouth cancer who are not surgical candidates can be treated with brachytherapy (with EBRT), but only if bone involvement is limited.

Doses for definitive and postoperative treatment are given in Table 1. Postoperative treatment to these structures should be somewhat less than definitive treatment. The exact dose may vary with the clinical circumstances (close versus microscopic versus grossly positive margins).

Lymph Nodes Nodes are either managed by active surveillance for T1N0 (small T2) or by planned surgery or radiation therapy or by both modalities for more extensive disease. The location of lymph nodes at risk are site specific, but doses are in the range of 50–60 Gy for N0 necks and higher under other circumstances. Salvage brachytherapy in previously irradiated patients for oral cavity tumors may be treated with approximately LDR equivalent to 60–65 Gy.

Complications are mainly soft tissue necrosis (STN) within the volume of the implant and bone injury (BI) (descried variously and progressively up through bone necrosis requiring surgery). The previous rates of bone necrosis listed in Table 1 are probably higher than expected using modern techniques. Bone injury can be prevented with proper tissue displacement, shielding, good dental management, and the use of dwell time adjustments with HDR brachytherapy. In most cases, the STN or BI heals with conservative measures, which may include hyperbaric oxygen treatment. Surgery is required in <5 % of cases depending upon the lesion and clinical circumstances. Mandible reconstruction is a rarely needed and morbid intervention after EBRT. It may be less so after brachytherapy alone [2, 25, 117, 118].

Pharynx Treatment of lesions in the oropharynx must include assessment and treatment of the lymphatics, which are involved in a large proportion of patients [2, 28–30, 102, 110, 116]. Management of gross adenopathy after 45–50 Gy EBRT for microscopic disease (author suggests 55–60 Gy in cases with extensive adenopathy) may consist of more EBRT, brachytherapy, or surgery. GEC-ESTRO indicates that lesions up to 5 cm can be treated (but the author believes such a limit is conservative). They also exclude lesions of the retromolar trigone, larynx, hypopharynx, and widespread adenopathy or those that involve the bone. Tracheostomy is apparently used somewhat more conservatively in Europe than in the author's practice. It is applied "if the vallecula is invaded by a large tumor." Mandibular protection is used if the lesion extends into the oral cavity. The implant margin is larger in oropharynx (>1 cm) than oral cavity due to the nature of the disease, lower accessibility of the lesion, and difficulties with delineation of the gross disease. The implant for base of tongue may include the entire structure if there is uncertainty about the extent of disease. Suggested doses (LDR equivalent) for a generous CTV are 20–25 Gy (total 70–75 Gy), and the GTV is given a boost to 30–35 Gy (total 80–85 Gy). Selected cases (mostly tonsil) with exophytic T1N0 lesion might be treated with brachytherapy alone.

Table 1 GEC-ESTRO site specific recommendations

Primary site	BT alone	BT+EBRT	BT Dose as LDR equivalent (lower dose if postoperative)	Local control	STN or BI
Lip [2, 112–114]	<5 cm	>5 cm	BT only T1 60–65 Gy T2 65–70 Gy T3 75+Gy	90–95 % T1-2 BT alone T3 not given	2–10 % STN
Buccal [2, 70, 115]	T1-2 N0	T3	BT only T1-2 65–70 Gy EBRT 45–50 Gy+BT 25–30 Gy	80–90 % BT alone	<10 % STN
Oral tongue [2, 25, 117, 118]	T1-2 N0	T3-4	BT only 65–70 Gy EBRT 45–50 Gy+BT 25–30 Gy Or Postop EBRT 50–60 Gy+BT 10–25 Gy	90 % T1-2 BT alone Lower with BT+EBRT	10–20 % STN 5–10 % BI
Floor of mouth [2, 118]	T1-2 N0 <3 cm	T2>3 cm, T3-4 N0	BT only 65Gy EBRT 45–50 Gy+BT 15–25 Gy Or Postoperative as above	90 % BT alone Postop similar	10–30 % STN 5–10 % BI
Oropharynx [2, 28–30, 102, 110, 116]	T1N0 highly selected	T1-4 N+ <5 cm	EBRT 45–50 Gy + BT 25-30Gy Tonsil/30-35Gy BOT	T1-2 80–90 % BT+EBRT T3-4 65–80 %	20–25 % STN Low rate BI
Nasopharynx [2, 119]	NR	T1-2	T1 EBRT 60+HDR 3Gy x 6 T2 EBRT 70+HDR 3Gy x6	90 % EBRT+BT	NR
Paranasal Sinus [120–124]	T1 (Small T2)	T2-4	EBRT 40-50Gy+BT (tentative recommendation) BT only for margins	NR	NR
Salvage [36, 103, 104, 125]	Common	Variable	BT only 50–60+Gy	50–70 % BT alone, but highly variable	5–25 %

The data in the tables are given either explicitly as provided in the references or they are the best estimates based upon the author's interpretation of the article

n number of patients in study, *Prim* primary tumor or mucosal site, *Rec* recurrent cancer, *Persist* persistent cancer, *LC* local control, *LRC* local & regional control, *Mo. f/u* months follow up, *LR* local recurrence, *RR* regional recurrence, *DM* distant metastasis, *CSS* cause specific survival, *DFS* disease free survival, *OS* overall survival, *OC* oral cavity, *OT* oral tongue, *FOM* floor of mouth, *RMT* retromolar trigone, *BA* bucco-alveolar, *OP* oropharynx, *BOT* base of tongue, *SP* soft palate, *T* tonsil, *NPC* nasopharynx, *LN* lymph node, *N+* node positive, *%LN only* cases of neck disease without primary site recurrence, *BT* brachytherapy, *EBRT* external beam radiation therapy, *chemo* chemotherapy, *S* surgery, *SS* surgical salvage, *CT* computer tomography, *MRI* magnetic resonance imaging, *Gy* Grey radiation dose unit, *LDR* low dose rate, *MDR* medium dose rate, *HDR* high dose rate, *PDR* pulsed dose rate, *LDR eq.* LDR equivalent dose comparable to HDR dose, *NR* not reported, *STN* soft tissue necrosis (ranges from superficial ulceration to deep necrosis), *BI* bone injury (ranges from simple exposure to necrosis, which in most instances does not involve surgical intervention),*BN* bone necrosis, *Tx sites* treatment sites, *fx* fraction(s), *IS* interstitial, *IC* intracavitary, *NS* not significant, *Grp* group, *f/u* follow up, *Est.* estimate (by author)

Nasopharynx Almost all patients with nasopharynx cancer are treated with EBRT and chemotherapy [2, 30, 119]. The nasopharynx presents access challenges but brachytherapy may still have a favorable impact. GEC-ESTRO suggests that only endocavitary brachytherapy can be performed (the author does not entirely agree, as noted above). Since the target depth is limited to <1.0 cm, they point out that endocavitary brachytherapy is most suitable for tumors with limited depth of invasion or those with good response to chemoradiation therapy. Relative contraindications are bone involvement, deep invasion into the infratemporal fossa or nasal cavity, or intracranial extension. The applicators should be properly fitted and standardized (e.g., Rotterdam), or a custom mold can be constructed. Since GTV definition can be challenging, a large safety margin is recommended. Dosimetry with the Rotterdam method was originally based upon 2D orthogonal films and dose points at 0.5–1.0 cm deep to bony anatomy. Such approaches have given way to CT-based dosimetry. When brachytherapy is applied with the Rotterdam applicator, recommended doses are T1 EBRT 60 Gy plus 18 Gy in 6 fractions in 3 days and T2+ 70 Gy plus 12 Gy in 4 fractions in 2 days.

More recently, stereotactic radiation has been used to boost T3–T4 disease. In the context of salvage radiation with brachytherapy, dose in the range of 60+ Gy (LDR equivalent) is delivered in approximately 6–7 days.

Nasal Cavity and Paranasal Sinus Nasal cavity and paranasal sinus cancer is an uncommon but challenging, cancer [86–88, 119, 198]. It typically presents as locally advanced disease without lymph node metastasis. External beam may be given before or after surgery, but surgery is the primary treatment. At the time of surgery, a cavity may be developed into which a brachytherapy device may be fitted for dose escalation in tumors where local control is problematic. Combined surgery and radiation therapy (including brachytherapy) offer the possibility of organ and functional preservation in stages I and II and in some stage III tumors with orbital invasion. Brachytherapy alone may be used for smaller lesions after surgery if surgical margins are in question, there is no proximal perineural invasion, and the sites at risk are accessible. It can also be used for recurrent disease either alone, with surgery, or with EBRT depending upon the clinical circumstances. Earlier LDR techniques consisted of packing of sinuses with radiation sources after surgery. In the modern era, molds with embedded brachytherapy catheters can be custom fitted and afterloaded using HDR techniques. Target definition should be based upon 3D imaging and surgical pathologic findings. More data are needed for unequivocal dose recommendations. At least one study favors EBRT with brachytherapy over EBRT alone and specifically noted reduced side effects with selected subtotal sinus treatment volumes. Although bony confines make interstitial brachytherapy difficult, there is evidence to suggest a role for interstitial implants to improve disease control and better preserve visual function.

6.2   Salvage

Brachytherapy has been extensively used for salvage of previously irradiated cancers of the head and neck [36, 103, 104, 125]. The surgical option should always be considered as well, and treatment recommendations should always be made in a multidisciplinary setting. Salvage implants can be complex and potentially morbid. Doses are usually in the range of 50–60+ Gy LDR equivalent. HDR fraction size recommended by GEC-ESTRO is limited to 4.5 Gy (slightly higher than mentioned above). The author notes that such fraction sizes mean that the radiation course must be on the order of 10 fractions, which means the patient must have the implant catheters in place sometimes more than 1 week. Larger fraction sizes may be a practical necessity.

7   ABS Recommendations for High Dose Rate Head and Neck Brachytherapy

The ABS indicated that HDR could be used alone or with EBRT with similar indications as LDR. HDR has radiation safety benefits for unrestricted nursing care and the technical advantage of dose optimization. It is also conveniently adapted for intracavitary brachytherapy as a safe radiation outpatient procedure. The brachytherapy applicator insertions are the same for HDR as LDR except that looping catheters with acute angles may obstruct passage of the HDR source and are generally not recommended for HDR application. The ABS recommended against concomitant chemotherapy during brachytherapy but indicated that it can be given during the EBRT portion of the treatment.

Treatment parameters for HDR are similar to LDR except dose per fraction and total dose are different. There is also greater opportunity to control dose distributions with HDR than LDR through dwell time modification. Tip and other dwell times can be adjusted to optimize the isodose distributions for the desired CTV coverage, dose uniformity, and OAR dose constraints. HDR may be delivered twice daily with 6 h between fractions, but it is not always practical (or necessary) to meet this recommendation. The author considers 4 hours an absolute minimum. The skin and normal tissue dose should always be lower than the tumor dose except when the normal structure is involved with tumor.

HDR brachytherapy can be done in conjunction with surgery to take advantage of tumor resection and exposure of tissues at risk for residual disease. One approach is to lay the catheters in the open wound, close, and then allow one or more days for wound healing before starting treatment delivery. The advantage of this approach is to allow time for wound healing to begin, to gain access to pathological data, to utilize 3D image-based dosimetry, and to allow fractionation. Another option is to do intraoperative radiation therapy (IORT) with brachytherapy in a single fraction. It can be done with HDR, if the operating room is properly shielded, or more recently (the author notes), it can be done with a low-energy electronic radiation source, which can be done in most standard operating rooms. Both methods require radiation safety protocols and proper attention to treatment delivery details since large doses of radiation are applied in just a few sessions. The electronic source has significant functional limitations for head and neck applications because of the relatively large source size, the restricted number of channels, and the limited source path length.

Recommendations for the use of HDR in oral cavity cancer are similar to LDR. In HDR, monotherapy should be used for early stage, and combined therapy is used for more extensive disease. HDR results for oropharynx are also similar to LDR. The ABS recommended a typical course consists of EBRT 45–50 and 7–10 fractions of 3 Gy or 4–6 fractions of 4 Gy. Higher doses were recommended for larger tumors. Recommendations for the use of brachytherapy in various forms for nasopharyngeal cancers were based upon local control rates of >90% [181–186]. HDR-IORT for paranasal sinus tumors has been developed in the context of an operating room shielded for HDR. It is most successful in cases where gross tumor has been completely resected [126].

HDR can also be used as salvage therapy in previously irradiated cases. Recurrences are generally better prevented than treated, so it is recommended that brachytherapy be considered as part of the initial treatment strategy. A complete restaging workup is needed, and the physicians should be aware of and notify the patients that complication risks are increased over primary treatment especially with prior surgery, skin involvement, deep necrosis, or bone exposure. Larger margins (clinical treatment volumes) are advisable, particularly if no EBRT is planned. A review of previous radiation doses and fields will help guide treatment planning. It is difficult to make specific fraction recommendations, but doses of 50–60 Gy LDR equivalent were suggested. A summary of the GEC-ESTRO and ABS site-specific recommendations can be found in Table 2.

8 Quality and Reporting Standards for Head and Neck Brachytherapy

These recommendations are based, in part, on the American College of Radiology Guidelines and Technical Standards for Brachytherapy, 2008 [127].

8.1 Pretreatment Standards

Brachytherapy of the head and neck is a complex multistep process administered by a group of qualified professionals. The radiation oncologist and medical physicist must be certified to perform brachytherapy, and the physician must be a duly authorized to use therapeutic radionuclides. Dosimetry calculations, treatment delivery, and nursing persons must be similarly appropriately qualified. Standards for delivery of head and neck brachytherapy require a history and physical examination, review of relevant operations and pathology reports, and review of imaging studies. A summary of the consultation should be provided to the patient's other physicians. Site-specific TNM staging must be performed, and a lesion diagram must be created. The therapeutic intent (curative, palliative, local tumor control, etc.) should be established, and treatment options should be reviewed with the patient. Informed consent must be obtained and documented. The

Table 2 Summary ABS and GEC-ESTRO guidelines

Work up	H&P, endoscopy, biopsy
Imaging	CT, MRI, PET-CT
Dental	Pretreatment evaluation and follow up
Mandible shields	Oral cavity/lip or other sites as needed
Sequence	EBRT then BT (GEC-ESTRO), ABS not stated
Antibiotics, steroids	Optional (antibiotics always used by author)
Techniques	Tube and button, guide gutter, intracavitary applicators
Catheter spacing	1.0–1.5 cm
Chemotherapy with BT	No – except salvage (preferably neoadjuvant or adjuvant)
Target volumes	CTV = PTV (see references for discussion of target volumes)
Treatment parameters	DVH, DHI, CTV, and OAR
Total treatment course	<8 weeks (<9 weeks chemo)
HDR fraction size	3–4 Gy (max 4.5 Gy) These fractions sizes are not always practical
Oral cavity T1-2 N0	LDR equivalent 60–70 Gy BT only
Oral cavity T3-4 or N+	EBRT 45–60 Gy + HDR 25–30 Gy (consider surgery and postop EBRT + BT)
Oropharynx	EBRT 45–60 Gy + HDR 20–30 Gy
Nasopharynx Intracavitary	T1 EBRT 60 + 3Gy × 6, T2 + EBRT 70 Gy + 4 Gy × 3
Nasal and paranasal	EBRT 45–50 Gy + BT or IORT (doses not standardized)
Salvage	BT usually interstitial EqD2 50–60 Gy

See Table 1 for abbreviations

need for tracheostomy and special medical needs related to the implant should be coordinated with anesthesia and head and neck surgeons and other physicians in advance of the procedure.

8.2 Preoperative Brachytherapy Checklist

1. Consultation sent to referring physicians
2. Pathology documentation in chart

3. Imaging study reports in chart
4. Relevant operative reports in chart
5. Lesion diagram
6. AJCC (or comparable) staging
7. Current medication list (including allergies)
8. Preoperative assessment should include:
    (a) Preoperative medical evaluation for anesthesia according to patient needs and facility standards
    (b) Evaluation of recent smoking and drinking history
    (c) Assessment of bleeding risk, history of DVT, or anticoagulation
    (d) Physical examination
    (e) Results of recent EKG, CXR, basic blood counts, and chemistry panel

8.3 Brachytherapy Treatment Planning

Planning consists of determination of the type and extent of the procedure. The risk to the airway and the risk of vascular injury and bleeding associated with the procedure are of primary interest. A plan for intubation and airway management is coordinated with anesthesia, and standardized preoperative and postoperative order sets are recommended. Coordination with the nursing staff and arrangements for radiation safety on the wards is required. The use of remote afterloading has markedly improved the ability of nurses to care for head and neck brachytherapy patients.

8.4 The Procedure, Prescription, and Treatment Delivery

The applicator insertion is done in the operating room or another appropriately prepared procedure room. Simulation radiography is subsequently required to obtain an image dataset of the relationship of the applicator to the target and normal anatomy. The image dataset is imported into the treatment planning system (TPS). The radiation oncologist must provide a written, signed, and dated prescription before treatment planning commences [128]. It must designate:

HDR brachytherapy: patient name, the radionuclide, treatment site, dose per fraction, number of fractions, and total dose

LDR brachytherapy: treatment site, the radionuclide, and dose (before implantation) and (after implantation but before completion of the procedure) the radionuclide, treatment site, number of sources, and total source strength and exposure time or total dose

The physician contours the CTV (±GTV) and organs at risk (OAR) on the CT images. The 3D locations of the brachytherapy catheters are digitized and reconstructed in the TPS. The medical physicist or supervised dosimetrist performs dosimetry calculations on the treatment planning computer and generates a dose volume histogram, target coverage (isodose volumes), and dose uniformity parameters. Dose optimization techniques should be described and, if possible, target coverage and OAR dose constraint parameters should be delineated. An independent dosimetry verification calculation must be performed to confirm the primary dosimetry calculations. The physicist and physician check the plan parameters, target coverage, and OAR dose constraints to ensure they are satisfactory and that the treatment meets the objectives of the written directive. Hardware such as HDR source transfer tube connections are made and verified by the radiation therapist, physicist, and physician.

Brachytherapy delivery can be manual or robotic and HDR or LDR, but it must be monitored and properly documented, along with any modifications during the course of treatment. Permanent seed applications should be in accordance with all standards set forth for permanent seed brachytherapy [129]. Patients with permanent seed implants should be provided with written descriptions of the home radiation protection guidelines. The medical physicist and radiation safety officer design institutional brachytherapy safety guidelines, consistent with governmental regulations for brachytherapy.

8.5 Treatment Monitoring

The radiation oncologist should regularly evaluate the patient during treatment. The applicator should be checked for position accuracy and stability. The patient's medical condition (vital signs, nutritional status, airway, wound condition, urine output, laboratory results, medications, etc.) should be reviewed and adjusted daily or more often as needed. Due to radiation safety consideration, HDR (and PDR) facilitates the care of head and neck brachytherapy patients who typically require frequent and close nursing attention. Plans should be made for implant removal either on the ward under controlled conditions (sitting up, good suction, preparation for airway problems and bleeding) or in the operating room. It is advisable to have an emergency tracheostomy tray at the bedside in some cases. Removal of the implant in the operating room requires preparations for anesthesia (i.e., nothing by mouth, consent, laboratory determinations, etc.). Operating room removal facilitates airway control, management of bleeding, and patient comfort.

8.6 Treatment Summary

At the completion of LDR brachytherapy and after each HDR fraction, a radiation safety survey should be performed. A written summary of the treatment delivery parameters should include description of:

1. Total brachytherapy dose
2. Brachytherapy dates
3. Total radiation dose including EBRT, if it was administered
4. Technique (intracavitary, interstitial)
5. Target volume
6. Clinical course during treatment
7. Disposition (source accounting, follow-up plan, coordination with chemoradiation physicians)

8.7 Follow-Up

A follow-up plan should be made to assess disease control and to manage side effects. The radiation oncologist should routinely see the patient at 1–2-week and then at 2–4-week intervals for 3 months. Subsequent follow-up may vary from case to case; it should be carefully coordinated with other physicians to monitor disease, manage reactions and complications, guide nutritional support, and encourage regular dental care. Monthly physician visits are reasonable for the first year and thereafter at regular intervals as indicated by the individual patient needs and circumstances.

8.8 Program Requirements

Brachytherapy supplies, equipment, and devices are diverse, complex, and often unfamiliar to most medical personnel. Prior to taking the patient to the operating room, the needles, catheters, templates, and other brachytherapy supplies must be checked for availability and for proper preparation. Ward facility arrangements are necessary for LDR applications. Admission to the intensive care unit is recommended whenever there is a fresh tracheostomy, if re-intubation might be difficult, or in cases with significant comorbid conditions. The author recommends liberal use of intensive care units in the management of head and neck brachytherapy patients.

A physics quality assurance program with regularly scheduled inspections, testing, and maintenance of the technical devices such as simulators, survey monitors, and the remote afterloader is required. Treatment planning computers must be up to date and in good working order. Standards for dosimetry, treatment delivery, and brachytherapy documentation must be set and maintained. Routine leak testing of all sealed sources is required by regulatory agencies, and the radiation safety officer must create and supervise a radiation safety and personnel protection program. The radiation oncologist and medical physicist must have a system to independently verify brachytherapy parameters such as source model, radionuclide type, source strength, dose rate, total dose, and treatment duration. Continuing education of the brachytherapy team and hospital personnel who work with radionuclides is also required.

8.9 HDR Remote Afterloading

Prior to each treatment, the medical physicist or radiation oncologist should verify the correctness of connections of the source transfer tubes from the HDR afterloader to the applicator. The medical physicist must verify that the treatment parameters at the HDR console correspond to those created at the treatment planning computer. Source decay calculations must be performed for each and every treatment delivery. Independent verifications of physics and dosimetry parameters (prescription, fraction number, current activity or air kerma strength, decay-corrected radiation time, total reference air kerma (TRAK), and indexer length) just prior to source insertion are essential for HDR brachytherapy. Applicator position and integrity should also be verified just before each HDR fraction.

The radiation therapist and nurses perform auditory, visual, and vital status monitoring throughout treatment. The radiation oncologist and medical physicist must supervise HDR afterloading and prepare for emergency procedures. The progress of treatment is displayed and followed on the HDR remote afterloading treatment console. At the end of treatment, a radiation survey is performed to confirm that the radiation source has been safely retracted into the afterloading device. A brachytherapy charting system specifically designed for HDR clinical management and for continuing medical physics should be employed. It should record target dose, dose per fraction, date and time of delivery, and normal tissue dose monitoring. Special physics evaluation before or during treatment may be used to evaluate or coordinate prior external beam or other complexities that may impact decisions about the current HDR brachytherapy program or affect the patient in any meaningful way.

9 Results

9.1 How to Read Tables

(Tables 3, 4, 5, 6, 7, 8, and 9)

A review of the literature was performed, and summary tables were created. Studies published after 1985 were selected, if they had at least 20 cases and at least two years of follow up. The results of brachytherapy alone or in combination with EBRT are presented. They are divided into (1) LDR oral cavity and oropharynx, (2) HDR oral cavity and oropharynx, (3) LDR versus HDR oral cavity and oropharynx, (4) lip and buccal mucosa, (5) nasal cavity and paranasal sinus, (6) nasopharynx, and (7) salvage brachytherapy. The T-stages or stage groupings are presented (for N0 cases stage I = T1 and stage II = T2), and the percentage of cases with positive lymph nodes are described as "%N+." The table specifies whether brachytherapy was used alone or with EBRT. Median follow-up times are provided for each study. Outcomes (ranging from 2 to 5 years) are described in terms of local control (LC) at the primary site, regional control (RC), or locoregional control (LRC). Management of the neck (observation or planned neck dissection) is presented, and RC with and without surgical salvage is given if the information was available. Survival is presented as disease-free survival (DFS), cause-specific survival (CSS), or overall survival (OS). The morbidity grading systems were too varied to attempt a direct tabular comparison. Complications are categorized as soft tissue necrosis (STN) and bone injury (BI). The severity and duration of STN and BI were sometimes difficult to gauge. Transient STN of limited severity (grade 1) may or may not have been included or described in the articles. Bone injury may also have ranged from simple bone exposure to frank osteonecrosis, but most reports suggest that only a small fraction of cases of BI required major surgical intervention. Other less common complications such as cranial neuropathies are not listed, and there was insufficient information about speech, swallowing, oral dryness, or taste acuity to describe them. The outcomes with brachytherapy are, for the most part, published before the epidemic of HPV or knowledge of its prognostic significance. References are listed in the tables.

9.2 Oral Cavity – Low Dose Rate

The largest experience with LDR brachytherapy comes from Europe and Asia. Early reports describe the use of radium-226 or cesium-137 needles, and a few centers used radium-222 or gold-198 permanent seeds. Iridium-192, iodine-125, and palladium-103 became the standard in the 1980s. The outcomes for LDR brachytherapy of the oral cavity fall into two categories: those that are done after surgery for close or positive margins (shaded in the table) and those that are done primarily.

Numerous studies address the use of brachytherapy alone versus those used in combination with EBRT for T1–T2 N0 cancers of the oral cavity or the floor of the mouth. The uniform conclusion is that brachytherapy alone provides higher control rates and fewer complications than when used with EBRT. Doses for brachytherapy alone are 60–70 Gy. When brachytherapy is used as a boost, the does is more variable because EBRT doses ranged from 30 to 60 Gy. The brachytherapy dose administered with 45–50 Gy EBRT was typically 20–30 Gy. Local control rates are 80–90 % for T1 and 70–80 % for T2 with a reasonable expectation for surgical salvage at the primary site for isolated recurrences. Management of the neck was frequently expectant where regional control was about 75 % without surgery and 80–90 % with surgery or surgical salvage or radiation therapy to the neck. It is doubtful if neck dissection or external beam irradiation is routinely required for favorable T1N0 or small T2N0 cancers of the oral cavity. Surgical salvage of isolated neck recurrence with or without radiation is successful in more than half of the cases depending upon the extent of disease. Simultaneous failure of the neck and primary is more ominous. Cause-specific survival approximates an LRC of 70–80 % because few patients have distant metastasis without persistent disease in the head and neck region. Overall survival is

Table 3 Low dose rate (LDR) brachytherapy oral cavity and oropharynx (bolded) – no prior irradiation

Author	n	Primary	Stage	EBRT dose	LDR BT dose	Mo. f/u	LC, RC, LRC 2–5 years	[a]Overall survival 2–5 years	STN	BI	Comments
Mazeron 1990 France [74]	168	OT	45% T1 55% T2 8% N+	None	60–70 Gy	120	78% LC ≤60 Gy 90% 65 Gy 94% ≥70 Gy 79% RC N0	52% T1N0 44% T2N0 8% T1-2 N1-3	16% T1 28% T2	12%	N–: 23% EBRT alone, 77% neck surgery+EBRT
Wendt 1990 USA [131]	95	OT	18% T1N0 82%T2N0	19% No EBRT EBRT Variable	20–55 Gy depending on EBRT dose	159	64–92% LC 56–93% RC	Est 50% DFS Est 75% with SS	5%	10%	91% Ra-226 needles LC better with BT (also high surgical salvage) RC better with more EBRT
Hareyama 1993 Japan [132]	130	OT	68% T1-2 32% T3 24% N+	40 Gy (10–50) 24% EBRT	52–170 Gy BT only 30–96 Gy EBRT+BT	60	91–94% T1-2 LC 71% T3 LC	65–85% Stage I/II 40% Stage III/IV	23%	13%	Cs-137 needles Neck surgery in N+ cases only (OS 52%) Neck SS 39% (OS 56%) Mandibular complications doubled with EBRT
Pernot 1992 France [133]	147	OT	T2N0	20–50 Gy Prim 36–50 Gy LN 52% EBRT	58–79 Gy BT only 31 Gy EBRT+BT	36	51% LC EBRT+BT 90% LC BT alone 47% LRC EBRT+BT 68% LRC BT alone	51% BT alone 33% EBRT+BT	11% BT 12% EBRT+BT	1%	21% neck dissection Increased complications in BT alone if dose >75 Gy
Simon 1993 France [65]	274	65% OT 35% FOM	49% T1 52% T2 9% N+	None	60–70 Gy BT only	35	88% LC T1 84% LC T2 82% OT, 86% FOM	NR	22%	22%	77% guide gutter/23% plastic tubes More complications if source spacing >15 mm (FOM>OT) Neck management not stated

Study	n	Site	Stage	EBRT dose	BT dose	Follow-up (months)	LC/LRC	Survival	%	%	Comments
Shibuya 1993 Japan [134]	370	OT	24 % T1N0 53 % T2aN0 23 % T2bN0	27 Gy (20–40) 19 % EBRT	70–95 Gy only	24–288	85 % LC	84 % T1 78 % T2a 72 % T2b	3 %	8 %	Same BT dose when EBRT given 9 % chemo
Bachaud 1994 France [135]	94	OT FOM	55 % T1N0 45 % T2N0	48 Gy (45–54) 72 % EBRT	66 Gy (60–70) BT only 26 Gy EBRT + BT	44	75 % LC T1 51 % LC T2	43 % 45 % DFS	3 %	3 %	No surgery No chemo
Pernot 1995 France [136]	97	47 % OT 50 % FOM 3 % Gingiva	65 % pT1–T2 31 % pT3–T4 23 % N+	Dose NR 53 % EBRT	NR	NR	89 % LC 82 % LRC	67 % 74 % CSS	6 %	5 %	Postop BT ± EBRT for close or positive margins
Takeda 1996 Japan [137]	27	OC	8 % T1N0 80 % T2N0 12 % T3N0	60 % EBRT 15–42.5 Gy	58–94 Gy	>24	73 % LC (89 % with SS) 63 % RC (96 % with SS)	82 %	30 %	30 %	Au198 mold technique with EBRT for lesions >5 mm thick 10 % underwent surgery for BN Assume all cases N0 – not specified
Chao 1996 USA [138]	55	OT	35 % pT1 65 % pT2 18 % N+	55–69 Gy EBRT 50 Gy (15–50)+ BT 94 % EBRT	57 Gy (18–60) BT only 26 Gy EBRT + BT	48	82 % LC EBRT 77 % LC EBRT + BT 67 % LC BT alone	68 % 70 % DFS	25 %	0 %	Postop BT for close or positive margins 71 % EBRT alone, 29 % neck surgery 13 BT + EBRT + 3 BT only (positive margins)
Pernot 1996 France [18]	1344	OC	48 % T1-2 13 % T3-4 14 % N+	40–50 Gy 54 % EBRT	60–75 BT only 20–30 BT + EBRT	≥60	50–97 % LC 38–85 % LRC	29–71 % 28–88 % CSS	NR	NR	Results given as a range of OC and OP sub-sites Better outcome with BT only T1-2 N0 Some cases received EBRT to LNs Complications: 9 % Grade 2 and 3 % Grade 3 (slightly higher for postop BT)
		Postop OC	7 % T1-4 2 % N+	NR	50–60 Gy BT only 10–15 Gy EBRT + BT		90 LC 80 % LRC	67 % 74 % CSS			
		OP	**20 % T1-2 12 % T3-4 14 % N+**	**40–60 Gy 96 % EBRT**	**60–75 BT only 20–30 EBRT + BT**		**46–94 % LC 43–89 % & LRC**	**27–65 % 27–88 % CSS**			

(continued)

Table 3 (continued)

Author	n	Primary	Stage	EBRT dose	LDR BT dose	Mo. f/u	LC, RC, LRC 2–5 years	[a]Overall survival 2–5 years	STN	BI	Comments
Yamazaki 1997 Japan [139]	254	OT	52 % T1N0 48 % T2N0	None	70 Gy (53–93) Ra226 70 Gy (62–85) Ir192	108	80 % LC T1, 67 % LC T2 75 % RC T1, 58 % RC T2	75 % T1, 68 % T2 CSS	NR	5 %	No surgery No chemo Same outcome Ra226 to Ir192
Matsuura 1998 Japan [140]	173	OT	43 % T1N0 57 % T2N0	30 Gy (18–50) 38 % EBRT	69 Gy (60–84) BT only 60 Gy (38–136) EBRT + BT	>24	93 % LC T1 78 % LC T2 85 % RC T1 71 % RC T2	84 % T1 69 % T2	NR	NR	Ra226 needles or Ir192 hairpins T <8 mm thick did better than ≥8 mm thick
Beitler 1998 USA [95]	29	Various	NR	60 Gy (50–65)	120–160 Gy I-125 seeds	26	93 % LC	59 %	10 %	3 %	Postop BT for close or positive margins 23 % developed DM
Yoshida 1999 Japan [141]	70	OT <40 y/o	T1-2 N0	30 Gy 36 % EBRT	70 Gy (50–98) +EBRT cases total 70 Gy	156	91 % LC T1 71 % LC T2 52 % LRC T1-2	80 % CSS	4 %	28 %	Various radionuclides Outcomes same as 40–65 y/o, slightly better LC than >65 y/o Increase BI only with EBRT + BT, not with BT only
Grabenbauer 2001 Germany [142]	236	62 % OC 28 % OP 10 % Other	42 % Stage I–II 58 % Stage III–IV N+ not specified	50–60 Gy 75 % EBRT	45 Gy (36–90) BT only 23 Gy (14–26) EBRT + BT	30	74 % LC 86 % Stage I-II 62 % Stage III–IV	50 % 64 % vs. 39 % Stage I–II vs. III–IV 62 % CSS	9 %	9 %	Postop BT 77 %, 13 % chemo, 10 % hyperthermia Article does not give TNM, combines Primary (74 %) and Recurrent (26 %) – see salvage Table 9 estimates OC=OP for OS (includes 26 % salvage cases)

Marsiglia 2002 Italy [143]	160	FOM	49% T1 51% T2 21% N+	50 Gy if N+	70 Gy (58–80)	>120	90% LC	89% DFS	14%	18%	Neck dissection T2 or N1/surveillance in 41% (lesions <3 cm) SS successful in 50% of T or N failures 2.5% BN required surgery, 30% developed 2nd primary
Nakagawa 2003 Japan [21]	616	OT	28% T1N0 72% T2N0	30 Gy (10–50) 23% EBRT	70 Gy (50–100) BT only	65	86% LC (94% with SS) 62% RC	77% CSS 87% T1, 73% T2	NR	NR	No T surgery, Neck SS only, No chemo 50% Cs-137/Ra226 needles and 28% Ir192 22% Au198/Ra222 permanent seeds older infirm patients No difference RC ±EBRT (20% R-failures also had L-failure)
Lapeyre 2004 France [25]	82	45% OT 55% FOM	71% T1-2 29% T3-4 23% N+	48 Gy (40–52) 56% EBRT	60 Gy BT only 24 Gy EBRT+BT	60	90% LC T1-2pN- 78% LC T1-2 N+ 80% LC T3N- 57% LC T3N+	68% 30% if N+ 80% CSS	NR	NR	Postop BT for close or positive margins Neck surgery 71% (28% pN+) Neck recurrence 15%, second primary 25% Morbidity G3 15% with BT+EBRT vs. 3% BT only
Bourgier 2005 France [22]	279	OT	T2N0 5% N+	None	60 (8–72) BT only	45	79% LC (89% with SS) 70% RC (78% with SS)	74% 2 y 47% 5 y	NR	NR	11% prior H&N cancer Neck surgery 67% (48% of operated cases were pN+) (EBRT neck given in 77% of pN+) Morbidity G1 12%, G2 1.4%, G3 2.9% (surgery needed)

(continued)

Table 3 (continued)

Author	n	Primary	Stage	EBRT dose	LDR BT dose	Mo. f/u	LC, RC, LRC 2–5 years	[a]Overall survival 2–5 years	STN	BI	Comments
Yamazaki 2010 Japan [145]	21	OT >80 y/o	10% T1N0 70% T2N0 20% T3N0	30 Gy 40% EBRT	32–85 Gy	30	91% LC 84% RC	83% CSS	10%	5%	20% HDR/80% various LDR source No major BI Results similar to younger patients
Yoshimura 2011 Japan [146]	180	68% OT 14% FOM 17% Other	T1-2 N0	30–40 Gy Est. <20% EBRT	70–90 Gy	26	79% LC 56% LRC	83% 87% CSS	NR	3%	No chemo, no surgery (i.e., BT ±EBRT) Cs137 or Ir192 IS, some Au-198, some molds No correlation complications and pre-existing comorbidity
Khalilur 2011 Japan [147]	127	OT >75 y/o	24% T1N0 76% T2N0	None	70 Gy	24–218	86% LC 63% RC (75% with SS)	57% 74% CSS	2%	1%	Au198/Rn222 seeds;Ra226/Cs137 needles;Ir192 pins Mandibular spacers used Outcomes worse for patients >80 years old
Strnad 2013 Germany [148]	385	78% Lip-OC 22% OP	91% T1-2 8% T3-4 30% N+	55 Gy 37% EBRT	57 Gy BT only 24 Gy EBRT+BT	63	86% LC 92% N0-1 v 74% N2	69% 81% CSS	10%	5%	Pulsed dose rate BT preceded by surgery (326/385, 85%) 3% had surgery for complications
Stannard 2014 South Africa [56]	114	47% Tongue 18% FOM 26% SP 9% Tonsil	89% T1-2 11% T3 11% N+	50 Gy (42–70) 37% EBRT	59 (27–64) BT only 23 (10–30) EBRT+BT	39	81% LC 61% LRC	57% 74% CSS	18%	0%	I-125 afterloading (instead of Ir 192) 11% cases had recurrent cancer 41% primary surgery, 15% neck surgery, 20% chemo
Puthawala 1988 USA [78]	**70**	**BOT**	**26% T1-2 74% T3-4 73% N+**	**45–50 Gy 100% EBRT**	**20–25 Gy T1-2 EBRT+BT 30–40 Gy T3-4 EBRT+BT**	**60**	**83% LC 77% LRC**	**67% DFS**	**6%**	**3%**	**No surgery No Chemo**

Study	n	Site	Stage	EBRT	BT	n	LC	Survival			Comments
Harrison 1992 USA [149]	36	BOT	69 % T1-2 31 % T3-4 86 % N+	50–54 Gy 100 % EBRT	20–30 Gy EBRT+BT	22	88 % LC	88 % 2y	22 %	3 %	N0: 50-54 Gy EBRT to neck N+: EBRT 60 Gy+post-RT neck dissection 22 % chemo
Demanes 2000 USA [90]	25	BOT	52 % T1-2 48 % T3-4 84 % N+	54 Gy (50–63)	19–37 EBRT+BT	55	92 % LC 86 % LRC	36 % 68 % DFS	4 %	0 %	No chemo No neck surgery Bone exposure in one case required soft tissue graft
Barrett 2002 USA [151]	20	BOT	65 % T1-2 35 % T3-4 85 % N+	50–54 Gy 100 % EBRT	25 Gy (20–30) EBRT+BT	45	87 % LC 84 % LRC	30 % 41 % DFS	20 %	0 %	4 cases excluded BT only for re-irradiation No chemo, 80 % neck surgery STN resolved without major intervention
Gibbs 2003 USA [152]	41	BOT	51 % T1-2 49 % T3-4 68 % N+	50 Gy (49–68) 100 % EBRT	26 Gy (20–30) EBRT+BT	62	85 % LC T1-2 79 % LC T3-4	66 % 79 % CSS	7 %	5 %	5 % chemo Neck surgery 82 % (of 28 N+ cases) LC 87 % with SS

See Table 1 for abbreviations

[a]Overall Survival (OS) unless specified otherwise

Table 4 High dose rate (HDR) brachytherapy oral cavity and oropharynx (bolded) – no prior irradiation

Author	n	Primary	Stage	EBRT dose	BT dose	Mo. f/u	LC, RC, LRC 2–5 years	[a]Overall survival 2–5 years	STN	BI	Comment
Lau 1996 Canada [159]	27	OT	93% T1-2 N0 7% T3N0	None	45.5 Gy 6.5 Gy/fx	36	53% LC (93% with SS) 89% RC with SS	66% 92% CSS	29%	15%	SS successful 11/12 cases T1-2 with L-recurrence SS successful 8/11 with RR 3/4 BN with SS). STN 7 G2 and 1 G3
Leung 2002 China [76]	19	OC	53% T1N0 47% T2N0	None	55 Gy (45–64) 5.5 Gy/fx	43	95% LC	74% 85% CSS	5%	5%	No chemo 7 cases elective neck dissection 3 cases salvage neck dissection 2 cases LN+ neck received postop neck EBRT
Kakimoto 2006 Japan [130]	71	OT	39% T1N0 61% T2N0	None	54–60 Gy 6Gy/fx	39	87% LC 63% RC	81% 84% CSS	13%	14%	72% single plane implants 65% successful SS of neck recurrence ±EBRT STN/BI resolved without surgery except 1 case
Patra 2009 India [61]	33	61% OC 39% OP	79% T1-2 21% T3 59% N+	50 Gy (46–66) 100% EBRT	17.5 Gy (14–21) 3–3.5Gy/fx	18–40	100% LC T1-2 61% Stage III–IV with SS	NR	0%	0%	6 cases speech and swallow toxicity (1 PEG) 78% LRC with surgical salvage
Guinot 2010 Spain [75]	50	OT	84% T1-2 16% T3 32% N+	50 Gy (40–70) 66% EBRT	44 Gy (42–49) 10 fx 18 Gy (12–25) 3Gy/fx	44	91% LC T1-2 43% LC T3 85% RC	74% DFS	16%	4%	24% chemo 82% postoperative RT 100% LC in BT only cases
Akiyama 2012 Japan [111]	17 34	OT	T1-2 N0	None	54 Gy (6 Gy/fx) (33%) 60 Gy (6 Gy/fx) (67%)	44 52	88% LC 85% LC	77% OS 85% OS	6% 3%	12% 9%	Matched pair analysis 54 Gy=60 Gy RC=65% (60Gy) and 47% (54 Gy) Bone "exposure" – not necrosis

Matsumoto 2013 Japan [160]	67	OT	36 % T1N0 64 % T2N0	20 Gy (8–38) 51 % EBRT	50 Gy (40–65) 4–6.5Gy/fx	59	90 % LC 72 % LRC	88 % 92 % CSS	22 %	0 %	54 % chemo Successful SS in 5/5 LR and 9/11 RR STN 7 % grade 2 and 15 % grade 3
Levendag 1997 Netherlands [33]	38	OP	71 % T1-2 29 % T3-4 53 % N+	46 Gy 100 % EBRT	Variable HDR/PDR Est. 24 Gy LDR eq.	31	87 % LC	Est. 60 % OS	NR	NR	50 % tonsil/50 % soft palate 6 % BT only Same outcome tonsil and soft palate
Rudoltz 1999 USA [161]	55	29 % OC 71 % OP	76 % T1-2 24 % T3-4 53 % N+	55 Gy (45–70) 100 % EBRT	17 Gy (12–30) 1.2–2.5 Gy/fx	31	79 % LC 87 % LC T1-2	NR	9 %	7 %	No chemo N+ treated with hyperthermia and EBRT 55 Gy SS successful in 5/10 L-recurrence
Nose 2004 Japan [60]	82	OP	65 % T1-2 35 % T3-4 51 % N+	46 Gy 83 % EBRT	21 Gy (18–36) 3.5 Gy/fx 48 Gy (48–54) 6 Gy/fx	26	82 % LC 68 % LRC 86 % LRC SS + EBRT	64 % 88 % CSS	29 %	0 %	No chemo, 7 % cases Rec or 2nd Prim 41 N+ Neck Surgery + 24Gy (18–30) EBRT boost STN healed 20/24 cases <12 months
Cano 2009 USA [79]	88	BOT	42 % T1-2 58 % T3-4 81 % N+	62 (50–70) 100 % EBRT	25 Gy (18–30) 3–3.5 Gy/fx	36	82 % LC 80 % LRC	81 % 70 % DFS	5 %	0 %	100 % chemo, BT (11LDR + 77HDR) SS in 7 cases for R-recurrence 3 % tracheostomy and 2 % G-tube dependent
Takacsi-Nagy 2013 Hungary [162]	60	BOT	11 % T1-2 89 % T3-4 70 % N+	62 Gy (50–70) 100 % EBRT	17 Gy (12–30) 5 Gy/fx	121	57 % LC 50 % LRC	47 % 61 % CSS	12 %	2 %	28 % chemo (OS 69 % with vs. 39 % without) 93 % cases Stage III–IV

See Table 1 for abbreviations
[a]Overall Survival (OS) unless specified otherwise

Table 5 Lip and buccal (bolded) brachytherapy – no prior irradiation

Author	n	Primary	Stage	Dose rate	Dose	Mo. f/u	LC, RC, LRC 2–5 years	[a]Overall survival 2–5 years	STN	BI	Comments
Mazeron 1984 [114]	1896	Lip	T1-4	LDR	NR	NR	89% LC Ra/Cs 97% LC Ir192	NR	NR	NR	In: Gerbaulet A, Potter R, Mazeron JJ, et al., editors. The GEC-ESTRO handbook of brachytherapy. Leuven, Belgium: ACCO; 2002. p. 227–236
Cowen 1990 [163]	248	Lip	T1-4	LDR	60–81 Gy	NR	96% LC	NR	NR	NR	
Orecchia 1991 [164]	47	Lip	T1-2	LDR	60–80 Gy	NR	94% LC	NR	NR	NR	
Van Limbergen 1993 [165]	2794	Lip	T1-4 and rec T	LDR	40–90 Gy	NR	90% LC Cs137 96% LC Ir192 80% LC rec cases	NR	NR	NR	
Gerbaulet 1994 [166]	231	Lip	NR	LDR	70–85 Gy		94% LC	NR	NR	NR	
Beauvois 1994 France [167]	237	Lip	66% T1N0 25% T2N0 6% T3N0+ 3% N+	LDR	65–68 Gy	72	95% LC 91% RC	74% 91% CCC	10%	<1%	39% T1N0, 63% T2N0 neck observed and Surgical salvage LC 99% RC 94% Most STN heal without complication in <3 mo
Farrus 1996 Spain [112]	72	Lip	54% T1N0 19% T2No 6% T3N0 and 21% rec	LDR	62–67 Gy	NR	89% LC	NR	NR	NR	Outcome comparisons: initial vs. later cases and implant quality BT only
Conill 2007 Spain [168]	54	Lip	61% T1N0 39% T2N0	LDR	61.5 Gy (60–65)		98% LRC	70% 100% DFS	0%	0%	No surgery or EBRT

Study	N	Site	Stage	Type	Dose	Follow-up (months)	LC/RC	DFS/CSS			Comments
Johansson 2011 Sweden [169]	43	Lip	51% T1N0 37% T2N0 12% T3N0	PDR	60 Gy (55–>60)	54	95% LC 93% RC	59% 86% DFS	2%	2%	79% previously untreated, 21% recurrent; 69% macroscopic, 31% microscopic (postoperative); BN case had previously received EBRT for tongue Ca
Guibert 2011 France [66]	161	Lip	Mean 1.5 cm	LDR	65 Gy (55–77)	64	90% LC 97% RC	84% DFS	3%	0%	Similar outcome for skin and vermillion/mucosal lesions 79% SCC and 21% Basal Cell; Good cosmetic and functional results
Lock 2011 Canada [98]	51	Lip	90% T1N0 10% T2N0 24% Rec s/p surgery	LDR Au198 Seeds	55 Gy	27	98% LC	88% 94% CSS	2%	0%	Good cosmetic and functional results no G3 or G4 toxicity
Rio 2013 France [170]	89	Lip	50% T1N0 37% T2N0 3% T3N0/10% Postop	LDR	58 Gy (50–62)	36	95% LC 93% RC	82% DFS	NR	NR	Neck surgery and RT for salvage only; Cosmetic and functional outcome inferior for large tumors or with prior surgery
Serkies 2013 Poland [171]	32	Lip	29% T1N0 58% T2N0 13% T3-4	PDR	66 Gy (66–70)	NR	94% LC 88% RC	NR	3%	0%	Pulsed dose rate 15% BT for post-surgical recurrence
Guinot 2014 Spain [113]	102	Lip	53% T1N0 47% T2-4 N+ 5%	HDR	5 Gy (5.5–6 Gy)×9 fx	45	95% LC 90% RC (95% with SS)	93% CSS	0%	0%	20% postop, 80% definitive BT (3 cases+EBRT); Neck RT 11%, neck surgery 12%; Good cosmetic and functional outcomes

(continued)

Table 5 (continued)

Author	n	Primary	Stage	Dose rate	Dose	Mo. f/u	LC, RC, LRC 2–5 years	[a]Overall survival 2–5 years	STN	BI	Comments
Nair 1988 India [172]	**234**	**Buccal**	**19 % T1-3 N0 BT only 2 % EBRT + BT 35 Gy 79% EBRT only**	**LDR Ra-226**	**65Gy BT only 50 Gy EBRT+ 35 Gy BT 50–60 Gy EBRT only**	**36**	**100 % LC T1-2**	**42 % DFS 57 % N0 DFS 31 % N1 DFS**			**Single plane Radium implants Similar survival Radium implants and small field EBRT**
Shibuya 1993 [99]	**45**	**Buccal – mixed**	**18 % T1N0 67 % T2N0 15 % T3N0 84 % EBRT**	**LDR-seeds**	**89 Gy BT only 20–50 Gy EBRT + 80 Gy BT**	**Est. 48**	**87 % LC**	**85 % OS 100 % T1 v 83 % T2**	**22 %**	**20 %**	**Au198 or Rn222 permanent seeds with EBRT 21 buccal, 14 RMT, 10 BA Neck mgmt. = observation Less BI for buccal vs. RMT or BA – 4 required surgery**
Lapeyre 1995 France [70]	**42**	**Buccal**	**71 % T1-2 N0 29 % T3-4-X 7 % N+**	**LDR**	**66 Gy BT only (67 %) 45 Gy EBRT + 34Gy BT**	**51**	**81 % LC 57 % LRC**	**48 % 74 % CSS**	**7 %**	**3 %**	**Better LC with loop tech; Successful SS in 5/7 LR Neck T1N0 observed – T2 or N+ either surgery or RT Successful SS in 3/9 RR Dental shield used in 79 % cases**

Study	N	Site	T stage	BT	Dose/protocol	OS	LC	LC %			Notes
Tayier 2011 Japan [100]	133	Buccal – mixed	27 % T1N0 73 % T2N0	LDR-seeds	70 Gy BT only (56 %) 28 Gy EBT+60 Gy BT	71	75 % LC (87 % with SS)	76–81 % buccal 100 % lip	11 %	6 %	Au198 permanent seeds/variable EBRT 77 buccal, 18 RMT, 23 BA, 15 lip No difference in outcome ± EBRT Only 1 patient needed surgery for BI
Gerbaulet 2002 [2]	748	Buccal	14 % T1, 28 % T2 24 % T3, T4 34 %	LDR	BT only EBRT+BT EBRT only Surgery+EBRT	NR	81 % LC 65 % LC 45 % LC 78 % LC	64 % 41 % 26 % 66 %	NR	NR	Book chapter referenced above Ra-226, Au-198, Ir-192 More complications with EBRT+BT than BT only
Ngan 2005 Hong Kong [64]	13	7 Buccal 4 Lip 2 Nasal	85 % T1-2 N0 15 %T2-3 or N+	LDR	70 Gy BT only (54 %) 50 Gy EBRT+ 35 Gy BT	43	75 % LC (92 % with SS)	89 %	0 %	0 %	4 patient also had surgery for adverse histology or positive margins

See Table 1 for abbreviations

[a]Overall Survival (OS) unless specified otherwise

Table 6 High dose rate versus low dose rate brachytherapy lip and oral cavity – no prior irradiation

Author	n	Site	Stage	EBRT dose (% cases)	BT dose	Mo. f/u	LC, RC, LRC 2–5 years	[a]Overall survival 2–5 years	STN	BI	Comment
Inoue 2001 Japan [144]	15 LDR	OT	54% T1N0 46% T2N0	None	70 Gy (65–75)	85	84% LC 85% RC	86% CSS	0%	0%	Phase III (single plane lesions ≤1 cm thick)
	14 HDR	OT			60 Gy 10 fx	78	87% LC 78% RC	88% CSS	7%	7%	Successful SS in 4/5 Neck failures No outcome difference
Kakimoto 2003 Japan [24]	61 LDR	OT	79% T3N0 21% T3N+	30 Gy (13–60) 87% EBRT	68 Gy (50–112) boost 72 Gy (59–94) BT only	49	67% LC	58% 64% CSS	5%	20%	Historical controls Younger patients did better No outcome difference
	14 HDR			36 Gy (27–48) 95% EBRT	48 Gy (32–60) 8–10 fx 60 Gy 10 fx BT only	21	71% LC	46% 57% CSS	21%	0%	
Umeda 2005 Japan [174]	78 LDR	OT	T1–T2N0	None	61 Gy Ra-226/C-137	98	83% LC 67% RC	84% T1 72% T2	NR	NR	HDR had more T2 lesions Elective neck dissection 4 cases only
	26 HDR				59 Gy 9–10 fx	61	65% LC 85% RC	73% T1 52% T2	NR	NR	SS successful in 69% (28/41) R-recurrence
	71 Surg				None	57	94% LC 84% RC	95% T1 94% T2	NR	NR	Surgery preferable according to author
Yamazaki 2007 Japan [175]	217 LDR-a	OT	33% T1N0 54% T2N0 13% T3N0	25–35 Gy 47% EBRT	70 Gy (55–93) Ra-226	156	75% LC 63% RC	86% CSS	8%	8%	All implants local anesthesia LC T1≈85%, T2≈75%, T3≈65%
	351 LDR-b			25–40 Gy 34% EBRT	70 Gy (61–85) Ir-192		75% LC 67% RC	81% CSS	7%	9%	Neck managed by observation with prn salvage
	80 HDR			30–40 Gy 26% EBRT	60 Gy (32–60) 6–10 fx	48	82% LC 66% RC	89% CSS	6%	15%	EBRT doubled complication rate (11% vs. 26%) No outcome difference
Ayerra 2010 Spain [176]	100 LDR	Lip	55% T1N0 36% T2N0 9% T4 or Tx	None	60–70 Gy	32	90% LC 92% RC	90% 98% CSS	0%	0%	Guide needles 90% and plastic tubes 10%
	21 HDR				45–50 Gy				0%	0%	HDR equivalent to LDR
Ghadjar 2012 Switzerland [177]	70 LDR	Lip	61% T1 33% T2 5% T3 1% N+	None	60 Gy (48–66)	37	93% LC 87% RC	77%	0%	0%	33% postop BT for positive surgical margins
	33 HDR				36 Gy (32–29) 9 fx		93% LC 96% RC	77%	0%	0%	55% acute G3 toxicity – resolved No outcome difference

See Table 1 for abbreviations
[a]Overall Survival (OS) unless specified otherwise

Table 7 Nasopharynx–no prior irradiation and recurrent-persistent nasopharynx – i.e., prior irradiation (bolded)

Author	n	Stage	Dose rate	EBRT dose	BT dose	Mo. f/u	LC, RC, LRC 2–5 years	*Overall survival 2–5 years	STN	BI	Comments
Teo 1989 Hong Kong [178]	403	T1-3 65 % N+	LDR-IC	60–62.5 Gy	18–24 Gy (3 fx)	NR	Est. 85 % LC T1-2 Est. 70 % LC T3	NR	NR	NR	Tables difficult to interpret
Wang 1991 USA [179]	76	84 % T1-2 16 % T3 ? N+	LDR-IC	60–64 Gy	7–10 Gy	NR	91 % LC	NR	NR	NR	Compared to 70 Cases EBRT (65–70 Gy) only – LC = 60 % Many with accelerated hypofractionation, No chemo
Chang 1996 Taiwan [180]	133	T1-2 N0	LDC – IC	46.8 Gy+cone down 64.8–68.4 Gy	5–16.5 Gy (1–3 fx)	72	74 % LC Grp I 94 % LC Grp II 80 % LC Grp III	77 % CSS Grp I 96 % CSS Grp II 82 % CSS Grp III	1.9 % 4.2 % 13.8 %	3 %	50 cases Grp I no BT <72.5 Gy 71 cases Grp II+BT 72.5–75 Gy 58 cases Grp III+BT >75 Gy
Teo 2000 Hong Kong [181]	163	T1-2 (nasal) 45 % EBRT+BT N+ vs. 65 % EBRT N+	HDR – IC	60 Gy EBRT+BT (32 %) EBRT only 75 Gy (68 %) (See comment)	18–24 Gy	80+	95 % LC BT versus 90 % LC no BT	90 % CSS BT vs. 84 % CSS no BT	6 %	0 %	Comparison 346 EBRT only to 163 with EBRT+BT 101 BT cases incomplete responders and 62 BT as adjuvant 10–15 % chemo EBRT+BT>EBRT only for LC (> STN with EBRT+BT)
Lee 2003 USA [182]	55	T1-3 78 % prim/22 % rec 51 % N+	56 % LDR –IC 44 % HDR –IC	66 Gy (50–72) prim 30–42 Gy rec	5–7 Gy HDR 10–54 Gy LDR	36 prim 50 rec	89 % LC prim 64 % LC rec	86 % 91 %	0 %	2 %	33 % chemo BI in 1 of the recurrent cases
Lu 2004 Singapore [183]	33	67 % T1 33 % T2 50 % N2-3+	HDR – IC	66 Gy 70 Gy bulky disease	10 Gy (2 fx)	29	94 % LC	74 % 82 % DFS	0 %	0 %	50 % chemo no diff in disease control/ more toxicity

(continued)

Table 7 (continued)

Author	n	Stage	Dose rate	EBRT dose	BT dose	Mo. f/u	LC, RC, LRC 2–5 years	[a]Overall survival 2–5 years	STN	BI	Comments
Ng 2005 USA [184]	38	87% T1-2, 37% N+	HDR – IC	60 Gy	6–15 Gy (2–5 fx)	47	96% LC	93%, 81% DFS	0%	0%	82% chemo; OS higher than DFS reflects salvage or alive with disease
Leung 2008 Hong Kong [185]	145	94% T1-2a, 40% N+	HDR – IC	66 Gy EBRT, 66 Gy EBRT+BT	10–12 Gy (2 fx)	65	96% LC EBRT+BT, 88% LC EBRT only	91% vs. 80%, 95% vs. 83% CSS	1%	0%	No chemo; Matched pair (n = 142) EBRT 66 Gy alone vs. EBRT+BT; Better outcome with EBRT+BT than EBRT only
Wu 2013 China [186]	175	18% T1N0, 82% T2N0	HDR – IC	58 Gy EBRT+BT, 72 Gy EBRT only	20 Gy	120	94% vs. 85% LC	72% vs. 50%S	2%	0%	Compared with 173 EBRT only (EBRT+BT better LC/OS); More chemo with EBRT only vs. EBRT+BT (42% vs. 25%); Slightly more STN (NS) but less neck fibrosis with BT
Levendag 2013 Netherlands [187]	280	50% T1-2 N+	HDR or LDR – IC	70 Gy (±11 Gy SBRT)	11 Gy (3–4 fx)	NR	100% LC HDR, 86% LC no HDR	NR	NR	NR	3 centers pooled boost data for chemoradiation ± boost; T1-2 N0: HDR vs. no boost (significant benefit to boost)
		50% T3-4 N0					90% LC HDR/SBRT, 85% LC no boost	NR	NR	NR	T3-4 N0: HDR or SBRT vs. no boost (ns)
Rosenblatt 2014 [188]	274	75% "Others", 25% T3-4 N2-3+	HDR or LDR – IC	51% 70 Gy EBRT only, 49% 70 Gy EBRT+BT	HDR 9 Gy (3 fx) LDR 11 Gy	29	61% LC no BT, 54% LC BT (ns)	63% no BT, 63% BT	NR	0%	Randomized trial chemoradiation ± BT boost; No difference even in T1-2 N+ cases; Grade 3–4 toxicity not significantly different (22% vs. 24%)

Study	N	Patient	Modality	EBRT	BT	N	LC	DFS	%	%	Comments
Wang 1987 USA [35]	38	100 Rec NPC	LDR – IC	40 Gy	20 Gy	NR	NR	38 % T1-2 15 % T3-4	0 %	3 %	IC Cs-137 ± EBRT (T3-4 EBRT only 66 Gy) Study patients RT ≥60 Gy
Choy 1993 Hong Kong [189]	43	23 % persist 77 % rec	LDR – IS Permanent seeds (Au198)	None	60 Gy	39	80 % LC persist Est. 67 % rec	Est. 50 % Est. 70 % DFS	16 %	0 %	Persistent = disease identified <4 months after RT Trans-palatal exposure (7 cases took 1 year to heal wound) Better LC if no base skull involvement (81 % vs. 44 %)
Syed 2000 USA [81]	56	Grp I 67 % T3-4 Grp II/III 80 % mod-adv.	LDR – IS (Ir-192)	Gp I 50-60 Gy Gp II/III None	49 Gy	84	93 % LC Grp I 59 % LC Grp II/III	74 % DFS Grp I 47 % DFS Grp II/III	14 %	2 %	27 % Grp I primary 61 % Grp II recurrent-persistent 12 % Grp III new primary (prior RT) More complications in Grp II/III
Koutcher 2010 USA [190]	29	84 % T1-2 (EBRT+BT) 31 % T1-2 (EBRT only)	LDR – IC (I-125)	45 % 45 Gy EBRT+BT 55 % 59.4Gy EBRT only	20Gy	45	52 % LC vs. 53 % LC	60 % vs. 57 % 41 % vs. 44 % DFS	NR	NR	Recurrence treated EBRT only or EBRT + BT 93 % chemo Equal LC/OS Complications 78 % EBRT vs. 8 % EBRT + BT
Ren 2013 China [191]	32	57 % T1-2 43 % T3-4 62.5 % N+	HDR – IC	60 Gy	12-20 Gy (4 fx)	39	94 % LC	97 % 78 % DFS	6 %	0 %	Locally persistent (biopsy proven) >10-16 weeks after IMRT
Wan 2014 China [82]	213	T1-2 55 % N+	171 HDR –IC 42 HDR –IS	62 Gy (50-70)	8-14 Gy IC 13.6-18 Gy (3-5 fx)	53	94 % LC vs. 97 % LC 97 % RC vs. 95 % RC	94 % vs. 97 % 87 % vs. 92 % DFS	NR	NR	Locally persistent (biopsy proven) after 10+ weeks Chemoradiation doses similar (30 % chemo) Higher stage group for IS No difference in RTOG toxicity (G3-4 = 2-5 %)

See Table 1 for abbreviations

[a] Overall Survival (OS) unless specified otherwise

Table 8 Nasal and paranasal sinuses (bolded) brachytherapy – no prior irradiation

Author	n	Primary	Stage	Dose rate	EBRT dose	BT dose	Mo. f/u	LC, RC, LRC 2–5 years	[a]Overall survival 2–5 years	STN	BI	Comment
Karim 1990 Netherlands [195]	**15**	**Upper Nasal & Sinus**	**NR most T2-4**	**LDR-IC**	**64 Gy**	**56–100 Gy BT only 62 Gy EBRT+20 Gy BT**	**NR**	**70 % LC all cases (see comment)**	**68 % DFS**	**12 %**	**NR**	**N=45 (30 EBRT, 4 BT only, 11 EBRT+BT) 93 % postoperative Most complications eye related**
McCollough 1993 USA [196]	18	Nasal Vestibule	41 % T1-2 33 % T4 26 % recurrent 5 % N+	LDR-IS	(65–75) Gy 50 Gy EBRT+BT	Est. 25 Gy	>24	100 % LC BT only 75 % LC EBRT+BT 73 % LC EBRT only	75 % Est. 87 % CSS	22 %	0 %	N=39 (12 EBRT, 9 BT only, 18 EBRT+BT) 100 % definitive RT (26 % rec after surgery) STN healed without surgery, no cartilage necrosis
Tawari 1999 Netherlands [197]	**20**	**Ethmoid Sinus**	**18 % T1-2 N0 82 % T3-4 N0**	**LDR-IC**	**54–70 Gy**	**12–28 Gy**	**NR**	**62 % LC**	**65 % OS**	**NR**	**NR**	**N=50 postoperative EBRT (+BT 40 %)**
Evensen 1994 Norway [84]	23	Nasal Vestibule	87 % T1-2 N0 13 % T4N0	LDR-IS	55 Gy (50–70)	55 Gy (50–60) S+BT 59Gy (47–65) BT only 30 Gy (25–39) EBRT+BT	>24	100 % LC S+BT 92 % LC BT only 86 % LC EBRT+BT	87 % DFS	17 %	0 %	N=23 (4 S+BT, 12 BT only, 7 EBRT+BT) 2 STN=cartilage necrosis
Langendijk 2004 Netherlands [85]	47	Nasal Vestibule	100 % T1-2 N0	MDR HDR	53 Gy EBRT+MDR 50 Gy EBRT+HDR 67.5 Gy EBRT only	16 Gy (8–40) MDR 18Gy (3Gy/fx)	>24	79& LC (95 % SS)	66 % 87 % DFS	6 %	0 %	N=47 (32 EBRT+MDR, 9 EBRT, 15 EBRT+HDR STN healed without surgery, no cartilage necrosis 8 patients developed second primaries

Study	N	Site	Stage	Dose rate	EBRT dose	BT dose	N	LC	Survival	%	%	Comments
Nag 2004 USA [87]	34	Paranasal Sinus	79% T2-4 21% recurrent N+ not specified	HDR-IORT	45–50 Gy EBRT+BT	15–20 Gy BT only 10–12.5 Gy EBRT+BT	50	68% LC	62% 50% DFS	0%	0%	N=34 (11 HDR alone, 23 EBRT+HDR) 21 new primaries received EBRT+HDR Gross residual disease poor prognosis
Levendag 2006 Netherlands [86]	64	Nasal Vestibule	69% T1N0 31% T2N0	HDR	None	44 Gy (3 Gy/fx)	NR	92% LC (100% SS)	58%	NR	NR	N=64 (78% BT only, 22% incomplete S+BT) Study of complications, cosmesis, cost analysis
Allen 2007 USA [198]	9	Nasal Cavity and Septum	60% T1-2 34% T3-4 9% N+	LDR	65–70 Gy EBRT only	65 Gy BT only	132	86% LC	82% 86% CSS	4%	1%	N=68 (35% EBRT, 12% EBRT+BT, 53% EBRT+S) BT vs. EBRT not separately reported Results no different with RT alone vs. S+RT Failures continue after 5 years
Teudt 2014 Germany [88]	35	Nasal and Paranasal	37% T1-2 N0 63% T3-4 or N+ 37% recurrent	HDR	43% BT only 57% EBRT+BT 50 Gy (40–63)	23 Gy (10–35) 2.5 Gy/fx	28	67% LC All Cases 91% if primary	72% 83% CSS	14%	NR	Surgery with intraop BT catheter insertion N=35 (54% R0, 37% R1, 3% R2) 32% prior surgery and 12% prior chemo Detailed description of complications

See Table 1 for abbreviations
[a]Overall Survival (OS) unless specified otherwise

Table 9 Salvage of primary site recurrences (excluding nasopharynx) and cervical lymph node recurrences (bolded)

Author	n	Treatment sites	Prior RT	Secondary EBRT	Dose rate	BT dose	Mo. f/u	LC, RC, LRC 2–5 years	[a]Overall survival 2–5 years	STN	BI	Comment
Park 1991 USA [37]	35	56 % Prim rec 44 % LN only	None	60 Gy (50–70)	LDR	83 Gy	28	40 % LRC	20 % 41 % DFS	NR	3 %	BT – surgery Iodine-125 seeds (mean 13.4 mCi) More complications with flap reconstruction
Peiffert 1994 France [38]	73	100 % Prim rec Various	100 % Dose NR	None	LDR	60 Gy	NR "Long"	86 % LC 79 % LRC	30 % 65 % CSS	10 %	0 %	No surgery Ir-192 BT alone to 60 Gy
Vikram 1985 USA [94]	21	48 % Prim rec 52 % LN only	100 % Dose NR	None	LDR Ir-192/I-125	48 Gy Ir-192 75 Gy I-125	35	81 % LC	55 % DFS	14 %	0 %	BT + surgery Ir-192 (11 cases) (40–56 Gy) I-125 (10 cases) (60–85 Gy)
Nag 1996 USA [199]	29	Various	29 % 50–75 Gy	71 % 45–50 Gy	HDR	15 Gy BT only 7.5– 12.5 Gy EBRT + BT	21	67 % LC –All 89 % LC if no prior RT	72 %	NR	NR	Locally advanced or recurrent disease
Zelefsky 1998 USA [39]	**100**	**100 % LN**	**76 % 54 Gy (30–80)**	**16 % Dose NR**	**LDR**	**171 Gy I-125 40 Gy Ir-192**	**10**	**25 % (2 yr LRC)**	**20 %**	**7 %**	**0 %**	**BT ± neck surgery 84 I-125 (gross) and 33 Ir-192 (micro) Prior neck surgery 55 %**
Klein 1998 Germany [200]	34	62 % Prim rec 72 % T3-4 41 % N+	59 % Dose NR	Est. 50 % 58 Gy (5–99)	HDR	12–15 Gy (1–7 fx)	12–69	65 % (CR + PR) (Prim cases 77 %)	38 %	0 %	3 %	No surgery 38 % "inoperable" Difficult to quantify EBRT
Puthawala 2001 USA [40]	220	70 % Prim rec 54 % N+ 30 % LN only	100 % 57 Gy (39–74)	None	LDR	53 Gy	NR "Long"	51 % (5 yr LRC)	20 % 33 % DFS	13 %	8 %	No surgery Prior surgery 52 % 60 % hyperthermia, 40 % chemo

Ashamalla 2002 USA [97]	37	76% Prim rec 16% persist/8% new 5% LN only	100% 60 Gy	None	LDR seeds	100 Gy (80–220)	NR "Long"	33% LC 11% LC for T>2.5 cm 64% LC T<2.5 cm	DFS Median 12 mo.	0%	0%	Au-198 seeds BT palliation in 76%
Glatzel 2002 Germany [42]	90	57% Prim rec 35% Persist Prim 8% BT only pall	92% Dose NR	57% 30–70 Gy	HDR	17.6 Gy (12.9–23.9) (3–7.5 Gy/fx)	NR	77% CR+PR Rec 100% Persist	1–25 mo.	3%	1%	No surgery 68 IS and 22 IC (NPC) Persist cases did better than recurrent cases
Grabenbauer 2001 Germany [142]	82	Est. 62% OC 28% OP 10% Other	"Few"	72% 50–60 Gy	LDR	55 Gy BT only 29 Gy (14–62) EBRT+BT	30	57% LC 63% vs. 60% Stage I–II vs. III–IV	29% 57% vs. 15% Stage I–II vs. III–IV	9%	9%	Primary site percentages are estimates Morbidity rates – from LDR Primary Table
Hepel 2005 USA [43]	30	100% Prim	100% 59 Gy (23–75)	6% Dose NR	HDR	34 Gy (18–48) (3–4 Gy/fx)	20	67% LC	45% (2 yr CSS) 37% (2 yr OS)	7%	3%	36% R2 surgery; 64% No surgery 43% chemo, 36% hyperthermia
Pellizzon 2005 Brazil [201]	**42**	**100% LN**	**83% 52 Gy (30–65)**	**38% Dose NR**	**HDR**	**24 Gy (12–24) (3–14 fx)**	**36**	**57% LRC**	**53%**	**0%**	**0%**	**BT+surgery Negative surgical margins better 3 severe ulcers and 1 neck fibrosis**
Nutting 2006 England [41]	**74**	**100% LN**	**100% ≥50 Gy**	**None**	**LDR**	**60 Gy**	**1–176**	**37% LRC**	**31% 28% CSS**	**0%**	**0%**	**BT+surgery 92% of cases Fistula 9%, Bleed 4%, Wound 8%**

(continued)

Table 9 (continued)

Author	n	Treatment sites	Prior RT	Secondary EBRT	Dose rate	BT dose	Mo. f/u	LC, RC, LRC 2–5 years	[a]Overall survival 2–5 years	STN	BI	Comment
Narayana 2007 USA [44]	30	66% Prim 33% LN only	77% Dose NR	10% 40–50 Gy	HDR	20–40 Gy (5–10 fx)	12	71% LC	63%	0%	3%	60% BT+surgery, 30% BT only, 10% BT+EBRT 6% neck fibrosis, 3% persistent pain
Kupferman 2007 USA [202]	**22**	**100% LN**	**100% 65 Gy (50–72)**	**None**	**LDR**	**60 Gy (20–60)**	**30**	**67% LRC**	**57%**	**0%**	**5%**	**BT+surgery (46% prior neck dissection)**
Schiefke 2008 Germany [203]	13	54% Prim rec 46% N+ 15% LN only	62% 61 Gy (60–70)	None	HDR	30 Gy (15–44.8) (1.5–3.5 Gy/fx)	25	85% LC 62% LRC	60% 65% CSS	15%	15%	77% BT+surgery 62% included neck dissection
Perry 2010 USA [204]	34	100% Prim rec 50% N+	100% 63 Gy (24–74)	None	HDR IORT	15 Gy (1 fx)	23	56% LC	55%	10	3%	Intraoperative radiation with multichannel open tumor bed surface applicator
Tselis 2011 Germany [205]	**74**	**100% LN**	**100% 60 Gy (22–72)**	**12% 40 Gy (20–70)**	**HDR**	**30 Gy (12–36)**	**14**	**37% LC**	**19%**	**5%**	**0%**	**Inoperable cervical adenopathy 58% prior surgery (45% with neck dissection) STN estimated**
Martinez-Monge 2011 Spain [206]	103	51% Prim rec 49% New prim 50% N+	55% 45 Gy (45–74)	55% 45 Gy	HDR	24 (16–24) 40 Gy (32–40) (4–10 fx)	52	86% LC 78% LRC	52%	5%	6%	BT+surgery±EBRT 49% Stage III–IV 63% chemo
Bartochowska 2012 Poland [45]	156	32% Prim rec 14% Paratracheal 54% LN only	91% Dose NR	None	106 PDR 50 HDR	PDR 20–40 Gy HDR 12–30 Gy (3–10 fx)	6	38% (6mo) LRC	17%	15%	1%	No surgery 5% chemo, 10% hyperthermia

Study	N											
Rudzianskas 2012 Lithuania [207]	30	56% Prim rec 44% LN	30% 66 Gy (50–72)	None	HDR	30 Gy (12 fx)	28	67% LC	47% 53% DFS	0%	3%	43% BT+surgery, 57% BT alone 70% prior surgery BT+surgery better outcome than BT only
Scala 2013 USA [208]	76	53% Prim rec 47% LN	100% Dose NR	24% 45 Gy (30–69)	HDR IORT	12.5–17.5 (1 fx)	11	62% LC	37% DFS	0%	0%	HAM applicator after gross total resection Negative surgical margins better LC/DFS BT+EBRT better
Teckie 2013 USA [93]	57	29% Prim rec 71% LN	98% 66 Gy (24–74)	21% 50 Gy (30–70)	HDR IORT	15 Gy (10–20) (1 fx)	NR	57% LC	43%	NR	0%	HAM applicator after gross total resection LC associate with improved OS Complications presented in detail
Zhu 2013 China [96]	19	100% Prim rec	100% 64 Gy (35–145)	None	LDR seeds I-125	131 Gy D90	11	68% LC	18%	0%	0%	Prior surgery and EBRT Median LC 24 months
Strnad 2014 Germany [209]	51	78% Prim rec 22% New Prim 25% N+	100% 65 Gy (60–76)	22% EBRT 46 Gy (28–67)	PDR	60 Gy 27 Gy if+EBRT	58	57% LC (5 yr) CT 79% v no CT 39%	26% 60% DFS	18%	12%	No surgery 69% chemo, 33% hyperthermia Chemo (CT)>STN

See Table 1 for abbreviations

aOverall Survival (OS) unless specified otherwise

often determined not only by cancer control but also comorbidity. Functional outcomes are better with brachytherapy alone than with the combination of brachytherapy and EBRT. Soft tissue necrosis, varying severity and duration, occurs in 15–20 % of cases, but it generally heals with conservative management. The occurrence of transient bone exposure is different from frank bone necrosis, but the literature does not always make the distinction. A reasonable estimate of BI is about 10 % without a mandible shield and 5 % with a shield. Relatively few patients require major surgery for osteonecrosis. It is the author's opinion that remedial measures should be instituted early for STN or bone exposure to prevent progression to osteonecrosis. Brachytherapy catheter spacing, technique, and dose significantly affect the morbidity rates.

More advanced oral cavity cancers (T3–T4 or N+) are usually treated with the combination of brachytherapy and EBRT because larger lesion can be difficult to implant and there is a greater chance for regional spread. The type of lesion (superficial spreading, exophytic, endophytic, etc.) and the baseline condition of the mucosa (i.e. leukoplakia) affect the LC rates and the long-term prognosis (mucosal field defects). According to the relatively sparse literature, the LC rates for T3 and T4 (defined by involvement of extrinsic tongue musculature) are 50–70%. The LC rate for T4 with bone involvement or extension to adjacent structures is less than 50%. Surgery (with radiation therapy) is warranted for lesions that involve bone. In the author's opinion, surgery probably increases LC over radiation alone for these locally advanced and deeply infiltrative lesions. Brachytherapy can also be used for close or positive margins if care is taken to minimize injury to flap wound closures.

9.3 Oropharynx – Low Dose Rate

Low dose rate (LDR) brachytherapy has been successfully employed in the treatment of oropharyngeal cancer (base of tongue, tonsil, and soft palate). Management strategy and outcomes are dominated by lymphatic involvement and the responsiveness of the disease to radiation and chemotherapy. Brachytherapy is most commonly used in conjunction with EBRT. Most patients are node-positive stage III or IV. When brachytherapy is used, local control is achieved in 80–90 % of T1–T3 cases. Control of T4 lesions again depends upon the definition of T4 (T4a LC 75–80 % and T4b 50–60 %). The functional outcomes (speech and swallowing) after EBRT and brachytherapy are relatively good compared to traditional surgery and postoperative radiation therapy. Chronic side effects of dry mouth and decreased taste acuity continue to be problematic occurrences after chemoradiation therapy. They are probably reduced when brachytherapy is used, but documentation of these somewhat subjective parameters is difficult.

The precise role of brachytherapy for oropharynx cancer remains unsettled. Relatively few physicians have the skill and training to perform these procedures, but that does not define the usefulness of the modality. There are those who believe EBRT alone is sufficient and those who think brachytherapy should be a routine part of radiation therapy of oropharynx cancer. With the advent of intensity-modulated radiation therapy and chemoradiation therapy, the questions have only deepened. Since implantation in the oropharynx requires specific procedural expertise, it may not be readily available for all patients. There are no randomized trials or even good historical comparisons to address questions about the comparative effectiveness of chemoradiation therapy with and without brachytherapy.

It has been discovered that the association of HPV virus (P16 positivity) with squamous cell carcinoma of the oropharynx significantly improves the prognosis [16, 153–156]. Standard doses of chemoradiation therapy without brachytherapy commonly results in hospitalization for acute toxicity and the adverse effects on pharyngeal muscular function and swallowing. In an attempt to maintain efficacy but decrease morbidity, dose de-escalation trials for HPV-positive patients have been performed or are currently underway. Treatment of oropharynx cancer should be stratified according to HPV status. Initial results of studies using EBRT dose (chemoradiation) to the primary tumor of 60 Gy in HPV-positive patients have resulted in comparable outcomes to 70 Gy [17].

Morbidity reduction might also be accomplished by a combination of decreased EBRT doses (50–55 Gy) alone with use of TORS or brachytherapy (Table 3 LDR) [31, 157, 158]. Advantages of TORS include avoiding morbidity related to surgical access to the oropharynx and there is usually no need for trachcostomy. The advantage of brachytherapy is that deep margins can be achieved with no tissue removal and there is less radiation to the pharyngeal constrictors and/or major blood vessels. In the author's opinion, this strategy should be applied regularly in HPV-negative patients. Brachytherapy can also be used in some HPV-positive patients, but the incremental benefit may be less. Although specific indications have yet to be defined, brachytherapy should be used in patients with deeply infiltrative disease or with gross residual or positive margins after TORS. The use of brachytherapy in soft palate cancer has the advantage of preserving the structure and function, which, if successful, eliminates the need for a palatal prosthesis. Chemoradiation is often sufficient to control the even bulky adenopathy in cancer of the oropharynx. Neck dissection can be used for persistent disease, or the adenopathy can be implanted in conjunction with the primary. Brachytherapy of adenopathy is challenging due to proximity to major blood vessels, but with proper technique, it is safe and effective.

9.4 Oral Cavity with High Dose Rate Brachytherapy

HDR has replaced LDR in many centers because of its radiation safety advantages and the need for close proximity to patients by medical personnel for better care. HDR outcome reports began appearing in the middle 1990s; therefore, the HDR cohorts are fewer and smaller than the ones for LDR. The patterns of care for early oral cav-

ity cancer, however, are similar. HDR-brachytherapy alone doses are 44–60 Gy in 9–10 fractions, but the optimal dose is unknown. One study showed no difference in outcome between 54 and 60 Gy [111]. The 6 Gy fraction size used commonly in Japan is a response to the practical concerns about how long to leave the implant in the patient versus normal tissue tolerance benefits of smaller fractions. The GEC-ESTRO recommendations are for doses of 3–4.5 Gy per fraction.

When brachytherapy is used as a boost with external beam, smaller fraction sizes are more feasible than when performing brachytherapy alone. The administration of 20–40 Gy EBRT, in some Japanese studies for example, was probably a mechanism to reduce brachytherapy fraction size rather than an attempt to control regional microscopic disease [140, 141, 145, 146, 160]. Implant volume, catheter spacing, disease location (oral tongue versus floor of mouth), and the use of mandible shields also affect the outcomes. There are no systematic studies to define the optimal number or size of HDR fractions. Local control rates for early oral cavity cancer are similar to LDR, namely, T1 80–90 % and T2 70–80 %.

9.5 Oropharynx – High Dose Rate

HDR brachytherapy results for cancer of the oropharynx are presented in the tables. Chemotherapy was used in some cases but not others because most reports antedate the era of routine use of chemoradiation. The EBRT course typically consists of 50–60 Gy to the primary and lymphatics followed by brachytherapy. Gross adenopathy is treated either with EBRT alone (≈70 Gy), surgery plus EBRT (50–60 Gy), or EBRT (50–60 Gy) with brachytherapy. These guidelines do not take into consideration possible dose de-escalation based on HPV status. Local tumor control rates for T1–T2 are approximately 90 %, T3 80 %, and T4 variable. Cause-specific survival rates are 60–80 %. Morbidity rates and preservation of function are comparable to LDR brachytherapy.

9.6 Lip and Buccal – Low Dose Rate and High Dose Rate

Perioral cancer is subdivided into those of the moist mucosal surface, the dry lip or vermillion region, and the perioral skin, which is probably similar to other skin cancers and only anatomically related to the mouth. Most lip cancers are either basal or squamous cell carcinomas that occur in sun-exposed area. They are more common in men than women and they occur more commonly on the lower lip. The upper lip is more subject to basal cell than the lower lip. The prognosis is worse for lesions greater than 3 cm, poorly differentiated squamous cell cancer, those that involve the upper lip or commissure, and those with lymph node involvement. Treatment becomes anatomically and functionally more complicated if the lesion involves the commissure [173]. Lip cancer lends itself to early diagnosis, so most cases are T1–T2 N0. Early lip cancers have a low risk of spreading to lymph nodes, a small chance of distant metastasis, and excellent prognosis. Most lip brachytherapy is interstitial and may be done with rigid needles or soft plastic catheters. However, some custom mold applicators have been designed to simplify the treatment and reduce the dose to the mandible [2, 54, 69].

All types of source loading and dose rates (LDR, HDR, and PDR) appear to result in similarly good outcomes and excellent functional results in perioral cancer. HDR lends itself to outpatient treatment. Local control and CSS rates for T1–T2 lesions are 95 % of cases. Surgical salvage is feasible and can be used to treat the recurrence at the primary or lymph nodes. External radiation can be selectively used as definitive or postoperative therapy to lymph nodes, or it can be used in the form of an electron beam to treat the primary. However, a course of electron beam radiation is usually longer than a course of brachytherapy. Brachytherapy can also be successfully employed for closing of positive surgical margins. Radiation-induced acute desquamation is common, but long-term functional outcomes are typically good. Soft tissue and bone necrosis are unusual.

Buccal cancer is more aggressive than lip cancer, and it has a distinctly worse prognosis. It is typically a well- to moderately differentiated squamous cell carcinoma, and it has a higher propensity for lymph node metastasis especially with locally advanced disease. It can be treated with surgery alone, radiation alone, or with combined therapy. The optimal management strategy is not clear, but brachytherapy alone is an acceptable option for early lesions whereas combined therapy including EBRT and surgery or brachytherapy or both is more suitable for locally advanced disease. A variety of brachytherapy methods have been used including interstitial tube and button afterloading and permanent seeds. The largest reported experiences are with LDR brachytherapy from France, India, and Japan [100, 165, 172]. Local control for early disease is approximately 80 % but is significantly less for locally advanced disease. Survival correlates directly with local control and regional spread. The published results are summarized in Table 5.

Comparisons of HDR and LDR within the same institution come mostly from Japan [144, 174, 175]. Cohort comparisons with historical controls in T1–T2 oral cavity cancers and one small randomized prospective trial showed no difference between HDR and LDR [144]. Another small study of T3N0 cases revealed 67 % LC and 64 % CSS, which was not significantly different between source loading methods [24]. Other studies from Europe have drawn similar conclusions [176]. Due to the radiation safety advantages, it seems unlikely that randomized comparison studies will ever be performed.

9.7 Nasopharynx – Low Dose Rate and High Dose Rate

The outcomes with radiation therapy of NPC are dose dependent. Doses ≥ 70 Gy give better results than doses of 66 Gy [192]. The addition of chemotherapy significantly improves local control and survival, and chemoradiation is the standard for NPC [193]. The role of brachytherapy depends upon the extent of disease; however, the use of intracavitary brachytherapy as initial treatment is most suitable for patients with primary T1–T2a lesions preferably with less bulky adenopathy. Lesions with disease invading the base of skull or with intracranial extension are beyond the range of brachytherapy applicators, and most studies take these circumstances into consideration when reporting their outcomes. Technology has migrated from LDR to HDR for practical reasons to allow outpatient treatment and to avoid radiation exposure to medical personnel. Local control is achieved in approximately 90 % of T1–T2 cases. Also, there have been significant advancements in applicator design [119]. Improved local control as retrospectively compared to EBRT alone has been reported with the HDR brachytherapy using the Rotterdam applicator in T1–T2 disease. However, a randomized controlled trial of locally or regionally advanced disease, under the auspices of the International Atomic Energy Commission (IAEC), failed to demonstrate additional benefit with a low dose of brachytherapy after 70 Gy of EBRT [188]. Criticism of the study included failure to perform brachytherapy in approximately 20 % of the cases randomized to the brachytherapy arm, and the relatively low local tumor rate in T1–T2 N2–N3 cases. Chemoradiation with EBRT doses of 70 Gy and stereotactic boost have been shown to be an effective alternative [187, 194].

Brachytherapy has also been used to treat recurrent NPC where clinical circumstances are usually complicated. Interstitial afterloading and permanent seed methods have been used. The results of IS implants have been reported to achieve 57 % local control and 47 % disease-free survival in presumably selected recurrent disease and new primaries in previously irradiated patients [81]. Effective palliation can be achieved with permanent seeds, but such treatment is unlikely to be curative [94, 97].

The results of brachytherapy for lesions of the nasal vestibule have been favorable for T1 and T2 lesions. A 92 % 5-year local control was achieved in 64 patients with T1–T2 N0 tumors using 44 Gy HDR brachytherapy [86]. T3 patients were treated with surgery and postoperative radiation therapy, while local failures were surgically salvaged. There were no lymph node recurrences in untreated necks. Others have achieved similarly good results using similar brachytherapy techniques and policies [84]. EBRT alone has also been used effectively [196]. The relative efficacy of surgery, brachytherapy alone, EBRT alone, or in various combinations has not been directly compared for this cancer. This disease, when treated early, is effectively controlled with brachytherapy alone.

9.8 Salvage Brachytherapy – Low Dose Rate and High Dose Rate

Recurrent and persistent cancers of the head and neck are serious illnesses with a high potential for morbidity. Recurrence may involve the primary site only, the neck only, or both. Persistent disease is typically defined as residual disease within some defined period after completion of therapy (usually less than 3 months). New primary cancers involving the head and neck also occur in approximately 20 % of patients cured of their original disease [210–213]. Salvage therapy then encompasses a heterogeneous group of patients who may have been treated with surgery, radiation, and chemotherapy in various combinations. The extent of the disease at presentation, the disease-free interval, prior treatment, and comorbidities all impact treatment selection, prognosis, and complication rates. Treatment intent may be curative or palliative.

Two basic requirements for previously irradiated patients to receive surgery include a through consultation with an appropriately skilled physician and a robust support system within the operating facility. Brachytherapy should be viewed as a valid alternative to surgery that entails an attempt to preserve the structure and function of the involved structures. There are no studies that directly compare outcomes of brachytherapy with surgery in recurrent cancer of the head and neck, and the complexity and variety of circumstances make a direct comparison difficult. Bone involvement would strongly increase the indications for surgery. Re-irradiation may consist of brachytherapy, external beam, or a combination with or without chemotherapy.

In patients who have had surgery alone, brachytherapy and EBRT are often used as salvage whereas brachytherapy alone may be more suitable for previously irradiated patients. Brachytherapy with or without EBRT can be combined with re-resection. The extent of the disease should be carefully assessed by physical examination and imaging studies before proceeding with salvage brachytherapy. Biopsy confirmation is a prerequisite.

Tumor control and morbidity rates with brachytherapy salvage depend upon case selection and clinical circumstances. Local control rates up to 75–80 % have been reported, but more realistic percentages are 50–60 %. Survival rates after salvage brachytherapy ranges from about 20 to 50 %. The author believes that soft tissue and bone necrosis risks are greater with salvage treatment than with primary therapy, but the numbers in the literature appear to be similar to primary treatment.

Isolated neck recurrence in patients with early cancer of the oral cavity whose necks were managed expectantly can often be effectively managed by surgery, with or without postoperative radiation therapy. Neck irradiation alone is used for patients with diffuse nodal involvement or unresectable disease. In previously irradiated patients, the use of brachytherapy with neck dissection is a useful strategy to reduce morbidity. Disease control in the previously irradiated neck largely depends upon whether the disease is resectable or not. Ideally, all gross disease should be removed, and brachytherapy can be used for residual microscopic disease. Brachytherapy without surgery may be used in patients with unresectable disease, but these neck implants require the skill and knowledge to perform implants in and around major vasculature. Image guidance is helpful. Disease that invades or fully encircles the carotid, prior neck dissection, and lesions invading the skin carry considerably more risk or acute and chronic complications. Patients, families, and other physicians should be counseled accordingly. Disease control rates in the neck range from 25 to 70 % among cases selected for treatment. Simultaneous recurrence at the primary site confers a poorer prognosis.

10 Complications and Management

Complications may be divided into those associated with the brachytherapy procedure and those associated with the radiation. The measures for avoidance of procedural complications (bleeding, infection, airway issues, venous thrombosis, decubiti, etc.) have in large part been described earlier in the chapter. In general, procedure related complications are unusual. Oral rinses, nutritional support, frequent suctioning, catheter cleaning, and proper airway management are important measures for avoiding procedural complications. Acute radiation reactions do not emerge until several days after the brachytherapy. The patient and the family need to be informed about the course of the radiation effects and optimal home care measures. Home care recommendations include:

1. Oral rinses with 1–2 % bicarbonate every 1–2 h while awake.
2. Keep implant exit sites clean and dry; avoid lotions and salves.
3. Washing and showering face and neck starting 24 h after implant removal.
4. Oral intake – advance as tolerated for patients who can swallow.
5. Dietary supplementation and feeding tube support as needed.
6. Tracheostomy site – keep clean and dry; dress daily or more often if needed.
7. Prophylaxis for trismus – preferably with specifically designed commercial devices.
8. Make arrangements for speech and swallow evaluation.
9. Make arrangements for follow-up dental care.
10. Call brachytherapy physician for questions or acute concerns.
11. Emergency room referral for urgent concerns (breathing, bleeding, acute infections, etc.).

12. Scheduled follow-up with all relevant physicians (primary care, head and neck, medical, and radiation oncologists).

Chronic complications of head and neck brachytherapy such as soft tissue necrosis (STN) and bone injury (BI) have already been discussed in the context of each disease site. Microvascular injury is thought to be underlying mechanism [214]. More recently, the complex pathophysiology has been described [215]. The predisposing factors and standard treatment have also been summarized [150, 215]. The rates of STN and BI are presented in the tables included. However, the extent and consequences of these occurrences are not apparent from the figures. Importantly, the rate of BI requiring surgery is relatively low, and it can be significantly reduced by proper implant techniques and the use of mandibular protection devices. There may be a greater incidence of soft tissue necrosis with brachytherapy than with EBRT, but it usually heals without permanent effects. Cranial neuropathy, although uncommon, may also be somewhat more common with brachytherapy than with EBRT. The nerves at most risk are the hypoglossal for tongue implants and the vagus, glossopharyngeal nerves, and sympathetic chain for neck implants.

The use of medical measures such as pentoxifylline 400 mg and vitamin E 400 mg three times daily has been shown to significantly improve the rate of healing in cases of soft tissue and bone injury [216]. The author recommends early administration of these medications for any apparent soft tissue injury because the rate of side effects from the medication is low.

Hyperbaric oxygen (HBO) therapy may also aid in the healing of soft tissue and bone injury [51, 52, 217, 218]. A multicenter French randomized trial of HBO, however, stopped enrollment at only 68 cases because of concerns about worse outcomes in the HBO arm [219]. The study concluded there was no benefit of HBO for osteonecrosis of the mandible. The author does not believe that one such study is definitive and wonders if perhaps medications and HBO may have an additive benefit in patients with osteonecrosis. Another setting for the use of HBO is in a preventive protocol for patients who have scheduled dental procedures. HBO treatments are recommended before and after the invasive procedures [220]. Regardless of the debate about treatment efficacy, measures to prevent necrosis are preferable. Cessation of smoking is another key factor in avoidance of complications.

Brachytherapy as the sole modality for lip and oral cavity cancer simultaneously enhances disease control and reduces morbidity. Relatively more radiation is given to the target, and less radiation is delivered to adjacent normal structures which thus limits the side effects of radiation on saliva production and taste acuity. Brachytherapy similarly improves the dosimetry index (relative tumor to normal tissue dose) when it is used to supplement EBRT. Dose reduction to adjacent mucosa, salivary tissue, taste buds, the pharyngeal constrictors, and muscles of mastication reduces acute and late morbidity, particularly when chemotherapy is administered with EBRT. A review of the late complications gives an account of the expected complication rates for radiation therapy of head and neck cancer [221]. One important example is accelerated carotid artery atherosclerosis [222, 223]. The dose-dependent rate and the severity of vascular injury could be reduced by the employment of brachytherapy. Similarly, reduction of dose and injury to pharyngeal constrictors could improve long-term swallowing function. Despite these and other potential morbidity reduction advantages, there are no outcome comparisons between chemoradiation alone and chemoradiation with brachytherapy.

Secondary aerodigestive malignancies occur in a relatively large percentage ($\approx 20\%$) of patients with head and neck cancers. Lung, esophagus, and head and neck sites must be monitored second primary cancers [211]. The patients must be followed carefully for life, screened, and evaluated for recurrence of the original primary, which tends to occur earlier, and a second new primary cancers, which tend to occur later than recurrences. The distinction may be difficult in patients with adjacent recurrences, similar histology, and moderately long disease-free intervals. While hypopharynx has the highest rate for second malignancy, larynx has the lowest rate. However, both sites have the propensity to be associated with bronchogenic carcinoma. On the other hand, the most common site for the second primary cancers for oral cavity and oropharynx primaries is a new head and neck cancer. The complication rates are markedly higher for patients who continue smoking and conversely are significantly lower in patients who stop smoking. Measures to help the patient avoid smoking, drinking, and HPV exposure are general health improvements that favorably impact on outcome.

11 Conclusions and Future Developments

Brachytherapy is an integral part of the treatment of head and neck cancer. It may be used alone or in combination with EBRT. T1N0 and small T2N0 lesions of the lip, nasal vestibule, buccal, and oral cavity are often successfully treated with brachytherapy alone. LDR equivalent doses of 65–70 Gy and dose rates of 0.3–0.6 Gy/h are recommended. Mandible spacers and shields are used to improve dosimetry. T3–T4 lip and oral cavity lesions are more difficult to control; however, brachytherapy can be used as a boost to EBRT, or it can be administered after surgery for lesions with close or positive margins, with or without EBRT depending upon the status of lymph nodes. Brachytherapy is also used as a boost to EBRT for oropharynx cancer. Combined doses are 50–60 Gy of EBRT and 25–30 Gy LDR equivalent brachytherapy. Such treatment is as effective as radical surgery and postoperative radiation therapy, but preservation of structure and function results in improved quality of life. Transoral robotic surgery is a new surgical paradigm, which has similar advantages for selected patients. The discovery of HPV-associated head and neck cancer has altered the management and prognosis for these patients. Finally, intracavitary brachytherapy in T1–T2 nasopharynx cancer has shown to improve local control. The routine use of chemoradiation, however, has probably reduced the impact. A recent

randomized trial did not demonstrate a difference from chemoradiation without brachytherapy, but the study can be criticized for randomization deficiencies and poor local control compared to previous reports. Brachytherapy has been used extensively as the salvage treatment for previously irradiated patients. The recommended dose is in the range of 50–60 Gy LDR equivalent.

HDR, LDR, and PDR source loading appear to be equally effective, but there are few direct comparisons. The advantage of HDR and PDR relates to radiation safety. HDR involves once- or twice-daily treatment, so it is the most convenient in terms of nursing and patient management. The recommended doses of HDR are still being determined. HDR fraction sizes are preferably in the 3–4.5 Gy range, but it is not always practical. The author often uses HDR 3.5–4.0 Gy × 5–6 fractions (i.e., 17.5–24 Gy) when combined with EBRT. Additionally, HDR monotherapy (5–6 Gy × 9–10 fractions) has been used in Asia (the author prefers 4–4.5 Gy × 10–12 fractions); lower can be used for patients with postoperative margins and perhaps for safety reason, in the treatment of patients with prior radiation. There is no consensus or uniformly accepted standard of HDR dose and fractionation for most head and neck cancers. Brachytherapy can also be done with surgery to improve outcomes and to reduce radiation morbidity. Intraoperative brachytherapy consists of the placement of brachytherapy catheters or devices during surgery followed either by immediate single fraction source loading (if there is a shielded operating room or low-energy source) or by fractionated dose delivery after wound healing and 3D dosimetry calculation. The potential of intraoperative brachytherapy has yet to be fully explored.

An experienced team of physicians, physicists, nurses, and therapists are needed to perform head and neck brachytherapy. Coordination with hospital personnel, operating room and ward staff members, and other treating physicians is a key factor in establishing a successful service. Strong radiation safety practices, quality assurance, and standard operating procedures are needed for the program to succeed. Physicians and other persons must have proper training and experience to perform these complicated procedures.

Technically improved and more consistent implants can be achieved with image guidance. Ultrasound, in its current form, has limited value, and CT scan simulation is usually performed after the implant procedure is completed. However, it would be better if there was image guidance of catheter placement during the procedure, and the simulation radiography is obtained at the end of the procedure so improvement in the implants could be made while the patient is still under anesthesia. A new generation of portable CT scanners is being developed which will serve this purpose. Although CT scanning does not permit true real-time needle guidance, there is clear potential for improvement in both implant quality and efficiency of the brachytherapy with this imaging modality. MRI scanning is another image guidance option, but the needle images are not as distinct and catheter relationships are more difficult to appreciate. MRI-ready operating rooms are also not readily available.

Another guidance approach with excellent potential is the use of navigation technology. In this system, fiducial tracking devices are affixed to the patient's head and to the implant needles. Optical and electoral magnetic navigation tools can then be used to guide the insertion of the implant needles. A 3D image (CT, PET/CT or MRI) can be fused with the navigation technology, so the tumor target and normal tissue anatomy was virtually displayed during the procedure. Such relationships can be coordinated with a preoperative CT, PET-CT, or MRI datasets and fused for optimal display of the disease and relevant anatomy. This system is similar to those used in neurosurgery and orthopedics. The challenge for brachytherapy is that soft tissue and vascular structures may be deformed and displaced during the implant. The use of intraoperative CT with navigation allows iterative accounting of changing anatomy and catheter relationships. This image guidance will surely improve the quality, efficiency, and effectiveness of brachytherapy.

References

1. Pierquin B, Wilson JF, Chassagne D (1987) Modern brachytherapy. Masson, New York
2. Gerbaulet A, Potter P, Mazeron JJ et al (2002) The GEC ESTRO handbook of brachytherapy, 1st edn. Brussels, ESTRO
3. Harrison LB, Sessions RB, Kies MS (2013) Head and neck cancer: a multidisciplinary approach. Philadelphia, PA, USA: Wolters Kluwer Health
4. Devlin PM (2007) Brachytherapy: applications and techniques. Philadelphia, PA, USA: Lippincott Williams & Wilkins
5. James AG, Henschke UK, Myers WG (1953) The clinical use of radioactive gold (Au-198) seeds. Cancer 6(5):1034–1039
6. Aronowitz JN (2015) Afterloading: the technique that rescued brachytherapy. Inj Radiat Oncol Biol Phys 92(3):479–487
7. Glasser O, Quimby E, Taylor L et al (1961) Physical foundations of radiology, 3rd edn. Harper & Row, New York
8. Quimby E (1932) The grouping of radium tubes in pack on plaques to produce the desired distribution of radiation. Am J Roentgenol Radium Ther 27:18
9. Quimby E (1941) The specification of dosage in radium therapy. Am J Roentgenol Radium Ther 45:16
10. Paterson R, Parker H (1995) A dosage system for gamma ray therapy. 1934. Br J Radiol 68(808): H60–H100
11. Meredith WJ (1967) Radium dosage: the manchester system, 2nd edn. Edinburgh, E & S Livingstone Ltd
12. Paterson R (1952) Studies in optimum dosage. Br J Radiol 25(298):505–516
13. Pierquin B, Dutreix A, Paine CH et al (1978) The Paris system in interstitial radiation therapy. Acta Radiol Oncol Radiat Phys Biol 17(1):33–48
14. Aronowitz JN, Rivard MJ (2014) The evolution of computerized treatment planning for brachytherapy: American contributions. J Contemp Brachyther 6(2):185–190
15. Lessard E, Pouliot J (2001) Inverse planning anatomy-based dose optimization for HDR-brachytherapy of the prostate using fast simulated annealing algorithm and dedicated objective function. Med Phys 28(5):773–779
16. Ang KK, Harris J, Wheeler R et al (2010) Human papillomavirus and survival of patients with oropharyngeal cancer. N Engl J Med 363(1):24–35
17. Masterson L, Moualed D, Liu ZW et al (2014) De-escalation treatment protocols for human papillomavirus-associated oropharyngeal squamous cell carcinoma: a systematic review and meta-analysis of current clinical trials. Eur J Cancer 50(15):2636–2648
18. Pernot M, Hoffstetter S, Peiffert D et al (1996) Role of interstitial brachytherapy in oral and oropharyngeal carcinoma: reflection of a series of 1344

patients treated at the time of initial presentation. Otolaryngol Head Neck Surg 115(6):519–526

19. Jackel MC, Ambrosch P, Christiansen H et al (2008) Value of postoperative radiotherapy in patients with pathologic N1 neck disease. Head Neck 30(7):875–882

20. Decroix Y, Ghossein NA (1981) Experience of the Curie Institute in treatment of cancer of the mobile tongue: II. Management of the neck nodes. Cancer 47(3):503–508

21. Nakagawa T, Shibuya H, Yoshimura R et al (2003) Neck node metastasis after successful brachytherapy for early stage tongue carcinoma. Radiother Oncol 68(2):129–135

22. Bourgier C, Coche-Déquéant B, Fournier C et al (2005) Exclusive low-dose-rate brachytherapy in 279 patients with T2N0 mobile tongue carcinoma. Int J Radiat Oncol Biol Phys 63(2):434–440

23. Pignol JP, le Maitre A, Maillard E et al (2009) Meta-analysis of chemotherapy in head and neck cancer (MACH-NC): an update on 93 randomised trials and 17,346 patients. Radiother Oncol 92(1):4–14

24. Kakimoto N, Inoue T, Inoue T et al (2003) Results of low- and high-dose-rate interstitial brachytherapy for T3 mobile tongue cancer. Radiother Oncol 68(2):123–128

25. Lapeyre M, Bollet MA, Racadot S et al (2004) Postoperative brachytherapy alone and combined postoperative radiotherapy and brachytherapy boost for squamous cell carcinoma of the oral cavity, with positive or close margins. Head Neck 26(3):216–223

26. Cooper JS, Zhang Q, Pajak TF et al (2012) Long-term follow-up of the RTOG 9501/intergroup phase III trial: postoperative concurrent radiation therapy and chemotherapy in high-risk squamous cell carcinoma of the head and neck. Int J Radiat Oncol Biol Phys 84(5):1198–1205

27. Harrison LB, Zelefsky MJ, Sessions RB et al (1992) Base-of-tongue cancer treated with external beam irradiation plus brachytherapy: oncologic and functional outcome. Radiology 184(1):267–270

28. Levendag P, Nijdam W, Noever I et al (2004) Brachytherapy versus surgery in carcinoma of tonsillar fossa and/or soft palate: late adverse sequelae and performance status: can we be more selective and obtain better tissue sparing? Int J Radiat Oncol Biol Phys 59(3):713–724

29. Pernot M, Malissard L, Hoffstetter S et al (1994) Influence of tumoral, radiobiological, and general factors on local control and survival of a series of 361 tumors of the velotonsillar area treated by exclusive irradiation (external beam irradiation+brachytherapy or brachytherapy alone). Int J Radiat Oncol Biol Phys 30(5):1051–1057

30. Mazeron JJ, Belkacemi Y, Simon JM et al (1993) Place of Iridium 192 implantation in definitive irradiation of faucial arch squamous cell carcinomas. Int J Radiat Oncol Biol Phys 27(2):251–257

31. Maan ZN, Gibbins N, Al-Jabri T et al (2012) The use of robotics in otolaryngology-head and neck

surgery: a systematic review. Am J Otolaryngol 33(1):137–146

32. Huncharek M, Kupelnick B (2002) Combined chemoradiation versus radiation therapy alone in locally advanced nasopharyngeal carcinoma: results of a meta-analysis of 1,528 patients from six randomized trials. Am J Clin Oncol 25(3):219–223

33. Levendag PC, Schmitz PI, Jansen PP et al (1997) Fractionated high-dose-rate and pulsed-dose-rate brachytherapy: first clinical experience in squamous cell carcinoma of the tonsillar fossa and soft palate. Int J Radiat Oncol Biol Phys 38(3):497–506

34. Levendag PC, Lagerwaard FJ, Noever I et al (2002) Role of endocavitary brachytherapy with or without chemotherapy in cancer of the nasopharynx. Int J Radiat Oncol Biol Phys 52(3):755–768

35. Wang CC (1987) Re-irradiation of recurrent nasopharyngeal carcinoma–treatment techniques and results. Int J Radiat Oncol Biol Phys 13(7):953–956

36. Langlois D, Hoffstetter S, Malissard L et al (1988) Salvage irradiation of oropharynx and mobile tongue about 192 iridium brachytherapy in Centre Alexis Vautrin. Int J Radiat Oncol Biol Phys 14(5):849–853

37. Park RI, Liberman FZ, Lee DJ et al (1991) Iodine-125 seed implantation as an adjunct to surgery in advanced recurrent squamous cell cancer of the head and neck. Laryngoscope 101(4 Pt 1):405–410

38. Peiffert D, Pernot M, Malissard L et al (1994) Salvage irradiation by brachytherapy of velotonsillar squamous cell carcinoma in a previously irradiated field: results in 73 cases. Int J Radiat Oncol Biol Phys 29(4):681–686

39. Zelefsky M, Zimberg S, Raben A et al (1998) Brachytherapy for locally advanced and recurrent lymph node metastases. J Brachyther Int 14:123

40. Puthawala A, Nisar Syed AM, Gamie S et al (2001) Interstitial low-dose-rate brachytherapy as a salvage treatment for recurrent head-and-neck cancers: long-term results. Int J Radiat Oncol Biol Phys 51(2):354–362

41. Nutting C, Horlock N, A'Hern R et al (2006) Manually after-loaded 192Ir low-dose rate brachytherapy after subtotal excision and flap reconstruction of recurrent cervical lymphadenopathy from head and neck cancer. Radiother Oncol 80(1):39–42

42. Glatzel M, Buntzel J, Schroder D et al (2002) High-dose-rate brachytherapy in the treatment of recurrent and residual head and neck cancer. Laryngoscope 112(8 Pt 1):1366–1371

43. Hepel JT, Syed AM, Puthawala A et al (2005) Salvage high-dose-rate (HDR) brachytherapy for recurrent head-and-neck cancer. Int J Radiat Oncol Biol Phys 62(5):1444–1450

44. Narayana A, Cohen GN, Zaider M et al (2007) High-dose-rate interstitial brachytherapy in recurrent and previously irradiated head and neck cancers—preliminary results. Brachytherapy 6(2):157–163

45. Bartochowska A, Wierzbicka M, Skowronek J et al (2012) High-dose-rate and pulsed-dose-rate brachy-

therapy in palliative treatment of head and neck cancers. Brachytherapy 11(2):137–143

46. Miura M, Takeda M, Sasaki T et al (1998) Factors affecting mandibular complications in low dose rate brachytherapy for oral tongue carcinoma with special reference to spacer. Int J Radiat Oncol Biol Phys 41(4):763–770

47. Fujita M, Hirokawa Y, Kashiwado K et al (1999) Interstitial brachytherapy for stage I and II squamous cell carcinoma of the oral tongue: factors influencing local control and soft tissue complications. Int J Radiat Oncol Biol Phys 44(4):767–775

48. Libby B, Sheng K, McLawhorn R et al (2011) Use of megavoltage computed tomography with image registration for high–dose rate treatment planning of an oral tongue cancer using a custom oral mold applicator with embedded lead shielding. Brachytherapy 10(4):340–344

49. Tamamoto M, Fujita M, Yamamoto T et al (1996) Techniques for making spacers in interstitial brachytherapy for tongue cancer. Int J Prosthodont 9(1):95–98

50. Marx RE, Johnson RP, Kline SN (1985) Prevention of osteoradionecrosis: a randomized prospective clinical trial of hyperbaric oxygen versus penicillin. J Am Dent Assoc 111(1):49–54

51. Hampson NB, Holm JR, Wreford-Brown CE et al (2012) Prospective assessment of outcomes in 411 patients treated with hyperbaric oxygen for chronic radiation tissue injury. Cancer 118(15):3860–3868

52. Bennett MH, Feldmeier J, Hampson N et al (2012) Hyperbaric oxygen therapy for late radiation tissue injury. Cochrane Database Syst Rev 16(5)

53. Kudoh T, Ikushima H, Kudoh K et al (2010) High-dose-rate brachytherapy for patients with maxillary gingival carcinoma using a novel customized intraoral mold technique. Oral Surg Oral Med Oral Pathol Oral Radiol Endodontol 109(2):e102–e108

54. Matsuzaki H, Takemoto M, Hara M et al (2012) Two-piece customized mold technique for high-dose-rate brachytherapy on cancers of the buccal mucosa and lip. Oral Surg Oral Med Oral Pathol Oral Radiol 113(1):118–125

55. Obinata K, Ohmori K, Shirato II et al (2007) Experience of high-dose-rate brachytherapy for head and neck cancer treated by a customized intraoral mold technique. Radiat Med 25(4):181–186

56. Stannard C, Maree G, Tovey S et al (2014) Iodine-125 brachytherapy in the management of squamous cell carcinoma of the oral cavity and oropharynx. Brachytherapy 13(4):405–412

57. Weinberg BD, Jiang H, Aguilera N et al (2013) A novel endocavitary HDR brachytherapy applicator for treatment of the deep oropharynx, posterior pharyngeal wall, supraglottic larynx, and hypopharynx. Brachytherapy 12:S36–S37

58. Doyle LA, Harrison AS, Cognetti D et al (2011) Reirradiation of head and neck cancer with high-dose-rate brachytherapy: a customizable intraluminal solution for postoperative treatment of tracheal mucosa recurrence. Brachytherapy 10(2):154–158

59. Demanes D, Rodriguez R, Syed AM et al (1997) Wire in leader technique: a method for loading implant catheters in inaccessible sites. J Brachyther Int 13(4):123

60. Nose T, Koizumi M, Nishiyama K (2004) High-dose-rate interstitial brachytherapy for oropharyngeal carcinoma: results of 83 lesions in 82 patients. Int J Radiat Oncol Biol Phys 59(4):983–991

61. Patra NB, Goswami J, Basu S et al (2009) Outcomes of high dose rate interstitial boost brachytherapy after external beam radiation therapy in head and neck cancer—an Indian (single institutional) learning experience. Brachytherapy 8(2):248–254

62. Sethi T, Ash DV, Flynn A et al (1996) Replacement of hairpin and loop implants by optimised straight line sources. Radiother Oncol 39(2):117–121

63. Demanes DJ, Friedman JM, Park SJ et al (2012) Brachytherapy catheter spacing and stabilization technique. Brachytherapy 11(5):392–397

64. Ngan RK, Wong RK, Tang FN et al (2005) Curative radiotherapy for early cancers of the lip, buccal mucosa, and nose–a simple interstitial brachytherapy technique employing angiocatheters as carriers for Iridium-192 wire implants. Hong Kong Med J 11(5):351–359

65. Simon JM, Mazeron JJ, Pohar S et al (1993) Effect of intersource spacing on local control and complications in brachytherapy of mobile tongue and floor of mouth. Radiother Oncol 26(1):19–25

66. Guibert M, David I, Vergez S et al (2011) Brachytherapy in lip carcinoma: long-term results. Int J Radiat Oncol Biol Phys 81(5):14

67. Guinot J-L, Arribas L, Tortajada MI et al (2013) From low-dose-rate to high-dose-rate brachytherapy in lip carcinoma: equivalent results but fewer complications. Brachytherapy 12(6):528–534

68. Guinot JL, Arribas L, Vendrell JB et al (2014) Prognostic factors in squamous cell lip carcinoma treated with high-dose-rate brachytherapy. Head Neck 36(12):1737–1742

69. Feldman J, Appelbaum L, Sela M et al (2014) Novel high dose rate lip brachytherapy technique to improve dose homogeneity and reduce toxicity by customized mold. Radiat Oncol 9(271):014–0271

70. Lapeyre M, Peiffert D, Malissard L et al (1995) An original technique of brachytherapy in the treatment of epidermoid carcinomas of the buccal mucosa. Int J Radiat Oncol Biol Phys 33(2):447–454

71. Prisciandaro JI, Foote RL, Herman MG et al (2005) A buccal mucosa carcinoma treated with high dose rate brachytherapy. J Appl Clin Med Phys 6(1):8–12

72. Diaz EM Jr, Holsinger FC, Zuniga ER, Roberts DB, Sorensen DM (2003) Squamous cell carcinoma of the buccal mucosa: one institution's experience with 119 previously untreated patients. Head Neck 25(4):267–273

73. Vavassori A, Gherardi F, Colangione SP et al (2012) High-dose-rate interstitial brachytherapy in early stage buccal mucosa and lip cancer: report on 12

consecutive patients and review of the literature. Tumori 98(4):471–477

74. Mazeron JJ, Crook JM, Benck V et al (1990) Iridium 192 implantation of T1 and T2 carcinomas of the mobile tongue. Int J Radiat Oncol Biol Phys 19(6):1369–1376

75. Guinot JL, Santos M, Tortajada MI et al (2010) Efficacy of high-dose-rate interstitial brachytherapy in patients with oral tongue carcinoma. Brachytherapy 9(3):227–234

76. Leung TW, Wong VY, Kwan KH et al (2002) High dose rate brachytherapy for early stage oral tongue cancer. Head Neck 24(3):274–281

77. Lapeyre M, Hoffstetter S, Peiffert D et al (2000) Postoperative brachytherapy alone for T1-2 N0 squamous cell carcinomas of the oral tongue and floor of mouth with close or positive margins. Int J Radiat Oncol Biol Phys 48(1):37–42

78. Puthawala AA, Syed AM, Eads DL et al (1988) Limited external beam and interstitial 192iridium irradiation in the treatment of carcinoma of the base of the tongue: a ten year experience. Int J Radiat Oncol Biol Phys 14(5):839–848

79. Cano ER, Lai SY, Caylakli F et al (2009) Management of squamous cell carcinoma of the base of tongue with chemoradiation and brachytherapy. Head Neck 31(11):1431–1438

80. Karakoyun-Celik O, Norris CM, Tishler R et al (2005) Definitive radiotherapy with interstitial implant boost for squamous cell carcinoma of the tongue base. Head Neck 27(5):353–361

81. Syed AM, Puthawala AA, Damore SJ et al (2000) Brachytherapy for primary and recurrent nasopharyngeal carcinoma: 20 years' experience at Long Beach Memorial. Int J Radiat Oncol Biol Phys 47(5):1311–1321

82. Wan XB, Jiang R, Xie FY et al (2014) Endoscope-guided interstitial intensity-modulated brachytherapy and intracavitary brachytherapy as boost radiation for primary early T stage nasopharyngeal carcinoma. PLoS One 9(3):e90048. doi:10.1371/journal.pone.0090048

83. Kremer B, Klimek L, Andreopoulos D et al (1999) A new method for the placement of brachytherapy probes in paranasal sinus and nasopharynx neoplasms. Int J Radiat Oncol Biol Phys 43(5):995–1000

84. Evensen JF, Jacobsen AB, Tausjo JE (1996) Brachytherapy of squamous cell carcinoma of the nasal vestibule. Acta Oncol 8:87–92

85. Langendijk JA, Poorter R, Leemans CR et al (2004) Radiotherapy of squamous cell carcinoma of the nasal vestibule. Int J Radiat Oncol Biol Phys 59(5):1319–1325

86. Levendag PC, Nijdam WM, van Moolenburgh SE et al (2006) Interstitial radiation therapy for early-stage nasal vestibule cancer: a continuing quest for optimal tumor control and cosmesis. Int J Radiat Oncol Biol Phys 66(1):160–169

87. Nag S, Tippin D, Grecula J, Schuller D (2004) Intraoperative high-dose-rate brachytherapy for paranasal sinus tumors. Int J Radiat Oncol Biol Phys 58(1):155–160

88. Teudt IU, Meyer JE, Ritter M et al (2014) Perioperative image-adapted brachytherapy for the treatment of paranasal sinus and nasal cavity malignancies. Brachytherapy 13(2):178–186

89. Bartochowska A, Skowronek J, Wierzbicka M et al (2013) The role of high-dose-rate and pulsed-dose-rate brachytherapy in the management of recurrent or residual stomal tumor after total laryngectomy. Laryngoscope 123(3):657–661

90. Demanes D, Ruwanthi P, Cmelak A et al (2000) Brachytherapy and external radiation for carcinoma of the base of tongue: implantation of the primary tumor and cervical adenopathy. Int J Brachyther 16:211–223

91. Nag S, Schuller D, Pak V et al (1997) IORT using electron beam or HDR brachytherapy for previously unirradiated head and neck cancers. Front Radiat Ther Oncol 31:112–116

92. Morikawa LK, Zelefsky MJ, Cohen GN et al (2013) Intraoperative high-dose-rate brachytherapy using dose painting technique: evaluation of safety and preliminary clinical outcomes. Brachytherapy 12(1):1–7

93. Teckie S, Scala LM, Ho F et al (2013) High-dose-rate intraoperative brachytherapy and radical surgical resection in the management of recurrent head-and-neck cancer. Brachytherapy 12(3):228–234

94. Vikram B, Strong EW, Shah JP et al (1985) Intraoperative radiotherapy in patients with recurrent head and neck cancer. Am J Surg 150(4):485–487

95. Beitler JJ, Smith RV, Silver CE et al (1998) Close or positive margins after surgical resection for the head and neck cancer patient: the addition of brachytherapy improves local control. Int J Radiat Oncol Biol Phys 40(2):313–317

96. Zhu L, Jiang Y, Wang J et al (2013) An investigation of 125I seed permanent implantation for recurrent carcinoma in the head and neck after surgery and external beam radiotherapy. World J Surg Oncol 11(60):1477–7819

97. Ashamalla H, Rafla S, Zaki B et al (2002) Radioactive gold grain implants in recurrent and locally advanced head-and-neck cancers. Brachytherapy 1(3):161–166

98. Lock M, Cao JQ, D'Souza DP et al (2011) Brachytherapy with permanent gold grain seeds for squamous cell carcinoma of the lip. Radiother Oncol 98(3):352–356

99. Shibuya H, Takeda M, Matsumoto S et al (1993) The efficacy of radiation therapy for a malignant melanoma in the mucosa of the upper jaw: an analytic study. Int J Radiat Oncol Biol Phys 25(1):35–39

100. Tayier A, Hayashi K, Yoshimura R (2011) Low-dose-rate interstitial brachytherapy preserves good quality of life in buccal mucosa cancer patients. J Radiat Res 52(5):655–659

101. Mazeron J-J, Ardiet J-M, Haie-Méder C et al (2009) GEC-ESTRO recommendations for brachytherapy for head and neck squamous cell carcinomas. Radiother Oncol 91(2):150–156

102. Prevost JB, de Boer H, Poll J et al (2008) Analysis of the motion of oropharyngeal tumors and consequences in planning target volume determination. Radiother Oncol 87(2):268–273

103. Geiger M, Strnad V, Lotter M et al (2002) Pulsed-dose rate brachytherapy with concomitant chemotherapy and interstitial hyperthermia in patients with recurrent head-and-neck cancer. Brachytherapy 1(3):149–153

104. Strnad V, Geiger M, Lotter M et al (2003) The role of pulsed-dose-rate brachytherapy in previously irradiated head-and-neck cancer. Brachytherapy 2(3):158–163

105. Das RK (1998) ICRU 58 (dose and volume specification for reporting interstitial therapy), by International Commission on Radiation Units and Measurements. Med Phys 25(7):1225–25

106. Melzner WJ, Lotter M, Sauer R et al (2007) Quality of interstitial PDR-brachytherapy-implants of head-and-neck-cancers: predictive factors for local control and late toxicity? Radiother Oncol 82(2):167–173

107. Mazeron JJ, Simon JM, Le Pechoux C et al (1991) Effect of dose rate on local control and complications in definitive irradiation of T1-2 squamous cell carcinomas of mobile tongue and floor of mouth with interstitial iridium-192. Radiother Oncol 21(1):39–47

108. Brenner DJ, Schiff PB, Huang Y, Hall EJ (1997) Pulsed-dose-rate brachytherapy: design of convenient (daytime-only) schedules. Int J Radiat Oncol Biol Phys 39(4):809–815

109. Visser AG, van den Aardweg GJ, Levendag PC (1996) Pulsed dose rate and fractionated high dose rate brachytherapy: choice of brachytherapy schedules to replace low dose rate treatments. Int J Radiat Oncol Biol Phys 34(2):497–505

110. Nag S, Cano ER, Demanes DJ et al (2001) The American Brachytherapy Society recommendations for high-dose-rate brachytherapy for head-and-neck carcinoma. Int J Radiat Oncol Biol Phys 50(5):1190–1198

111. Akiyama H, Yoshida K, Shimizutani K et al (2012) Dose reduction trial from 60 Gy in 10 fractions to 54 Gy in 9 fractions schedule in high-dose-rate interstitial brachytherapy for early oral tongue cancer. J Radiat Res 53(5):722–726

112. Farrus B, Pons F, Sanchez-Reyes A et al (1996) Quality assurance of interstitial brachytherapy technique in lip cancer: comparison of actual performance with the Paris System recommendations. Radiother Oncol 38(2):145–151

113. Guinot JL, Arribas L, Chust ML et al (2003) Lip cancer treatment with high dose rate brachytherapy. Radiother Oncol 69(1):113–115

114. Mazeron JJ, Richaud P (1984) Lip cancer, report of the 18th annual meeting of the European Curietherapy Group, May 1981. J Eur Radiother 5:50–56

115. Gerbaulet A, Pernot M (1985) Le carcinome épidermoïde de la face interne de joue. A propos de 748 malades. J Eur Radiother 6:1–4

116. Harrison LB, Zelefsky MJ, Armstrong JG, Carper E, Gaynor JJ, Sessions RB (1994) Performance status after treatment for squamous cell cancer of the base of tongue–a comparison of primary radiation therapy versus primary surgery. Int J Radiat Oncol Biol Phys 30(4):953–957

117. Pernot M, Luporsi E, Hoffstetter S et al (1997) Complications following definitive irradiation for cancers of the oral cavity and the oropharynx (in a series of 1134 patients). Int J Radiat Oncol Biol Phys 37(3):577–585

118. Strnad V, Melzner W, Geiger M et al (2005) Role of interstitial PDR brachytherapy in the treatment of oral and oropharyngeal cancer. A single-institute experience of 236 patients. Strahlenther Onkol 181(12):762–767

119. Levendag PC, Peters R, Meeuwis CA et al (1997) A new applicator design for endocavitary brachytherapy of cancer in the nasopharynx. Radiother Oncol 45(1):95–98

120. Strege RJ, Kovács G, Lamcke P et al (2007) Role of perioperative brachytherapy in the treatment of malignancies involving the skull base and orbit. Neurosurg Q 17(3):193–207

121. Werner J, Rochels R, Kovacs G et al (1997) Therapieprinzipien bei malignen Nasennebenhöhlentumoren mit Orbitabeteiligung. In: Rochels R, Behrendt S (eds) Orbita–chirurgie. Einhorn Presse Verlag, Reinbeck, pp 93–101

122. Kovács G, Rochels R, Mehdorn H et al (1997) Eye preservation brachytherapy for orbital and adjacent tumors: preliminary results. In: Wiegel T, Bornfeld N, Hinkelbein W (eds) Radiotherapy of ocular disease, vol 30. Front Radiat Ther Oncol Basel, Karge, pp 56–64

123. Tyl JW, Blank LE, Koornneef L (1997) Brachytherapy in orbital tumors. Ophthalmology 104(9):1475–1479

124. Naszaly A, Nemeth G (1982) Therapy result of malignant tumors of the paranasal sinuses in patients treated at the metropolitan onco-radiologic centre of Budapest. Period under review: 1946–1974 (author's transl). Strahlentherapie 158(5):270–4

125. Mazeron JJ, Langlois D, Glaubiger D et al (1987) Salvage irradiation of oropharyngeal cancers using iridium 192 wire implants: 5-year results of 70 cases. Int J Radiat Oncol Biol Phys 13(7):957–962

126. Nag S, Schuller DE, Rodriguez-Villalba S et al (1999) Intraoperative high dose rate brachytherapy can be used to salvage patients with previously irradiated head and neck recurrences. Rev Med Univ Navarra 43(2):56–61

127. ACR technical standard for the performance of brachytherapy physics: remotely loaded HDR sources (2008) Practice Guidelines and Technical Standards. American College of Radiology, Reston, Virginia pp 1197–1201

128. Title 10 of the Code of Federal Regulations (10 CFR) Part 35 (2011) "Medical Use of Byproduct

Material," for permanent implant brachytherapy programs pp 682–683

129. Nath R, Anderson LL, Meli JA et al (1997) Code of practice for brachytherapy physics: report of the AAPM Radiation Therapy Committee Task Group No. 56. American Association of Physicists in Medicine. Med Phys 24(10):1557–1598

130. Kakimoto N, Inoue T, Inoue T et al (2006) High-dose-rate interstitial brachytherapy for mobile tongue cancer: influence of the non-irradiated period. Antican Res 26(5):2933–2937

131. Wendt CD, Peters LJ, Delclos L et al (1990) Primary radiotherapy in the treatment of stage I and II oral tongue cancers: importance of the proportion of therapy delivered with interstitial therapy. Int J Radiat Oncol Biol Phys 18(6):1287–1292

132. Hareyama M, Nishio M, Saito A et al (1993) Results of cesium needle interstitial implantation for carcinoma of the oral tongue. Int J Radiat Oncol Biol Phys 25(1):29–34

133. Pernot M, Malissard L, Aletti P et al (1992) Iridium-192 brachytherapy in the management of 147 T2N0 oral tongue carcinomas treated with irradiation alone: comparison of two treatment techniques. Radiother Oncol 23(4):223–228

134. Shibuya H, Hoshina M, Takeda M et al (1993) Brachytherapy for stage I & II oral tongue cancer: an analysis of past cases focusing on control and complications. Int J Radiat Oncol Biol Phys 26(1):51–58

135. Bachaud JM, Delannes M, Allouache N et al (1994) Radiotherapy of stage I and II carcinomas of the mobile tongue and/or floor of the mouth. Radiother Oncol 31(3):199–206

136. Pernot M, Aletti P, Carolus JM et al (1995) Indications, techniques and results of postoperative brachytherapy in cancer of the oral cavity. Radiother Oncol 35(3):186–192

137. Takeda M, Shibuya H, Inoue T (1996) The efficacy of gold-198 grain mold therapy for mucosal carcinomas of the oral cavity. Acta Oncol 35(4):463–467

138. Chao KS, Emami B, Akhileswaran R et al (1996) The impact of surgical margin status and use of an interstitial implant on T1, T2 oral tongue cancers after surgery. Int J Radiat Oncol Biol Phys 36(5):1039–1043

139. Yamazaki H, Inoue T, Koizumi M et al (1997) Comparison of the long-term results of brachytherapy for T1-2N0 oral tongue cancer treated with Ir-192 and Ra-226. Anticancer Res 17(4A):2819–2822

140. Matsuura K, Hirokawa Y, Fujita M et al (1998) Treatment results of stage I and II oral tongue cancer with interstitial brachytherapy: maximum tumor thickness is prognostic of nodal metastasis. Int J Radiat Oncol Biol Phys 40(3):535–539

141. Yoshida K, Koizumi M, Inoue T et al (1999) Radiotherapy of early tongue cancer in patients less than 40 years old. Int J Radiat Oncol Biol Phys 45(2):367–371

142. Grabenbauer GG, Rodel C, Brunner T et al (2001) Interstitial brachytherapy with Ir-192 low-dose-rate in the treatment of primary and recurrent cancer of the oral cavity and oropharynx. Review of 318 patients treated between 1985 and 1997. Strahlenther Onkol 177(7):338–344

143. Marsiglia H, Haie-Meder C, Sasso G et al (2002) Brachytherapy for T1-T2 floor-of-the-mouth cancers: the Gustave-Roussy Institute experience. Int J Radiat Oncol Biol Phys 52(5):1257–1263

144. Inoue T, Yoshida K, Yoshioka Y et al (2001) Phase III trial of high- vs. low-dose-rate interstitial radiotherapy for early mobile tongue cancer. Int J Radiat Oncol Biol Phys 51(1):171–175

145. Yamazaki H, Yoshida K, Kotsuma T et al (2010) Age is not a limiting factor for brachytherapy for carcinoma of the node negative oral tongue in patients aged eighty or older. Radiat Oncol 5(1):116

146. Yoshimura R, Shibuya H, Hayashi K et al (2011) Disease control using low-dose-rate brachytherapy is unaffected by comorbid severity in oral cancer patients. Br J Radiol 84(1006):930–938

147. Khalilur R, Hayashi K, Shibuya H (2011) Brachytherapy for tongue cancer in the very elderly is an alternative to external beam radiation. Br J Radiol 84(1004):747–749

148. Strnad V, Lotter M, Kreppner S et al (2013) Interstitial pulsed-dose-rate brachytherapy for head and neck cancer—single-institution long-term results of 385 patients. Brachytherapy 12(6):521–527

149. Harrison LB, Sessions RB, Fass DE, Armstrong JG, Hunt M, Spiro RH (1992) Nasopharyngeal brachytherapy with access via a transpalatal flap. Am J Surg 164(2):173–175

150. Beumer J, Harrison R, Sanders B et al (1984) Osteoradionecrosis: predisposing factors and outcomes of therapy. Head Neck Surg 6(4):819–827

151. Barrett WL, Gleich L, Wilson K et al (2002) Organ preservation with interstitial radiation for base of tongue cancer. Am J Clin Oncol 25(5):485–488

152. Gibbs IC, Le Q-T, Shah RD et al (2003) Long-term outcomes after external beam irradiation and brachytherapy boost for base-of-tongue cancers. Int J Radiat Oncol Biol Phys 57(2):489–494

153. Tornesello ML, Perri F, Buonaguro L et al (2014) HPV-related oropharyngeal cancers: from pathogenesis to new therapeutic approaches. Cancer Lett 351(2):198–205

154. Chenevert J, Chiosea S (2012) Incidence of human papillomavirus in oropharyngeal squamous cell carcinomas: now and 50 years ago. Hum Pathol 43(1):17–22

155. Fakhry C, Westra WH, Li S et al (2008) Improved survival of patients with human papillomavirus-positive head and neck squamous cell carcinoma in a prospective clinical trial. J Natl Cancer Inst 100(4):261–269

156. Ang KK, Zhang Q, Rosenthal DI et al (2014) Randomized phase III trial of concurrent accelerated

radiation plus cisplatin with or without cetuximab for stage III to IV head and neck carcinoma: RTOG 0522. J Clin Oncol 32(27):2940–2950

157. Schmitt NC, Duvvuri U (2015) Transoral robotic surgery for oropharyngeal squamous cell carcinoma. Curr Opin Otolaryngol Head Neck Surg 23(2):127–131

158. Hutcheson KA, Holsinger FC, Kupferman ME et al (2014) Functional outcomes after TORS for oropharyngeal cancer: a systematic review. Eur Arch Otorhinolaryngol 272(2):463–471

159. Lau HY, Hay JH, Flores AD et al (1996) Seven fractions of twice daily high dose-rate brachytherapy for node-negative carcinoma of the mobile tongue results in loss of therapeutic ratio. Radiother Oncol 39(1):15–18

160. Matsumoto K, Sasaki T, Shioyama Y et al (2013) Treatment outcome of high-dose-rate interstitial radiation therapy for patients with stage I and II mobile tongue cancer. Jpn J Clin Oncol 43(10):1012–1017

161. Rudoltz MS, Perkins RS, Luthmann RW et al (1999) High-dose-rate brachytherapy for primary carcinomas of the oral cavity and oropharynx. Laryngoscope 109(12):1967–1973

162. Takácsi-Nagy Z, Oberna F, Koltai P et al (2013) Long-term outcomes with high-dose-rate brachytherapy for the management of base of tongue cancer. Brachytherapy 12(6):535–541

163. Cowen D, Thomas L, Richaud P et al (1990) Cancer des lèvres. Résultas du traitement de 299 patients. Ann Oto-Laryngol 107:121–126

164. Orecchia R, Rampino M, Gribaudo S et al (1991) Interstitial brachytherapy for carcinomas of the lower lip. Results of treatment. Tumori 77:336–338

165. Van Limbergen E, Ding W, Haustermans K et al (1993) Lip cancer: local control results of low dose rate brachytherapy. The GEC-ESTRO 1993 survey on 2800 cases. Annual GEC ESTRO meeting. Venice

166. Gerbaulet A, Grande C, Chirat E et al (1994) Braquiterapia intersticial con iridio 192 en el carcinoma del labio: analysis de 231 casos tratados en el Institut Gustave Roussy. Oncologia 17:45–49

167. Beauvois S, Hoffstetter S, Peiffert D et al (1994) Brachytherapy for lower lip epidermoid cancer: tumoral and treatment factors influencing recurrences and complications. Radiother Oncol 33(3):195–203

168. Conill C, Verger E, Marruecos J et al (2007) Low dose rate brachytherapy in lip carcinoma. Clin Transl Oncol 9(4):251–254

169. Johansson B, Karlsson L, Hardell L et al (2011) Clinical investigations long term results of PDR brachytherapy for lip cancer. J Contemp Brachyther 2:65–69

170. Rio E, Bardet E, Mervoyer A et al (2013) Interstitial brachytherapy for lower lip carcinoma: global assessment in a retrospective study of 89 cases. Head Neck 35(3):350–353

171. Serkies K, Ziemlewski A, Sawicki T et al (2013) Pulsed dose rate brachytherapy of lip cancer. J Contemp Brachyther 3:144–147

172. Nair MK, Sankaranarayanan R, Padmanabhan TK (1988) Evaluation of the role of radiotherapy in the management of carcinoma of the buccal mucosa. Cancer 61(7):1326–1331

173. Zitsch RP, Park CW, Renner GJ et al (1995) Outcome analysis for lip carcinoma. Otolaryngol Head Neck Surg 113(5):589–596

174. Umeda M, Komatsubara H, Ojima Y et al (2005) A comparison of brachytherapy and surgery for the treatment of stage I–II squamous cell carcinoma of the tongue. Int J Oral Maxillofac Surg 34(7):739–744

175. Yamazaki H, Inoue T, Yoshida K et al (2007) Comparison of three major radioactive sources for brachytherapy used in the treatment of node negative T1-T3 oral tongue cancer: influence of age on outcome. Anticancer Res 27(1B):491–497

176. Ayerra AQ, Mena EP, Fabregas JP et al (2010) Clinical investigations HDR and LDR brachytherapy in the treatment of lip cancer: the experience of the Catalan Institute of Oncology. J Contemp Brachyther 2(1):9–13

177. Ghadjar P, Bojaxhiu B, Simcock M et al (2012) High dose-rate versus low dose-rate brachytherapy for lip cancer. Int J Radiat Oncol Biol Phys 83(4):1205–1212

178. Teo P, Tsao SY, Shiu W et al (1989) A clinical study of 407 cases of nasopharyngeal carcinoma in Hong Kong. Int J Radiat Oncol Biol Phys 17(3):515–530

179. Wang CC (1991) Improved local control of nasopharyngeal carcinoma after intracavitary brachytherapy boost. Am J Clin Oncol 14(1):5–8

180. Chang JT, See LC, Tang SG et al (1996) The role of brachytherapy in early-stage nasopharyngeal carcinoma. Int J Radiat Oncol Biol Phys 36(5):1019–1024

181. Teo PM, Leung SF, Lee WY et al (2000) Intracavitary brachytherapy significantly enhances local control of early T-stage nasopharyngeal carcinoma: the existence of a dose-tumor-control relationship above conventional tumoricidal dose. Int J Radiat Oncol Biol Phys 46(2):445–458

182. Lee AW (2003) Contribution of radiotherapy to function preservation and cancer outcome in primary treatment of nasopharyngeal carcinoma. World J Surg 27(7):838–843

183. Lu JJ, Shakespeare TP, Kim Siang Tan L et al (2004) Adjuvant fractionated high-dose-rate intracavitary brachytherapy after external beam radiotherapy in T1 and T2 nasopharyngeal carcinoma. Head Neck 26(5):389–395

184. Ng T, Richards GM, Emery RS et al (2005) Customized conformal high-dose-rate brachytherapy boost for limited-volume nasopharyngeal cancer. Int J Radiat Oncol Biol Phys 61(3):754–761

185. Leung T-W, Wong VY, Sze W-K et al (2008) High-dose-rate intracavitary brachytherapy boost for early

T stage nasopharyngeal carcinoma{PRIVATE}. Int J Radiat Oncol Biol Phys 70(2):361–367

186. Wu J, Guo Q, Lu JJ et al (2013) Addition of intracavitary brachytherapy to external beam radiation therapy for T1–T2 nasopharyngeal carcinoma. Brachytherapy 12(5):479–486

187. Levendag PC, Keskin-Cambay F, de Pan C et al (2013) Local control in advanced cancer of the nasopharynx: is a boost dose by endocavitary brachytherapy of prognostic significance? Brachytherapy 12(1):84–89

188. Rosenblatt E, Abdel-Wahab M, El-Gantiry M et al (2014) Brachytherapy boost in loco-regionally advanced nasopharyngeal carcinoma: a prospective randomized trial of the International Atomic Energy Agency. Radiat Oncol 9(67):9–67

189. Choy D, Sham JS, Wei WI et al (1993) Transpalatal insertion of radioactive gold grain for the treatment of persistent and recurrent nasopharyngeal carcinoma. Int J Radiat Oncol Biol Phys 25(3):505–512

190. Koutcher L, Lee N, Zelefsky M et al (2010) Reirradiation of locally recurrent nasopharynx cancer with external beam radiotherapy with or without brachytherapy. Int J Radiat Oncol Biol Phys 76(1):130–137

191. Ren YF, Cao XP, Xu J et al (2013) 3D-image-guided high-dose-rate intracavitary brachytherapy for salvage treatment of locally persistent nasopharyngeal carcinoma. Radiat Oncol 8(165):8–165

192. Teo PM, Leung SF, Tung SY et al (2006) Dose–response relationship of nasopharyngeal carcinoma above conventional tumoricidal level: A study by the Hong Kong nasopharyngeal carcinoma study group (HKNPCSG). Radiother Oncol 79(1):27–33

193. Al-Sarraf M, LeBlanc M, Giri PG et al (1998) Chemoradiotherapy versus radiotherapy in patients with advanced nasopharyngeal cancer: phase III randomized Intergroup study 0099. J Clin Oncol 16(4):1310–1317

194. Chen HH, Tsai S-T, Wang M-S et al (2006) Experience in fractionated stereotactic body radiation therapy boost for newly diagnosed nasopharyngeal carcinoma. Int J Radiat Oncol Biol Phys 66(5):1408–1414

195. Karim AB, Kralendonk JH, Njo KH et al (1990) Ethmoid and upper nasal cavity carcinoma: treatment, results and complications. Radiother Oncol 19(2):109–120

196. McCollough WM, Mendenhall NP, Parsons JT et al (1993) Radiotherapy alone for squamous cell carcinoma of the nasal vestibule: management of the primary site and regional lymphatics. Int J Radiat Oncol Biol Phys 26(1):73–79

197. Tiwari R, Hardillo JA, Tobi H et al (1999) Carcinoma of the ethmoid: results of treatment with conventional surgery and post-operative radiotherapy. Eur J Surg Oncol 25(4):401–405

198. Allen MW, Schwartz DL, Rana V et al (2008) Long-term radiotherapy outcomes for nasal cavity and septal cancers. Int J Radiat Oncol Biol Phys 71(2):401–406

199. Nag S, Schuller D, Pak V et al (1996) Pilot study of intraoperative high dose rate brachytherapy for head and neck cancer. Radiother Oncol 41(2):125–130

200. Klein M, Menneking H, Langford A et al (1998) Treatment of squamous cell carcinomas of the floor of the mouth and tongue by interstitial high-dose-rate irradiation using iridium-192. Int J Oral Maxillofac Surg 27(1):45–48

201. Pellizzon AC, dos Santos Novaes PE, Conte Maia MA et al (2005) Interstitial high-dose-rate brachytherapy combined with cervical dissection on head and neck cancer. Head Neck 27(12):1035–1041

202. Kupferman ME, Morrison WH, Santillan AA et al (2007) The role of interstitial brachytherapy with salvage surgery for the management of recurrent head and neck cancers. Cancer 109(10):2052–2057

203. Schiefke F, Hildebrandt G, Pohlmann S et al (2008) Combination of surgical resection and HDR-brachytherapy in patients with recurrent or advanced head and neck carcinomas. J Craniomaxillofac Surg 36(5):285–292

204. Perry DJ, Chan K, Wolden S et al (2010) High-dose-rate intraoperative radiation therapy for recurrent head-and-neck cancer. Int J Radiat Oncol Biol Phys 76(4):1140–1146

205. Tselis N, Ratka M, Vogt H-G et al (2011) Hypofractionated accelerated CT-guided interstitial 192Ir-HDR-Brachytherapy as re-irradiation in inoperable recurrent cervical lymphadenopathy from head and neck cancer. Radiother Oncol 98(1):57–62

206. Martínez-Monge R, Pagola Divassón M, Cambeiro M et al (2011) Determinants of complications and outcome in high-risk squamous cell head-and-neck cancer treated with Perioperative High–Dose Rate Brachytherapy (PHDRB). Int J Radiat Oncol Biol Phys 81(4):e245–e254

207. Rudzianskas V, Inciura A, Juozaityte E et al (2012) Reirradiation of recurrent head and neck cancer using high-dose-rate brachytherapy. Acta Otorhinolaryngol Ital 32(5):297–303

208. Scala LM, Hu K, Urken ML et al (2013) Intraoperative high-dose-rate radiotherapy in the management of locoregionally recurrent head and neck cancer. Head Neck 35(4):485–492

209. Strnad V, Lotter M, Kreppner S et al (2014) Re-irradiation with interstitial pulsed-dose-rate brachytherapy for unresectable recurrent head and neck carcinoma. Brachytherapy 13(2):187–195

210. Chuang SC, Scelo G, Tonita JM et al (2008) Risk of second primary cancer among patients with head and neck cancers: a pooled analysis of 13 cancer registries. Int J Cancer 123(10):2390–2396

211. Morris LG, Sikora AG, Patel SG et al (2011) Second primary cancers after an index head and neck cancer: subsite-specific trends in the era of human papillomavirus-associated oropharyngeal cancer. J Clin Oncol 29(6):739–746

212. Chaturvedi AK, Engels EA, Pfeiffer RM et al (2011) Human papillomavirus and rising oropharyngeal cancer incidence in the United States. J Clin Oncol 29(32):4294–4301

213. Mroz EA, Forastiere AA, Rocco JW (2011) Implications of the oropharyngeal cancer epidemic. J Clin Oncol 29(32):4222–4223. doi:10.1200/JCO.2011.37.8893, Epub 2011 Oct 3

214. Marx RE (1983) Osteoradionecrosis: a new concept of its pathophysiology. J Oral Maxillofac Surg 41(5):283–288

215. Suryawanshi A, Pawar V, Singh M et al (2014) Maxillofacial osteoradionecrosis. J Dent Res Rev 1(1):42

216. Delanian S, Chatel C, Porcher R et al (2011) Complete restoration of refractory mandibular osteoradionecrosis by prolonged treatment with a pentoxifylline-tocopherol-clodronate combination (PENTOCLO): a phase II trial. Int J Radiat Oncol Biol Phys 80(3):832–839

217. Shaw RJ, Butterworth C (2011) Hyperbaric oxygen in the management of late radiation injury to the head and neck. Part II: prevention. Br J Oral Maxillofac Surg 49(1):9–13

218. Shaw RJ, Dhanda J (2011) Hyperbaric oxygen in the management of late radiation injury to the head and neck. Part I: treatment. Br J Oral Maxillofac Surg 49(1):2–8

219. Annane D, Depondt J, Aubert P et al (2004) Hyperbaric oxygen therapy for radionecrosis of the jaw: a randomized, placebo-controlled, double-blind trial from the ORN96 study group. J Clin Oncol 22(24):4893–4900

220. Fritz GW, Gunsolley JC, Abubaker O et al (2010) Efficacy of pre- and post-irradiation hyperbaric oxygen therapy in the prevention of post-extraction osteoradionecrosis: a systematic review. J Oral Maxillofac Surg 68(11):2653–2660

221. Bhandare N, Mendenhall WM (2012) A literature review of late complications of radiation therapy for head and neck cancers: incidence and dose response. Nucl Med Radiat Ther S2:009

222. Xu J, Cao Y (2014) Radiation-induced carotid artery stenosis: a comprehensive review of the literature. Intervent Neurol 2(4):183–192

223. Scott AS, Parr LA, Johnstone PA (2009) Risk of cerebrovascular events after neck and supraclavicular radiotherapy: a systematic review. Radiother Oncol 90(2):163–165

224. Marineloo G, Wilson JF, Pierquin B et al (1985) The guide gutter or loop techniques of interstitial implantation and the Paris system of dosimetry. Radiother Oncol 4:265–273

Breast Brachytherapy: Interstitial Breast Brachytherapy

Csaba Polgár and Tibor Major

Abstract

Interstitial brachytherapy used in the management of breast cancer has enjoyed broad acceptance among many in the field. It is a complex technical procedure that requires great skill and significant experience to be properly performed. We present a detailed and thorough discussion of the technique, evidence, and results in this chapter.

1 Introduction

Before the era of breast-conserving therapy, interstitial brachytherapy (BT) implants (with or without external-beam irradiation) were used to treat large, inoperable tumors [1, 2]. Later interstitial BT with rigid needles or multiple flexible catheters was used to deliver an additional (boost) dose to the tumor bed after breast-conserving surgery (BCS) and whole-breast irradiation (WBI) [3–6]. In the last two decades, the new concept of accelerated partial-breast irradiation (APBI) opened a new perspective for breast BT [7–9]. APBI is an attractive treatment approach that shortens the 5–7-week course of conventional postoperative radiotherapy (RT) to 4–5 days. The acceleration of RT eliminates some of the disadvantages of the extended treatment period, especially for elderly patients, working women, and those who live at a significant distance from the RT facility. The rationale for APBI is that the majority of local recurrences (LRs) occur in close proximity to the tumor bed [3, 7, 9]. Less than 20 % of LRs appear "elsewhere" in the breast, and the absolute number of such failures is very low (e.g., far less than 1 % per year and similar to the rate of new contralateral tumors) [10, 11]. In addition, some elsewhere failures are likely to be new primary breast cancers that arose after initial therapy and hence would not have been prevented by WBI. Thus, in the last two decades, APBI using low-dose-rate (LDR), high-dose-rate (HDR), or pulsed-dose-rate (PDR) interstitial implants has been intensively evaluated in phase I–II (and later in phase III) studies as a possible alternative to conventional WBI [7–9].

C. Polgár, MD, PhD, MSc (✉)
Center of Radiotherapy, National Institute of
Oncology, Budapest, Hungary
e-mail: polgar@oncol.hu

T. Major, PhD
Department of Medical Physics, Center of
Radiotherapy, National Institute of Oncology,
Budapest, Hungary

© Springer International Publishing Switzerland 2016
P. Montemaggi et al. (eds.), *Brachytherapy: An International Perspective*, Medical Radiology,
DOI 10.1007/978-3-319-26791-3_8

The first technique utilized in early APBI studies was multicatheter interstitial BT [12–18]. The implementation of all other techniques (including 3-D conformal external-beam irradiation and intraoperative radiotherapy) to deliver APBI was based on the success of these phase I–II clinical studies using multicatheter breast implants. Beyond classical interstitial BT, recently new intracavitary balloon applicators have been developed to decrease the existing barrier against the widespread use of multicatheter BT [19, 20]. Furthermore, permanent breast seed implants have been also implemented as an alternative for stepping-source multicatheter BT [21]. However in this chapter, we will give an overview on interstitial breast BT used as a boost or sole postoperative irradiation after BCS. Management of ipsilateral breast tumor recurrence (IBTR) as well as breast intracavitary and seed techniques will be reported in other chapters of this text.

2   Indications for Interstitial Breast Brachytherapy

2.1   Indications for Tumor Bed Boost

The standard technique of RT after BCS is to treat the whole breast by teletherapy via tangential fields up to a total dose of 45–50 Gy. The main rationale to give an additional dose of 10–25 Gy to the tumor bed after WBI was based on the clinical observation that 67–100 % of ipsilateral breast recurrences originated from the vicinity of the original index lesion [3]. Based on the analysis of dose-response curves, Van Limbergen et al. [6] reported that above 50 Gy, an increase of 15 Gy would reduce the LR rate by a factor of 2. To date, multiple randomized trials have confirmed that a boost dose of 10–16 Gy after 50 Gy WBI significantly decreased the LR rate (Table 1) [3, 22–25]. Patient age less than 50 years; close, microscopically positive, or unknown surgical margins; and the presence of an extensive intraductal component (EIC) are generally accepted as indications for boost

irradiation [3, 6, 8]. Other factors (e.g., lympho-vascular invasion (LVI), high-grade tumors, and large tumor size >3 cm) can be also considered for the indication of a tumor bed boost.

Traditionally LDR BT, electrons, or photons have been used to deliver the boost dose to the tumor bed [1, 22, 25–29]. Later HDR BT has been also accepted as a safe alternative boost modality [5, 30–39]. However, a controversy still exists regarding the optimal boost technique. Interstitial BT is preferable in some anatomical situations, especially in cases of deep-seated tumor beds in large-volume breasts. Obviously, BT offers the practical advantage of more conformal treatment of small volumes to higher doses and lower doses to the skin [6, 40]. Van Limbergen [6] compared dose distributions of 4.5–15 MeV electron boosts to different settings of interstitial implants. He found that for target depths reaching beyond 2.8 cm under the skin, interstitial implants had a ballistic advantage delivering significantly lower skin doses than electron beams. Thus, in addition to external-beam boost modalities, interstitial BT is a standard treatment option to deliver an additional dose to the tumor bed after BCS and WBI.

2.2   Indications for APBI

Patient selection in early APBI clinical trials was flawed or absolutely inadequate [12–15, 41–43]. In later studies patient selection criteria were refined excluding patients with high risk for multicentricity from APBI protocols [17, 18, 45–53] Based on the limited scientific evidence obtained mainly from phase I–II prospective clinical trials, professional scientific organizations both in the USA and Europe have generated and published their recommendations on patient selection for APBI Table 2 [4, 54–57]. These recommendations provide conservative and useful clinical guidance regarding the safe use of APBI outside the context of a clinical trial. In addition to the ASTRO "suitable" and GEC-ESTRO "good candidate" groups, both the ASTRO consensus guidelines and the GEC-ESTRO recommendations

Table 1 Results of randomized "boost versus no boost" trials

Clinical trial	Patient no.	Technique	Boost dose (Gy)	Median FUP (years)	5-year LR boost vs. no boost (%)	20-year LR boost vs. no boost (%)	p-value
EORTC [22]	5318	EBI/LDR BT	15–16	17.2	4.3 vs. 7.3	12.0 vs. 16.4	<0.0001
Budapest [3, 23, 24]	627	ELE/HDR BT	12–16	5	6.3 vs. 13.3	NR	0.0017
Lyon [25]	1024	ELE	10	3.3	3.6 vs. 4.5	NR	0.044

EORTC European Organisation for Research and Treatment of Cancer, *FUP* follow-up period, *LR* local recurrence, *EBI* external-beam irradiation (photons or electrons), *ELE* electrons, *LDR* low dose rate, *HDR* high dose rate, *BT* brachytherapy

Table 2 ASTRO, GEC-ESTRO, ABS, and DEGRO patient selection criteria for the routine use of APBI outside of clinical trials

Characteristic	ASTRO [56]	GEC-ESTRO [4]	ABS [56]	DEGRO [54]
Patient age (years)	≥60	>50	≥50	>70
Tumor size (cm)	≤2	≤3	≤3	<2
Surgical margins (cm)	≥0.2	≥0.2	Negative	Negative
Nodal status	pN0 (SNB or AD)	pN0 (SNB or AD)	pN0 (SNB or AD)	pN0 (SNB or AD)
Histology	IDC or other favorable subtypes	IDC, mucinous, tubular, medullary, and colloid cc.	All invasive subtypes + DCIS	IDC luminal A type
ILC	Not allowed	Not allowed	Allowed	Not allowed
DCIS	Not allowed	Not allowed	Allowed	Not allowed
Multicentricity	Unicentric only	Unicentric only	NS	NS
Multifocality	Clinically unifocal with total size ≤2 cm	Unifocal only	NS	NS
EIC	Not allowed	Not allowed	NS	Not allowed
LVI	Not allowed	Not allowed	Not allowed	NS
Receptor status	ER positive	Any	Any	ER and PR pos., HER2 neg.
HG	Any	Any	NS	1–2
Neoadjuvant therapy	Not allowed	Not allowed	NS	NS

ASTRO American Society for Radiation Oncology, *GEC-ESTRO* Groupe Européen de Curiethérapie-European Society for Therapeutic Radiology and Oncology, *ABS* American Brachytherapy Society, *DEGRO* Deutsche Gesellschaft für Radiotherapie, *SNB* sentinel node biopsy, *AD* axillary dissection, *IDC* invasive ductal carcinoma, *ILC* invasive lobular carcinoma, *DCIS* ductal carcinoma in situ, *LVI* lympho-vascular invasion, *EIC* extensive intraductal carcinoma, *ER* estrogen receptor, *PR* progesterone receptor, *HG* histologic grade, *NS* no statement

defined an intermediate group of patients (the so-called ASTRO "cautionary" and GEC-ESTRO "possible candidate" groups) for whom APBI considered acceptable only with caution or preferably in the context of prospective clinical trials [4, 56]. The third group of women (defined as the ASTRO "unsuitable" and GEC-ESTRO "high-risk" groups) should not be treated with APBI, as there is enough evidence against the use of APBI for such patients. The validity of these recommendations has been tested in several studies and highlighted the limitations of such guidelines [52, 57, 58]. However, until large-scale randomized clinical trial outcome data become available, these guidelines serve as clinically useful tools for the selection of patients for APBI and promote further clinical research focusing on controversial issues in the radiation therapy of early-stage breast carcinoma.

2.3 Techniques

Technically there is no difference between whether the treatment is a boost or sole postoperative irradiation after (BCS). Different techniques exist, but the implantation is always performed using stainless steel needles with sharply beveled tips (trocars) which are then exchanged with flexible plastic catheters. Then, the catheters are fixed to skin with locking buttons without skin sutures and are trimmed at a consistent length. Using the comfort catheter system (Elekta AB, Stockholm, Sweden), which is a "catheter-within-a-catheter" system, there is no catheter protruding past the fixation buttons and therefore it is very comfortable for the patient. Just for the irradiation, another thin inner catheter is temporarily inserted into the outer one (Fig. 1) in which the ^{192}Ir source can be advanced after connecting it to the afterloader.

There are centers where the boost dose is delivered only with one or two to three fractions. In this case the rigid needles are used not only for insertion but also for the irradiation. The needles are inserted under ultrasound (US) guidance by freehand technique or using a template [59].

Whatever dose delivery method is used, the most important goal during implantation is to place the catheters in an appropriate distribution in order to geometrically cover the target volume. In the intraoperative setting only, visual inspection of the lumpectomy cavity helps to place the needles, but when the implantation is performed a few weeks after cavity closure, image guidance is always needed for proper implantation. Different types of imaging modalities can be used, including US, mammography, and CT.

2.4 Freehand Catheter Insertion

Historically, this was the first breast BT technique. The catheters are inserted into the breast in the operating room while the skin incision is open. The edges of the lumpectomy cavity are marked on the skin, and under visual inspection, needles are inserted manually with appropriate geometry in order to cover the target volume and ensure homogeneous dose distribution. When all catheters are in place, the surgeon closes the wound cavity. A few days later, postimplant CT scans are taken for treatment planning. This technique requires thorough skill and experience from the radiation oncologist. Moreover, without

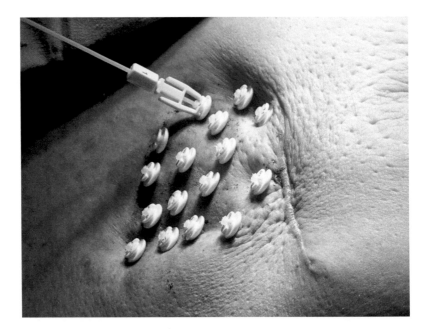

Fig. 1 The Comfort catheter system with the implanted outer catheters and one inner catheter. The outer catheters are fixed to skin with locking buttons

imaging, it is difficult to determine the target volume related to the catheters. For these reasons this technique is less commonly used.

When the BT treatment is performed postoperatively with closed cavity in a separate procedure, all needles can be inserted under US guidance, provided that the excision cavity is readily seen. First, the cavity is projected and marked on the skin and then each needle, one by one, is inserted using real-time US guidance [60]. This technique is also very skill dependent, since holding the US probe and inserting a needle at the same time is quite challenging and requires extensive knowledge and much experience.

2.5 Image-Guided Catheter Implantation

When performing implantation a few weeks after the lumpectomy, some kind of imaging before or during the insertions is necessary for placing the adequate number of catheters in the correct geometry in relation to the cavity volume. The use of a template around the involved breast is of great help to achieve this. However, the template with the holes has to be visualized on an image together with the cavity geometry in order to select the appropriate holes to be used for needle insertions.

2.6 Implantation with Mammography

Generally, but not exclusively, the implantation of catheters in breast BT is performed in the supine position which is the standard patient positioning in RT. However, the implantation can be done in the prone position as well. An advantage of this technique is that the breast tissue pulls away from the chest wall, pectoral muscles, and ribs which makes the deep-plane implantation easier. The patient is lying on a stereotactic core needle breast biopsy table, and with a template and built-in mammography equipment, the catheters can be placed accurately in relation to the target volume [61]. To help the cavity

localization, contrast medium is injected into lumpectomy cavity by US guidance for better visualization. Having taken a mammographic image, the cavity and the holes of the templates are clearly seen on the superimposed image, and the template coordinates of the needles covering the target volume can be easily identified. Since the breast hangs by gravity, the template can be pushed up against the chest wall, and in this way adequate deep-plane position can be achieved. Finally, when all needles are in place, they are replaced with plastic catheters, and the treatment planning is done the next day. The CT image acquisition and the dose delivery are done in the supine position.

2.7 Implantation with US Guidance

Ultrasound imaging is an effective method to localize the surgical cavity, define the target volume, and guide the implantation [61, 62]. As a first step, the dimensions of the cavity are defined as the largest extension of the hypoechoic region in the three cardinal directions. The distance between the superior cavity wall and skin and the depth of chest wall can be also measured. After target volume localization, the implant geometry is designed and the entry and exit points of the needles are marked on the skin. Then, under real-time US guidance, the superficial needles are inserted one by one. For intermediate- and deep-plane needles, a template can be used which makes the insertions of the remaining needles easier.

2.8 Implantation with CT Guidance

Various CT-based techniques exist for interstitial brachytherapy, but the entrance and exit planes or points of the catheters on the skin are always determined using the 3-D rendering of the target volume and patient anatomy. When the implantation and the imaging are done in the same room after placement of a few needles (e.g., in the deep plane), a CT image can be used for initial evaluation of target coverage. Then, the remaining needles are inserted manually in a standard pattern with 1.0–1.5-cm separation [63]. If needed, additional CT imaging can be performed, and with frequent imaging, the optimal catheter placement is ensured. Planning the catheter positions on the skin can be done with radiopaque angiographic catheters placed on the involved breast [64] or using a plastic template during preimplant CT imaging [7, 65]. Then, using 3-D rendering of patient anatomy and virtual simulation, the appropriate catheter positions can be defined. A few needles (e.g., deep plane) can be inserted freehand with or without real-time intraoperative US guidance. The remainder should be guided by a template. Alternately, all needle insertions are performed via template. When the imaging and insertion are performed in one session, a CT-compatible template is placed on the involved breast after the radiation oncologist locates the scar and palpates the seroma. For template fixation, catheters or needles can be used in a few template holes, and these can also help orient the template in a 3-D view [61]. Contrast material can then be injected directly into lumpectomy cavity to help in contouring the cavity. With 3-D rendering and creating a "needle's eye view," visualization of the proposed needle holes can be identified. In another technique, two CT image series (pre and post implant) are used for implantation and planning [7, 65]. First, one day before the implantation, a CT-compatible plastic template is placed proximate to the involved breast taking into account the scar position on the skin and other relevant clinical information about the tumor location. Geometrical parameters of the template are recorded and its position is marked on the skin (Fig. 2). Preimplant CT imaging is performed, and the cavity is outlined in axial slices and the target volume is created according to the contouring protocol. Then, using 3-D rendering, the patient is rotated in the "needle's eye view", and the target volume is projected on the rendered

template with the holes. By visual inspection, the holes covering the target volume are identified, and their coordinates recorded (Fig. 3). The next day, another more rigid template, geometrically identical to the first, is placed proximate to the breast in the same position using the skin marks and template parameters. Then, using the predefined coordinates, the needles are inserted into the breast and are later replaced with plastic catheters. Additional CT images are acquired for planning, and the cavity, target volume, and organs at risk are outlined. The catheters are reconstructed using the CT and dose planning is performed. According to the target definition rules used in the GEC-ESTRO APBI trial, the PTV is defined as the expansion of the contoured cavity (including surgical clips) in each direction with an individual margin of 2.0 cm minus the actual width of the pathological surgical margin. The expansion of the PTV is limited to 0.5 cm below the skin and at the pectoral fascia (Figs. 4 and 5). When inadequate target coverage is obtained by the catheters, a few additional catheters are implanted manually by freehand technique. Obviously, in this case new CT imaging is taken for planning.

3   Quality and Reporting Standards

A good implant in interstitial BT is characterized by adequate dose coverage, high-dose homogeneity inside and steep dose falloff outside the target volume. The evaluation of a plan can be done in qualitative and quantitative manner. In classical BT, the plan evaluation was limited to having dose values in reference points and looking at 2-D dose distributions related to catheters/applicators. The use of these evaluation methods is still recommended, but in modern BT additional tools are now available to assess the quality of the implant. The 3-D dose calculation algorithm and real 3-D anatomical information about the patient make it possible to use the target- and organ-related DVH and volumetric

Fig. 2 CT-compatible plastic template on the breast (**a**) and its marked position on the skin (**b**)

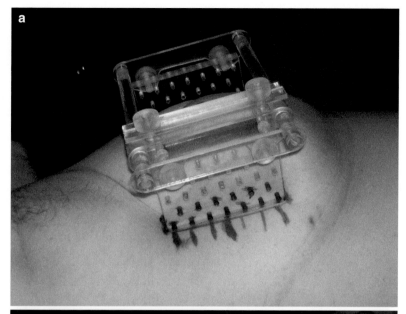

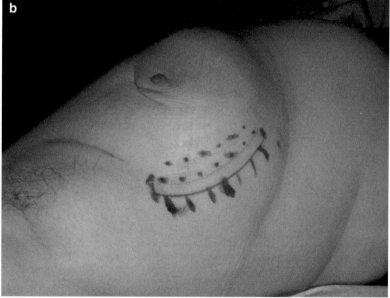

parameters. This means that the treatment planning and plan evaluation have to be based on the real 3-D volume of the PTV and organs at risk. From the DVH, a given amount of a volume receiving a certain dose can be quantitatively calculated and from those data different quality indices can be determined, which serve as objective and quantitative measures of the accuracy and quality of the implant.

3.1 Parameters Related to Implant Geometry

In interstitial BT, high-dose regions occur in proximity of the radioactive source(s), which is a consequence of a basic geometrical phenomenon: the inverse-square law. Due to the high-dose gradient around the sources, it is difficult to achieve a uniform dose distribution in the

Fig. 3 Needle's eye view of the template with patient anatomy. The projection of the target volume (*red wire frames*) to the front side of the template helps to identify the holes to be used for inserting needles.

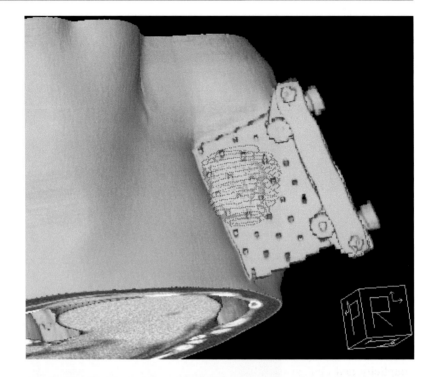

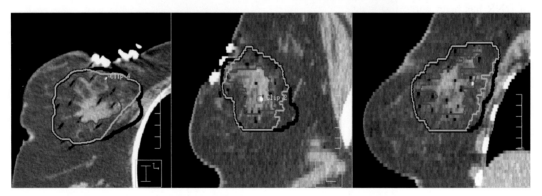

Fig. 4 PTV definition on postimplant CT images for multicatheter APBI. Cavity, *red line*; expanded tumor bed, *black line*; final PTV, *green line*. The final PTV is defined excluding the pectoral muscle and a 0.5-cm rim of tissue below the skin

target volume, however with appropriate source placement; a relatively uniform dose distribution can be obtained. For quantitative dose assessment of interstitial implants, the dose nonuniformity ratio (DNR) was introduced [66] as the ratio of the high-dose volume to the reference volume. By definition, $DNR = V_{1.5 \times PD}/V_{PD}$, where the reference volume (V_{PD}) is the volume receiving equal to or greater dose than the prescribed dose (PD), the high-dose volume ($V_{1.5 \times PD}$) is a volume that receives equal to or greater dose than the $1.5 \times PD$. For a specific implant configuration, the reference isodose can be selected in such a way that the DNR is minimal, resulting in an optimal dose distribution in terms of dose uniformity. The DNR as a quantitative parameter for evaluating dose uniformity is always specific to the implant configuration

Fig. 5 Dose distribution on postimplant CT image. PTV, *Thick red line*; 100 % (reference) isodose, *thin red line*; 50 % isodose, *green line*; 150 % isodose, *yellow line*; 200 % isodose, *blue line*

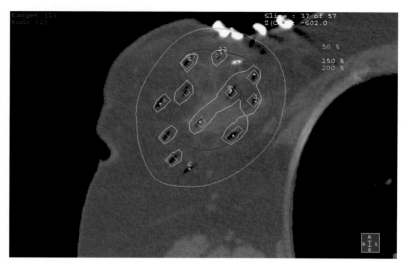

and the relative isodose line selected for prescription, but it does not depend on the absolute value of the dose prescription. Because of its simplicity and clinical usefulness, the concept of DNR has been widely accepted and used. In breast implants, the DNR is expected to be in the range of 0.2–0.35.

3.2 Parameters Related to Target Volume

For a CT-based plan, after delineation of the target volume and critical organs, a target- and organ-related DVH can be calculated, and additional parameters can be defined for plan evaluation [65, 66]. By definition Vxx is the volume of tissue treated to at least xx% of the prescribed dose. Note that the volume can be of the PTV, the breast, or normal tissue. The coverage index (CI) is the fraction of the PTV receiving a dose equal to or greater than the PD. From this definition it follows that $V100 = 100 \times CI$, if $V100$ relates to the target volume. The homogeneity index (HI) is the fraction of the PTV receiving a dose between 100 and 150 % of the PD. In case the homogeneity is not restricted to target volume, but to the whole implant, the term of dose homogeneity index (DHI) is used instead of HI [66].

By definition, $DHI = (V100–V150)/V100$. Sometimes the overdose volume index (OI) is also reported, which is the fraction of the PTV receiving a dose equal to or greater than twice the PD. Additional dose parameters (e.g., D100, D90) are recommended to use for quantitative plan evaluation. D100 is the maximal percentage dose that irradiates the full PTV (same as minimal target dose); D90 is the percentage dose that irradiates 90 % of the PTV.

For quantifying the conformality of dose distribution, the conformal index (COIN) was defined [67] as follows: $COIN = c_1 \times c_2$, where $c_1 = PTV_{ref}/V_{PTV}$ and $c_2 = PTV_{ref}/V_{ref}$. The PTV_{ref} is the volume of the PTV receiving a dose equal to or greater than the reference dose (prescribed dose). The V_{PTV} is the volume of the PTV and V_{ref} is the volume receiving a dose equal to or greater than the reference dose. The COIN takes into consideration the coverage of the PTV by the reference dose (c_1) and also the unwanted irradiation of normal tissue outside the PTV (c_2). In an ideal case, both coefficients (c_1 and c_2) are equal to 1. In real situations, this never happens and therefore the COIN value is less than 1. The best dose distribution, in terms of conformality, is obtained when the COIN is maximal. In breast implants the COIN for a good implant is expected to be larger than 0.5.

3.3 Plan Evaluation in Clinical Studies

No commonly accepted parameters exist for evaluating interstitial breast implants. Various metrics and indices are used in the literature depending on the complexity of the planning method. Table 3 shows the parameters used for reporting dosimetry of breast implants in two large, multicentric, randomized APBI studies. Note that in the GEC-ESTRO study, the DHI is calculated for the target volume. According to the definition of the DNR and the DHI, they are complementary parameters $(DNR = 1 - DHI)$. The use of mean central dose (MCD) and $V_{1.5 \times MCD}$ (high-dose volume) is recommended by ICRU 58 [68].

Although the quantitative dosimetric measures of implants are frequently used in clinical trials, their correlation to clinical outcome (local control, late side effects) is still unclarified. More clinical research is needed to find which parameters should be calculated and reported to characterize the optimal implant. Furthermore, due to the diversity of dose prescriptions (to reference point/points, isodose line or DVH-based), any comparison of the dosimetric and clinical results from different institutions has to be made cautiously.

4 Results

4.1 Results of Interstitial Implants as a Boost After WBI

Only a few reports compared the outcome in patients treated with interstitial BT or external-beam boost (Table 4) [1, 22–24, 26, 28–30, 35–37, 69]. In the classical trial of the Institut Curie, women with 3–7-cm breast cancer treated by irradiation alone were randomized to ^{192}Ir BT versus ^{60}Co teletherapy boost after WBI [1]. The 8-year LR rate was significantly lower with LDR BT compared to external-beam boost (24 % vs. 39 %; $p = 0.02$). However, in the postoperative setting, similar local control and cosmetic results have been reported for women boosted either

Table 3 Quantitative dose and volume parameters used for reporting multicatheter breast brachytherapy implants in the American and European multicentric randomized APBI trials

	NSABP B-39/RTOG 0413	GEC-ESTRO
For implant	DHI	DNR, MCD, $V_{1.5 \times MCD}$
For PTV_EVAL	V90	V90, V100, V150, DHI, COIN
For skin	D_{max}	D_{max}
For breast	V50, V150, V200	–

DHI dose homogeneity index, *DNR* dose nonuniformity ratio, *MCD* mean central dose, *COIN* conformal index

with interstitial implants or electrons/photons. In the EORTC boost trial, the 20-year cumulative incidence of LR was 9.9 % for the 1640 patients who received an electron boost, 7.8 % in the 753 patients who received a photon boost, and only 6.2 % in the 225 patients who had an interstitial LDR BT boost [22]. The difference was not significant ($p = 0.094$); however the trial was not powered to detect the possible difference in local control between different boost modalities.

Recently, Knauerhase et al. [36] reported that a median dose of 10 Gy HDR BT boost yielded significantly lower 10-year actuarial LR rate compared to external-beam boost (5.9 % vs. 12.5 %; $p = 0.023$). The long-term results of several other (mainly European) clinical studies proved that HDR BT used either as a single fraction of 7–12 Gy or as a fractionated boost was safe and yielded excellent local control [30–39, 47, 70, 71] (Table 5).

4.2 Results of Interstitial Implants as Sole APBI

4.2.1 Early APBI Brachytherapy Trials

Several European and American centers pioneered the use of different APBI regimens for unselected patients in the 1980s and early 1990s [12–15, 41–43]. However, results in all but one of these early studies were poor, with high LR rates (Table 6). The high rates of local failure seen in these early APBI studies

Table 4 Results of comparative studies with different boost (brachytherapy vs. external beam) techniques after whole-breast irradiation

Institution/study	Technique	Patient no.	Boost dose (Gy)	Median FUP (years)	5-year LR % (n)	p-value	Exc./good cosmesis %	p-value
Saarbrücken [35]	HDR	202	12–15	>3	6.4[a]	NR	85	NA
	ELE	91	12–15	>3	8.8[a]		NR	
Institut Curie, Paris [1]	LDR	126	20–25	8.1	24 (8-year)[b]	0.02	71	0.6
	Cobalt-60	129	11–36	8.1	39 (8-year)[b]		75	
Thomas Jefferson [26]	LDR	654	15–20	3.3	7	0.21	91	NS
	ELE	416	20	3.3	8		95	
Hôpital Tenon, Paris [26]	LDR	169	15–25	6.7	8.1 (10-year)	0.32	61	0.001
	ELE	161	5–20	6.9	13.5 (10-year)		83	
Mallinckrodt Institute of Radiology [69]	LDR	119	10–20	5.6	6.7	NS	82	NS
	ELE	487	10–20	5.6	6.2		80	
WBH, Michigan [28]	LDR (I-125)	87	15	3.8	3 (8-year)	0.46	94	0.59
	LDR (Ir-192)	190	15	6.3	9 (8-year)		88	
	ELE	108	10–15	4.2	9 (8-year)		90	
	Photons	15	10–15	4.5	0 (8-year)		82	
Tufts University [29]	LDR	127	20	>6	3.9	0.62	90	0.001
	ELE	87	20	>6	3.2		78	
Budapest [23, 24]	HDR	66	8–14.25	5	8.5	0.43	90	0.29
	ELE	237	16	5	5.6		86	
EORTC [22]	LDR	225	15	17.2	6.2[a]	0.094	NR	NA
	ELE	1640	16	17.2	9.9[a]		NR	
	Photons	753	16	17.2	7.8[a]		NR	
TMH, Mumbai [30]	HDR	153	10	3	8	0.43	83	<0.001
	LDR	383	15–20	6	10		84	<0.00001
	ELE	460	15	2.75	7		69	
University of Rostock [36]	HDR	75	8–12	7.8	5.9 (10-year)	0.023	NR	NA
	ELE + photons	181	6–14	7.8	12.5 (10-year)		NR	

FUP follow-up period, *LR* local recurrence, *LDR* low dose rate, *HDR* high dose rate, *ELE* electrons, *EORTC* European Organisation for Research and Treatment of Cancer, *TMH* Tata Memorial Hospital, *WBH* William Beaumont Hospital, *NS* not significant, *NR* not reported, *NA* not applicable

[a]Crude rate

[b]Patients treated with radiotherapy alone

reflect inadequate patient selection criteria and/or suboptimal treatment technique and lack of appropriate quality assurance (QA) procedures.

Uzsoki Hospital's Cobalt-Needle APBI Study

One of the first prospective APBI studies using interstitial implants was conducted in Hungary at

Table 5 Results of HDR brachytherapy boost series

Institution	Patient no.	RT scheme (dose [Gy]×fraction no.)	Median FUP (years)	5-year LR %	Annual LR %	Exc./good cosmesis %
Saarbrücken [35]	202	12–15×1	>3	6.4[a]	NA	85
Linz [32]	212	10×1	5.2	4.6	0.92	78
Paris [33]	108	5×2	3.75	5.1	1.02	63
Virginia C. University [37]	18	2.5×6	4.2	0	0	67
Barcelona [34]	294	2–2.5×8–11	5.8	9 (9-year)	1.00	96
Wien [39]	274	7–12×1	8.7	3.9 (10-year)	0.39	38
TMH, Mumbai [30]	153	10×1	3	8	1.6	83
Valencia [70]	125	4.4×3	7	4.2	0.84	77
Brno [38]	215	8–12×1	5.8	1.5	0.30	73
Rostock [36]	75	8–12×1	7.8	5.9 (10-year)	0.59	NR
Budapest [5]	100	4-4.75×3; 6.4×2; 8–10.35×1	7.8	7 (8-year)	0.87	57
Madrid [71]	210	7x1	7.1	5.3 (10-year)	0.53	85
Valencia [70]	167	7×1	7.7	4.9 (10-year)	0.49	97
All patients	2153		3–8.7	0–9	0–1.6	38–97

RT radiotherapy, *FUP* follow-up period, *LR* local recurrence, *TMH* Tata Memorial Hospital, *NA* not applicable, *NR* not reported

[a]Crude rate

Table 6 Results of early interstitial brachytherapy APBI trials

Institution	Dose rate	RT scheme (dose [Gy]×fraction no.)	Median FUP (years)	Crude LR % (n)	Annual LR %	Cosmesis exc./good %
Uzsoki Hospital [43]	MDR	50×1	12	24 (17 of 70)	2	50
Guy's Hospital I [13, 14]	LDR	55×1	6	37 (10 of 27)	6.2	83
Guy's Hospital II [15]	MDR	11×4	6.3	18 (9 of 49)	2.9	81
Florence Hospital [12]	LDR	50–60×1	4.2	6 (7 of 115)	1.4	NR
Royal Devon/Exeter Hospital [41]	HDR	20×2; 8×4; 6×6	1.5	16 (7 of 45)	10.7	95
London Regional Cancer Center [42]	HDR	3.72×10	7.6	15 (6 of 39)	2	100
All patients			1.5–12	16 (56 of 345)	1.4–10.7	50–100

APBI accelerated partial-breast irradiation, *RT* radiotherapy, *FUP* follow-up period, *LR* local recurrence, *MDR* medium dose rate, *LDR* low dose rate, *HDR* high dose rate, *NR* not reported

the Uzsoki Hospital between 1987 and 1992 [43]. Due to the limited availability of modern teletherapy equipment and the lack of ^{192}Ir wires in Hungary, special ^{60}Co sources were designed and manufactured to allow manual afterloading of interstitial BT catheters. During this period, 70 patients were treated with these needles following BCS, without use of WBI. Any patient with a pathological T1 or T2 tumor that was clinically unifocal was eligible. Two to eight (median 5) catheters with a fixed 4-cm active length were implanted into the tumor bed in a single plane. A dose of 50 Gy was prescribed at 0.5 cm from the surface of the sources, given in a single session of 10–22 h at a dose rate of 2.3–5.0 Gy per hour. The volume included within the reference iso-dose surface was quite small (median: 36 cm³). Updated 12-year results of this series showed that the crude LR rate was 24 %, with 59 % of patients having grade 3 or 4 complications. Unfortunately, at that era most patients did not have preoperative mammographic evaluation, and the vast majority of pathology reports did not contain such important information as pathological tumor size and the presence of multifocality. Other important pathological factors were not assessed, such as pathological axillary node status (unknown for 80 % of patients) and microscopic marginal status (unknown for all patients). Hence, perhaps most of the patients treated in this study would not at all be considered eligible for breast-conserving therapy today. Therefore, it is likely that the high rate of LR in this study was due to having persistent (not recurrent!) tumor due to inadequate patient selection criteria and radiological and pathological evaluation, as well as a very small and inadequate implant volume [72]. The high rate of toxicity may have resulted from giving a high total dose (86–134 Gy LDR equivalent dose) delivered within a short overall treatment time without fractionation. Thus, indeed it was an unfortunate use of unfractionated medium-dose-rate (MDR) BT. Despite its obvious limitations, the pioneering experience of the Uzsoki Hospital subsequently served as a basis for the development of more successful APBI series at the Hungarian National Institute of Oncology, Budapest, carried out subsequently [46–48].

Guy's Hospital Studies

Fentiman et al. [13–15] also explored the feasibility and limitations of partial-breast BT in two consecutive pilot trials performed at the Guy's Hospital, London, UK. In the first study, conducted in 1987–1988, 27 patients were treated with LDR implants using rigid needles [13, 14]. The target volume included a 2-cm margin around the tumor bed. The dose prescription was based on the Paris dosimetry system with a dose of 55 Gy given over 5–6 days using manually afterloaded ¹⁹²Ir wires. With a median follow-up of 6 years, 10 of 27 patients (37 %) experienced recurrence in the treated breast [14].

A second Guy's Hospital study enrolled 50 patients between 1990 and 1992 [15]. Patient selection criteria and surgical and implant techniques were similar to the first series. An MDR remote-controlled afterloading system employing ¹³⁷cesium was used to give a total dose of 45 Gy in 4 fractions over 4 days. At a median follow-up of 6.3 years, 8 of 49 patients (18 %) developed an in-breast relapse.

It is to be noted that the surgical technique and patient selection criteria used in these studies were far from optimal. No attempt was made to achieve a wide excision either grossly or microscopically. As a consequence, the surgical margins were involved in 56 % of patients in the first study and in 43 % of patients in the second one. Furthermore, in the first study, 41 % of patients had tumors containing EIC, and in both studies 44 % had positive axillary lymph nodes.

Florence Series

Between 1989 and 1993, Cionini et al. [12] in Florence, Italy, treated 115 patients with T1–2 N0–1 tumors with quadrantectomy, axillary dissection, and LDR BT to the entire quadrant, giving a dose of 50–60 Gy using ¹⁹²Ir implants. Young patients, patients with positive or unknown margins, and patients with infiltrating lobular carcinoma were included in the study. Patients with positive axillary nodes (38 %) received chemotherapy or tamoxifen. The 5-year actuarial LR rate was 6 %.

Royal Devon/Exeter Hospital Series

In a pilot study performed at the Royal Devon and Exeter Hospital in the United Kingdom, fractionated HDR interstitial BT was used to treat the involved quadrant after tumor excision in 45 patients [41]. Patients selected for BT alone had tumors smaller than 4 cm, grade 1 or 2 tumors, and clear or close margins. Three different fractionation schedules were used: 20 Gy given in 2 fractions, 28 Gy given in 4 fractions, and 32 Gy given in 6 fractions. The crude LR rate was 15.6 % at a short follow-up of 18 months. However, this study was also limited by the surgical techniques and pathological reports used, as axillary dissection was not performed routinely, and in many cases detailed histologic findings were not available.

London Regional Cancer Center's Pilot Study
One of the first APBI studies utilizing fractionated HDR BT was conducted in Canada [42]. Between 1992 and 1996, 39 patients with T1–2 breast cancers received 37.2 Gy in 10 fractions over 1 week prescribed to a small volume (median: 30 cm^3) encompassing the surgical clips only. With a median follow-up of 91 months, the 5-year actuarial LR rate was 16.2 %. There were 6 breast recurrences, of which 3 occurred outside the implanted volume. However, this study has been criticized for inappropriately limiting the target volume to the boundaries of the excision cavity without adding any safety margin to sterilize possible residual tumor foci in the 1–2-cm vicinity of the tumor bed [73].

4.2.2   Contemporary APBI Brachytherapy Trials
Based on the controversial results of earlier studies, several groups created APBI trial protocols incorporating more strict patient selection criteria and systematic QA procedures. As a result, the outcomes of these studies have been much improved (Table 7) [4, 16–18, 40, 44–46, 48–50, 56, 74–80].

Ochsner Clinic Experience
The first group in the USA to evaluate the feasibility of APBI using multicatheter BT was King et al. [17] at the Ochsner Clinic in New Orleans. Between 1992 and 1993, 50 patients (with 51 breast cancers) were treated with either 45 Gy LDR BT (n=25) or 32 Gy HDR BT (n=26) given in 8 fractions of 4 Gy. All patients had tumors <4 cm with negative margins. Patients with negative or up to 3 positive axillary nodes were eligible. Wide-volume implants were used

to encompass the excision cavity with 2-cm margins in each direction. At a median follow-up of 75 months, only 1 breast recurrence (2 %) and 3 regional nodal failures (6 %) were observed. The authors compared the outcome of their patients with a matched control group of 94 patients who met the eligibility criteria for APBI but were treated with conventional WBI during the same time period. The two groups were similar for LR rates, cosmetic results, and grade 3 side effects.

William Beaumont Hospital (WBH) Experience
One of the largest experiences using multicatheter BT to deliver APBI was published by the WBH group from Royal Oak, Michigan [9, 51]. Between 1993 and 2001, 199 consecutive patients were treated with 50 Gy interstitial LDR (n=120) or HDR (n=79) BT. In the latter group, a total dose of 32 Gy in 8 fractions (n=71) or 34 Gy in 10 fractions (n=8) was delivered. Eligibility criteria included age greater than 40 years, infiltrating ductal carcinoma less than 3 cm in diameter, negative surgical margins, and up to 1–3 positive axillary nodes. Patients with an EIC, pure infiltrating lobular histology, pure ductal carcinoma in situ (DCIS), or clinically significant areas of lobular carcinoma (LCIS) in situ were excluded. All implants were designed to irradiate the lumpectomy cavity plus at least a surrounding 1–2-cm margin. According to the last updated report, at a median follow-up of 10.7 years, a total of 10 ipsilateral breast failures (5 %) were observed, translating into a 10-year actuarial LR rate of 5 % [51]. The results of BT patients were compared with those in a matched cohort of 199 patients treated with conventional WBI at the same institution. There were no statistically significant differences in the 5- and 10-year actuarial rates of LR or regional recurrence.

Hungarian National Institute of Oncology (HNIO) Studies
Between 1996 and 1998, 45 selected patients with early-stage invasive breast cancer were treated with APBI using interstitial HDR implants at the HNIO, Budapest [40, 46, 47]. Patients were

Table 7 Results of contemporary interstitial brachytherapy APBI trials with a median FUP of ≥4 years

Institution/study	Dose rate	RT scheme (dose [Gy]×fraction no.)	Median FUP (years)	Crude LR % (n)	Annual LR %
Budapest phase II [40, 47]	HDR	4.33×7; 5.2×7	13.8	11.1 (5 of 45)	0.80
Massachusetts General Hospital [77]	LDR	50–60×1	11.2	12.0 (6 of 50)	1.07
WBH, Michigan [55]	LDR/HDR	50×1/4×8; 3.4×10	10.7	5.0 (10 of 199)	0.47
Budapest phase III [48]	HDR	5.2×7	10.2	5.7 (5 of 88)	0.56
Örebro Medical Centre [45]	PDR	50/0.83[a]	7.2	6.0 (3 of 50)	0.83
Tufts University, Boston [16]	HDR	3.4×10	7	9.1 (3 of 33)	1.30
RTOG 95–17 [44]	LDR/HDR	45×1/3.4×10	6.7	6.1 (6 of 99)	0.91
Ochsner Clinic [17]	LDR/HDR	45×1/4×8	6.25	2 (1 of 51)	0.32
Ninewells Hospital [51]	LDR	46–55×1	5.6	0 (0 of 11)	0
German-Austrian phase II [18]	PDR/HDR	50/0.6[a]/4×8	5.25	2.9 (8 of 274)	0.55
University of Nice Sophia Antipolis [75]	HDR	3.4×10; 4×8	5.1	1.4 (1 of 70)	0.27
University of Perugia [74]	HDR	4×8	5	3.0 (3 of 100)	0.60
University of Navarra [76]	HDR	3.4×10	4.4	3.8 (1 of 26)	0.86
Osaka Medical Center [78]	HDR	6×6; 6×7	4.3	5.0 (1 of 20)	1.15
Wisconsin University [49]	HDR[b]	4×8; 3.4×10	4	2.9 (8 of 273)	0.72
All patients			4–13.8	4.4 (61 of 1389)	0–1.30

APBI accelerated partial-breast irradiation, *FUP* follow-up period, *LR* local recurrence, *HDR* high dose rate, *LDR* low dose rate, *PDR* pulsed dose rate, *WBH* William Beaumont Hospital, *RTOG* Radiation Therapy Oncology Group *NR* not reported
[a]Total dose/pulse dose
[b]26 pts. (9.5 %) were treated with the MammoSite® applicator

eligible for sole BT if they met all of the following conditions: unifocal tumor, tumor size ≤2.0 cm (pT1), microscopically clear surgical margins, pathologically negative axillary nodes or only axillary micrometastases (pN1mi), histologic grade 1 or 2, and technical suitability for breast implantation. Exclusion criteria were pure DCIS or LCIS (pTis), invasive lobular carcinoma, and the presence of EIC. The planning target volume (PTV) was defined as the excision cavity plus a margin of 1–2 cm. A total dose of 30.3 Gy (n=8) or 36.4 Gy (n=37) in 7 fractions over 4 days was delivered to the PTV. The 7-year results (and later the 12- and 15-year update) of this study were reported, including comparison with results of a control group treated during the same time period with conventional breast-conserving therapy [40, 46, 47]. The control group comprised 80 consecutive patients who met the eligibility criteria for APBI, but were treated with 50 Gy

WBI with (n=36) or without (n=44) 10–16 Gy tumor bed boost. The 12-year actuarial rate of LR was not significantly different between patients treated with APBI (9.3 %) and WBI (11.1 %). There were no significant differences in either the 12-year probability of disease-free survival (75 % and 74 %, respectively), or cancer-specific survival (91 % and 89 %, respectively).

Based on the encouraging results of the first HNIO study, a randomized study was conducted between 1998 and 2004 at the same institution in Budapest [48]. Initial eligibility criteria were similar to those for the previous study, although following the publication of the EORTC boost trial in 2001, patients aged 40 years or younger were excluded. In addition, the trial allowed patients with breasts technically unsuitable for performing interstitial implantation to enroll and be treated with an external-beam (EB) approach. By May 2004, 258 eligible patients had been randomized to receive either 50 Gy WBI ($n=130$) or partial-breast irradiation (PBI, $n=128$). The latter consisted of either 36.4 Gy (given over 4 days using 7 fractions of 5.2 Gy) with HDR multicatheter BT ($n=88$) or limited-field electron irradiation ($n=40$) giving a dose of 50 Gy in 25 fractions. According to the last updated report, there has been no significant difference in the 10-year actuarial rate of LR (APBI: 5.9 % vs. WBI: 5.1 %), disease-free (85 % vs. 84 %), cancer-specific (94 % vs. 92 %), or overall survival (80 % vs. 82 %) between the two treatment arms [48].

Örebro Series

The first APBI study using PDR BT was begun in December 1993 at the Örebro Medical Centre in Sweden [45]. Inclusion criteria included age 40 years or older with a unifocal breast cancer measuring 5 cm or less without an EIC which was excised with clear inked margins and up to three positive axillary lymph nodes. Freehand plastic tube implants were used to cover the PTV defined as the excision cavity plus 3-cm margins. Fifty patients were treated to a total dose of 50 Gy using pulses of 0.83 Gy delivered over 5 days. At a median follow-up time of 86 months, the 7-year actuarial LR rate was 4 %.

German-Austrian Multicentric APBI Trial

In the year 2000, two German (Erlangen and Leipzig) and two Austrian (Vienna and Linz) institutions decided to start the first European multi-institutional phase II trial to investigate the efficacy and safety of HDR/PDR multicatheter APBI [18]. The four participating centers recruited 274 patients between 2000 and 2005. Patients were eligible for APBI, if they had a tumor diameter ≤3 cm, complete resection with clear margins ≥0.2 cm, pathologically negative axillary lymph nodes or singular nodal micrometastasis (pN1mi), hormone receptor-positive tumors, and patient age ≥35 years. Patients were excluded from the protocol if they showed a multicentric invasive growth pattern and had poorly differentiated tumors, residual microcalcifications, EIC, or lymph vessel invasion. Among the 274 patients, 175 (64 %)

received PDR and 99 (36 %) HDR BT. Prescribed dose in the PDR BT group was 49.8 Gy in 83 pulses of 0.6 Gy each hour. Prescribed dose for HDR BT was 32 Gy in 8 fractions of 4 Gy, twice daily. Total treatment time for both groups was 5 days. The PTV was confined to the tumor bed plus a safety margin of 2–3 cm in each direction. According to the last update of this study, 8 patients (2.9 %) had developed ipsilateral breast recurrence after a median follow-up of 63 months, yielding a 5- and 8-year actuarial LR rate of 2.3 % and 5.0 %, respectively.

Radiation Therapy Oncology Group (RTOG) 95–17 Phase II APBI Trial

Based on the success of single-institution phase I–II APBI studies, the RTOG conducted a multi-institutional phase II trial investigating the use of multicatheter BT as the sole method of RT after BCS [44]. Eligibility criteria included unicentric infiltrating non-lobular breast carcinomas ≤3 cm that had been resected with clear margins, with 0–3 positive axillary nodes without extracapsular extension. Ineligibility criteria included evidence of EIC or any lobular component. Between 1997 and 2000, 99 eligible patients have been enrolled from 11 institutions. Two-thirds of patients ($n=66$) received HDR BT with a prescribed dose of 34 Gy in 10 fractions, and one-third ($n=33$) were treated with 45 Gy LDR BT. The PTV was defined as a 2-cm margin peripheral to the cavity and 1 cm anteriorly and posteriorly. At a median follow-up of 6.7 years, the estimated 5-year LR rate for the entire cohort was 4 % (3 % in the HDR and 6 % in the LDR groups). It is to be noted that patients with all ages were eligible for the study. Out of the six LRs, four occurred in patients younger than 50 years. The crude rate of LR for patients below and above the age of 50 years was 19 % and 2.6 %, respectively.

University of Wisconsin Experience

In the prospective APBI study of the University of Wisconsin, eligibility criteria similar to the RTOG 95–17 trial were used [49]. Between 2000 and 2005, 273 patients were treated with a total dose of 32–34 Gy in 8–10 twice-daily fractions within 4–5 days using HDR BT. The majority of patients ($n = 247$) were treated using multicatheter BT, while the others ($n = 26$) with the MammoSite® applicator. For study purposes, the authors separated their patients into two groups: high-risk patients, who satisfied one or more of the so-called "high-risk" criteria as age <50 years, estrogen receptor negative, and/or positive lymph nodes ($n = 90$), and low-risk patients, who comprised the remainder of the cohort ($n = 183$). At a median follow-up of 4 years, the actuarial 5-year LR rate in the high- and low-risk groups was 6.4 % and 2.2 %, respectively ($p = 0.29$).

Other Multicatheter APBI Experiences

Additional experiences with multicatheter APBI have been published by other groups with smaller sample sizes and/or less mature follow-up [16, 50, 74–79] (see Table 7). In the majority of these trials, similar local tumor control rates were achieved as in other breast-conserving series using conventional WBI.

4.2.3 Multicentric Randomized APBI Trials

In addition to the Hungarian randomized APBI study, to date seven prospective phase III clinical trials have been activated to compare the efficacy of APBI to conventional WBI. Among these, two protocols (the European GEC-ESTRO and the American NSABP/RTOG trials) use BT for the delivery of APBI in the investigational arm [7, 9].

The GEC-ESTRO Multicentric Randomized APBI Trial

Based on the success of the Hungarian and German-Austrian APBI studies, a multicentric phase III APBI protocol has been developed by the Breast Cancer Working Group of the GEC-ESTRO [7]. Only interstitial HDR or PDR BT was allowed for the APBI arm of this European multicentric phase III trial. Between April 2004 and July 2009, 1188 patients were enrolled at 16 centers from 7 European countries. Patients in the control group were treated with 50 Gy WBI plus a 10 Gy electron boost. Patients in the APBI arm were treated with HDR or PDR multicatheter BT. The primary end point of the study is LR as a first event within 5 years. The scientific hypothesis

to be assessed and statistically tested is "non-relevant non-inferiority" of the experimental treatment. Secondary end points address overall, disease-free, and distant metastasis-free survival, contralateral breast cancer, early and late side effects, cosmesis, and quality of life. Eligibility criteria included unifocal DCIS or invasive carcinoma of the breast, tumor size ≤ 3 cm, microscopic negative margins of at least 0.2 cm (0.5 cm for DCIS or invasive lobular carcinoma), no EIC, no lymphovascular invasion, no more than one micrometastasis in axillary lymph nodes (pN1mi), and patient age ≥ 40 years. Patients were stratified before randomization according to the treatment center, having DCIS or invasive carcinoma, and menopausal status. The QA program for partial-breast BT included preimplant PTV definition by surgical clips and/or preimplant CT image-based preplanning of the implant geometry. The PTV was defined as the excision cavity plus 2-cm margin minus the minimum clear pathological margin. Postimplant CT scans were mandatory for the documentation of target coverage and dose homogeneity. Acceptable treatment parameters for CT image-based treatment planning included:

- DVH analysis of target coverage confirming that the prescribed dose covers ≥ 90 % of the PTV (coverage index ≥ 0.9)
- DNR ≤ 0.35
- Maximum skin dose <70 % of the prescribed dose

The GEC-ESTRO APBI trial is financially supported by the grant from German Cancer Aid (Deutsche Krebshilfe) for a study period of 4 years between 2005 and 2009. It is anticipated that the 5-year results will be published in late 2015.

NSABP B-39/RTOG 0413 Multicentric Randomized APBI Trial

The American multicentric phase III trial investigating APBI was initiated in March 2005 by the National Surgical Adjuvant Breast and Bowel Project (NSABP) together with the RTOG [9]. Patients were randomized between standard

WBI and APBI. The latter was delivered with any of the three techniques: multicatheter HDR BT, MammoSite® BT, or 3-dimensional external-beam RT. Eligibility criteria included unicentric DCIS or invasive carcinoma allowing microscopical multifocality confined to one quadrant of the breast, tumor size ≤3 cm, microscopically negative margins by the NSABP criteria (no tumor on inked margins), and no more than 3 positive axillary lymph nodes (pN0-1a) without extracapsular extension. In contrast to the GEC-ESTRO trial, patients below the age of 40 years with tumors excised with close (but clear) surgical margins or containing an EIC as well as patients with 1–3 positive nodes were eligible for the NSABP/RTOG trial. Due to the rapid enrollment of low-risk patients by multiple American centers, the original accrual goal (3000 patients) was increased to 4300. In December 2006, the trial closed enrollment to low-risk patients, thereby limiting further accrual to patients satisfying one or more of the high-risk criteria including age <50 years, estrogen receptor negativity, or 1–3 positive nodes [49]. The enrollment of 4300 patients concluded in 2013 and the first results are to be published in 2017 (personal communication; Vicini FA). Unfortunately, only 29 % of patients randomized to APBI have been treated with BT (23.3 % with MammoSite® BT, and only 5.7 % with interstitial HDR BT).

5 Side Effects and Management

5.1 Acute Side Effects

Acute side effects of interstitial breast BT include hematoma formation, edema, infection, acute radiation dermatitis (mainly limited to the needle puncture sites), and mastalgia [18, 45, 77, 80, 81]. However, the rate and severity of these early complications are low and clinically negligible. The rate of perioperative breast infection was reported in the range of 0–11 % [45, 47, 48, 80, 81] In the William Beaumont series, 22 of 199 patients (11 %) developed infections, but only 5

of them (2 % of all patients) required surgical intervention including incision and drainage or debridement [80]. It is to be noted that a significantly lower rate of infections occurred following closed-cavity implant placement (4.9 %) compared to intraoperative open-cavity placement (17.5 %; $p=0.005$). In other series using postoperative catheter implantation and prophylactic antibiotics, breast infections rarely occurred [18, 47, 48, 81].

5.2 Late Side Effects and Cosmetic Results

Late side effects of interstitial breast BT include skin and subcutaneous toxicities [16–18, 40, 42, 45, 47, 48, 74–77, 79, 82–86]. Among these, skin telangiectasia >1 cm^2, moderate and severe subcutaneous fibrosis, and symptomatic fat necrosis are clinically relevant which have been reported in wide ranges in different series (Table 8).

The rate of telangiectasia is highly dependent on the dose delivered to the subcutaneous small vessels beneath the skin [6, 42, 87]. A higher incidence of late skin side effects occurred in early BT studies not using any skin dose constraints or dose optimization [42, 43, 45, 77, 79]. However using strict skin dose constraints (e.g., <60–70 % of prescription dose), the rate of telangiectasia was reported far below 10 % [18, 40, 47, 84].

Moderate to severe subcutaneous fibrosis was reported in the range of 4–54 % in contemporary series of interstitial breast BT (see Table 8). The rate of subcutaneous toxicities primarily depends on the total dose, dose fractionation, dose rate, overall implant volume (V100 %), and dose homogeneity (represented by the DNR). Other factors playing critical roles in the development of late parenchymal side effects and ultimate cosmetic results include chemotherapy and particularly surgery [87]. On the other hand, asymptomatic fat necrosis is a common adverse event after breast-conserving therapy, having no significant clinical relevance in the majority of cases [16, 83, 85, 86]. In the Budapest randomized

Table 8 Late side effects and cosmetic results of contemporary interstitial brachytherapy APBI trials with a median FUP of ≥4 years

Institution/study	Dose rate	Median FUP (years)	≥G2 telangiectasia % (n)	≥G2 fibrosis % (n)	Symptomatic fat necrosis %	Exc./good cosmesis %
Budapest phase II [40]	HDR	13.8	4 (2 of 45)	9 (4 of 45)	22 (10 of 45)	80
Massachusetts General Hospital [77]	LDR	11.2	35 (16 of 46)	54 (25 of 46)	35[a] (16 of 46)	67
Budapest phase III [84]	HDR	10.2	8 (7 of 85)	19 (16 of 85)	1.2 (1 of 85)	85
Örebro Medical Centre [45]	PDR	7.2	22 (11 of 50)	26 (13 of 50)	12 (6 of 50)	56
Tufts University, Boston [16]	HDR	7	7 (2 of 28)	36 (10 of 28)	52[a] (17 of 33)	93
WBH, Michigan [82]	LDR/HDR	6.4	1.3 (1 of 79)	8 (6 of 79)	14 (11 of 79)	99
Ochsner Clinic [17]	LDR/HDR	6.25	NR	NR	4 (2 of 51)	75
Tufts and Virginia C. Universities [86]	HDR	6.1	4 (3 of 75)	17 (13 of 75)	13[a] (10 of 75)	91
German-Austrian phase II [18]	PDR/HDR	5.25	8 (21 of 274)	14 (39 of 274)	5 (14 of 274)	90
University of Nice Sophia Antipolis [75]	HDR	5.1	1.4 (1 of 70)	6 (4 of 70)	NR	96
RTOG 95–17 [79]	LDR/HDR	5	10 (10 of 98)	31 (30 of 98)	15 (15 of 98)	68
University of Perugia [74]	HDR	5	7 (7 of 100)	4 (4 of 100)	1 (1 of 100)	98
London Regional Cancer Center [42]	HDR	5	22 (6 of 27)	37 (10 of 27)	19[a] (5 of 27)	100
University of Navarra [76]	HDR	4.4	4 (1 of 26)	4 (1 of 26)	NR	87.5
All patients		4.4–13.8	9 (88 of 1003)	17 (175 of 1003)	11 (108 of 963)	56–100

APBI accelerated partial-breast irradiation, *FUP* follow-up period, *HDR* high dose rate, *LDR* low dose rate, *PDR* pulsed dose rate, *WBH* William Beaumont Hospital, *RTOG* Radiation Therapy Oncology Group, *NR* not reported
[a]Symptomatic and asymptomatic fat necroses were reported together

APBI trial, the incidence of fat necrosis was similar after HDR APBI BT and WBI [83]. Among the evaluated patient-, tumor-, and treatment-related variables, only larger bra cup size was significantly associated with the incidence of fat necrosis. They also concluded that routine follow-up examinations (including mammography, US, aspiration cytology, and ultimately breast MRI) are sufficient for the differential diagnosis of fat necrosis. They also warned that open biopsy should be avoided when possible, as core biopsy and MRI are useful for differentiating fat necrosis from LR.

To keep the rate of subcutaneous toxicities (including fibrosis and symptomatic fat necrosis) low, the overall implant volume should be limited, and more importantly the high-dose volume (e.g., V150 % and V200 %) should be minimized keeping the dose distribution as homogenous as possible (e.g., keeping the DNR below 0.30 or DHI above 0.70) [47, 48, 66, 85, 86, 88]. Within the range of small- to intermediate-volume implants (up to 160 cm³), neither implant volume (V100 %), volume of high-dose region (V150 %, V200 %), or dose inhomogeneity is associated with an increased risk of subcutaneous toxicities [45, 47, 83, 84]. However with large-volume implants (>160 cm³), larger high-dose regions are correlated with a higher incidence of fat necrosis, and the absolute volume of the high-dose region seems to be associated with the risk of subsequent fat necrosis [85, 86]. As a conclusion, to minimize late subcutaneous toxicities, image-guided BT and 3-D CT-based planning are suggested to minimize the overall volume of breast implants and control the volume of hot spots.

6   Summary and Future Perspectives of Interstitial Breast Brachytherapy

Before the era of breast-conserving therapy, BT implants were used to treat large inoperable breast tumors. More recently, interstitial BT has been used to deliver an additional dose to the tumor bed after BCS and WBI. Based on the obvious dosimetric advantages of interstitial breast implants (over external-beam techniques) supported by the encouraging results of modern boost series utilizing stepping-source afterloading technology, multicatheter HDR/PDR BT remains a standard treatment option for boosting the tumor bed after BCS and WBI.

APBI is an attractive treatment approach with considerable advantages over conventional WBI opening new prospects for interstitial breast BT. Contemporary APBI trials using interstitial BT with strict patient selection criteria and systematic strict QA procedures resulted in an annual LR rate of <1 %. Issues of patient selection, PTV definition, total dose, and fractionation will be addressed and refined by the experience obtained from the eagerly awaited results of the GEC-ESTRO and NSABP/RTOG multicentric randomized APBI trials.

Development of new standards for 3-D CT image-based BT treatment planning together with the implementation of inverse dose planning will further improve the conformity of dose distribution delivered by multicatheter implants maximizing the advantage of interstitial breast BT.

References

1. Forquet A, Campana F, Mosseri V et al (1995) Iridium-192 versus cobalt-60 boost in 3–7 cm breast cancer treated by irradiation alone: final results of a randomized trial. Radiother Oncol 34:114–120
2. Keynes G (1929) The treatment of primary carcinoma of the breast with radium. Acta Radiol 10:393–402
3. Polgar C, Fodor J, Major T et al (2001) The role of boost irradiation in the conservative treatment of stage I-II breast cancer. Pathol Oncol Res 7:241–250
4. Polgar C, Van Limbergen E, Pötter R et al (2010) Patient selection for accelerated partial-breast irradiation (APBI) after breast-conserving surgery: Recommendations of the Groupe Européen de Curiethérapie – European Society for Therapeutic Radiology and Oncology (GEC-ESTRO) Breast Cancer Working Group based on clinical evidence (2009). Radiother Oncol 94:264–273
5. Polgar C, Jánváry L, Major T et al (2010) The role of high-dose-rate brachytherapy boost in breast-conserving therapy: long-term results of the Hungarian National Institute of Oncology. Rep Pract Oncol Radiother 15:1–7
6. Van Limbergen E (2007) Indications and technical aspects of brachytherapy in breast conserving treatment of breast cancer. Cancer Radiother 7:107–120
7. Polgar C, Strnad V, Major T (2005) Brachytherapy for partial breast irradiation: the European experience. Semin Radiat Oncol 15:116–122
8. Polgar C, Major T (2009) Current status and perspectives of brachytherapy for breast cancer. Int J Clin Oncol 14:7–24
9. Vicini FA, Arthur DW (2005) Breast brachytherapy: north American experience. Semin Radiat Oncol 15:108–115
10. Morrow M (2002) Rational local therapy for breast cancer. N Engl J Med 347:1270–1271
11. Veronesi U, Cascinelli N, Mariani L et al (2002) Twenty-year follow-up of a randomized study comparing breast-conserving surgery with radical mastectomy for early breast cancer. N Engl J Med 347:1227–1232
12. Cionini L, Marzano S, Pacini P et al (1995) Iridium implant of the surgical bed as the sole radiotherapeutic treatment after conservative surgery for breast cancer. [Abstract]. Radiother Oncol 35(Suppl):S1
13. Fentiman IS, Poole C, Tong PJ et al (1991) Iridium implant treatment without external radiotherapy for operable breast cancer: a pilot study. Eur J Cancer 27:447–450
14. Fentiman IS, Poole C, Tong D et al (1996) Inadequacy of iridium implant as a sole radiation treatment for operable breast cancer. Eur J Cancer 32A:608–611
15. Fentiman IS, Deshmane V, Tong D et al (2004) Cesium137 implant as sole radiation therapy for operable breast cancer: a phase II trial. Radiother Oncol 71:281–285
16. Kaufman SA, DiPetrillo TA, Price LL et al (2007) Long-term outcome and toxicity in a phase I/II trial using high-dose-rate multicatheter interstitial brachytherapy for T1/T2 breast cancer. Brachytherapy 6:286–292
17. King TA, Bolton JS, Kuske RR et al (2000) Long-term results of wide-field brachytherapy as the sole method of radiation therapy after segmental mastectomy for Tis,1,2 breast cancer. Am J Surg 180:299–304

18. Strnad V, Hildebrandt G, Pötter R et al (2011) Accelerated partial breast irradiation: 5-year results of the German-Austrian multicenter phase II trial using interstitial multicatheter brachytherapy alone after breast-conserving surgery. Int J Radiat Oncol Biol Phys 80:17–24

19. Cuttino LW, Todor D, Rosu M et al (2011) A comparison of skin and chest wall dose delivered with multicatheter, Contura multilumen balloon, and MammoSite® breast brachytherapy. Int J Radiat Oncol Biol Phys 79:34–38

20. Edmundson GK, Vicini F, Chen P et al (2002) Dosimetric characteristics of the MammoSite® RTS, a new breast brachytherapy applicator. Int J Radiat Oncol Biol Phys 4:1132–1139

21. Pignol JP, Keller B, Rakovitch E et al (2006) First report of permanent breast 103Pd seed implant as adjuvant radiation treatment for early-stage breast cancer. Int J Radiat Oncol Biol Phys 64:176–181

22. Bartelink H, Maingon P, Weltens C et al (2015) Whole-breast irradiation with or without a boost for patients treated with breast-conserving surgery for early breast cancer: 20-year follow-up of a randomised phase 3 trial. Lancet Oncol 16:47–56

23. Polgar C, Fodor J, Orosz Z et al (2002) Electron and high dose rate brachytherapy boost in the conservative treatment of stage I-II breast cancer: first results of the randomized Budapest boost trial. Strahlenther Onkol 178:615–623

24. Polgar C, Fodor J, Orosz Z et al (2002) Electron and brachytherapy boost in the conservative treatment of stage I-II breast cancer: 5-year results of the randomized Budapest boost trial. [Abstract]. Radiother Oncol 64(Suppl 1):S15

25. Romestaing P, Lehingue Y, Carrie C et al (1997) Role of a 10-Gy boost in the conservative treatment of early breast cancer: results of a randomized clinical trial in Lyon, France. J Clin Oncol 15:963–968

26. Mansfield CM, Komarnicky LT, Schwartz GF et al (1995) Ten-year results in 1070 patients with stages I and II breast cancer treated by conservative surgery and radiation therapy. Cancer 75:2328–2336

27. Wazer DE, Kramer B, Schmid C et al (1997) Factors determining outcome in patients treated with interstitial implantation as a radiation boost for breast conservation therapy. Int J Radiat Oncol Biol Phys 39:381–393

28. Vicini FA, Horwitz EM, Lacerna MD et al (1997) Long-term outcome with interstitial brachytherapy in the management of patients with early-stage breast cancer treated with breast-conserving therapy. Int J Radiat Oncol Biol Phys 37:845–852

29. Moreno F, Guedea F, Lopez J et al (2000) External beam irradiation plus 192Ir implant after breast-preserving surgery in women with early breast cancer. Int J Radiat Oncol Biol Phys 48:757–765

30. Budrukkar AN, Sarin R, Shrivastava SK et al (2007) Cosmesis, late sequelae and local control after breast-conserving therapy: influence of type of tumour bed boost and adjuvant chemotherapy. Clin Oncol 19:596–603

31. Guinot JL, Roldan S, Maronas M et al (2007) Breast-conservative surgery with close or positive margins: can the breast be preserved with high-dose-rate brachytherapy boost? Int J Radiat Oncol Biol Phys 68:1381–1387

32. Hammer J, Seewald DH, Track C et al (1994) Breast cancer: primary treatment with external-beam radiation therapy and high-dose-rate iridium implantation. Radiology 193:573–577

33. Hennequin C, Durdux C, Espié M et al (1999) High-dose-rate brachytherapy for early breast cancer: an ambulatory technique. Int J Radiat Oncol Biol Phys 45:85–90

34. Henriquez I, Guix B, Tello JI et al (2001) Long term results of high-dose-rate (HDR) brachytherapy boost in preserving-breast cancer patients: the experience of Radiation Oncology Medical Institute (IMOR) of Barcelona. [Abstract]. Radiother Oncol 60(Suppl 1):S11

35. Jacobs H (1992) HDR afterloading experience in breast conservation therapy. Select Brachytherapy J 6:14–17

36. Knauerhase H, Strietzel M, Gerber B et al (2008) Tumor location, interval between surgery and radiotherapy, and boost technique influence local control after breast-conserving surgery and radiation: retrospective analysis of mono-institutional long-term results. Int J Radiat Oncol Biol Phys 72:1048–1055

37. Manning MA, Arthur DW, Schmidt-Ullrich RK et al (2000) Interstitial high-dose-rate brachytherapy boost: the feasibility and cosmetic outcome of a fractionated outpatient delivery scheme. Int J Radiat Oncol Biol Phys 48:1301–1306

38. Neumanova R, Petera J, Frgala T et al (2008) Long-term outcome with interstitial brachytherapy boost in the treatment of women with early-stage breast cancer. Neoplasma 54:413–423

39. Resch A, Pötter R, van Limbergen E et al (2002) Long-term results (10 years) of intensive breast conserving therapy including a high-dose and large-volume interstitial brachytherapy boost (LDR/HDR) for T1/T2 breast cancer. Radiother Oncol 63:47–58

40. Polgar C, Major T, Fodor J et al (2011) Accelerated partial breast irradiation with multicatheter brachytherapy: 15-year results of a Phase II clinical trial. Acta Medica Marisiensis 57:717–720

41. Clarke DH, Vicini F, Jacobs H et al (1994) High dose rate brachytherapy for breast cancer. In: Nag S (ed) High dose rate brachytherapy: a textbook. Futura Publishing Company, Armonk-New York, pp 321–329

42. Perera F, Yu E, Engel J et al (2003) Patterns of breast recurrence in a pilot study of brachytherapy confined to the lumpectomy site for early breast cancer with six years' minimum follow-up. Int J Radiat Oncol Biol Phys 57:1239–1246

43. Póti Z, Nemeskéri C, Fekésházi A et al (2004) Partial breast irradiation with interstitial 60Co brachytherapy results in frequent grade 3 or 4 toxicity. Evidence based on a 12-year follow-up of 70 patients. Int J Radiat Oncol Biol Phys 58:1022–1033

44. Arthur DW, Winter K, Kuske RR et al (2008) A phase II trial of brachytherapy alone after lumpectomy for select breast cancer: tumor control and survival outcomes of RTOG 95-17. Int J Radiat Oncol Biol Phys 72:467–473

45. Johansson B, Karlsson L, Liljegren G et al (2009) Pulsed dose rate brachytherapy as the sole adjuvant radiotherapy after breast-conserving surgery of T1-T2 breast cancer: first long time results from a clinical study. Radiother Oncol 90:30–35

46. Polgar C, Major T, Fodor J et al (2004) HDR brachytherapy alone versus whole breast radiotherapy with or without tumor bed boost after breast conserving surgery: seven-year results of a comparative study. Int J Radiat Oncol Biol Phys 60:1173–1181

47. Polgar C, Major T, Fodor J et al (2010) Accelerated partial breast irradiation using high-dose-rate interstitial brachytherapy: 12-year update of a prospective clinical study. Radiother Oncol 94:274–279

48. Polgar C, Fodor J, Major T et al (2013) Breast-conserving therapy with partial or whole breast irradiation: ten-year results of the Budapest randomized trial. Radiother Oncol 108:197–202

49. Patel RR, Christensen ME, Hodge C et al (2008) Clinical outcome analysis in "high-risk" versus "low-risk" patients eligible for National Surgical Adjuvant Breast and Bowel B-39/Radiation Therapy Oncology Group 0413 trial: five-year results. Int J Radiat Oncol Biol Phys 70:970–973

50. Samuel LM, Dewar JA, Preece PE et al (1999) A pilot study of radical radiotherapy using a perioperative implant following wide local excision for carcinoma of the breast. Breast 8:95–97

51. Shah C, Antonucci JV, Wilkinson JB et al (2011) Twelve-year clinical outcomes and patterns of failure with accelerated partial breast irradiation versus whole-breast irradiation: results of a matched-pair analysis. Radiother Oncol 100:210–214

52. Vicini F, Arthur D, Wazer D et al (2011) Limitations of the american society of therapeutic radiology and oncology consensus panel guidelines on the use of accelerated partial breast irradiation. Int J Radiat Oncol Biol Phys 79:977–984

53. Yoshida K, Nose T, Masuda N et al (2009) Preliminary result of accelerated partial breast irradiation after breast-conserving surgery. Breast Cancer 16: 105–112

54. Sedlmayer F, Sautter-Bihl M-L, Budach W et al (2013) DEGRO practical guidelines: radiotherapy of breast cancer I: radiotherapy following breast conserving therapy for invasive breast cancer. Strahlenther Onkol 189:825–833

55. Shah C, Vicini F, Wazer DE et al (2013) The American Brachytherapy Society consensus statement for accelerated partial breast irradiation. Brachytherapy 12:267–277

56. Smith BD, Arthur DW, Buchholz TA et al (2009) Accelerated partial breast irradiation consensus statement from the American Society for Radiation Oncology (ASTRO). Int J Radiat Oncol Biol Phys 74:987–1001

57. Leonardi MC, Maisonneuve P, Mastropasqua MG et al (2013) Accelerated partial breast irradiation with intraoperative electrons: using GEC-ESTRO recommendations as guidance for patient selection. Radiother Oncol 106:21–27

58. Wilkinson JB, Beitsch PD, Shah C et al (2013) Evaluation of current consensus statement recommendations for accelerated partial breast irradiation: a pooled analysis of William Beaumont Hospital and American Society of Breast Surgeon MammoSite Registry Trial Data. Int J Radiat Oncol Biol Phys 85:1179–1185

59. Gutiérez C, Najjari D, Martinez E et al (2014) The use of an interstitial boost in the conservative treatment of breast cancer: how to perform it routinely in a radiotherapy department. J Contemp Brachytherapy 6:397–403

60. Kuske RR (2006) Brachytherapy techniques: the university of Wisconsin/Arizona approach. In: Wazer DE, Arthur DW, Vicini FA (eds) Accelerated partial breast irradiation, techniques and clinical implementation. Springer, Berlin/Heidelberg, pp 105–127

61. Chen PY, Edmundson G (2006) The William Beaumont hospital technique of interstitial brachytherapy. In: Wazer DE, Arthur DW, Vicini FA (eds) Accelerated partial breast irradiation, techniques and clinical implementation. Springer, Berlin/Heidelberg, pp 91–103

62. Polo A, Guedea F (2006) Ultrasound-based implant technique. In: Strnad V, Ott OJ (eds) Partial breast irradiation using multicatheter brachytherapy. W. Zuckschwerdt Verlag, München, pp 83–90

63. Cuttino LW, Todor D, Arthur DW (2005) CT-guided multi-catheter insertion technique for partial breast brachytherapy: reliable target coverage and dose homogeneity. Brachytherapy 4:10–17

64. Vicini FA, Jaffray DA, Horwitz EM et al (1998) Implementation of 3D-virtual brachytherapy in the management of breast cancer: a description of a new method of interstitial brachytherapy. Int J Radiat Oncol Biol Phys 40:629–635

65. Major T, Fröhlich G, Lövey K et al (2009) Dosimetric experience with accelerated partial breast irradiation using image-guided interstitial brachytherapy. Radiother Oncol 90:48–55

66. Saw CB, Suntharalingam N, Wu A (1993) Concept of dose non-uniformity in interstitial brachytherapy. Int J Radiat Oncol Biol Phys 26:519–527

67. Baltas D, Kolotas C, Geramani K et al (1998) A conformal index (COIN) to evaluate implant quality and dose specification in brachytherapy. Int J Radiat Oncol Biol Phys 40:515–524

68. ICRU (1997) Dose and volume specification for reporting interstitial therapy, ICRU report 58. ICRU, Bethesda
69. Perez CA, Taylor ME, Halverson K et al (1996) Brachytherapy or electron beam boost in conservation therapy of carcinoma of the breast: a nonrandomized comparison. Int J Radiat Oncol Biol Phys 34:995–1007
70. Guinot JL, Baixauli-Perez C, Soler P et al (2015) High-dose-rate brachytherapy boost effect on local tumor control in young women with breast cancer. Int J Radiat Oncol Biol Phys 91:165–171
71. Rodríguez Pérez A, Samper Ots PM, López Carrizosa MC et al (2012) Early-stage breast cancer conservative treatment: high-dose-rate brachytherapy boost in a single fraction of 700 cGy to the tumour bed. Clin Transl Oncol 14:362–368
72. Polgar C, Major T, Strnad V et al (2004) What can we conclude from the results of an out-of-date breast brachytherapy study? In regard to Póti Z, Nemeskéri C, Fekeshazy A, et al: (Int J Radiat Oncol Biol Phys 2004 58:1022–1033). Int J Radiat Oncol Biol Phys 60:342–343
73. Vicini F, Arthur D, Polgar C et al (2003) Defining the efficacy of accelerated partial breast irradiation: the importance of proper patient selection, adequate quality assurance and common sense. Int J Radiat Oncol Biol Phys 57:1210–1213, Editorial
74. Aristei C, Palumbo I, Capezzali G et al (2013) Outcome of a phase II prospective study on partial breast irradiation with interstitial multi-catheter high-dose-rate brachytherapy. Radiother Oncol 108:236–241
75. Genebes C, Chand ME, Gal J et al (2014) Accelerated partial breast irradiation in the elderly: 5-year results of high-dose rate multi-catheter brachytherapy. Radiat Oncol 9:115
76. Gómez-Iturriaga A, Pina L, Cambeiro M et al (2008) Early breast cancer treated with conservative surgery, adjuvant chemotherapy, and delayed accelerated partial breast irradiation with high-dose-rate brachytherapy. Brachytherapy 7:310–315
77. Hattagandi JA, Powell SN, MacDonald SM et al (2012) Accelerated partial breast irradiation with low-dose-rate interstitial implant brachytherapy after wide local excision: 12-year outcomes from a prospective trial. Int J Radiat Oncol Biol Phys 83:791–800
78. Nose T, Komoike Y, Yoshida K et al (2006) A pilot study of wider use of accelerated partial breast irradiation: intraoperative margin-directed re-excision combined with sole high-dose-rate interstitial brachytherapy. Breast Cancer 13:289–299
79. Rabinovitch R, Winter K, Kuske R et al (2014) RTOG 95–17, a phase II trial to evaluate brachytherapy as the sole method of radiation therapy for stage I and II breast carcinoma: 5-year toxicity and cosmesis. Brachytherapy 13:17–22
80. Benitez PR, Chen PY, Vicini FA et al (2004) Partial breast irradiation in breast-conserving therapy by way of interstitial brachytherapy. Am J Surg 188:355–364
81. Kuske RR, Winter K, Arthur DW et al (2006) Phase II trial of brachytherapy alone after lumpectomy for select breast cancer: toxicity analysis of RTOG 95–17. Int J Radiat Oncol Biol Phys 65:45–51
82. Chen PY, Vicini FA, Benitez P et al (2006) Long-term cosmetic results and toxicity after accelerated partial-breast irradiation. Cancer 106:991–999
83. Lovey K, Fodor J, Major T et al (2007) Fat necrosis after partial-breast irradiation with brachytherapy or electron irradiation versus standard whole-breast radiotherapy – 4-year results of a randomized trial. Int J Radiat Oncol Biol Phys 69:724–731
84. Polgar C, Major T, Sulyok Z et al (2014) Toxicity and cosmetic results of partial vs whole breast irradiation: 10-year results of a randomized trial. [Abstract]. Radiother Oncol 111(Suppl 1):72
85. Wazer DE, Lowther D, Boyle T et al (2001) Clinically evident fat necrosis in women treated with high-dose-rate brachytherapy alone for early-stage breast cancer. Int J Radiat Oncol Biol Phys 50:107–111
86. Wazer DE, Kaufman S, Cuttino L et al (2006) Accelerated partial breast irradiation: an analysis of variables associated with late toxicity and long-term cosmetic outcome after high-dose-rate interstitial brachytherapy. Int J Radiat Oncol Biol Phys 64:489–495
87. Hepel J (2014) Late toxicity and cosmetic outcomes related to interstitial multicatheter brachytherapy for partial breast irradiation. [Editorial]. Brachytherapy 13:23–26
88. Major T, Fröhlich G, Polgar C (2011) Assessment of dose homogeneity in conformal interstitial breast brachytherapy with special respect to ICRU recommendations. J Contemp Brachytherapy 3:150–156

Breast Brachytherapy: Intracavitary Breast Brachytherapy

Jaroslaw T. Hepel, David E. Wazer, Frank A. Vicini, and Douglas W. Arthur

Abstract

Accelerated partial breast irradiation (APBI) represents a more conformal and convenient method to deliver adjuvant radiation as part of a breast-conserving therapy approach. Interstitial multi-catheter brachytherapy was the first technique developed to deliver APBI, however, the complexity of this implant procedure limited its widespread use to select high-volume centers. The intracavitary brachytherapy (ICB) technique was introduced to provide a less complex implant and resulted in adoption across a broader user's base. Studies of the initial single-lumen MammoSite® catheter have shown a high rate of local control and good-to-excellent cosmetic outcomes. However, the simplicity of this initial system limited any dosimetric modulation. As a result, implants that were close to the skin or chest wall were at an increased risk of toxicity and compromised cosmetic outcome. The next generation of ICB applicators (Contura®, MammoSite ML®, and SAVI®) utilizes multiple lumens, now allowing for optimization of the dose distribution resulting in improved normal tissue sparing.

J.T. Hepel, MD, FACRO (✉)
Department of Radiation Oncology, Rhode Island Hospital, Warren Alpert Medical School of Brown University, Providence, RI, USA
e-mail: jhepel@lifespan.org

D.E. Wazer, MD, FACRO, FACR, FASTRO
Departments of Radiation Oncology, Tufts Medical Center, Tufts University School of Medicine, Rhode Island Hospital, Alpert Medical School of Brown University, Boston, MA, USA
e-mail: dwazer@tuftsmedicalcenter.org

F.A. Vicini, MD, FACR
Department of Radiation Oncology, St. Joseph Mercy Oakland, Pontiac, MI, USA
e-mail: fvicini@rtsx.com

D.W. Arthur, MD
Department of Radiation Oncology, Virginia Commonwealth University School of Medicine, Richmond, VA, USA
e-mail: darthur@mcvh-vcu.edu

© Springer International Publishing Switzerland 2016
P. Montemaggi et al. (eds.), *Brachytherapy: An International Perspective*, Medical Radiology,
DOI 10.1007/978-3-319-26791-3_9

1 Introduction

The advent of breast-conserving therapy (BCT) marks a major advance in the management of early-stage breast cancer, sparing women the morbidity and psychosocial impact associated with mastectomy [1]. The equivalence of BCT consisting of breast-conserving surgery (BCS) and radiation therapy compared with more radical surgery has been demonstrated in several phase III trials [2–4]. Despite the undisputed efficacy of this treatment approach, the amount of clinically uninvolved breast tissue surrounding the lumpectomy cavity requiring irradiation has never been definitively established. Standard radiation therapy after BCS has consisted of elective treatment of the whole breast. The addition of this "prophylactic" treatment of uninvolved breast tissue with radiation is generally considered responsible, at least in a large part, for the acute and chronic toxicity associated with BCT and for the protracted time required to complete therapy.

In recognition of these limitations, accelerated partial breast irradiation (APBI) has been investigated as a possible option for the management of selected patients with an anticipated low risk of harboring in-breast microscopic disease remote from the lumpectomy cavity [5]. APBI incorporates both a reduction of the radiation field to the region of the surgical bed after BCS and of the overall radiation treatment time from 6 to 1 week or less. Thus APBI not only represents a logistically simpler and more practical method for radiation as part of BCT, but also has the potential advantages of reduced treatment-related toxicities and improved overall quality of life for early-stage breast cancer patients [6].

Interstitial multi-catheter brachytherapy was the first technique commonly employed to deliver APBI. As such, the studies using interstitial brachytherapy have provided the largest group of patients with the longest follow-up and have established APBI as an acceptable treatment option [7–9]. However, the complexity and reproducibility of the interstitial procedure have limited the widespread use of this technique, particularly for lower-volume centers. The intracavitary brachytherapy (ICB) technique was, therefore, introduced to provide a less complex implant with increased reproducibility of radiation delivery to the target volume. Since its introduction, ICB has become the most widely used brachytherapy technique for APBI.

2 Indications and Patient Selection

Although ICB is occasionally used for "boost" irradiation to the lumpectomy cavity as part of whole breast irradiation, the invasive nature of this technique as compared to other simpler methods limits its utility for this indication to select complex cases. ICB was developed to deliver APBI and this remains the predominant indication.

In addition to target delineation and dose coverage, one of the key components contributing to the successful application of APBI is patient selection. Patients with a significant risk of harboring microscopic disease within the breast, but located outside the stated treatment target (1 cm beyond the lumpectomy cavity), are not optimal candidates for APBI [10]. To date, conservative patient selection criteria have been employed until more definitive outcomes data become available. The National Surgical Adjuvant Breast and Bowel Project/Radiation Therapy Oncology Group (NSABP/RTOG) and Groupe Européen de Curiethérapie – European Society for Therapeutic Radiology and Oncology (GEC-ESTRO) are conducting phase III randomized trials evaluating APBI which will help determine which patients are appropriate for this approach and better define the breadth of application. Until mature data are available for these trials, several societies have endorsed conservative patient selection criteria with the goal of providing guidance and general consistency in selection of eligible patients [11–14]. These are summarized in Table 1.

Table 1 Guidelines for appropriate patient selection for APBI

American Society of Radiation Oncology (ASTRO) (2009)

"Suitable" group

Patient factors

    Age ≥60 years

    BRCA1/2 mutation not present

Pathologic factors

    Tumor size ≤2 cm

    T stage: T1

    Margins negative (by at least 2 mm)

    Any grade

    No LVSI

    ER +

    Unicentric and unifocal

    Histology: invasive ductal or other favorable subtypes

    Pure DCIS or EIC not allowed

    Associated LCIS is allowed

Nodal factors

    N stage: pN0 (i−, i+)

    Nodal surgery: SN Bx or ALND

Treatment factors

    Neoadjuvant chemotherapy not allowed

Groupe Européen de Curiethérapie-European Society for Therapeutic Radiology and Oncology (GEC-ESTRO) (2010)

Low risk group

Age ≥50 years

Histology: invasive ductal or other favorable subtypes

Invasive lobular carcinoma not allowed

Pure DCIS or EIC not allowed

Tumor size ≤3 cm

ER + or −

Margins negative (by at least 2 mm)

Unicentric and unifocal

No LVSI

Lymph node negative by SN Bx or ALND (pN0)

Neoadjuvant chemotherapy not allowed

American Society of Breast Surgeons (ABSB) (Update 2011)

Age ≥45 years

Invasive ductal carcinoma or DCIS

Tumor size ≤3 cm

Margins negative (no tumor at inked margin)

Lymph node negative by SN Bx or ALND (pN0)

American Brachytherapy Society (ABS) (Update 2013)

Age ≥50 years

Invasive carcinoma (any histology)

DCIS

Tumor size ≤3 cm

ER + or −

Margins negative (no tumor at inked margin)

No LVSI

Lymph node negative

The American Society of Radiation Oncology (ASTRO) appointed a task force to review available treatment outcomes data from APBI trials and determine the most appropriate patient selection criteria. This was first accomplished in 2009 and work toward reevaluation with a possible update has begun. The consensus statement published in 2009 consisted of three categories "suitable," "cautionary," and "unsuitable" [13]. These categories refer to appropriate patient selection for treatment outside the context of a clinical trial. Patients considered meeting the "suitable" criteria for APBI consist of age ≥60 years, lack of BRCA 1/2 germ line mutation, invasive ductal histology, tumor size ≤2 cm, margins microscopically negative by at least 2 mm, estrogen receptor (ER) positive, unicentric disease, and pathologically node negative. Patient and tumor characteristics falling outside these criteria were delegated to the "cautionary" or "unsuitable" categories. These criteria were based on available outcomes data from predominantly early treatment experiences which were highly selective. Several recent studies have called into question these conservative criteria showing no difference in ipsilateral breast tumor recurrence (IBTR) for patients in the "cautionary" and even "unsuitable" categories [15–17]. To incorporate recent data, the American Brachytherapy Society (ABS) released an update of their consensus statement [12]. According to the ABS criteria, patients deemed "acceptable" for APBI are patients who are age ≥50 years with tumors ≤3 cm of any invasive histology or DCIS that are either ER positive or negative, and who have negative margins (no ink on tumor), no LVSI, and negative lymph nodes. Although patients that do not meet these criteria have not been definitively shown to have inferior results with APBI, there is limited experience in treating such patients. Thus, employing conscrvative patient selection criteria as supported by the ABS, ASTRO, GEC-ESTRO, and American Society of Breast Surgeons (ASBS) remain prudent until definitive data are available.

In addition to patient selection for APBI in general, appropriate APBI technique selection in order to achieve optimal dosimetry is important in order to optimize outcomes [18]. The patient's comorbidities, body habitus, breast size, tumor location, and lumpectomy cavity geometric configuration should all be considered. For the ICB technique, it is important for the applicator to conform to the lumpectomy cavity. A collaboration with the breast surgeon is essential to help create a desirable target cavity and to avoid certain oncoplastic maneuvers that can transpose at-risk tissue to remote locations within the breast away from the lumpectomy cavity. Furthermore, the ability to control and limit the skin and rib dose is of paramount importance. Initially, with the use of a single-lumen balloon catheter, the spacing between the lumpectomy cavity and the skin and the resultant influence on skin dose, toxicity, and cosmetic outcome was the focus. With the use of the single-lumen catheter, a minimum skin spacing of 7 mm was required in order to meet recommended skin dose-volume constraints, and a lumpectomy cavity to rib spacing of 5 mm was required in order to meet recommended rib point dose constraints. With the transition to multilumen catheters, the focus has shifted away from physical spacing to limiting the dose through 3D planning platforms and therefore acceptable skin and rib doses can be achieved despite reduced distance to the skin and/or rib.

3   Technique and Catheter Systems

The ICB technique was introduced to provide a less complex implant technique over placement of multiple interstitial catheters. The first com-

mercially available device (MammoSite®) consisted of a balloon applicator with a single central lumen for delivery of radiation. The simple single-entry insertion coupled with simple treatment planning of this device made ICB widely popular in North America. However, the simplicity of this initial system possessed significant dosimetric limitations. This led to the evolution of more complex devices (Contura MLB®, MammoSite ML®, SAVI®) to help address these limitations yet maintain the ease of use of a single-entry applicator system. Each of these devices will be reviewed here.

3.1   Single-Lumen Intracavitary Balloon Catheter (MammoSite®)

The MammoSite® breast brachytherapy applicator (Hologic Inc., Bedford, MA, USA) received clearance by the FDA in 2002 and became one of the most used forms of APBI with more than 40,000 women implanted to date [19]. This device is a single-catheter system (Fig. 1) consisting of an outer lumen that allows for inflation of a balloon at the end of the shaft of the catheter and a single central lumen allowing the passage of a high-dose-rate (HDR) afterloaded ^{192}Ir source for the administration of radiation. The implantation of the MammoSite® device is relatively simple and reproducible. Implantation can be performed either at the time of surgery under direct visualization of the lumpectomy cavity (open technique) or postoperatively under image guidance (closed technique). The closed technique is recommended as the risk of infection, rate of persistent seroma formation, and resulting compromise in cosmetic outcome had been shown to be reduced with this approach [20]. The closed technique is typically performed 1–2 weeks postoperatively. Although placement at longer delays is possible, organization and contracture of the lumpectomy cavity may result in difficulty of cavity identification, catheter insertion, and/or balloon to cavity conformance. Using the closed technique, the catheter is inserted using image guidance via ultrasound (US), computed tomog-

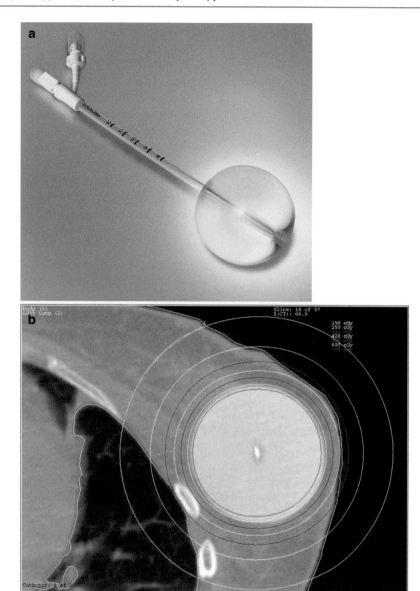

Fig. 1 (**a**) MammoSite® single-lumen intracavitary balloon catheter. (**b**) Near-spherical dose distribution prescribed to 1.0 cm from the balloon surface

raphy (CT), or both (Fig. 2). Based on measurements of the lumpectomy cavity on imaging, an appropriately sized applicator is selected. A variety of balloon sizes in both spherical and elliptical shapes have been available for optimal conformity. Using sterile technique and local anesthesia, the device is inserted utilizing an accompanying trocar. Insertion can be performed via the lumpectomy scar or via a remote site. Although less common, the scar-entry tech-

nique provides safe, direct access to the cavity and provides an ideal orientation, perpendicular to the skin and chest wall, for the single-lumen catheter. This orientation allows for the effect of anisotropy and a degree of dwell position manipulation to protect the skin and rib from excessive dose if the distance is close [21]. More commonly, the entry point is selected so that the balloon orientation is parallel to the skin and chest wall. Regardless of preferred style, the entry

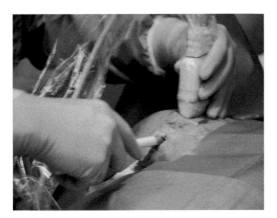

Fig. 2 Closed cavity balloon catheter insertion technique using real-time ultrasound guidance and a lateral entry approach

point should be individualized to the patient and selected so as to minimize the distance between insertion site and cavity, allow for optimal geometric conformity of the cavity to the balloon, and result in a comfortable applicator position for the patient for the duration of therapy.

After insertion, the balloon is inflated using saline and radiographic contrast. A planning CT scan is then performed to evaluate the adequacy of device placement. This should include conformality of the balloon surface to the lumpectomy cavity (>90 %), symmetry of the balloon applicator (<0.2 cm deviation in any dimensions), and the adequacy of skin spacing (≥0.7 cm). Once proper applicator and balloon position is established, CT imaging is acquired for 3D planning. The balloon, skin, chest wall, and target volume should be contoured. Likewise the central lumen and source dwell positions should be identified for planning. The target volume or planning tumor volume (PTV) consists of the 1 cm rim of breast tissue around the inflated balloon applicator. With adequate applicator placement, this will correspond to the tissue surrounding the lumpectomy cavity. The PTV should not extend into the chest wall and should be limited by 0.5 cm from the skin surface. Source dwell positions and times are then determined in order to deliver the prescription dose to the PTV. Treatment can either be delivered via a single central source dwell position or via

multiple source dwell positions along the central lumen. The use of multiple dwell positions reduces the dose heterogeneity across the implant, but the clinical implications of this have not been established [22]. Using either method, the resulting dose distribution is a near-symmetric sphere or ellipse. The simplicity of this catheter system makes treatment planning simple but also allows virtually no ability to modulate the dose distribution. Thus, the dose to the skin and chest wall is purely a function of applicator position and skin or chest wall spacing. Once the treatment plan is generated, treatment is delivered using a HDR Ir-192 source via a remote afterloader. Prior to each fraction of treatment, the balloon position and volume should be verified using US, CT, or fluoroscopic imaging.

3.2 Multi-lumen Balloon Intracavitary Catheters (Contura; MammoSite Multi-Lumen®)

The next generation of balloon applicators sought to improve upon the limitations of the single-lumen MammoSite® system's fixed geometry and inflexibility to sculpt dose. By introducing multiple lumens, these new applicators have a greater capacity to shape dose through optimization of source dwell time and position. Two similar multi-lumen balloon catheters are currently available: Contura MLB® (SenoRx Inc, Aliso Viejo, CA) and MammoSite Multi-Lumen® (ML) (Hologic Inc, Bedford, MA). The Contura catheter has one central lumen surrounded by four peripheral arched lumens at a 0.5 cm central offset (Fig. 3). The MammoSite Multi-Lumen® has one central lumen surrounded by three peripheral parallel lumens (Fig. 4).

The insertion technique for the MammoSite ML® and Contura MLB® are essentially similar to that of the single-lumen MammoSite® described above. The Contura® catheter does have an additionally vacuum port which can eliminate seroma fluid or air pockets surrounding the inflated balloon improving conformality of the lumpectomy cavity to the balloon [23]. Treatment planning for

Fig. 3 Contura® multi-lumen balloon catheter

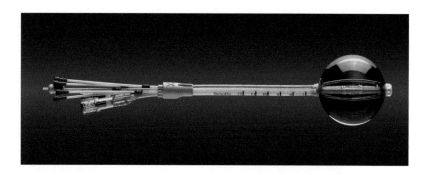

Fig. 4 MammoSite® multi-lumen balloon catheter

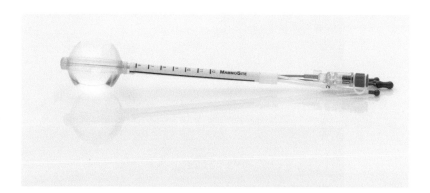

these two multi-lumen catheters allows for optimization of source dwell times among the 4–5 lumens and thus allows asymmetric dose distributions. This results in the ability to reduce skin or chest wall dose despite close applicator spacing.

The dosimetric advantages of the Contura MLB® catheter have been evaluated by several investigators and have been consistently shown to improve skin and chest wall dose sparing compared to a single-lumen MammoSite® catheter (Fig. 5) [24–27]. Arthur et al. performed a preliminary dosimetric analysis of a phase IV trial evaluating the Contura® catheter [26]. They reviewed 144 cases and found that 92 % and 89 % of case met dose restriction to the skin (<125 %) and chest wall (<145 %), respectively. Even in cases with <7 mm of skin spacing and <5 mm of chest wall spacing, most plans met these constraints.

For the multi-lumen catheters, prior to each treatment, not only is it important to verify balloon position and fill volume, but the rotational position of the applicator needs to be verified. This is typically done using alignment of a skin and catheter mark which has been shown to result in a reproducible applicator position [28].

3.3 Multi-lumen Non-balloon Intracavitary Catheter (SAVI)

The strut-adjusted volume implant or SAVI® (Cianna Medical, Aliso Viejo, CA) is a hybrid, non-balloon-based, intracavitary brachytherapy catheter system. This system combines the dosimetric flexibility of interstitial implants with the simplicity of a single-catheter entry into the breast. The SAVI® consisting of a central lumen surrounded by 6–10 peripherally positioned lumens depending on the selected applicator size (Fig. 6). When initially inserted into the breast, all the lumens are collapsed together and catheter insertion is identical to the balloon-based ICB catheters. Upon placement into the lumpectomy cavity, the peripheral lumens are expanded to form a cage-like structure that conforms to the lumpectomy cavity. The multiple

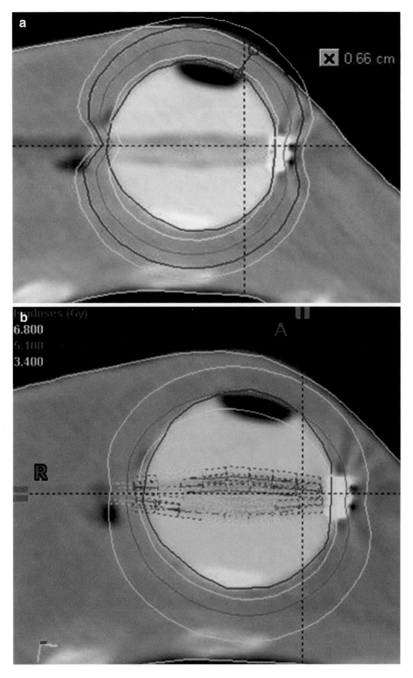

Fig. 5 Dosimetric comparison of single-lumen versus multi-lumen balloon catheters for treatment of a lumpectomy cavity with 0.66 cm skin spacing. (**a**) MammoSite® single-lumen catheter with 95 % coverage of the PTV with 95 % of prescription dose resulting in a maximum skin dose of 4.6 Gy (126 % of prescription).

(**b**) Contura® (MLB) demonstrating the ability to modulate the dose distribution via source dwell positions and times within the five lumens resulting in 95 % of the PTV covered by 95 % of prescription dose while reducing the maximum skin dose to 2.9 Gy (85 % of prescription)

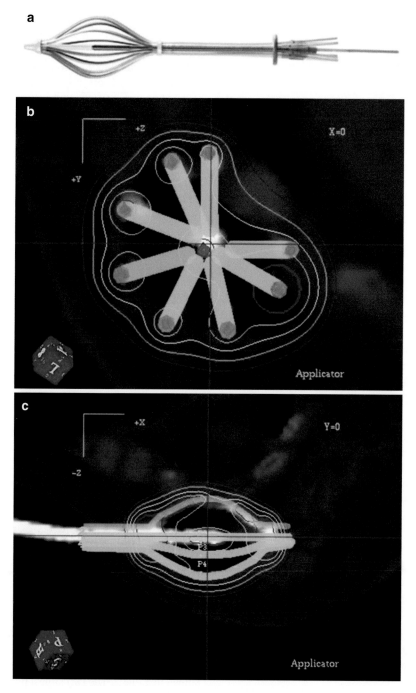

Fig. 6 Strut-adjusted volume implant. (**a**) SAVI® multi-lumen intracavitary catheter. Dosimetry images in the (**b**) coronal and (**c**) sagittal planes demonstrating ability to modulate dose distribution to conform to the lumpectomy cavity

lumens of the SAVI® catheter abut the tissue surrounding the lumpectomy cavity and allow great flexibility in dosimetric geometry. This allows for dose distribution that can conform to irregular target volume configurations and allows for a greater ability to restrict dose to the skin and chest wall [29]. However, it is important to note that the SAVI® catheter has distinct dosimetry compared with the balloon-based ICB systems resulting in distinct dosimetric and radiobiological consideration for normal tissue effects. The dosimetry of the SAVI® catheter is in some ways similar to that which is achieved with interstitial brachytherapy. However, unlike interstitial implants, the multiple lumens of the SAVI catheter line the lumpectomy cavity rather than being positioned with even spacing throughout the entire target volume. Thus, the distance from the lumens to the edge of the PTV is greater with the SAVI catheter than when using the interstitial catheters. This can result in higher dose hotspots. Mean V150 (volume of target receiving 150 % of prescribed dose) and V200 (volume of target receiving 200 % of prescribed dose) have been reported to be 22.7–30.8 cc and 11.6–14.9 cc, respectively [30, 31]. These values of V150 and V200 are higher than what is typically seen with balloon-based ICB catheters but in most cases do not exceed the values associated with suboptimal cosmetic outcomes in the interstitial brachytherapy experience [32]. Early clinical experience has been encouraging, but mature clinical data is needed for the SAVI® catheter to understand the clinical implications of the distinct radiobiology of this catheter system [33, 34].

4   Dosimetric Constraints and Quality Metrics

The most commonly prescribed dose with ICB is 34.0 Gy in 10 fraction delivered twice daily at least 6 h apart over 1 week. Shorter treatment courses delivered in an even more convenient schedule over 2 days (4 fractions) and even 1 day (2 fractions) are being explored [35, 36]. The intended dose is prescribed to the PTV

margin which consists of the 1 cm rim of tissue around the applicator or lumpectomy cavity limited by the chest wall and 0.5 cm from the skin. An acceptable plan will have >90 % of the prescription dose encompassing >90 % of the PTV. However, >95 % of the prescription dose encompassing >95 % of the PTV is desirable. The maximum skin surface dose and chest wall dose should be reported. These should be <100–125 % and <145 % of prescription dose, respectively, particularly when using the multi-lumen catheters. The V150 and V200 should also be reported. The optimal V150 and V200 have not been well established for the ICB technique. Empiric V150 and V200 constraints of <50 cc and <10 cc are recommended for the balloon-based techniques and <50 cc and <20 cc for the SAVI device.

5   Treatment Outcomes

A multi-institutional trial designed to evaluate the safety and performance of the single-lumen MammoSite® catheter was performed as part of the regulatory approval process in the United States. The initial report by Keisch et al. [19] showed the feasibility and acceptable acute toxicity of this approach in a cohort of 43 patients. As data matured, results at 5-year follow-up were reported demonstrating no local or regional failures. The rates of implant-related infection (9 %) and fat necrosis (9 %) were acceptable. Seroma formation occurred in 33 % of patients, of which 12 % were symptomatic requiring aspiration. Overall, good-excellent cosmetic outcome was observed in 83.3 % of patients [37]. This trial led to the United States Food and Drug Administration (FDA) clearance of the MammoSite® device for use in the United States.

A summary of clinical experience with ICB is shown in Table 2. The two largest published experiences come from a multi-institutional cohort compiled at Virginia Commonwealth University (VCU) and the American Society of Breast Surgeons (ASBS) MammoSite® registry trial [20, 38]. The VCU group reported on 483 patients with a median follow-up of 24 months [20]. Ipsilateral breast tumor recurrence (IBTR) was

Table 2 Intracavitary brachytherapy (ICB) single and multi-institutional trials

Institution/study	Device	Number of patients	Median follow-up (months)	IBTR (%)	Cosmesis (% excellent/good)
FDA trial [37]	MammoSite	43	66	0 (at 5 years)	81.3
ASBS registry trial [38]	MammoSite	1440	63	3.8 (at 5 years)	90.6
Magee-Women's Hosp. [51]	MammoSite	92	30	0	NR
St. Luke's Cancer Inst. [52]	MammoSite	93	29	1.3 (at 3 years)	NR
Rush Univ. [53]	MammoSite	70	26	5.7	NR
VCU multi-institutional [20]	MammoSite	483	24	1.2	91
MUSC [54]	MammoSite	90	24	2.2	90
WBH [43]	MammoSite	80	22	2.9	88.2
Multi-institutional [39]	Contura	342	36	2.2 (at 3 years)	88
WellStar Kennestone Hosp. [55]	Contura	46	36	2	97
UCSD/ABCS [33]	SAVI	102	21	1	NR

IBTR ipsilateral breast tumor recurrence, *NR* not reported, *FDA* Federal Drug Administration, *ASBS* American Society of Breast Surgeons, *VCU* Virginia Commonwealth University, *MUSC* Medical University of South Carolina, *WBH* William Beaumont Hospital, *UCSD* University of California, San Diego, *ABCS* Arizona Breast Cancer Specialists

1.2 %. The infection rate was 9 % overall but only 4.8 % when the implant was performed as a closed procedure. Any telangiectasia was seen in 17 % and significant telangiectasia in 5 % of patients. Overall good-excellent cosmetic outcome was 91 %. The final results of the ASBS MammoSite® registry trial were recently presented consisting of 1440 patients and 1449 cases [38]. With a median follow-up of 63 months, the actuarial IBTR at 5 years was 3.8 %. The rates of fat necrosis, infections, and symptomatic seroma were 2.5 %, 9.6 %, and 13.4 %, respectively, with few toxicity events occurring beyond 2 years of follow-up. The overall good-excellent cosmetic outcome was 91.3 % at 5 years and 90.6 % at 7 years.

Although the outcomes of the single-lumen MammoSite® catheter have been good, it became clear that simplicity of the device limited any kind of dosimetric modulation leading to suboptimal outcomes in patient with close lumpectomy cavity to skin distance. This led to the development of multi-lumen devices as described above. The Contura® catheter is currently being evaluated in a multi-institutional, phase IV trial. Initial results were presented by Cuttino et al. consisting of 342 treated patients with median follow-up of 36 months [39]. The local recurrence-free survival at 3 years was 97.8 %. Treatment was well tolerated, with implant-related infection observed in 8.5 %, fat

necrosis in 6.8 %, telangiectasia (grade 1) in 8.2 %, and symptomatic seroma in 4.4 %. There was no grade 2–4 telangiectasia or fibrosis observed. Overall cosmetic outcome was good or excellent in 88 % of patients. Furthermore, patients treated at high-volume centers appeared to have improved outcomes with 3-year local recurrence-free survival of 98.1 %, infection rate of 2.9 %, symptomatic seroma rate of 1.9 %, and good-to-excellent cosmesis rate of 95 %.

Very early results with the SAVI® catheter have also been reported and are likewise encouraging [33, 34]. Yashar et al. [34] reported on 102 patients with a median follow-up of 21 months. Toxicity was minimal with 1.9 % symptomatic seroma, 1.9 % grade 2 fibrosis, and 1.9 % asymptomatic fat necrosis. In-breast failure was seen in only 1 % of patients. More clinical experience and longer follow-up are needed to confirm these early results.

6 Toxicity Prevention and Management

The success of an ICB implant should be evaluated not only on the success of prevention of disease recurrence but also with regard to treatment-related toxicity and the ultimate cosmetic outcome. Adverse outcomes of the ICB technique can broadly be grouped into two categories: insertion-related adverse events and dosimetry/radiation-related toxicity.

Insertion-related complications include infection, hemorrhage, and implant failure from nonconformance of the applicator to the excision cavity or balloon rupture/device failure. Prevention of post-procedural infection is of particular importance as this has been shown to compromise the ultimate cosmetic outcome [20]. Measures to minimize this risk should be taken. Insertion should be performed with scrutiny to sterile technique. Meticulous attention should be paid to wound care during the time the applicator remains in place. Prophylactic antibiotics have been used and may be helpful but are not universally employed [20, 40, 41]. Analysis from the VCU experience has also shown that a closed insertion approach as opposed to intraoperative placement significantly reduced the risk of infection by nearly half [20]. It appears that by employing these simple measures, the infection rate can be kept acceptably low even when assessed among a broad base of users. In a report of the ASBS MammoSite® registry trial, the device-related infection rate of 793 patients was only 5.9 % [41].

Although we have learned much from the early interstitial brachytherapy experience about the dosimetric factors that lead to late toxicity, ICB implants have distinctly different dosimetry with distinctly different radiobiologic implication with regard to normal tissue toxicity. Shah et al. [42] reported a series of interstitial and MammoSite® implants and found significant differences in critical dosimetric parameters. MammoSite® implants are associated with significantly less irradiated tissue and smaller volume "hotspots" as compared to interstitial brachytherapy. In contrast, the global uniformity as reflected in the calculated dose homogeneity index (DHI) is superior with an interstitial implant. As a result, the lessons we learned from interstitial brachytherapy with regard to late tissue affects do not necessarily apply to ICB. Clinical experience has taught us a host of new factors that are important.

The initial single-lumen MammoSite® device had simple and predictable dosimetry with a near-symmetric geometrical dose distribution. As such, spacing between the applicator surface and the normal tissue at risk is critical to determining normal tissue toxicity. This has been most clearly shown with regard to skin toxicity. Benitez et al. [37] evaluated the initial MammoSite® FDA trial showing a correlation with suboptimal results when skin spacing was ≤0.7 cm. Chao et al. [43] evaluated the William Beaumont Hospital experience consisting of 80 patients with a median follow-up of 22.1 months and found a similar correlate of lower rates of good-excellent cosmetic outcome with skin spacing of <0.7 cm. Cuttino et al. [20] in the VCU analysis also showed the importance of skin spacing with a statistically significant correlation between skin spacing of <0.6 cm and the rate of severe acute skin reaction and late telangiectasia. Based on these data, it is recommended for an applicator to skin spacing of ≥0.7 cm which corresponds to a maximum skin surface dose of <145 % of prescription. With the simple design of the initial single-lumen MammoSite® catheter, little can be done for patients with inadequate skin spacing. These patients are either not candidates for treatment or subject to increase risk of toxicity. The new multi-lumen catheters were designed to allow for 3D planning and customization of the dose distribution. This has allowed for sparing of skin dose in patients with close lumpectomy cavity to skin distances. As a result, significantly lower skin doses can be achieved and a more conservative maximum skin dose constraint is recommended, <100–125 % of prescription. This more conservative skin constraint may further reduce the likelihood of late skin toxicity. In addition, patients with skin spacing between 0.5 and 0.7 cm are considered good candidates for treatment.

Other observed late toxicities include fat necrosis, persistent seroma, chest wall pain, and rib fracture. Seroma rates of 21–68 % have been reported [43–47], but only one third of these are symptomatic [47]. The ASBS MammoSite® registry trial found that seromas were reported more often with intraoperative placement rather than when employing the closed placement approach (30 % vs. 19 %) and with the use of larger balloons [20, 48]. Chest wall pain and rib fraction can be a significant complication of the ICB technique and are likely dependent on dose and irradiated volumes [49, 50]. With the initial MammoSite®, a maximum dose to the chest wall of <145 % of prescription was recommended. A more conservative recommendation is used with the newer multi-catheter devices of <125 % of prescription.

Conclusion

ICB represents a simplified brachytherapy approach for APBI. Mature clinical experience has shown excellent outcomes in terms of both prevention of tumor recurrence within the breast as well as the overall cosmetic outcome. The newer multi-lumen catheter systems allow for flexibility in dose modulation to allow for skin and chest wall sparing and will likely improve outcomes in regard to toxicity endpoints. As with all APBI techniques, the results of ongoing randomized trials will definitively prove whether APBI is equivalent to whole breast irradiation and will define the optimal patient population for this approach. Until mature data from these trials are available, the current clinical experience support continued use of APBI delivered using ICB for select patients.

References

1. Janni W, Rjosk D, Dimpfl TH et al (2001) Quality of life influenced by primary surgical treatment for stage I-III breast cancer-long-term follow-up of a matched-pair analysis. Ann Surg Oncol 8(6):542–548
2. Early Breast Cancer Trialists' Collaborative Group (EBCTCG), Darby S S, McGale P, Correa C et al (2011) Effect of radiotherapy after breast-conserving surgery on 10-year recurrence and 15-year breast cancer death: meta-analysis of individual patient data for 10,801 women in 17 randomized trials. Lancet 378(9804):1707–1716
3. Fisher B, Anderson S, Bryant J et al (2002) Twenty-year follow-up of a randomized trial comparing total mastectomy, lumpectomy, and lumpectomy plus irradiation for the treatment of invasive breast cancer. N Engl J Med 347:1233–1241
4. Veronesi U, Cascinelli N, Mariani L et al (2002) Twenty-year follow-up of a randomized study comparing breast-conserving surgery with radical mastectomy for early breast cancer. N Engl J Med 347:1227–1232
5. Arthur DW, Vicini FA (2005) Accelerated partial breast irradiation as a part of breast conservation therapy. J Clin Oncol 23:1726–1735
6. Athas WF, Adams-Cameron M, Hunt WC et al (2000) Travel distance to radiation therapy and receipt of radiotherapy following breast-conserving surgery. J Natl Cancer Inst 92:269–271
7. Arthur DW, Winter K, Kuske RR et al (2008) A phase II trial of brachytherapy alone after lumpectomy for select breast cancer: tumor control and survival outcomes of RTOG 95-17. Int J Radiat Oncol Biol Phys 72:467–473
8. Chen PY, Vicini FA, Benitez P et al (2006) Long-term cosmetic results and toxicity after accelerated partial-breast irradiation: a method of radiation delivery by interstitial brachytherapy for the treatment of early-stage breast carcinoma. Cancer 106:991–999
9. Shah C, Antonucci JV, Wilkinson JB et al (2011) Twelve-year clinical outcomes and patterns of failure with accelerated partial breast irradiation versus whole-breast irradiation: results of a matched-pair analysis. Radiother Oncol
10. Vicini FA, Kestin LL, Goldstein NS et al (2004) Defining the clinical target volume for patients with early-stage breast cancer treated with lumpectomy and accelerated partial breast irradiation: a pathologic analysis. Int J Radiat Oncol Biol Phys 60:722–730
11. Polgár C, Van Limbergen E, Pötter R et al (2010) Patient selection for accelerated partial-breast irradiation (APBI) after breast-conserving surgery: recommendations of the Groupe Européen de Curiethérapie-European Society for Therapeutic Radiology and Oncology (GEC-ESTRO) breast cancer working group based on clinical evidence (2009). Radiother Oncol 94(3):264–273
12. Shah C, Vicini F, Wazer DE et al (2013) The American Brachytherapy Society consensus statement for accelerated partial breast irradiation. Brachytherapy 12(4):267–277
13. Smith BD, Arthur DW, Buchholz TA et al (2009) Accelerated partial breast irradiation consensus statement from the American Society for Radiation Oncology (ASTRO). Int J Radiat Oncol Biol Phys 74(4):987–1001
14. http://www.breastsurgeons.org/statements/PDF_Statements/APBI_statement_revised_100708.pdf. Accessed 13 Mar 2015.
15. Shaitelman SF, Vicini FA, Beitsch P et al (2010) Five-year outcome of patients classified using the American Society for Radiation Oncology consensus statement guidelines for the application of accelerated partial breast irradiation: an analysis of patients treated on the American Society of Breast Surgeons MammoSite Registry Trial. Cancer 116(20):4677–4685
16. Vicini F, Arthur D, Wazer D et al (2011) Limitations of the American Society of Therapeutic Radiology and Oncology Consensus Panel guidelines on the use of accelerated partial breast irradiation. Int J Radiat Oncol Biol Phys 79(4):977–984

17. Wilkinson JB, Beitsch PD, Shah C et al (2013) Evaluation of current consensus statement recommendations for accelerated partial breast irradiation: a pooled analysis of William Beaumont Hospital and American Society of Breast Surgeon MammoSite Registry Trial Data. Int J Radiat Oncol Biol Phys 85(5):1179–1185

18. Hepel JT, Wazer DE (2012) A comparison of brachytherapy techniques for partial breast irradiation. Brachytherapy 11(3):163–175

19. Keisch M, Vicini F, Kuske RR et al (2003) Initial clinical experience with the MammoSite breast brachytherapy applicator in women with early-stage breast cancer treated with breast-conserving therapy. Int J Radiat Oncol Biol Phys 55:289–293

20. Cuttino LW, Keisch M, Jenrette JM et al (2008) Multi-institutional experience using the MammoSite radiation therapy system in the treatment of early-stage breast cancer: 2-year results. Int J Radiat Oncol Biol Phys 71:107–114

21. Edmundson GK, Vicini FA, Chen PY et al (2002) Dosimetric characteristics of the MammoSite RTS, a new breast brachytherapy applicator. Int J Radiat Oncol Biol Phys 52(4):1132–1139

22. Stewart AJ, Hepel JT, O'Farrell DA et al (2013) Equivalent uniform dose for accelerated partial breast irradiation using the MammoSite applicator. Radiother Oncol 108(2):232–235

23. Tokita KM, Cuttino LW, Vicini FA et al (2011) Optimal application of the Contura multilumen balloon breast brachytherapy catheter vacuum port to deliver accelerated partial breast irradiation. Brachytherapy 10(3):184–189

24. Arthur DW, Vicini FA, Todor DA et al (2011) Improvements in critical dosimetric endpoints using the Contura multilumen balloon breast brachytherapy catheter to deliver accelerated partial breast irradiation: preliminary dosimetric findings of a phase IV trial. Int J Radiat Oncol Biol Phys 79:26–33

25. Brown S, McLaughlin M, Pope DK et al (2011) A dosimetric comparison of the Contura multilumen balloon breast brachytherapy catheter vs. the single-lumen MammoSite balloon device in patients treated with accelerated partial breast irradiation at a single institution. Brachytherapy 10:68–73

26. Cuttino LW, Todor D, Rosu M et al (2011) A comparison of skin and chest wall dose delivered with multicatheter, Contura multilumen balloon, and MammoSite breast brachytherapy. Int J Radiat Oncol Biol Phys 79:34–38

27. Wilder RB, Curcio LD, Khanijou RK et al (2009) A Contura catheter offers dosimetric advantages over a MammoSite catheter that increase the applicability of accelerated partial breast irradiation. Brachytherapy 8:373–378

28. Ouhib Z, Benda R, Kasper M et al (2011) Accurate verification of balloon rotation correction for the Contura multilumen device for accelerated partial breast irradiation. Brachytherapy 10(4):325–330

29. Manoharan SR, Rodriguez RR, Bobba VS et al (2010) Dosimetry evaluation of SAVI-based HDR brachytherapy for partial breast irradiation. J Med Phys 35:131–136

30. Bloom ES, Kirsner S, Mason BE et al (2011) Accelerated partial breast irradiation using the strut-adjusted volume implant single-entry hybrid catheter in brachytherapy for breast cancer in the setting of breast augmentation. Brachytherapy 10(3):178–183

31. Gurdalli S, Kuske RR Jr, Quiet CA et al (2011) Dosimetric performance of Strut-Adjusted Volume Implant: a new single-entry multicatheter breast brachytherapy applicator. Brachytherapy 10(2):128–135

32. Wazer DE, Kaufman S, Cuttino L et al (2006) Accelerated partial breast irradiation: an analysis of variables associated with late toxicity and long-term cosmetic outcome after high-dose-rate interstitial brachytherapy. Int J Radiat Oncol Biol Phys 64:489–495

33. Yashar CM, Blair S, Wallace A et al (2009) Initial clinical experience with the Strut-Adjusted Volume Implant brachytherapy applicator for accelerated partial breast irradiation. Brachytherapy 8:367–372

34. Yashar C, Scanderbeg D, Kuske R et al (2011) Initial Clinical Experience With the Strut-Adjusted Volume Implant (SAVI) Breast Brachytherapy Device for Accelerated Partial-Breast Irradiation (APBI): First 100 Patients With More Than 1 Year of Follow-Up. Int J Radiat Oncol Biol Phys 80(3):765–770

35. Khan AJ, Vicini FA, Brown S et al (2013) Dosimetric feasibility and acute toxicity in a prospective trial of ultrashort-course accelerated partial breast irradiation (APBI) using a multi-lumen balloon brachytherapy device. Ann Surg Oncol 20(4):1295–1301

36. Wallace M, Martinez A, Mitchell C et al (2010) Phase I/II study evaluating early tolerance in breast cancer patients undergoing accelerated partial breast irradiation treated with the mammosite balloon breast brachytherapy catheter using a 2-day dose schedule. Int J Radiat Oncol Biol Phys 77:531–536

37. Benitez PR, Keisch ME, Vicini F et al (2007) Five-year results: the initial clinical trial of MammoSite balloon brachytherapy for partial breast irradiation in early-stage breast cancer. Am J Surg 194:456–462

38. Shah C, Badiyan S, Ben Wilkinson J et al (2013) Treatment efficacy with accelerated partial breast irradiation (APBI): final analysis of the American Society of Breast Surgeons MammoSite(®) breast brachytherapy registry trial. Ann Surg Oncol 20(10):3279–3285

39. Cuttino LW, Arthur DW, Vicini F et al (2014) Long-term results from the Contura multilumen balloon breast brachytherapy catheter phase 4 registry trial. Int J Radiat Oncol Biol Phys 90(5):1025–1029

40. Harper JL, Jenrette JM, Vanek KN et al (2005) Acute complications of MammoSite brachytherapy: a single institution's initial clinical experience. Int J Radiat Oncol Biol Phys 61:169–174

41. Vicini F, Beitsch P, Quiet C et al (2005) First analysis of patient demographics, technical reproducibility, cosmesis and early toxicity by the American Society of

Breast Surgeons MammoSite breast brachytherapy registry trial in 793 patients treated with accelerated partial breast irradiation (APBI). Cancer 104:1138–1148

42. Shah NM, Tennenholz T, Arthur D et al (2004) MammoSite and interstitial brachytherapy for accelerated partial breast irradiation: factors that affect toxicity and cosmesis. Cancer 101:727–734

43. Chao KK, Vicini FA, Wallace M et al (2007) Analysis of treatment efficacy, cosmesis, and toxicity using the MammoSite breast brachytherapy catheter to deliver accelerated partial-breast irradiation: the William Beaumont hospital experience. Int J Radiat Oncol Biol Phys 69:32–40

44. Evans SB, Kaufman SA, Price LL et al (2006) Persistent seroma after intraoperative placement of MammoSite for accelerated partial breast irradiation: incidence, pathologic anatomy, and contributing factors. Int J Radiat Oncol Biol Phys 65:333–339

45. Haley ML, Beriwal S, Heron DE et al (2007) Accelerated partial breast irradiation (APBI) with Mammosite: an interim outcome analysis with two years follow-up. Int J Radiat Oncol Biol Phys 69:S236

46. Vicini F, Beitsch P, Quiet C et al (2011) Five-year analysis of treatment efficacy and cosmesis by the American Society of Breast Surgeons MammoSite Breast Brachytherapy Registry Trial in patients treated with accelerated partial breast irradiation. Int J Radiat Oncol Biol Phys 79:808–817

47. Watkins JM, Harper JL, Dragun AE et al (2008) Incidence and prognostic factors for seroma development after MammoSite breast brachytherapy. Brachytherapy 7:305–309

48. Vicini F, Beitsch PD, Quiet CA et al (2007) Three year analysis of treatment efficacy, cosmesis, and toxicity by the American Society of Breast Surgeons MammoSite Breast Brachytherapy Registry Trial in patients treated with Accelerated Partial Breast Irradiation (APBI). Cancer 112:758–766

49. Brashears JH, Dragun AE, Jenrette JM (2009) Late chest wall toxicity after MammoSite breast brachytherapy. Brachytherapy 8:19–25

50. Cuttino LW, Todor D, Rosu M et al (2009) Skin and chest wall dose with multi-catheter and MammoSite breast brachytherapy: implications for late toxicity. Brachytherapy 8:223–226

51. Soran A, Evrensel T, Beriwal S et al (2007) Placement technique and the early complications of balloon breast brachytherapy: Magee-Womens Hospital experience. Am J Clin Oncol 30:152–155

52. Edwards JM, Herzberg SM, Shook JW et al (2013) Breast Conservation Therapy Utilizing Partial Breast Brachytherapy for Early-stage Cancer of the Breast: A Retrospective Review From the Saint Luke's Cancer Institute. Am J Clin Oncol [Epub ahead of print]

53. Chen S, Dickler A, Kirk M et al (2007) Patterns of failure after MammoSite brachytherapy partial breast irradiation: a detailed analysis. Int J Radiat Oncol Biol Phys 69:25–31

54. Dragun AE, Harper JL, Jenrette JM et al (2007) Predictors of cosmetic outcome following MammoSite breast brachytherapy: a single-institution experience of 100 patients with two years of follow-up. Int J Radiat Oncol Biol Phys 68:354–358

55. Israel PZ, Robbins A, Shroff P et al (2012) Three-year clinical outcome using the Contura multilumen balloon breast brachytherapy catheter to deliver accelerated partial breast irradiation (APBI): improving radiation standards for the optimal application of APBI. Brachytherapy 11(4):316–321

Breast Brachytherapy: Permanent Breast Seed Implants – How and Why?

Jean-Philippe Pignol and Juanita Crook

Abstract

This chapter reports patient selection criteria, planning, technique, and results of permanent breast seed implant. In a single 1 h procedure, this technique uses stereotactic localization to permanently implant stranded ^{103}Pd seeds in and around the seroma cavity after lumpectomy for early stage breast cancer. Five-year results for a cohort of 137 patients are excellent in terms of both local control and tolerance.

1   Introduction

Due to the widespread adoption of screening mammography, the majority of breast cancers are diagnosed at an early stage [1, 2]. These patients have a good prognosis, and the 10 year risk of dying of cancer is small [3]. The goals of therapy are therefore to ensure local control and breast preservation, to reduce long-term side effects, and to minimize the burden of care. The current standard of care is breast-conserving surgery, which is most frequently a lumpectomy with node sampling, followed by adjuvant whole breast irradiation (WBI) using small daily fractions of 5 days per week for 3–7 weeks [4–6].

Several reports have shown that for early stage breast cancer, the majority of recurrences occur in proximity to the surgical seroma [7]. Thus, limiting radiation to the postsurgical cavity with a margin may suffice to prevent local recurrence-free for carefully selected patients [8]. Irradiating a smaller volume of breast allows treatment to be delivered over a shorter period of time [9]. Accelerated partial breast irradiation (APBI) has been tested since 1992 in multiple studies, including several multicenter randomized controlled trials [10–13]. The oldest and most frequently used technique is brachytherapy, followed by 3D conformal external beam radiotherapy (EBRT) and intraoperative radiotherapy [14].

Historically, brachytherapy used low-dose-rate sources like iridium wires or iodine seeds [15], but more recently multi-catheter and balloon high-dose-rate (HDR) brachytherapy have become the techniques of choice [16]. A SEER

J.-P. Pignol, MD, PhD (✉)
Radiation Oncology Department, Erasmus Medical Center, Rotterdam, The Netherlands
e-mail: j.p.pignol@erasmusmc.nl

J. Crook, MD, FRCPC
Department of Radiation Oncology, University of British Columbia, British Columbia Cancer Agency Centre for the Southern Interior,
Kelowna, BC, Canada

© Springer International Publishing Switzerland 2016
P. Montemaggi et al. (eds.), *Brachytherapy: An International Perspective*, Medical Radiology,
DOI 10.1007/978-3-319-26791-3_10

database analysis has revealed that HDR brachytherapy patients may have a 1.5 % increased risk of mastectomy which is very unlikely to impact significantly on survival [17].

In 2006 the technique of permanent breast seed implant (PBSI) for APBI was initiated at the Sunnybrook Odette Cancer Centre [18]. This approach was derived from permanent prostate seed brachytherapy but required adaptation of ultrasound image guidance and the use of a "fiducial" needle to localize the target volume. To date, patients have been treated in seven centers in North America and enrolled in Phase I/II studies for early stage invasive cancers, a Phase II study for low-risk ductal carcinoma in situ (DCIS), and a prospective multicenter registry study. In Europe, one report described the use of iodine seeds for a radiation boost after whole breast radiotherapy [19].

This chapter describes patient selection, treatment planning and the implantation procedure, as well as the quality assurance process, and outcomes of PBSI.

2   Indications

2.1   Rationale of PBSI Eligibility Criteria

Initial APBI studies included some patients with aggressive clinical or pathologic features such as young age, nodal positivity, or close margins [10, 20]. In 2009 the American Society for Therapeutic Radiation and Oncology (ASTRO) published a consensus statement with relatively strict eligibility criteria for APBI [21]. Several other societies followed with similar guidelines and recommendations [22–24]. An appropriate patient for APBI has a low risk of locoregional or distant relapse and is node negative and hormone receptor positive, with a small infiltrating ductal carcinoma and no lobular features, extensive carcinoma in situ, or lymphovascular invasion. The Toronto experience was initiated prior to the publication of these guidelines and initially included patients as young as 40 years of age and with more aggressive

pathologic features such as one to three positive nodes and negative hormone receptors. Following the publication of the guidelines, the protocols were amended to be more restrictive, limiting the minimum age to 50 and restricting eligible patients to node negative with favorable pathology.

2.2   Currently Recommended Clinical Criteria for PBSI

Eligible patients should be 50 years of age or older and referred for adjuvant radiotherapy after breast-conserving surgery. We do not recommend PBSI for patients with a medical history of connective tissue disorder, poorly controlled or complicated diabetes, or those with post-lumpectomy complications such as abscess or delayed wound healing. At the first patient consultation, the technical feasibility of implantation is evaluated. With the patient supine, there must be enough breast tissue to implant or three planes of needles spaced 1 cm apart. In addition, seroma location in the lateral quadrants of the breast is preferable. Implanting the upper inner quadrant tends to be more challenging and can be associated with more skin toxicity since the breast skin in this region is in closer proximity to the chest wall, especially when the patient is standing.

2.3   Pathologic Selection Criteria

PBSI should be limited to patients with unifocal infiltrating ductal carcinoma of less than 3 cm in diameter, resected with at least a 0.2 cm clear margin or with negative re-excision margins. It is unclear if non-luminal pathology, with negative hormone receptors and overexpression of HER2, or triple negative tumors are suitable for APBI although some such patients were included in the Canadian series. Also, although experience is limited, there is no strong rationale for excluding DCIS. There is a general consensus to exclude multifocal tumors, lobular pathology, lymphovascular infiltration (LVI), extensive carcinoma in situ, and patients who are node positive. A 0.2 cm negative margin for APBI may be questioned given the recent data suggesting that no further surgery is required before WBI provided there is no tumor at the inked margin [25].

2.4   Planning Selection Criteria

The high dose of radiation delivered to the breast with PBSI is not homogenous. As the dose distribution cannot be optimized after the implant is done, several precautions are taken to avoid severe permanent side effects. Based on our experience, we do not recommend implanting volumes larger than 120 cc (corresponding to a sphere of 6 cm in diameter). The skin dose should be limited such that the maximum dose to an area of 1 cm^2 does not exceed 90 % of the prescribed dose [26]. A breast ultrasound is performed either during the first consultation or at the time of the planning CT to ensure the fluid cavity constituting the seroma is clearly visible and is not larger than 2.5 cm in the direction of the needle insertion. Larger seromas are associated with greater seed migration and possible accumulation of seeds at the inferior aspect of the seroma. Finally the shape of the implanted volume should permit the placement of a minimum of two superimposed planes of needles.

3   Technique

3.1   Planning

3.1.1   Computed Tomography (CT) Simulation

Although the implant procedure is ultrasound-guided (US), the planning is CT based. The CT simulation is performed with the patient lying supine on a breast board, with one (or both) arm abducted and supported above the head. The position is identical to that for EBRT simulation such that, in case the patient is found ineligible for PBSI at time of dosimetry, the CT images can be used for planning standard whole breast radiotherapy. The scar is identified using a thin metal wire, and a lead bead is placed on the inferior medial quadrant of the nipple (Fig. 1a, b). These markers are used at the time of implantation to help localize the seroma projection on the skin. Wire to mark the breast skin folds is not required.

The CT images are acquired with the finest spacing and thickness available to optimize the resolution of re-sliced images in the planning system. At this stage it is important to ensure the seroma is easily identifiable, of appropriate size, and sufficiently far from the skin surface. This is assessed by contouring the target volume on the horizontal image sets before the re-slicing. The

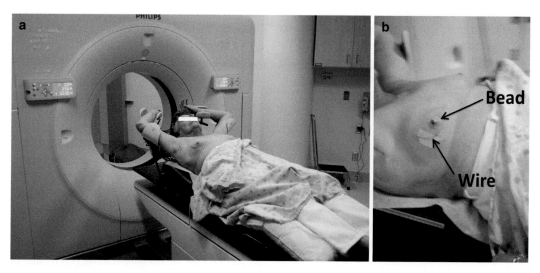

Fig. 1 (**a**, **b**) The CT simulation is performed with the patient lying supine on a breast board, with wire and beads placed on the surgical scar and the nipple

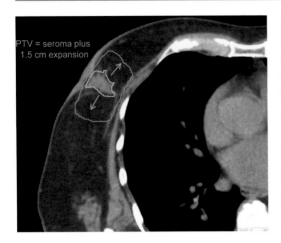

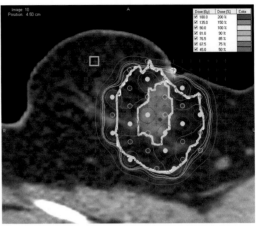

Fig. 2 The clinical target volume (CTV) is defined as the surgical cavity, the microscopic extension of the tumor, and a security margin. Practically this corresponds to the seroma with an additional expansion of 1.5 cm

Fig. 3 For planning optimization, the needles are inserted following a square or a triangular pattern, whichever fits better to the PTV shape on the most central slice

clinical target volume (CTV) is defined as the surgical cavity, the surrounding fibrosis, and suspected possible microscopic extension. Practically this corresponds to the surgical cavity and its surrounding fibrosis, which are visible on CT as the seroma, with an additional expansion of 1 cm (Fig. 2). This expansion is limited to 0.5 cm below the skin surface and to the surface of the *fascia pectoralis*. The planning target volume (PTV) incorporates an additional safety margin accounting for seed placement accuracy. In our experience this is an additional 0.5 cm expansion that is also limited to 0.5 cm below the skin surface and to the surface of the *fascia pectoralis*. Of note, the seroma on US is always smaller than that seen on CT as the US visualizes only the fluid-filled cavity and not the surrounding fibrotic rim.

An important planning step is the selection of the fiducial needle insertion point, angle, and direction. The fiducial needle should pass through the center of gravity (centroid) of the CTV. Its trajectory goes from an entry point on the posterolateral side of the breast and passes through the breast with an angle tangential to the chest wall to minimize the risk of lung perforation. The distance from the CTV centroid to the chest wall can be adjusted at this time to enable the first row of needles to be placed above the *fascia pectoralis*.

If the case meets the technical requirements, the CT images are then re-sliced in a plane perpendicular to the fiducial needle axis and evenly spaced by 0.5 cm. The new images are used for seed placement optimization in the planning process.

3.1.2 Planning

Seed placement optimization starts with localization of the template grid on the re-sliced images. The grid is superimposed on the central image of the PTV and the scale verified and adjusted if necessary. This grid enables the loaded needles to be spaced 1 cm apart. Needles are placed following a square or triangular pattern, whichever is a best fit, to the PTV shape on the central slice (Fig. 3). Unlike prostate implants where needles are not placed centrally because of the urethra, PBSI needles are evenly placed throughout the PTV. This generates a "hotter" implant but also prevents the occurrence of a "cold" spot in the center of the CTV where the implantation pattern may be stressed due to the natural motion of the breast.

Once the positions are defined in the grid, the needles are loaded with ^{103}Pd seeds and spacers. Seeds of 2.5 U of activity are initially selected and are loaded into the needles in a staggered fashion between adjacent needles to reduce hot spots. In the peripheral needles, the seeds are spaced every centimeter using alternating seeds and spacers. Central needles should use two spacers between each pair of seeds to minimize hot spots. The plan can be optimized by adjusting the seed activity within a range from 1.6–2.7 U and, when appropriate, by adding or removing seeds.

The preplanning optimization constraints are as follows [26]:

- The 90 % isodose line must not bulge through the skin surface on more than 1 cm^2.
- The relative amount of PTV receiving at least 90 % of the prescribed dose (V_{90}) is close to 100 %.
- The volume of the PTV enclosed by the 100 % isodose (V_{100}) is between 95 and 100 %, and the V_{200} is between 20 and 30 %.

When using low energy photon sources, breast density could have a major impact on the dose distribution. For example, dose calculation on the skin could be underestimated as much as 40 % when the density of fat is not accounted for using the TG43 protocol [27]. Since the skin is the main critical structure for PBSI, we recommend using a heterogeneity correction in planning. Heterogeneity correction algorithms that are suitable for low energy photon sources include Monte Carlo simulation and the inhomogeneity correction factor (ICF) [28, 29].

3.1.3 Dose Prescription

The biological equivalent dose to 50 Gy of external radiotherapy using a low-dose-rate source such as Pd 103 has been calculated from two radiobiological models of tissue response.

- *The time, dose, and fractionation (TDF) factor.* The TDF of an EBRT dose of 50 Gy in 25 fractions over 5 weeks is 82. This is equivalent to a PBSI dose of 90 Gy [30, 31].
- *The biological effective dose (BED)* for an α/β value of 3 Gy for late responding tissues is 76 for a 50 Gy EBRT in 25 fractions and 75 for 90 Gy PBSI [32, 33]. For α/β values of 10 Gy corresponding to acute reaction, the BED for EBRT is 52, but for PBSI it is 71, suggesting a higher risk of acute reactions.

When the plan is approved and the patient has consented, a preanesthetic assessment is performed, which includes an ECG, chest X-ray, and appropriate blood tests, depending on the patient's age and previous medical history. The implantation date is scheduled, and the prescription stranded seeds are then ordered.

3.2 PBSI Procedure

3.2.1 Patient Preparation

Patients are on liquid diet starting the evening before the procedure and fasting from midnight. They must stop any blood thinners prior to the implant, 5 days for warfarin and 8 days for ASA. On arriving in the brachytherapy suite, patients are asked to change into a gown, and an intravenous perfusion line is placed in the arm contralateral to the implant. After a last anesthesia evaluation, they are brought to the brachytherapy suite and placed supine on a breast board on a surgical table with the arms placed exactly as for the planning CT. The positioning step is critical as even minimal differences in the arm position have an impact on the seroma location.

After anesthesia induction, the breast skin is sterilized using chlorhexidine 0.5 % and sterile drapes are placed. The projected PTV and the surgical cavity are outlined on the skin surface using a sterile pen with the help of 3D reconstruction printouts from the CT planning (Fig. 4). The surgical scar, tattoos from the time of CT simulation, and the nipple marker are all used as references for the drawing. The skin drawing is carefully verified using ultrasound, ensuring that the surgical cavity is well centered within the drawing boundaries, which can be modified if needed.

3.2.2 Anesthesia

The preferred anesthesia protocol is light sedation that includes (i) Ketoprofen 200 mg PO BID for 48 h starting the day of implant and PRN for 15 days, (ii) Neuroleptic analgesia is induced with IV propofol or a mix of fentanyl 100 μg and midazolam 0.3 mg/kg, (iii) Skin freezing using a maximum of 30 ml of bupivacaine HCl 0.5 % is performed on the area where the needles will be

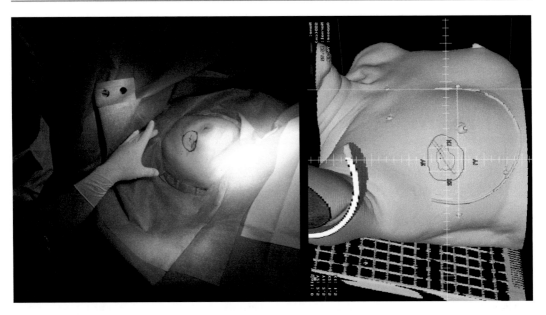

Fig. 4 After anesthesia induction, the projected PTV and the surgical cavity are outlined on the skin surface using a sterile pen with the help of 3D reconstruction printouts from the CT planning

inserted and the retroareolar complex using a longer needle if seeds will be implanted in this area. The skin area that has been anesthetized can be outlined using a skin marker. This protocol was validated prospectively and found effective on 31 patients using a visual analog pain scale (VAS) [18].

3.2.3 Fiducial Needle Placement

The most critical part of the implantation procedure is the accurate placement of the fiducial needle, which serves as a reference for seed placement. The needle must accurately reach the CTV centroid defined during planning, with the same direction and angle as dictated by the plan, and respecting the same distance to the skin and the chest wall. Accounting for the bevel distance and the bone wax, the tip of the needle is generally inserted 3–5 mm beyond the medial boundary of the drawing. US guidance for fiducial needle insertion is essential. US is used to verify the needle position relative to the seroma centroid projection marked on the skin and to verify the distance from the needle to the skin and to the *fascia pectoralis*. The needle direction and depth of penetration are verified using the skin projections and a ruler. The angle of penetration is verified using an inclinometer. When the

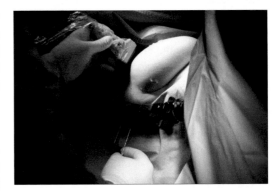

Fig. 5 A template is attached to the fiducial needle using the locking mechanism and immobilized using a medical articulated arm. This apparatus enables precise placement of the stranded seeds

fiducial needle position is deemed correct, a sterile template is attached using the locking mechanism and immobilized using a medical articulated arm (Fig. 5).

3.2.4 Alternate Approach to Fiducial Needle Placement, the Kelowna Technique

PBSI was introduced in British Columbia in 2012 according to the technique described supra. Although the general principles are the same, several modifications have been developed and introduced to facilitate reproducibility of the technique, shorten the learning curve, and enhance the confidence of a novice operator.

Just prior to the procedure, the patient is brought to the CT suite where she is positioned identically as for her prior CT simulation, on a breast board, with a headrest and with the ipsilateral arm abducted and supported above her head. This is accomplished by the attending radiation technologists, as if she were being set up for her first EBRT treatment. The nipple marker is then placed, and lateral tattoo height from the table is verified bilaterally to rule out any patient rotation. The translations from the nipple marker to the projection of the CTV centroid on the skin and to the fiducial entry point laterally are then carried out using the wall lasers and adjusting the couch. We find this much more reproducible than measuring with a ruler along a curved skin surface. These reference points are marked on the skin, and the seroma projection is drawn around the CTV centroid and verified with US. No CT imaging is required during this session.

The patient is then brought to the procedure room, and light anesthesia is induced using a laryngeal mask for airway protection. The same team of radiation technologists repeats the positioning and setup, verifying the lateral tattoos and fiducial entry height using portable table lasers. The articulated arm is then attached to the OR table side bar. The articulated arm is not sterile, but the template is, and the procedure must be carried out under sterile protocol. Due to logistic difficulties in trying to adjust the articulated arm to get the sterile template correctly positioned in a sterile field, we instituted an initial nonsterile "dummy run." We attach a nonsterile template to the articulated arm and maneuver it into position so that the blunt end of a needle can be placed through the template at exactly the right angle and hit the fiducial entry point marked on the skin. We then lock the articulated arm in this position, remove the template, cover the articulated arm with a sterile clear plastic "scope bag," sterilize the skin, drape the patient, and proceed with the sterile procedure. The sterile template is then slipped into position

on the articulated arm, and the fiducial needle is advanced through the template at the correct angle to encounter the entry point on the skin. The angle is verified with an inclinometer, and the needle is advanced under US guidance to its intended mid-seroma position. The rest of the implant continues as described below.

3.2.5 Seed Insertion and Verification

The seed-bearing needles are inserted using US guidance, starting with the deepest row closest to the chest wall. For the first few rows, each needle direction, distance to the *fascia pectoralis*, and parallelism to the fiducial needle are carefully verified using US. When the needle positioning is deemed correct within 0.1–0.2 cm of its planned position, the seeds are released by stabilizing the trocar and pulling the needle straight back along the trocar until the hubs meet. The seeds can be released after the insertion of each needle, or after the insertion of multiple needles depending on the preference of the operator. Inserting and positioning the needles one row at a time before depositing the seeds help to stabilize the breast and achieve parallelism. When the implantation of all sources is done, the skin is cleansed with chlorhexidine 0.5 % and gently rubbed to close the insertion holes, improve adhesion of the strands, and prevent expulsion.

3.3 Post-implant Recovery, QA, and Follow-Up

3.3.1 Radioprotection Measurements and Patient Instruction

After the implant, the patient is brought to the recovery room, and the exposure rate at one meter is measured in multiple directions. It is typically in the order of 2.5 mR/h and should be less than 5 mR/h in order to release the patient without additional radioprotection measures such as a breast shield. A breast shield is a flexible, circular flap of 0.06 cm-thick Xenoprene (0.0175 cm lead equivalent) encased in thin soft plastic [34]. When recommended, the breast shield is placed inside the bra next to the implanted area and can be worn for the first half-life of the seeds, or approximately 3 weeks.

Radioprotection measures reduce public exposure and more particularly exposure to the patient's partner and other family. Keller has estimated the effective dose received by the partner over the course of treatment using a general equation. To keep this dose at an acceptable level, we recommend the use of ^{103}Pd instead of ^{125}I as the radioisotope of choice [35]. These estimations were prospectively validated on a cohort of 36 patients whose partners were asked to wear radiation badges for the first month after the implant. The average measured partner dose was 0.97 mSv (range 0.06–5.1 mSv; SD = 1.0 mSv), which remains within the acceptable dose range of 5 mSv annual exposure as recommended by the National Council on Radiation Protection and Measurements Commentary #11 [36] for non-radiation workers. Additional radiation safety recommendations are given to the patient at time of discharge, including avoidance of close (within 1 m) and prolonged contact with pregnant women or young children for 2 months (~3 half-lives) and at least 6 months of strict pregnancy precautions.

3.3.2 Patient's Follow-Up
After the implantation, patients can return to normal activity. They are asked to keep the dressing dry and not to shower for 24 h. They are seen in follow-up 1 or 2 months after the implant, at a time when the acute skin reaction peaks. They also undergo a repeat planning CT for quality assurance purposes. Patients are followed clinically at 6 months then yearly and have annual mammograms. In our experience there have not been any negative issues for mammographic or MRI surveillance. In the uncommon event that targeted biopsies are recommended for calcifications in the implanted area, these can be undertaken without any special concerns.

4 Quality and Reporting Standards

A quality assurance postplan CT is performed 2 months after the implant. The seroma and its expansion into an evaluation CTV are contoured with the help of the pre-implant CT images. It is often a challenging task to identify the seroma in the implanted volume because of the artifact created by the seeds and associated fibrosis. The post-implant evaluation CTV should have the same volume in cc as the pre-implant CTV. Deformable image registration between pre and post-implant images facilitates and improves accuracy of the QA process [37]. Dose-volume histograms (DVH) are generated to calculate the evaluation CTV V_{100} and V_{200}.

In a review of 85 patients treated with PBSI, Keller reported a mean evaluation CTV coverage of 85.6 % ± 10.4 % SD for the V_{100} and 36.2 % ± 13.9 % SD for the V200 on CT scans performed immediately after the implant. Over time, the seeds seem to cluster together resulting in apparently hotter implants. At 2 months the mean V_{100} increased to 88.4 % ± 9.9 % SD and the V_{200} to 48.3 % ± 16.6 % SD, but by that time over 85 % of the radiation has already been delivered.

5 Results

5.1 Clinical Outcomes

5.1.1 Local Recurrence-Free, Disease-Free, and Overall Survival
Pooling together the patients from the first Phase I/II study for early stage invasive ductal carcinoma, the Phase II study for ductal carcinoma in situ, and the registry study, 88 % of the patients are without evidence of disease after a median follow-up of 58.6 months (unpublished data). The actuarial local recurrence-free survival at 5 years is 98.8 % (SD ± 1.20 %), overall survival 97.4 % (SD ± 1.91 %), and the disease-free survival 96.4 % (SD ± 2.07 %). These outcomes are similar to those expected for early stage breast cancer treated with breast-conserving surgery followed by whole breast EBRT.

5.1.2 Cosmetic Outcomes and Patient Satisfaction
PBSI cosmetic outcomes and patient satisfaction were reported for the patients accrued in the Phase I/II study [38]. Independent assessment by

a trained clinical research assistant found that 96.9 % of the patients had excellent (83.1 %) or good (13.8 %) cosmetic results at 3 years. The vast majority of the patients (92.5 %) were "totally satisfied with the treatment and result" 6 months after the implant.

5.2   PBSI Advantages

The precise role of APBI is still pending final results of several multicenter randomized controlled trials in Europe, the USA, and Canada [11]. There are also multiple techniques of partial breast irradiation, each having advantages and drawbacks. PBSI is a 1 h outpatient procedure, performed under light sedation. The treatment has minimal impact on the patient's daily activities. These are clear advantages over other brachytherapy or external beam APBI techniques. Only intraoperative radiotherapy (IORT) delivered at the time of surgery can compete for patient convenience. However, PBSI is offered when the final pathology report is available, ensuring appropriate patient selection and fully informed consent, whereas IORT is delivered before the final pathology and margin status are known. Also, compared to other techniques, PBSI delivers a very low dose to the heart and other body organs [39]. This is potentially a significant benefit for patients who have little chance of dying of their cancer and are receiving adjuvant radiotherapy because they chose a breast-conserving approach.

5.3   PBSI Drawbacks

The strict clinical, pathological, and technical selection criteria for PBSI render many motivated patients ineligible. We found that following our recommended pathology and age criteria reduced the number of eligible patients to only 20 % of those referred for adjuvant radiotherapy. Eventually issues around the seroma size and technical feasibility further reduce this number by another 50 %. However, many of the ineligible patients may be good candidates for other APBI techniques such as balloon HDR brachytherapy for patients with a large seroma, or interstitial HDR brachytherapy. PBSI could hence be part of a spectrum of therapeutic modalities where the appropriate technique can be selected for a specific clinic-pathological presentation.

Another drawback is that, although PBSI does not result in significant postprocedural pain or infection, it is still an invasive procedure which may deter some patients. Also, some have expressed concern about having material permanently implanted. To this end, current research on bioabsorbable seeds based on alginate implants of nanoparticles is justified. A final limitation is that, like all brachytherapy procedures, specific skills and training are essential. The implantation must be perfect since there is no possibility to correct a suboptimal implant. There is also a risk of injury to the lung or heart if an inexperienced radiation oncologist is implanting needles in the breast, especially left-sided. Participation in a training program is strongly advised, and experience in other US-guided interstitial implantation procedures such as prostate brachytherapy is clearly an advantage.

6   Complications and Management

6.1   Acute Tolerance

6.1.1   Pain

During the implant procedure, 56 % of 31 patients did not experience any pain and 25 % reported minimal pain (VAS score, 0.5–2). For three patients (10 %) the anesthesia protocol was modified using only skin freezing without sedation, but all experienced significant pain during the procedure (VAS score, 6.5–8), so neuroleptanalgesia was reintroduced and is deemed essential to the anesthesia protocol.

In the first week after the implant, one third of patients did not experience any pain, one third reported minimal pain, and one third moderate to significant pain (VAS score, 3–10). We observed two peaks in pain, the first within 48 h and the second at about 6 weeks. We interpret the first pain flare to be related to hematoma formation following needle insertion, and the second seems to be due to the radiation dose to the skin. While chronic pain after adjuvant WBI has been reported in 43 % of patients in two series [40, 41], we rarely observed pain after 2 months. In addition, no patient reported any increased discomfort during follow-up mammogram.

6.1.2   Skin Side Effects

Acute side effects have been collected prospectively for 127 patients in three prospective trials in Ontario, Canada. The most frequent acute toxicity is skin erythema in the region of the implant which occurred in 41.7 % of patients. Twenty percent of patients noticed a lump due to edema. Moist desquamation was seen in 15.9 % of patients, but had an impact on daily activities in only 5.6 %. In the multicenter randomized trial of breast IMRT that used the same impact scale, 31.2 % of patients treated with breast IMRT and 47.8 % of patients treated with a wedged technique experienced moist desquamation [42]. One patient with complications of type I diabetes developed skin ulceration which took 4 months to heal.

6.2   Long-Term Tolerance

The most frequent delayed side effect is induration, occurring in the vicinity of the seroma in 23.2 % of patients at 2 years, plateauing at 39.2 % at 5 years. This induration is generally asymptomatic and had no impact on the patient's daily activities or treatment satisfaction score. It could however sometimes impact on the cosmetic outcome, creating a breast dimple when the patient lifted her arm. This rate of induration is higher than the 10 % fat necrosis observed in the MammoSite® registry trial [43], but is similar to the rate of 39.5 % at 5 years rate reported by Ajkay using HDR brachytherapy APBI [44]. These rates may depend on the way fat necrosis is defined; however, it is likely that induration is a frequent side effect of PBSI. We have observed telangiectasia in 22.4 % of the patients at 2 years, and this rate remains stable at 24.3 % at 5 years. The telangiectasia was mostly grade I, limited

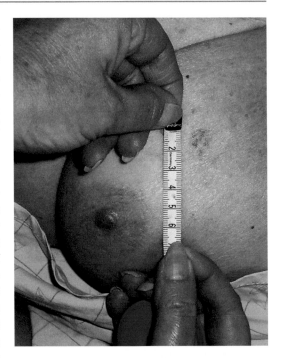

Fig. 6 Telangiectasia are typically limited in area and occurred more frequently when the patient had moist desquamation 6 weeks after the implant

in area, and occurred more frequently if there was prior moist desquamation [40] (Fig. 6). Interestingly, we observed that in four out of 11 patients the telangiectasia disappeared with follow-up longer than 5 years.

7   Summary

PBSI is an effective means of delivering partial breast irradiation for selected patients with favorable breast cancer following breast-conserving surgery and sentinel node evaluation. It compares favorably to alternate methods of partial breast radiation in terms of patient convenience, cosmesis, and limitation of dose to adjacent organs.

References

1. Peto R, Boreham J, Clarke M et al (2002) UK and USA breast cancer deaths down 25% in year 2000 at ages 20–69 years. Lancet 355:1822
2. Nystrom L, Andersson I, Bjurstam N et al (2002) Long-term effects of mammography screening:

updated overview of the Swedish randomised trials. Lancet 359:909–919

3. SEER. http://seer.cancer.gov/csr/1975_2011/results_merged/sect_04_breast.pdf

4. Early Breast Cancer Trialists' Collaborative Group (EBCTCG), Darby S, McGale P et al (2011) Effect of radiotherapy after breast-conserving surgery on 10 year recurrence and 15 year breast cancer death: meta-analysis of individual patient data for 10,801 women in 17 randomised trials. Lancet 378:1707–1716

5. Bartelink H, Horiot JC, Poortmans PM et al (2007) Impact of a higher radiation dose on local control and survival in breast-conserving therapy of early breast cancer: 10 year results of the randomized boost versus no boost EORTC 22881–10882 trial. J Clin Oncol 25(22):3259–3265

6. Whelan TJ, Pignol JP, Levine MN et al (2010) Long-term results of hypofractionated radiation therapy for breast cancer. N Engl J Med 362:513–520

7. Fisher ER, Sass R, Fisher B et al (1986) Pathologic findings from the National Surgical Adjuvant Breast and Bowel Project (Protocol 6). II. Relation of local breast recurrence to multicentricity. Cancer 57:1717–1724

8. Bethune WA (1991) Partial breast irradiation for early breast cancer. J Natl Med Assoc 83:768–800, 808

9. Pawlik TM, Bucholz TA, Kuerer HM (2004) The biologic rationale for and emerging role of accelerated partial breast irradiation for breast cancer. J Am Coll Surg 199:479–492

10. Vicini FA, Kestin L, Chen P et al (2003) Limited-field radiation therapy in the management of early stage breast cancer. J Natl Canc Inst 95:1205–1211

11. Mannino M, Yarnold J (2009) Accelerated partial breast irradiation trials: diversity in rationale and design. Radiother Oncol 91:16–22

12. Olivotto IA, Whelan TJ, Parpia S et al (2013) Interim cosmetic and toxicity results from RAPID: a randomized trial of accelerated partial breast irradiation using three-dimensional conformal external beam radiation therapy. J Clin Oncol 31:4038–4045

13. Vaidya JS, Wenz F, Bulsara M et al (2014) Risk-adapted targeted intraoperative radiotherapy versus whole-breast radiotherapy for breast cancer: 5 year results for local control and overall survival from the TARGIT-A randomised trial. Lancet 383:603–613

14. Beitsch PD, Shaitelman SF, Vicini FA (2011) Accelerated partial breast irradiation. J Surg Oncol 103:362–368

15. Clarke DH, Edmundson GK, Martinez A et al (1989) The clinical advantages of I-125 seeds as a substitute for Ir-192 seeds in temporary plastic tube implants. Int J Radiat Oncol Biol Phys 17:859–863

16. Nelson JC, Beitsch PD, Vicini FA et al (2009) Four-year clinical update from the American society of breast surgeons MammoSite® brachytherapy trial. Am J Surg 98:83–91

17. Smith BD, Arthur DW, Buchholz TA et al (2009) Accelerated partial breast irradiation consensus statement from the American Society for Radiation Oncology (ASTRO). Int J Radiat Oncol Biol Phys 74:987–1001

18. Pignol JP, Keller B, Rakovitch E et al (2006) First report of a permanent breast 103Pd seed implant as adjuvant radiation treatment for early-stage breast cancer. Int J Radiat Oncol Biol Phys 64:176–181

19. Jansen N, Deneufbourg JM, Nickers P (2007) Adjuvant stereotactic permanent seed breast implant: a boost series in view of partial breast irradiation. Int J Radiat Oncol Biol Phys 67:1052–1058

20. Wazer DE, Berle L, Graham R et al (2002) Preliminary results of a phase I/II study of HDR brachytherapy alone for T1/T2 breast cancer. Int J Radiat Oncol Biol Phys 53:889–897

21. Smith GL, Jiang J, Buchholz TA et al (2014) Benefit of adjuvant brachytherapy versus external beam radiation for early breast cancer: impact of patient stratification on breast preservation. Int J Radiat Oncol Biol Phys 88:274–284

22. Polgár C, Van Limbergen E, Pötter R et al (2009) Patient selection for accelerated partial-breast irradiation (APBI) after breast-conserving surgery: recommendations of the Groupe Européen de Curiethérapie-European Society for Therapeutic Radiology and Oncology (GEC-ESTRO) breast cancer working group based on clinical evidence. Radiother Oncol 94: 264–273

23. Shah C, Vicini F, Wazer DE et al (2013) The American Brachytherapy Society consensus statement for accelerated partial breast irradiation. Brachytherapy 12:267–277

24. ASBS. https://www.breastsurgeons.org/statements/PDF_Statements/APBI.pdf. Accessed on Feb 2015

25. Buchholz TA, Somerfield MR, Griggs JJ et al (2014) Margins for breast-conserving surgery with whole-breast irradiation in stage I and II invasive breast cancer: American Society of Clinical Oncology endorsement of the Society of Surgical Oncology/American Society for Radiation Oncology consensus guideline. J Clin Oncol 32:1502–1506

26. Keller BM, Ravi A, Sankreacha R et al (2012) Permanent breast seed implant dosimetry quality assurance. Int J Radiat Oncol Biol Phys 83:84–92

27. Afsharpour H, Pignol JP, Keller B et al (2010) Influence of breast composition and interseed attenuation in dose calculations for post-implant assessment of permanent breast 103Pd seed implant. Phys Med Biol 55:4547–4561

28. Furstoss C, Reniers B, Bertrand MJ et al (2009) Monte Carlo study of LDR seed dosimetry with an application in a clinical brachytherapy breast implant. Med Phys 36:1848–1858

29. Mashouf S, Lechtman E, Beaulieu L et al (2013) A simplified analytical dose calculation algorithm accounting for tissue heterogeneity for low-energy brachytherapy sources. Phys Med Biol 58: 6299–6315

30. Orton CG, Ellis F (1973) A simplification in the use of the NSD concept in practical radiotherapy. Br J Radiol 46:529–537

31. Orton CG, Webber BM (1977) Time-dose factor analysis of dose rate effects in permanent implant dosimetry. Int J Radiat Oncol Biol Phys 2:55–60

32. Fowler JF (1989) The linear-quadratic formula and progress in fractionated radiotherapy. Br J Radiol 62:679–694

33. Ling CC, Chui CS (1993) Stereotactic treatment of brain tumors with radioactive implants or external photon beams: radiobiophysical aspects. Radiother Oncol 26:11–18

34. Keller BM, Pignol JP, Rakovitch E et al (2008) A radiation badge survey for family members living with patients treated with a ^{103}Pd permanent breast seed implant. Int J Radiat Oncol Biol Phys 70: 267–271

35. Keller B, Sankreacha R, Rakovitch E et al (2005) A permanent breast seed implant as partial breast radiation therapy for early-stage patients: a comparison of palladium-103 and iodine-125 isotopes based on radiation safety considerations. Int J Radiat Oncol Biol Phys 62:358–365

36. NCRP Commentary #11. http://www.ncrponline.org/Publications/Commentaries/Comm11press.html. Accessed on Feb 2015

37. Hilts M, Batchelar D, Rose J et al (2015) Deformable image registration for defining the post-implant seroma in permanent breast seed implant brachytherapy. Brachytherapy 14(3):409–418

38. Pignol JP, Rakovitch E, Keller BM et al (2009) Tolerance and acceptance results of a palladium-103 permanent breast seed implant Phase I/II study. Int J Radiat Oncol Biol Phys 73:1482–1488

39. Pignol JP, Keller BM, Ravi A (2011) Doses to internal organs for various breast radiation techniques--implications on the risk of secondary cancers and cardiomyopathy. Radiat Oncol 6:5

40. Bentzen SM, Overgaard M (1991) Relationship between early and late normal-tissue injury after postmastectomy radiotherapy. Radiother Oncol 20:159–165

41. Amichetti M, Caffo O (2003) Pain after quadrantectomy and radiotherapy for early-stage breast cancer: incidence, characteristics and influence on quality of life. Oncology 65:23–28

42. Pignol JP, Olivotto I, Rakovitch E (2008) A multicenter randomized trial of breast intensity-modulated radiation therapy to reduce acute radiation dermatitis. J Clin Oncol 26:2085–2092

43. Vargo JA, Verma V, Kim H et al (2014) Extended (5-year) outcomes of accelerated partial breast irradiation using MammoSite balloon brachytherapy: patterns of failure, patient selection, and dosimetric correlates for late toxicity. Int J Radiat Oncol Biol Phys 88:285–291

44. Ajkay N, Collett AE, Bloomquist EV et al (2015) A comparison of complication rates in early-stage breast cancer patients treated with brachytherapy versus whole-breast irradiation. Ann Surg Oncol 22(4):1140–1145

Breast Brachytherapy: Brachytherapy in the Management of Ipsilateral Breast Tumor Recurrence

Mark Trombetta, Thomas B. Julian, and Jean-Michel Hannoun-Levi

Abstract

In this chapter, we present an alternative management of ipsilateral breast tumor recurrence following conservation therapy for early breast cancer. We will present the evidence to date and hope to establish this alternative approach as a plausible option for women affected by in-breast recurrence, but desirous of breast preservation. We discuss this option presenting the established standard of care and the alternatives, as well as the specific concerns related to retreatment.

1 Introduction

According to the World Health Organization, International Agency for Research on Cancer (IARC), more than 1.7 million women were diagnosed with breast cancer worldwide in 2012 (the most recent data reported to date), which accounts for approximately 12 % of all cancers [1]. Of that number, up to 70 % of patients will have selected breast conservation therapy [2], depending on global and local practice patterns. Unfortunately, it has now been replaced by less curable lung cancer as the most common malignancy in women. Additionally, the IARC noted that the breast cancer incidence had increased by more than 20 % since the 2008 estimates with an overall 14 % increase in mortality worldwide. Coincidently, the mortality rate in the developed countries (the United States, Europe, Canada, etc.) has fallen significantly [3]; hence, people affected by breast cancer in much of the world are living longer, adding to the potential for an increase in the rate of ipsilateral breast tumor recurrence (IBTR). The risk of breast cancer recurrence for a given subject depends on a variety of factors, including patient age, inherited susceptibility, tumor characteristics, type of treatment for original tumor (e.g., surgery and/or radi-

M. Trombetta, MD (✉)
Professor, Division of Radiation Oncology,
Allegheny Health Network Cancer Institute, Drexel University College of Medicine, 320 East North Avenue, Pittsburgh, PA, USA
e-mail: MTROMBET@wpahs.org

T.B. Julian, MD
Department of Surgery, Allegheny General Hospital, Temple University School of Medicine,
Drexel University College of Medicine,
Allegheny Health Network, Pittsburgh, PA, USA

J.-M. Hannoun-Levi, MD, PhD
Radiation Therapy Department, Antoine Lacassagne Cancer Center, Nice, France

© Springer International Publishing Switzerland 2016
P. Montemaggi et al. (eds.), *Brachytherapy: An International Perspective*, Medical Radiology,
DOI 10.1007/978-3-319-26791-3_11

ation therapy), and other lifestyle factors such as obesity and alcohol consumption. Currently, the local recurrence rates after completion of adjuvant therapy are still approximately 2–20 % (range 2–36 %) after a minimum 10-year follow-up [4, 5] depending on clinical and biologic factors, with a generally noted trend of increasing recurrence rates inversely proportional to age at diagnosis. When enhanced with hormonal manipulation, the recurrence rates drop to 2–20 % in lower risk and hormonally sensitive patients [4–6].

2   Paradigm Shift: The Era of Breast Conservation in Breast Cancer Management

2.1   Role of Retreatment

The concept of breast conservative treatment (BCT) as an alternative to the traditional Halsted radical mastectomy (and the subsequent modification of such) began to take shape in the 1970s. Seminal efforts by Veronesi et al. at the European Institute of Oncology (EIO) based in Milan, Italy, were nearly concurrent with the efforts of Fisher et al. at the National Surgical Breast and Bowel Project (NSABP) based in Pittsburgh, Pennsylvania, USA. From the beginning, the Italian and American teams faced difficult criticism in postulating that less than radical surgery was necessary to control or cure breast cancer. Halstedian surgeries had been the established standard of care for nearly 80 years. By the mid-1980s, initial reports from both groups demonstrated equivalence, and in 2002 both groups reported their 20-year follow-up which established BCT as the new standard local treatment for appropriately selected patients [7, 8].

The primary goal of such therapy is eradication of disease, but important secondary goals are cosmetic and functional preservation. For IBTR, the international standard of care for local recurrence following breast conservation therapy has been salvage mastectomy, which is physically well tolerated by most women and has demonstrated salvage local control rates of greater than 90 % [9, 10]. While the rate of local control is acceptable, these patients are often left with cosmetically and functionally suboptimal results [11, 12]. A number of studies have shown that mastectomy is displeasing and devastating to many women, especially when the acute post-therapeutic phase has past and patients have time to reflect [12, 13], but real functional problems can develop related to physical asymmetry and the resultant degenerative structural spinal disorders such as kyphosis and scoliosis. The interest in retreatment in the setting of IBTR is growing as evidenced by the fact that the Radiation Therapy Oncology Group (RTOG) has recently completed a retreatment protocol using hyperfractionated external beam radiotherapy [14].

2.2   Psychological Issues and Breast Conservation

The issue of mastectomy and the subsequent emotional and physical distress associated with this therapy have been well described. Ganz et al. [11] have demonstrated a clear cause-effect relationship between mastectomies and clothing difficulties as well as body self-image.

In the study by Rowland et al. [12], patients who underwent lumpectomy, modified radical mastectomy (MRM), and modified radical mastectomy with subsequent reconstruction surgery were evaluated. The post-analysis findings revealed that women who had undergone MRM with reconstruction had the highest incidence of negative impact upon their sex lives (45.4 % versus 29.8 % of women undergoing lumpectomy). Maunsell et al. [13] further subdivided groups of women noting that women under age 40 who had conservation surgery were significantly less negatively affected than those who had undergone MRM.

2.3   Indications

Patients with a significant surgical defect or limited remaining breast tissue should generally not be considered for conservation from a cosmetic standpoint, but even in this situation, a face-to-face discussion should be proposed to the patient who would be willing to accept a suboptimal cosmetic outcome as a consequence of a second conservative treatment. In these patients, mastectomy, the accepted standard of care must be discussed. We also recommend consideration of repeat conservation in patients with favorable recurrent tumor characteristics only according to the breast size, maximum tumor size between 2.0 and 3.0 cm, negative final margins of resection, no clinically apparent lymphadenopathy, and generally no evidence of metastatic disease. In rare cases of bone-only metastatic disease or when a suspected long-term survival is possible, or even in the situation of patient preference, retreatment lumpectomy and radiotherapy could be reasonable. Finally, the therapeutic endeavor must demonstrate equivalence in terms of overall life expectancy.

While salvage mastectomy following IBTR has long been the accepted standard, repeat breast preservation is possible in those women who:

(a) Are desirous of breast preservation
(b) Have recurrent disease limited to a single site of the breast
(c) Demonstrate no evidence for residual disease at the time of postoperative imaging
(d) Have enough projected residual breast tissue to warrant breast preservation
(e) Are well informed about the risks versus benefits of the procedure and the alternatives including the possibility of recurrence and resultant mastectomy with potentially additional healing concerns

3 Treatment Options for IBTR

3.1 Mastectomy Following IBTR

We have stated that mastectomy has been considered the standard of care for IBTR with local control rates of 2–36 % being reported [15–22]. However, when studies of only large numbers of patients (>100) are considered, local failure rates dramatically decline to less than 10 % overall [15, 17–19]. These excellent local control rates with mastectomy alone established salvage mastectomy as the standard of care for IBTR. Furthermore,

it is important to notice that the vast majority of those retrospective studies reported contain results from patients who presented with locally advanced stages at the time of IBTR.

In the study by Huang et al., nearly all patients recurred with similar characteristics related to invasiveness [17]. That is, nearly all of those patients initially presenting with invasive lesions re-presented with invasive lesions, whereas of those with an IBTR following conservative treatment for Ductal Carcinoma in Situ (DCIS) recurred with DCIS. The findings at the Allegheny General Hospital in Pittsburgh, PA (USA), differed in that there was less correlation between the original and recurrent pathology [23].

Many authors have described the synchronous presentation of IBTR with distant metastatic disease which may occur in 5–15 % of patients [18, 21, 22]. Management of these patients primarily concerns the management of the systemic failure. Therefore, these patients should not be considered for repeat breast conservation. A 5-year survival rate of only 37 % was identified in patients who underwent salvage mastectomy alone [20]. One patient in our original cohort of interstitial patients did have metastatic disease at the time of evaluation for repeat conservation therapy; however, she was treated in the era of high-dose chemotherapy and bone marrow salvage [23, 24], which was thought to be curative in such patients at the time. She was 2 years disease-free from her transplant when she developed an IBTR. She succumbed to disease approximately 2 years following retreatment, free of locally recurrent disease. In case of synchronous IBTR and metastatic disease, a second conservative treatment must be carefully discussed, taking into account the patient point of view.

3.2 Observation Only Following Repeat Lumpectomy for IBTR

Repeat lumpectomy without adjuvant local therapy following local recurrence has been reported by a number of authors. Multiple authors report local recurrence rates following IBTR treated by re-excision of 19–35 % compared to 2–4 % in patients treated with salvage mastectomy

[15, 22], with one group noting no difference in disease-free survival [15]. Komoike et al. [16] reviewed patients who developed IBTR in a sample of 979 patients evaluated. Fifty-three patients did not receive initial postoperative irradiation in the cohort. Of the entire group, 47 developed IBTR including 15 with positive margins at lumpectomy. With salvage mastectomy and repeat lumpectomy used in this group, the overall survival was in excess of 90 % [16]. Some authors have asked whether surgery alone even in de novo cases is enough. In general, the consensus for invasive cancers is that all patients should have follow-up radiotherapy. Since we know that adjuvant radiotherapy to the primary decreases significantly the rate of local recurrence (even if there is no change in terms of OS); it is probably hazardous to claim that it is possible to avoid breast re-irradiation in case of IBTR following conservation surgery [25–27].

For DCIS, the decision is less definitive. A number of authors and groups have proposed potential subsets of patients who may not require postoperative radiotherapy if they are appropriately counseled about the low absolute risk reduction of both local recurrence and overall survival in favorable subgroups [28–31], but to date, no study has demonstrated a clear subgroup in which radiotherapy does not reduce local recurrence. National Surgical Adjuvant Breast and Bowel Project (NSABP) and others have demonstrated the need for radiotherapy in all subsets of women [32, 33]. Silverstein et al. [30] demonstrated that for de novo DCIS patients undergoing local excision with negative final margins of resection, no further local therapy was required. However, the extensive pathologic assessment in this study is beyond that routinely practiced and may be impractical in most clinical settings. Also, the study required margins of resection of at least 2.0 cm to demonstrate a relative low risk of IBTR. As the volume of tissue excised increases exponentially with increasing linear resection margins [volume of a sphere $= (4/3)\ \pi\ r^3$], this marginal requirement may lead to suboptimal cosmesis. In patients who are undergoing repeat resection, even small volumetric increases may result in poor cosmetic out-

comes due to the extent of tissue defect from multiple surgeries. While the re-excision data noted above are not robust enough to give definitive correlation with the later referenced de novo data, local failure rates from re-excision seem to mirror local failure rates in de novo cases. Considering these data, it is likely that repeat surgical excision alone may result in suboptimal outcome.

3.3 Comparative Studies Between Salvage Radical Mastectomy and Second Breast-Conserving Surgery Alone

Four retrospective studies compared clinical outcomes obtained after salvage mastectomy or second BCT consisting of re-excision without re-irradiation [8, 13, 16, 23]. Kurtz et al. [22] retrospectively analyzed the clinical outcome of 118 patients treated either with salvage mastectomy (66 patients) or repeat BCT (52 patients). With a median follow-up of 84 months, the rate of second local recurrence was 12.1 % and 23 % for salvage mastectomy and repeat BCT, respectively. Salvadori et al. [15] retrospectively analyzed the clinical outcome of 191 patients who presented an IBTR after BCT for the primary. Among those patients, 134 underwent salvage mastectomy, while 57 were treated with re-excision alone. At a median follow-up of 73 months, the authors noticed a higher risk of second local recurrence in case of repeat BCT (19 % vs. 4 %), while the 5-year Overall Survival (OS) was 70 % and 85 % for mastectomy and re-excision, respectively (metastatic rates were 47 % and 20 % for salvage mastectomy and re-excision alone, respectively), and no significant difference was observed between the two salvage procedure in terms of Disease Free Survival (DFS). Alpert et al. [63] retrospectively analyzed the clinical outcome of 146 patients who presented with an IBTR after BCT for the primary. Among those patients, 116 underwent salvage mastectomy, while 30 were treated with salvage breast-conserving surgery. The rates of second local recurrence were 6.9 % and 6.7 % after mastectomy and salvage breast-conserving surgery, respectively, with the second IBTR tumor size significantly larger in the mastectomy group. There was no difference in terms of distant metastases between the mastectomy cohort (31.8 %) and the breast-conserving surgery cohort (23.9 %). Ten-year OS was not significantly different between mastectomy (65.7 %) and salvage breast-conserving surgery (58.0 %). Chen et al. [64] retrospectively analyzed the clinical outcomes of 747 patients who presented with an IBTR after a BCT. Among those patients, 568 underwent salvage mastectomy and 179 were treated with a salvage breast-conserving surgery. Five percent of patients with mastectomy and 21 % of patients with salvage breast-conserving surgery received postoperative irradiation. Patients in the mastectomy group were younger and had larger, high-grade, and hormone receptor-negative tumors. The authors observed a significantly better 5-year OS after salvage mastectomy compared to salvage breast-conserving surgery (78 % vs. 67 %, $p = 0.003$). This study is of interest due to the high number of patients. However, several data points were not specified (median follow-up, specific details regarding re-irradiation dose and technique applied), making the interpretation of this study debatable.

3.4 External Beam Radiotherapy Following Repeat Lumpectomy for IBTR

Very little has been published regarding the use of external irradiation in the management of IBTR following conservation surgery and postoperative irradiation. Recht et al. [20] reported on a single case of IBTR treated with wide excision and postoperative external irradiation that was disease-free 72 months postprocedure. Mullen et al. [36] published an initial report describing a series of patients retreated following IBTR, and Deutsch [37] later expanded this to 39 patients who developed IBTR after breast conservation therapy (BCT). In this study, all patients initially received 4500–5040 cGy at 180–200 cGy/frac-

tion following breast conservation surgery. The initial pathology was invasive ductal carcinoma in 31 and DCIS in 8 patients. When the recurrences were analyzed, 26 of the patients who originally had invasive cancer recurred with invasive cancer, whereas the eight patients who presented with DCIS recurred with DCIS [although two specimens demonstrated microinvasion]. Five patients had positive margins of resection at the time of re-irradiation. Re-irradiation consisted of 5000 cGy (200 cGy/fx) of photon or electron external beam therapy in all but a single patient who did not complete therapy. Eight of 39 patients (20.5 %) developed a second IBTR with three of these occurring in the same quadrant of the breast. Though not scored according to the NSABP criteria, cosmetic results roughly corresponded to NSABP category 1 or 2 for 15 patients, category 3 for 15 patients, and category 4 cosmesis for 9 patients. Each patient reported satisfaction with the cosmetic effect compared to mastectomy.

3.5 Interstitial Brachytherapy Following Repeat Lumpectomy for IBTR

Accelerated Partial Breast Irradiation (APBI) for in-breast recurrence following whole breast irradiation is denoted as APBrI. Currently, for APBI, different irradiation techniques are available with intra (electrons – IORT or 50 Kv X photons)- or postoperative radiation therapy (brachytherapy or external beam RT), while brachytherapy techniques are based on preoperative (balloon, multicatheter interstitial) or postoperative (multicatheter interstitial) techniques. In case of APBrI, all technical options are described in the literature (except IORT with e-), while interstitial brachytherapy remains one of the most popular methods. Interstitial brachytherapy can be performed intra- or postoperatively and can use low- [24, 38–40], pulsed [41] or high-dose rate (HDR) [42–44] radiation. Due to radioprotection and dose optimization considerations, HDR interstitial brachytherapy is currently considered as a standard of care. Furthermore, this technique allows for an outpatient procedure, leading to a more comfortable and acceptable treatment for the patient.

For APBI as well as for APBrI, the delineation of the target volume remains a critical point. Whatever the APBrI technique used, clips within the tumor bed represent an important point for this delineation. Recently, the Breast Cancer Working Group of GEC-ESTRO proposed some recommendations to define and delineate the target in case of APBI using multicatheter interstitial brachytherapy [34].

Briefly, five different steps are described:

1. Detailed knowledge about the primary surgical procedure (particularly about type of surgery, use/number and location of surgical clips, tumor bed-related position of the skin scar), details of the surgical pathology including size of resection margins in six directions, as well as the details of the preoperative imaging (mammography and/or MRI and/or ultrasound) is obligatory.
2. Identification of the tumor localization before breast-conserving surgery inside the breast and translation of this information into a current CT imaging data set.
3. Calculation of the size of safety margins needed to cover CTV in all six directions.
4. Definition of the target – clinical target volume (CTV)/planning target volume (PTV).
5. Delineation of the target – CTV/PTV according to defined rules.

For interstitial brachytherapy, the rules of implant must follow the Paris system recommendations [35]. It is important to implant (if possible) at least two planes with, in this case, a minimum number of 10–12 catheters. For Pulsed Dose Rate (APBI) or HDR brachytherapy, planification should be done based on a 3-D imaging approach (utilizing a CT scan). Dose-volume adaptation can be performed automatically with dedicated software using graphical optimization. Dose-volume histogram (DVH) analysis should confirm that the prescribed dose covers 90 % of the PTV, with a dose nonunifor-

mity ratio (DNR): V150/V100 ≤ 0.35 (preferably ≤ 0.30). The V150 is defined as the volume receiving 150 % of dose, with the V100 similarly identified for 100 % of dose. The maximum surface skin dose should be ≤70 % of prescribed. A confluence of two V200 % isodoses or a V200 % isodose diameter >10 mm must be avoided.

Regarding the prescribed dose for HDR brachytherapy, the protocols used for APBI were empirically reported for APBrI: 34 Gy (3.4 Gy/fraction over 5 consecutive days) or 32 Gy (4 Gy/fraction over 4 consecutive days), while for PDR brachytherapy, a total dose of 46–50 Gy can be delivered (0.50–0.80 Gy/h, 1 pulse/h, 24 h/day).

In case of re-irradiation for a second breast conservation therapy (BCT), interstitial brachytherapy was the most commonly applied technique using either low-dose rate (LDR) [24, 38–40], pulsed (PDR) [41] or high-dose rate (HDR) [42, 43]. In case of interstitial brachytherapy, whatever the dose rate used, vectors (needles or plastic tubes) were implanted intra- or postoperatively. The mean delivered dose was approximately 46 Gy (range 30–50 Gy) and 32 Gy (range 30–34 Gy) with LDR or HDR, respectively. The second local recurrence rate was 10 % (range 0–26 %). The 5-year DFS rate was 60 % (range 31–85 %), while the 5-year OS rate was 75 % (range 50–89 %). The grade 3–4 complication rate was 8 % (range 3–11 %), and cosmetic results were reported as excellent/good in 70 % (range 53–100 %). Maulard et al. [40] have retrospectively compared IBTR treated by salvage brachytherapy alone (LDR 60–70 Gy) with second BCT with postoperative brachytherapy (LDR 30 Gy). Tumors treated with salvage brachytherapy alone were statistically larger. The authors reported a second local recurrence rate of 26 % and 17 % after surgery plus brachytherapy and brachytherapy alone, respectively. Hannoun-Levi et al. [39] have retrospectively analyzed a series of 69 patients who underwent a second BCT for IBTR using LDR brachytherapy. Two groups of patients were compared regarding the delivered dose (30 vs. 46 Gy) and the number of plans used (1 vs. 2). The authors showed that the second local recurrence rate was lower in case of higher delivered dose and larger irradiated volume. Using PDR brachytherapy combined with a repeat lumpectomy for IBTR, Kauer-Dorner et al. [41] reported an actuarial 5-year second local control rate of 93 % with a mean follow-up of 57 months (two patients experienced a second local relapse). Five-year DFS and OS were 77 % and 87 %, respectively. Grade 3–4 late side effects were 7 %, while cosmetic outcome was excellent to fair in 76 %. Regarding quality of life, the authors reported that mean scores of scales and items of QLQ-BR23 were comparable to primary breast-conserving therapy. Guix et al. [42] have retrospectively analyzed a series of patients who were treated with second BCT and interstitial high-dose rate brachytherapy. With a median follow-up of 89 months which corresponds to the longest follow-up in this specific field, the authors reported 10-year DFS and OS rates of 64 % and 97 %, respectively. In this series, no grade 3–4 complications were observed. More recently, the GEC-ESTRO Breast Cancer Working Group presented the results of an international multicentric retrospective study of 217 patients with IBTR who underwent a second BCT for IBTR combining salvage lumpectomy plus interstitial brachytherapy [44]. The authors reported an actuarial 5- and 10-year second local recurrence rate of 5.6 % and 7.2 %, respectively, while the actuarial 5- and 10-year distant metastasis rates were 9.6 % and 19.1 %, respectively. Actuarial 5- and 10-year OS rates were 88.7 % and 76.4 %, respectively.

3.6 Intracavitary Brachytherapy

Balloon brachytherapy gained wide acceptance in the USA and Europe following its introduction in 2002. Since that time, hundreds of thousands of procedures have been performed. The longest trial to date was the MammoSite® (Hologic Inc., Bedford, MA) registry trial which was overseen by the American Society of Breast Surgeons. In 1449 patients with a median follow-up of 60 months, the IBTR rate was only 3.6 % which compared favorably with standard whole breast

radiotherapy [45]. In this study, "elsewhere failures" (tumors recurring outside of the original tumor bed and thought to be "new" tumors) (EF) were significantly higher (2.6 %) than "true recurrences" (tumor recurring in and around the original tumor bed) (TR) (1.1 %). Because TR results in lower survival rates [46], retreatment localized radiotherapy requires additional discussion with patients. Soon after approval, we published our original experience using the MammoSite® balloon catheter in IBTR retreatment [47]. Additional devices utilizing a "strut" construction are available and can be substituted. We prefer multilumen balloons due to ease of use, adjustability of size following implantation, and ease of explantation (Table 1).

Interstitial brachytherapy has enjoyed wide usage and acceptance since it was one of the seminal methods of radiotherapy. However, the significant learning curve and experience level needed to provide excellent therapy is often a dissuading influence for clinicians. Sadly, many training programs have fallen away from interstitial therapy as patients look for more convenience and clinicians look for ease of use and work flow advantages. The relatively small number of experts in this method and the small number of training sites that actively use

Table 1 Comparison of interstitial and intracavitary brachytherapy

| *Interstitial* |
| More experience overall worldwide |
| Most mature data |
| Better and more uniform dose distribution |
| Can be LDR or HDR |
| Requires significantly more technical skill |
| Does not require surgical assistance in many centers |
| *Intracavitary* |
| Ease of use |
| Improved workflow |
| Significantly less homogeneity |
| Requires surgical collaboration |
| May be better accepted by surgical community |
| Less trauma to the skin |
| Less wound risk for infection |
| Easier for patient compliance |

interstitial brachytherapy make for a dearth of interstitial brachytherapists in many countries. Intracavitary brachytherapy (ICB), whether by balloon device or strut, has filled this void in many professional communities. Originally driven by breast surgeons (and in some institutions, interventional radiologists), the devices have gained wide acceptance in a multidisciplinary setting. From a technical aspect, the single catheter devices are much easier to use than their multicatheter counterparts. For the surgeons, it is a simple additional procedure. For the brachytherapist, the ease of use following implantation adds to workflow efficiencies and does not require radiotherapist operative time. From a practical standpoint, the theoretical risk of infection is lessened with a single entrance wound as compared with multiple entrance and exit wounds with the interstitial approach. Although infection rates vary across many small sample sizes in the studies to date, the infection rate with balloon catheters tends to be reported at less than 5 %. We have noted an infection rate of 2 %. The overall trauma to the breast considering the lesser number of puncture sites is also reduced with potential improved overall cosmesis. Despite the large diameter difference between the single catheter, multilumen devices, and the smaller 17 or 18 gauge diameter of the interstitial approach, overall patient acceptance is quite good and the resultant incisional scar is many times imperceptible, especially considering the ominous appearance of the wound with the device in place.

Selection of the correct patient for strut or balloon brachytherapy in general and retreatment brachytherapy specifically is critical for good outcomes and patient safety. Generally we follow the consensus guidelines first authored by the American Society for Radiation Oncology (ASTRO) [48] and later updated and adopted by the American Brachytherapy Society (ABS) [49] (Table 2), although there is significant clinical latitude between investigators on what clinical features would make a patient fit for acceptable guidelines. Clinicians should use reasonable standards of care when selecting such patients.

Table 2 ABS guidelines for APBI

Age	>50 years
Size	<3.0 cm
Histology	All invasive and DCIS
Estrogen receptor status	Positive/negative
Surgical margins	Negative
Lymphovascular space invasion	Not present
Nodal status	Negative

• For retreatment, we do not limit prior subtypes or type of cancer
• For retreatment we have treated patients with 1–3 nodes positive at recent axillary sampling

3.7 Intracavitary Brachytherapy Technique

Following a complete history and physical examination, current discussion of the standard of care (including mastectomy), and multidisciplinary consultation, patients who are accepting of retreatment with balloon brachytherapy are admitted either to a surgical or radiologic suite, or in some cases a clinical office. Generally, ultrasound is used to guide the placement of the device, and we perform a pre-procedure sonogram to document the existence of a seroma cavity and verify appropriate cavity-to-skin distance (usual accepted minimum 0.3 cm). The pre-procedure sonogram also is helpful in determining balloon diameter and shape (spherical or ellipsoid) or strut size. Under sedation and local anesthetic, or in some cases, local anesthetic alone, a 1.5–2.0 cm incision is made in the lateral or inferior breast margin. Other pathways can be utilized, but we have found that, when possible, these entrance sites are most comfortable for the patients. We do not use the lumpectomy surgical incision entry technique as this may worsen cosmesis in a physically evident section of the breast. The entrance trocar is passed through the incision using constant guidance by ultrasound into the seroma cavity. If the balloon is placed following establishment of complete excision and obtainment of negative margins, the balloon catheter is placed and saline is infused into the balloon (or the strut is expanded and fixed). Five cc of a standard opacification solution is infused as part of the balloon fill. We have found that higher amounts of contrast obscure the balloon surface margin and sometimes surrounding structures. We use only multi-lumen catheters for therapy to provide maximum flexibility of dose distribution. If a catheter is placed at the time of definitive surgery, an interim cavity device should be used as a place holder until the final pathology can be confirmed as suitable for implant. Broad spectrum antibiotics are initiated intraoperatively and continued until day 2 post-explantation. Analgesia is generally not necessary or acetaminophen is recommended.

Following verification of pathology, a non-contrast CT planning scan should be performed with the device in place to allow for dosimetric calculations. We use 0.3 cm slice thickness and limit the scan to encompass organs at risk and minimize dose to the nonessential tissues. We limit the scan as well to the area of interest only to eliminate the inevitable potential nonsignificant findings that are sometimes seen on unenhanced scans or with suboptimal diagnostic techniques and may cause undue concern. Planning criteria are those used standardly for the devices and memorialized in NSABP protocol B-39 (RTOG 0413). For patients with brittle skin or other concerns, dose reduction has been utilized occasionally, both in dose per fraction and total dose. Caution must be utilized in reduced dose treatments as there has been a trend toward lesser local control rates with reduced total dose in LDR applications [39, 50].

The daily treatment with balloon catheters requires balloon integrity verification and catheter lumen integrity evaluation before each individual fraction is delivered, although some clinicians perform the verification procedures once daily. We recommend ultrasound verification as opposed to serial CT verification to minimize radiation dose to uninvolved organs. If ultrasound is not available, we recommend limited CT scanning in a manner similar to that used for initial dosimetric data capture. For diminished fluid volume findings in the balloon as evidenced by diameter variations of greater than 0.2 cm between fractions, saline can be added to the balloon to restore the initial diameter. Rotational variances of up to 15° in either the clockwise or counterclockwise direction

have shown to cause minimal and insignificant dosimetric variances [51], but care should be taken to check alignment and adjust the balloon rotation before each fraction if the variance is greater than these parameters. With severe and frequent variations in diameter, the balloon should be replaced. We recommend that catheter covers be used between treatment to prevent debris from entering the catheter lumens. Upon completion of therapy, the balloon is removed first by painting a germicidal solution on the skin around the catheter. The balloon is then deflated and then gently twisted 360° to loosen tissue adhesions. A constant firm but careful pull on the device usually frees it with minimal discomfort. The excess seroma fluid is then gently expressed following explantation, and the wound is covered with a small bandage. When the wound heals over, the patient is allowed to shower or bathe. Until that point, we recommend sponge bathing. The patient is instructed in post-operative wound care and expectations and discharged from the brachytherapy suite.

Dose distribution comparison example of single versus multilumen applications (0.8 cm skin to balloon surface distance) (Figs. 1 and 2).

3.7.1 Results

Twenty-two patients have been retreated with intracavitary brachytherapy at Allegheny General Hospital as of the time of this writing. The mean time to IBTR was 141 months (range 26–341 months). At a mean follow-up of 42.1 months (range 15–76 months), only two patients developed a local recurrence both successfully locally treated with salvage mastectomy. One patient recurred with "inflammatory" carcinoma within 1 year of treatment, raising suspicion of occult aggressive disease underlying what was originally thought to be a 2.0 cm moderately differentiated IDC with clearly negative (1.0 cm) margins. She expired 1 year later from extensive metastatic disease. No patient developed any acute reaction greater than grade II erythema as scored by the Common Terminology Criteria for Adverse Events scale (CTCAE v4.03) [52]. Cosmesis as graded by the NSABP/Harvard Scale [53] (Table 3) was grade I in eleven patients, grade II in six patients, and grade III in three

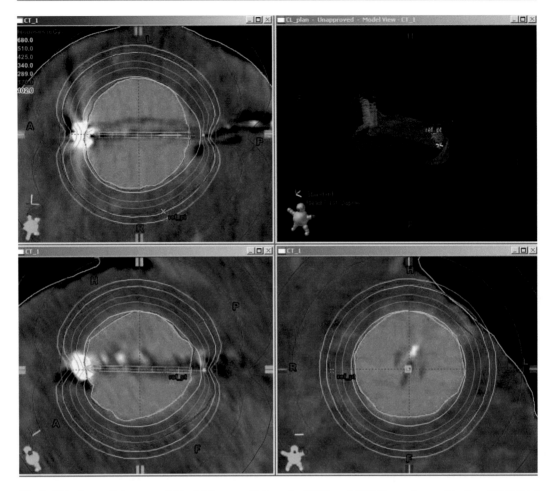

Fig. 1 Skin dose utilizing central (single) lumen catheter only. (PTV_eval 97.7 %; maximum skin dose 121.6 % of prescribed)

patients. The Harvard criteria, while reasonably good in describing de novo cosmetic outcomes following initial breast conservation therapy, are inadequate in describing cosmesis in the retreated breast as they do not allow for accurate description of the cosmetic effect of retreatment from a standard baseline. It cannot do so by definition. The Allegheny General Hospital (AGH) modification of the Harvard/NSABP scoring system allows more accurate standardization of the effects of repeat breast conservation by reestablishing a relative baseline. Cosmesis according to the AGH modification of the Harvard criteria [54] (Table 4) was more reflective of the changes related solely to the retreatment: grade (1) in ten patients, grade (2-2) in six patients, grade (3-3) in

two patients, grade (1-2) in one patient, and grade (2-3) in one patient. The AGH modification highlighted that only two patients demonstrated cosmetic downgrading from retreatment irradiation. Patient satisfaction was uniformly high as all patients, when queried, were happy that they chose the option of repeat preservation including those who required salvage mastectomy.

4   Importance of the AGH Modification

The Harvard criteria have been the most useful cosmesis criteria accepted in the literature to date. However, when trying to correlate outcomes

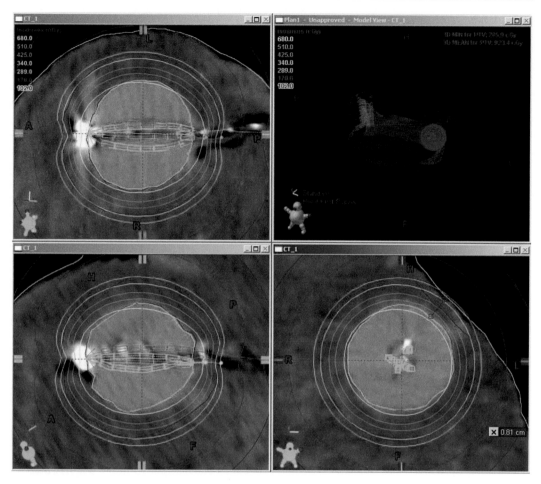

Fig. 2 Skin dose using multilumen catheter optimized for minimum skin dose (104 % of prescribed) and appropriate dose to PTV_eval (95.2 %)

Table 3 NSABP breast cosmesis grading scale (Harvard criteria)

I. Excellent: when compared to the untreated breast, there is minimal or no difference in the size or shape of the treated breast. The way the breasts feel (its texture) is the same or slightly different. There may be thickening, scar tissue, or fluid accumulation within the breast, but not enough to change the appearance
II. Good: there is a slight difference in the size or shape of the treated breast as compared to the opposite breast or the original appearance of the treated breast. There may be some mild reddening or darkening of the breast. The thickening or scar tissue within the breast causes only a mild change in the shape or size
III. Fair: obvious difference in the size and shape of the treated breast. This change involves one quarter or less of the breast. There can be moderate thickening or scar tissue of the skin and the breast, and there may be obvious color changes
IV. Poor: marked change in the appearance of the treated breast involving more than one quarter of the breast tissue. The skin changes may be obvious and detract from the appearance of the breast. Severe scarring and thickening of the breast, which clearly alters the appearance of the breast, may be found

NSABP Protocol B-39 Form COS [39]

relative to retreatment, the Harvard criteria are inadequate since they do not allow an adjustment for the original cosmesis following the first con-servation effort to set a standard for future com-parison. The comparison of cosmetic terminology between a surgically altered breast in the de novo

Table 4 Allegheny modification of the Harvard/RTOG/NSABP criteria for the re-irradiated breast

A-0 (X). Where X = the breast cosmesis grade according to the Harvard/RTOG/NSABP criteria prior to repeat surgical and radiotherapeutic intervention

A-1. When compared to the A-0 breast, there is minimal or no change in the size or shape of the retreated breast. The breast texture is the same or slightly different. There may be thickening, scar tissue, or fluid accumulation within the breast, but not enough to change the appearance

A-2. When compared to the A-0 breast, there is a slight difference in the size or shape of the treated breast as compared to the opposite breast or the original appearance of the retreated breast. There may be some mild reddening or darkening of the breast. The thickening or scar tissue within the breast causes only a mild change in the shape or size

A-3. When compared to the A-0 breast, there is an obvious difference in the size and shape of the treated breast. This change involves one quarter or less of the breast. There can be moderate thickening or scar tissue of the skin and the breast, and there may be obvious color changes

A-4. When compared to the A-0 breast, there is marked change in the appearance of the treated breast involving more than one quarter of the breast tissue. The skin changes may be obvious and detract from the appearance of the breast. Severe scarring and thickening of the breast, which clearly alters the appearance of the breast, may be found

The initial scoring should consist of the A0 (X) score and all subsequent scores should be graded A0(X) followed by the post-therapeutic A score [i.e., A (1-1) for excellent cosmesis pre- and postretreatment]. Initial scoring for this same example would be graded as A (1-X) to denote the unknown future scoring

setting compared to a breast evaluated years after surgery and postoperative irradiation followed by the retreatment effects of both a second surgical and radiotherapeutic intervention are intuitively not equivalent.

This may be even more important when one considers the variability in cosmetic outcomes among different surgeons and radiation oncologists. Since many of these patients are referred to and treated by tertiary and quaternary institutions, a wider variety of reported cosmetic outcomes is likely.

5 Complications and Management

5.1 Acute and Subacute

The most frequent acute complication is mild mastalgia at the balloon site which occurs between 1 and 2 weeks post-explantation and usually requires no therapeutic intervention. If analgesia is desired, nonsteroidal anti-inflammatory medications (NSAIDs) are preferred unless contraindicated. Wound infection or abscess formation occurs rarely. Our experience reflects approximately a 2 % rate of infection which is generally managed by changing the antibiotic coverage. Rare patients will develop a

non-healing wound which generally responds to conservative expectant management.

5.2 Long Term and Chronic

The most common chronic side effects are sinus tract formation and fat necrosis in the retreated breast. Sinus tract formation has occurred in two of our 22 patients, one of whom required mastectomy to remedy chronic pain and drainage. She remains disease-free at 6 years posttreatment, with very good postmastectomy healing and relative cosmesis. The second patient healed completely after 4 months with grade I cosmesis. Four patients developed fat necrosis visible on imaging studies, but asymptomatic. Fat necrosis infrequently requires therapeutic intervention [55]. When necessary, aspiration or, rarely, limited surgical resection will remedy the issue. Generally we recommend conservative management with expectant observation and NSAIDs with surgical management reserved only for the rare patient with persistent and refractory mastalgia. Chronic cardiac dysfunction, having been reported with external beam breast radiotherapy, has not been encountered with intracavitary brachytherapy and was shown to deliver minimal cardiac dose, even in left-sided lesions [56]. Balloon brachytherapy has also been shown to be safely used in patients with cardiac pacing and defibrillating devices [57, 58] as long as the approximate distance from balloon surface to the pacing device is approximately 14 cm.

We are currently in the process of reducing the total dose by reducing both the dose per fraction and the number of fractions as are being done in de novo single institutional trials. We do not believe that a further volume reduction would be safe or acceptable at this time; therefore, the volume parameters will remain unchanged.

6 Further Steps, Controversies, and Summary

One of the most important controversies of IBTR is the risk of systemic disease. This risk of systemic disease is correlated with the pathologic features of IBTR but also with the notion that the new breast event may be a true recurrence (TR) or a new primary (NP) tumor. The difference between the two entities is generally based on pathologic and location information of the IBTR compared to the original primary tumor but also considers the time interval between primary and recurrent tumor [59]. Indeed, this time interval was reported as an independent prognostic factor for DFS and OS with a cutoff ranging from 24 to 36 months [18, 60]. New molecular approaches are proposed to refine more precisely the IBTR features between NP and TR [61, 62]. However, because it is often difficult to determine if the IBTR is or is not a true recurrence, it is probably better to speak in terms of a second ipsilateral breast cancer event (IBCE) or a third IBCE, if any.

While there is a standard in terms of evidence-based medicine for considering conservative treatment option for primary breast cancer [7, 8], there is no significant proof for considering such treatment as well as considering salvage radical mastectomy as the standard treatment in the case of IBTR. Could the concept of breast conservative treatment be also considered for women presenting with IBTR taking into account the fact that the patient already underwent surgery, whole breast irradiation, and various systemic therapies for the primary? If a second BCT is proposed, in regard to the presented results, this treatment strategy should probably include re-irradiation of the tumor bed. Consequently, in terms of clinical research for achieving a high proof level, the appropriate approach could be a randomized trial comparing for IBTR, between salvage mastectomy and second BCT with re-irradiation of the tumor bed. However, for this type of prospective phase III trial, what could be the best statistical design: noninferiority or equivalence? What could be the best primary end point: second local recurrence rate, DFS, or OS? If such a phase III trial was designed, the number of needed patients for statistical significance would be high (1000–2000 patients) for a nevertheless rare event (IBTR) with the likelihood that patients would not accept randomization between salvage mastectomy and second BCT. Because a phase III trial appears difficult to manage, the Radiation Therapy Oncology Group (RTOG) proposed a phase II prospective trial [14] which recently closed due to complete completion of accrual [14]. This trial is investigating toxicity (grade 3+ treatment-related skin, fibrosis, and mastalgia) occurring within 1 year of re-irradiation (3-D external beam radiation therapy) of the tumor bed after salvage breast conservative surgery. The radiation treatment volume consists of the surgical cavity plus a 2.5 cm margin excluding the skin surface. Twice daily fractions of 1.5 Gy were administered to a total dose of 45 Gy. The study will secondarily evaluate end points of local control, freedom from mastectomy, cosmesis, and overall survival.

The development and promotion of phase II trials for second BCT represent a pragmatic and encouraging approach as it remains simple and feasible, with favorable inclusion criteria, a standard re-irradiation technique, and accepted tolerance. However, this clinical prospective research will not allow any rigorous comparison with salvage mastectomy. Matched-pair analysis between salvage mastectomy and second BCT could be a good compromise to provide consistent but retrospective realistic results. Currently, even if salvage mastectomy remains the historical local treatment, a case can easily be made for retreatment breast conservation in favorable patients with IBTR.

References

1. International Agency for Research on Cancer: Globocan 2012 http://globocan.iarc.fr/Default.aspx
2. Glass A, Lacey J, Carreon J et al (2007) Breast cancer incidence, 1980–2006: combined roles of menopausal hormone therapy, screening mammography, and estrogen receptor status. J Natl Cancer Inst 99:1152–1161
3. World Health Organization Global Health Initiative. 2014. http://who.int/cancer/detection/breastcancer/en/index1.html
4. Bartelink H, Horiot JC, Poortmans PM (2007) Impact of a higher radiation dose on local control and survival in breast conserving therapy of early breast cancer: 10 year results of the randomized boost versus no boost EORTC 22881-10882 trial. J Clin Oncol 25:3259–3265
5. Early Breast Cancer Trialists' Collaborative Group (EBCTCG), Darby S, McGale P, Correa C et al (2011) Early Breast Cancer Trialists' Collaborative Group (EBCTCG): effect of radiotherapy after breast-conserving surgery on 10-year recurrence and 15 year breast cancer death: meta-analysis of individual patient data for 10801 women in 17 randomized trials. Lancet 378(9804):1707–1716
6. Poetter R, Gnant M, Kwasny W et al (2007) Lumpectomy plus tamoxifen or anastrozole with or without whole breast radiation in women with favorable early breast cancer. Int J Radiat Oncol Biol Phys 68(2):334–340
7. Fisher B, Anderson S, Bryant J et al (2002) Twenty-year follow-up of a randomized trial comparing total mastectomy, lumpectomy. And lumpectomy plus irradiation for the treatment of invasive breast cancer. N Engl J Med 347:1233–1241
8. Veronesi U, Cascinelli N, Mariani L et al (2002) Twenty-year follow-up of a randomized study comparing breast-conserving surgery with radical mastectomy for early breast cancer. N Engl J Med 347:1227–1232
9. Abner AL, Recht A, Eberlein T et al (1993) Prognosis following salvage mastectomy for recurrence in the breast after conservative surgery and radiation therapy for early-stage breast cancer. J Clin Oncol 11:44–48
10. Ries LAG, Miller BA, Hankey BF et al (1994) SEER cancer statistics review, 1973-1991: tables and graphs. NIH publ no. 94-2789. USDHHS National Cancer Institute, Bethesda
11. Ganz P, Coscarelli A, Schag C et al (1992) Breast conservation versus mastectomy; is there a difference in psychological adjustment or quality of life in the year after surgery? Cancer 69:1729–1738
12. Rowland J, Desmond K, Meyerowitz B et al (2000) Role of breast reconstruction in physical and emotional outcomes among breast cancer survivors. J Natl Cancer Inst 92:1422–1429
13. Maunsell E, Brisson J, Deschhes L (1989) Psychological distress after initial treatment for breast cancer: a comparison of partial and total mastectomy. J Clin Epidemiol 42:765–771
14. RTOG 1014. Radiation therapy in treating women with locally recurrent breast cancer previously treated with repeat breast-preserving surgery. http://www.rtog.org/ClinicalTrials/ProtocolTable/StudyDetails.aspx?study=1014
15. Salvadori B, Marubini E, Miceli R et al (1999) Reoperation for locally recurrent breast cancer in patients previously treated with conservative surgery. Br J Surg 86:84–87
16. Komoike Y, Motomura K, Inaji H et al (2003) Repeat lumpectomy for patients with ipsilateral breast tumor recurrence after breast conserving surgery. Oncology 64:1–6
17. Huang E, Bucholz T, Meric F et al (2002) Classifying local disease recurrences after breast conservation therapy based on location and histology. Cancer 95(10):2059–2067
18. Doyle T, Schultz D, Peters C et al (2001) Long-term results of local recurrence after breast conservation treatment for invasive breast cancer. Int J Radiat Oncol Biol Phys 51(1):74–80
19. Cajucom C, Tsangaris T, Nemoto T et al (1993) Results of salvage mastectomy for local recurrence after breast-conserving surgery without radiation therapy. Cancer 57(5):1174–1779
20. Recht A, Schnitt SJ, Connolly JL et al (1989) Prognosis following local or regional recurrence after conservative surgery and radiotherapy for early stage breast cancer. Int J Radiat Oncol Biol Phys 16:3–9
21. Fowble B, Solin L, Schultz D et al (1990) Breast recurrence following conservative surgery and radiation: patterns of failure, prognosis, and pathologic findings from mastectomy specimens with implications for treatment. Int J Radiat Oncol Biol Phys 19:833–842
22. Kurtz JM, Spitalier JM, Amalric R (1988) Results of salvage surgery for mammary recurrence following breast conserving therapy. Ann Surg 207:347–351
23. Trombetta M, Julian TB, Bhandari T et al (2008) Breast conservation surgery and interstitial brachytherapy in the management of locally recurrent carcinoma of the breast: the Allegheny General Hospital experience. Brachytherapy 7(1):29–36
24. Trombetta M, Julian TB, Kim Y et al (2012) Mature follow-up of low dose rate brachytherapy following ipsilateral breast tumor recurrence in patients initially treated with breast conservation therapy. J Solid Tumors 2(1):8–15
25. Fyles AW, McCready DR, Manchul LA et al (2004) Tamoxifen with or without breast irradiation in women 50 years of age or older with early breast cancer. N Engl J Med 351:963–970
26. Hughes KS, Schnaper LS, Berry D et al (2004) Lumpectomy plus tamoxifen with or without irradiation in women 70 years of age or older with early breast cancer. N Engl J Med 351:971–977

27. Kunkler IH, Williams LJ, Jack WJ et al (2015) Breast conserving surgery with or without irradiation in women aged 65 years or older with early breast cancer (PRIME II): a randomized controlled trial. Lancet Oncol 16:266–273
28. Wong JS, Kaelin CM, Troyan SL et al (2006) Prospective study of wide excision alone for ductal carcinoma in situ of the breast. J Clin Oncol 24:1031–1036
29. Fong J, Kurniawan ED, Rose AK et al (2011) Outcomes of screening-detected ductal carcinoma in situ treated with wide excision alone. Ann Surg Oncol 18:3778–3784
30. Silverstein MJ, Poller DN, Waisman JR et al (1996) A prognostic index for ductal carcinoma of the breast. Cancer 77:2267–2274
31. Hughes LL, Wang M, Page DL et al (2009) Local excision alone without irradiation for ductal carcinoma in situ of the breast: a trial of the eastern Cooperative Group. J Clin Oncol 27(32):5319–5324
32. Wapnir I, Dignam J, Fisher E et al (2011) Long term outcomes of invasive ipsilateral breast tumor recurrences after lumpectomy in NSABP B-17 and B-24 clinical trials for DCIS. J Natl Cancer Inst 103(6):478–488
33. Correa C, McGale P, Taylor C et al (2010) Overview of the randomized trials of radiotherapy in ductal carcinoma in-situ of the breast. J Natl Cancer Inst Monogr 41:162–177
34. Strnad V, Van Limbergen E, Hannoun-Levi JM et al., on behalf of Working Group Breast Cancer of GEC-ESTRO (2015) Recommendations from GEC ESTRO Breast Cancer Working Group (I): target definition and target delineation for accelerated or boost Partial Breast Irradiation using multicatheter interstitial brachytherapy after breast conserving closed cavity surgery. Radiother Oncol. 115(3):342–348. doi: 10.1016/j.radonc.2015.06.010. Epub 2015 Jun 20
35. Pierquin B, Dutreix A, Paine CH et al (1978) The Paris system in interstitial radiation therapy. Acta Radiol Oncol Radiat Phys Biol 17:33–48
36. Mullen E, Deutsch M, Bloomer WD et al (1997) Salvage radiotherapy for local failures of lumpectomy and breast irradiation. Radiother Oncol 42:25–29
37. Deutsch M (2002) Repeat high-dose external beam irradiation for in-breast tumor recurrence after previous lumpectomy and whole breast irradiation. Int J Radiat Oncol Biol Phys 53(3):687–691
38. Chadha M, Feldman S, Boolbol S et al (2008) The feasibility of a second lumpectomy and breast brachytherapy for localized cancer in a breast previously treated with lumpectomy and radiation therapy for breast cancer. Brachytherapy 7:22–28
39. Hannoun-Levi JM, Houvenaeghel G, Ellis S et al (2004) Partial breast irradiation as second conservative treatment for local breast cancer recurrence. Int J Radiat Oncol Biol Phys 60(5):1385–1392
40. Maulard C, Housset M, Brunel P et al (1995) Use of perioperative or split-course interstitial brachytherapy techniques for salvage irradiation of isolated local recurrences after conservative management of breast cancer. Am J Clin Oncol 18:348–352
41. Kauer-Dorner D, Pötter R, Resch A et al (2012) Partial breast irradiation for locally recurrent breast cancer within a second breast conserving treatment: alternative to mastectomy? Results from a prospective trial. Radiother Oncol 102:96–101
42. Guix B, Lejárcegui JA, Tello JI et al (2010) Exeresis and brachytherapy as salvage treatment for local recurrence after conservative treatment for breast cancer: results of a ten-year pilot study. Int J Radiat Oncol Biol Phys 78:804–810
43. Hannoun-Levi JM, Castelli J, Plesu A et al (2011) Second conservative treatment for ipsilateral breast cancer recurrence using high-dose rate interstitial brachytherapy: preliminary clinical results and evaluation of patient satisfaction. Brachytherapy 10:171–177
44. Hannoun-Levi JM, Resch A, Gal J, Kauer-Dorner D, Strnad V, Niehoff P, Loessl K, Kovács G, Van Limbergen E, Polgár C, GEC-ESTRO Breast Cancer Working Group (2013) Accelerated partial breast irradiation with interstitial brachytherapy as second conservative treatment for ipsilateral breast tumour recurrence: multicentric study of the GEC-ESTRO Breast Cancer Working Group. Radiother Oncol 108:226–231
45. Beitch P, Wilkinson JB, Vicini F et al (2012) Tumor bed control with balloon-based accelerated partial breast irradiation: Incidence of true recurrence versus elsewhere failures in the American Society of Breast Surgery MammoSite® Registry trial. Ann Surg Oncol 19(10):3165–3170
46. Yi M, Buchholz TA, Meric-Bernstam F et al (2011) Classification of ipsilateral breast tumor recurrences after breast conservation therapy can predict patient prognosis and facilitate treatment planning. Ann Surg 253:572–579
47. Trombetta M, Julian TB, Miften M et al (2008) The use of the MammoSite® balloon applicator in re-irradiation of the breast. Brachytherapy 316–319
48. Smith B, Arthur D, Buchholz T et al (2009) Accelerated partial breast irradiation consensus statement from the American Society for radiation oncology. Int J Radiat Oncol Biol Phys 74(4):387–1001
49. Shah C, Vicini F, Wazer D et al (2013) The American brachytherapy society consensus statement for accelerated partial breast irradiation. Brachtherapy 12:267–277
50. Chadha M, Trombetta M, Boolbol S, Osborne M (2009) Managing a small recurrence in the previously irradiated breast: is there a second chance for breast conservation? Oncology 23(11):933–940
51. Kim Y, Trombetta M (2014) Dosimetric evaluation of multilumen intracavitary balloon rotation in HDR brachytherapy for breast cancer. J Appl Clin Med Phys 15(1):4429
52. Common Terminology Criteria for Adverse Events (version 4.03). http://evs.nci.nih.gov/ftp1/CTCAE_4.03_2010-06-14_QuickReference_5x7.pdf

53. NSABP protocol B-39 form COS. http://www.rtog.org/members/protocols/0413/0413.pdf58

54. Trombetta M, Julian TB, Kim Y, Werts D, Parda D (2009) The allegheny general modification of the harvard breast cosmesis scale for the retreated breast. Oncology 23(11):954–956

55. Trombetta M, Valakh V, Julian TB et al (2010) Mammary fat necrosis in the conservative management of localized breast cancer: does it matter? Radiother Oncol 97(1):92–94

56. Valakh V, Kim Y, Werts ED et al (2012) A comprehensive analysis of cardiac dose in balloon-based high dose rate brachytherapy for left sided breast cancer. Int J Radiat Oncol Biol Phys 82(5):1698–1705

57. Croshaw R, Kim Y, Kim E et al (2011) Avoiding Mastectomy: accelerated partial breast irradiation for breast cancer patients with pacemakers or defibrillators. Ann Surg Oncol 18(12):3500–3505

58. Kim Y, Arshoun Y, Trombetta M (2012) Pacemaker/implantable cardioverter/defibrillator dose in high dose rate brachytherapy for breast cancer. Brachytherapy 11:380–386

59. Panet-Raymond V, Truong PT, McDonald RE et al (2011) True recurrence versus new primary: an analysis of ipsilateral breast tumor recurrences after breast conserving therapy. Int J Radiat Oncol Biol Phys 81:409–417

60. Kurtz JM, Jacquemier J, Amalric R et al (1991) Is breast conservation after local recurrence feasible? Eur J Cancer 27:240–244

61. Bollet MA, Servant N, Neuvial P et al (2008) High-resolution mapping of DNA breakpoints to define true recurrences among ipsilateral breast cancers. J Natl Cancer Inst 100:48–58

62. Vicini FA, Antonucci JV, Goldstein N et al (2007) The use of molecular assays to establish definitively the clonality of ipsilateral breast tumor recurrences and patterns of in-breast failure in patients with early-stage breast cancer treated with breast-conserving therapy. Cancer 109:1264–1272

63. Alpert TE, Kuerer HM, Arthur DW et al (2005) Ipsilateral breast tumor recurrence after breast conservation therapy: outcomes of salvage mastectomy vs. salvage breast-conserving surgery and prognostic factors for salvage breast preservation. Int J Radiat Oncol Biol Phys 63:845–851

64. Chen SL, Martinez SR (2008) The survival impact of the choice of surgical procedure after ipsilateral breast cancer recurrence. Am J Surg 196:495–499

Thoracic Brachytherapy

Paul Renz, Matthew Van Deusen,
Rodney J. Landreneau, and Athanasios Colonias

Abstract

Brachytherapy for thoracic malignancies provides localized intrathoracic delivery of high-dose targeted radiotherapy, which can be very potent as a primary treatment, an adjuvant treatment, or a salvage treatment. We present our experience, data, and recommendations in this regard.

P. Renz, DO
Department of Oncology, Allegheny General Hospital, Pittsburgh, PA, USA

M. Van Deusen, MD
Department of Thoracic Surgery, Allegheny General Hospital, Allegheny Health Network, Pittsburgh, PA, USA

R.J. Landreneau, MD
Department of Thoracic Surgery, Allegheny General Hospital, Allegheny Health Network, Pittsburgh, PA, USA

A. Colonias, MD (✉)
Department of Radiation Oncology, Allegheny General Hospital, Allegheny Health Network, Pittsburgh, PA, USA
e-mail: acolonia@wpahs.org

1 Lung Cancer Brachytherapy

1.1 Incidence/Epidemiology

Lung cancer results in more cancer-related deaths than any other malignancy in men and women in the United States [1]. The American Cancer Society estimates 221,200 new cases of lung cancer will be diagnosed in the United States in 2015. Lung cancer is the second most common malignancy in men and women, following prostate and breast cancer, respectively, and will account for an estimated 158,040 deaths in the United States in 2015. Worldwide, lung cancer accounted for 1.6 million cancer-related deaths in 2012 [2].

Cigarette smoking is the most important risk factor in the development of lung cancer. It is estimated to be the likely causative factor in up to 90 % of patients [3]. Risk is increased with duration and quantity of tobacco use. Cigar and pipe smoking are also associated with increased risk of developing lung cancer, as is exposure to second hand smoke.

© Springer International Publishing Switzerland 2016
P. Montemaggi et al. (eds.), *Brachytherapy: An International Perspective*, Medical Radiology,
DOI 10.1007/978-3-319-26791-3_12

Environmental factors, including exposure to radon gas and various occupational exposures, also contribute to the development of lung cancer [3].

1.2 Diagnosis and Staging

Non-small cell lung cancer (NSCLC) accounts for approximately 80 % of all lung cancers. Adenocarcinoma, squamous cell carcinoma, and large-cell carcinoma are the most common types of non-small cell lung cancer. Small cell lung cancer (SCLC) accounts for approximately 15 % of all lung cancers. Accurate diagnosis and staging are of critical importance in the determination of staging, treatment, and prognosis.

Lung cancer is staged according to the American Joint Committee on Cancer (AJCC) seventh edition of the tumor-node-metastasis (TNM) classification system [4]. Clinical, radiographic, and pathologic criteria are utilized. Tumor status is primarily dependent on the size of the tumor. Other factors, including tumor location, involvement of visceral and parietal pleura, the presence of post-obstructive pneumonia, and the presence (and location) of satellite nodules, are considered. Nodal status is dependent on the location of involved nodal stations: hilar, ipsilateral mediastinal, contralateral mediastinal, and ipsilateral supraclavicular. Metastasis relates to the presence of distant disease or the presence of a malignant pleural effusion.

Appropriate imaging routinely includes CT and PET scan evaluations. These allow evaluation of the primary lung lesion and associated hilar and mediastinal adenopathy, as well as the presence of distant disease. Invasive testing is commonly performed to obtain an initial diagnosis of lung cancer. Typically, bronchoscopic evaluation and CT-guided needle biopsy are utilized. Additional modalities are considered in the assessment of hilar and mediastinal lymphadenopathy. These may include traditional bronchoscopy with transbronchial needle biopsies, endobronchial ultrasound, or endoscopic ultrasound-guided biopsies, as well as surgical procedures, including mediastinoscopy, anterior mediastinotomy, or thoracoscopic surgical evaluation. Distant disease, when suspected, generally requires pathologic confirmation. Depending on the presentation, invasive techniques may include image-guided percutaneous biopsy, drainage of associated pleural or pericardial effusion, or surgical evaluation of an extrathoracic lesion.

1.3 Treatment Overview

The TNM stage at presentation is the greatest determinant of prognosis. Early-stage disease is associated with favorable survival compared with later-stage disease. The changes to the seventh edition of the AJCC TNM staging guide reflect these survival differences [4].

For medically operable candidates with early-stage disease (stage I and II), the mainstay of therapy is surgical resection with lymph node staging. The extent of resection is dependent on the size and location of the lesion and the patient's cardiopulmonary status. It may include sublobar resection (nonanatomic wedge resection or anatomic segmentectomy), lobectomy, bilobectomy, or pneumonectomy. Various approaches to surgical resection are available, with comparable safety and oncologic outcomes. These include open thoracotomy approaches and minimally invasive, video-assisted techniques. Postoperative adjuvant platinum-based chemotherapy is routinely considered in patients with pathologic stage II disease and may be of benefit in some patients with pathologic stage Ib (patients with tumors >4 cm) [5–7]. Adjuvant radiation is a consideration in the setting of incomplete resection.

Medically inoperable candidates with early-stage disease (stage I) may be candidates for a variety of nonsurgical ablative therapies, including stereotactic body radiation therapy (SBRT) or stereotactic ablative body radiation (SABR), radio-frequency ablation (RFA), microwave ablation, or cryotherapy. Systemic platinum-based chemotherapy is offered to medically inoperable candidates with locally advanced disease (stage II), as these nonsurgical ablative therapies do not address hilar nodal disease.

For patients with advanced-stage disease (stage III), multimodality treatment with platinum-based chemotherapy and radiation therapy is typically recommended. This may be a definitive treatment strategy or a neoadjuvant (induction) treatment strategy followed by surgical resection in selected patients.

Patients with metastatic disease (stage IV) are treated medically with platinum-based chemotherapy. Palliative treatment of symptomatic disease is a consideration. This may include endobronchial therapies (airway stenting, laser therapy, photodynamic therapy, high-dose rate brachytherapy, and cryotherapy) for palliation of airway obstruction or bleeding, management of malignant pleural effusions (chemical pleurodesis or chronic pleural drainage) for palliation of dyspnea and shortness of breath, and radiation therapy for palliation of painful metastatic bone lesions or other indications.

2 Background/History of Thoracic Brachytherapy

Lung brachytherapy as a treatment technique for various stages of lung cancer dates back to the 1920s. In 1922, Yankauer published the first report on brachytherapy for lung cancer as they treated two patients with radium-226 [8]. Several years later in 1929, Kernan and Cracovaner further described lung brachytherapy with the implantation of three radon-222 seeds into a malignant endobronchial tumor in a 35-year-old woman [9]. He subsequently reported eight additional cases of endoluminal interstitial radon-222 seed implantation by rigid bronchoscopy and in conjunction with diathermy [10]. Remarkably, five of the eight patients lived beyond 2 years with this treatment.

In parallel with the cases reported by Kernan, his contemporaries were also performing this exciting new technique. Pool et al. reported their experience at the Memorial Hospital with 42 patients permanently implanted with hollow gold seeds filled with radon-222 gas from 1936 to 1960 in a variety of tracheobronchial locations as both an adjunct to surgery and as primary therapy [11]. In 1932, Graham and Sanger performed a radical pneumonectomy with mediastinal nodal dissection for a 1.0 cm left mainstem bronchus squamous cell carcinoma. They utilized the cutting edge technology of their time as they implanted seven radon seeds with activity of 10.5 mCi into the bronchial stump [12].

Despite some initial success with brachytherapy and rigid bronchoscopy, the technique was fraught with technical difficulty. Uniform dose distribution and precise geometric arrangement of sources was difficult to produce due to limited range of motion using rigid bronchoscopy. Seeds were often times placed superficially and expectorated or, conversely, placed too deep and within the chest cavity or lung parenchyma. In addition, perioperative hemorrhage and airway edema complicated the procedure as severe acute side effects [11–17]. Over time lung brachytherapy was refined as applicators for endoluminal brachytherapy were developed for use with flexible bronchoscopy. In the early 1980s, Mendiondo et al. described the first true endoluminal brachytherapy with a low-dose rate (LDR) afterloading system [18]. Further advances in remote afterloading systems and high-dose rate sources then ushered us into endoluminal treatments as most centers perform today [19, 20]. High-dose rate (HDR) endobronchial brachytherapy (EBBT) solved many shortcomings of its predecessors as a less invasive modality with decreased treatment times and lessened staff radiation exposure.

3 Endoluminal Brachytherapy in Lung Cancer

3.1 Low-Dose Rate (LDR) Versus High-Dose Rate (HDR) Brachytherapy

With the advent of computerized remote HDR (>2 Gy/min) afterloading systems, LDR (<2 Gy/h) endoluminal brachytherapy gave way to the enhanced patient convenience and radiation safety of HDR treatments [21]. HDR treatment could be performed on an outpatient basis and in an expedient fashion. Patient satisfaction and comfort were increased by the lack of need for indwelling endobronchial catheters for extended time periods of up to 48–72 h. Treatment was able to be performed in shielded vaults and did not pose the radiation safety hazards to hospital staff of LDR treatment. Needless to say, the question remained: Is HDR equivalent to LDR in terms of safety and efficacy for the treatment of lung cancer?

Lo et al. compared the outcomes of patients treated with LDR and HDR showing equal efficacy and toxicity [22, 23]. They compared their experience of 110 patients treated with LDR endoluminal brachytherapy for malignant airway obstruction prior to the advent of HDR treatments with a cohort of 110 patients treated with HDR endoluminal brachytherapy. Their results showed no significant difference in bronchoscopic response or complications between the two cohorts [22, 23].

With the available evidence showing equal response and toxicity, it is a reasonable conclusion that HDR endoluminal brachytherapy is the preferred brachytherapy modality (when available) given its ease of use, patient convenience, and better radiation safety profile.

3.2   HDR Technique

Endobronchial brachytherapy is performed on an outpatient or inpatient basis with the assistance of either a pulmonologist or thoracic surgeon. The patient is brought to either the bronchoscopy suite or operating room and sedated. In most situations, the patient is not intubated. A face mask with high-flow oxygen is placed over the patient's open mouth. A flexible bronchoscope is then placed into the patient's nostril and passed through the nasopharynx and into the patient's larynx. The true vocal cords are then anesthetized with lidocaine passed through the bronchoscope. It is also helpful to anesthetize the carina with additional lidocaine to prevent coughing in the recovery room and/or radiation oncology department. The patient's bronchial tree is then fully inspected by the bronchoscopist with particular attention to the endobronchial lesion to be treated.

The next step is crucial for accurate treatment planning. The bronchoscopist must then make

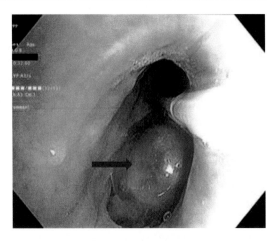

Fig. 1 Endobronchial lesion from renal cell carcinoma metastasis (*arrow*) with adjacent endobronchial catheter placed under bronchoscopic direct visualization

measurements of the length and width of the endobronchial disease as well as the distance from the proximal end of the lesion to the carina. Additional measurements that provide useful information include the distance from carina to the distal extent of the endobronchial lesion. These measurements must be obtained prior to insertion of brachytherapy catheter through the bronchoscope. It is also important to note any anatomical branch points of the secondary or tertiary bronchi in proximity to the lesion as a further reference point.

After appropriate measurements are made, the brachytherapy catheter is then placed. The brachytherapy catheter (5 or 6 French) is placed through a port in the bronchoscope. It is placed distal to the lesion under direct visualization (Fig. 1). The distal extent of the catheter is identified by a radiopaque plug at the end of the catheter. Fluoroscopic images are obtained to verify the desired final position of the catheter (Fig. 2). The catheter should be placed at least 3–4 cm past the distal extent of the lesion, yet special attention must be made to not pass the catheter onto the pleural surface as this may cause a pneumothorax or pleuritic chest pain. The catheter tip must not coil, and if so, a guide wire may be used to aid in placement and prevent coiling. In order to avoid the catheter laying directly onto the bronchial wall and especially when in close

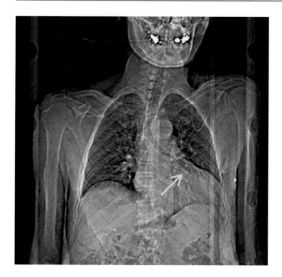

Fig. 2 Digitally reconstructed AP radiograph showing the brachytherapy catheter in the left lower lobe bronchus (*arrow*)

proximity to mediastinal vessels, the catheter may be placed inside a silicone tube such as a thin nasogastric tube which acts as a spacing buffer avoiding high dose to that immediate bronchial wall [24]. On occasion when treating endobronchial lesions at the bifurcation of two bronchi, a catheter may be placed within each bronchus to achieve better dose distribution to the target [24, 25]. When removing the bronchoscope, the brachytherapy catheter is then visualized under continuous fluoroscopy to verify that the catheter is not displaced and remains in the correct anatomic alignment.

The catheter is then fixed to the patient's nose with adhesive tape. Helpful techniques are using tincture of benzoin to add extra adhesive to the patient's nose and the catheter itself. The catheter is then marked at a length distal to the taping, and the distance from the tip of the patient's nose to that mark is recorded as the reference to assure the catheter position. The remaining length of the catheter is then taped to the patient's forehead or scalp. Special instructions/education should then be given to all involved personnel on the purpose of the catheter and the importance of its static fixation.

After recovery from anesthesia, the patient is then taken to the radiation oncology department.

Dummy sources are placed through the catheter and a simulation is performed with a CT scan of the neck and chest without contrast. Prior to the CT, the catheter length is verified using a guide wire and verifying that the actual length coincides with the manufacturers reported length. Medical physics and dosimetry then upload the CT simulation data set to a brachytherapy-based treatment planning system. The radiation oncologist prescribes a dose to a depth over the length of the lesion with a margin proximally and distally. Dosing varies dependent on numerous patient/tumor factors including location of lesion, prior treatment history, size of lesion, and occasionally diameter of the bronchial lumen. A commonly prescribed depth is 1 cm and a common margin is 2 cm proximal and distal to the lesion. The plan is then generated based on TG-43 (Fig. 3) and quality assurance is ascertained [26].

The patient is then ready for treatment and is taken to a shielded vault. The position of the catheter is verified. A remote afterloading HDR unit is then connected with the catheter (Fig. 4). Remote afterloading systems are extremely sensitive to detect the end of the catheter. This may be problematic if sharp angles, such as those seen with lesions in upper lobe bronchi, cause the system to detect the bend/angle at the end of the catheter. A computer-controlled HDR source, such as Ir-192, is then remotely passed by the afterloader to the desired location in the catheter, and treatment is delivered. The duration of treatment varies depending on the isotope used and its activity as well as the treatment length, depth, and dose. Usually the treatment is delivered over an approximately 5–10 min time period. Afterward the HDR source is remotely removed and stored within the afterloader. A radiation survey of the treatment room and patient is then conducted to insure the radioactive source is within the shielded afterloader. After successful treatment, the brachytherapy catheter is then removed and the patient is monitored for a brief period of time before being discharged for the next fraction of treatment. Auscultation of all lung fields and vital signs are checked after treatment and prior to discharge.

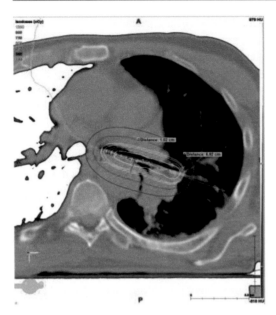

Fig. 3 Plan of an HDR treatment delivering 600 cGy to a 1 cm depth and a 7 cm treatment length to the left lower airway

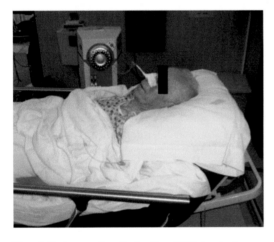

Fig. 4 Patient at the afterloading HDR brachytherapy unit ready to receive treatment

4 Indications for HDR Endoluminal Brachytherapy (EBBT)

4.1 Definitive EBBT

Endobronchial brachytherapy has been utilized in a definitive fashion in a number of settings. It is perhaps best described as an effective modality for the rare entity of roentgenograph-

ically occult endobronchial cancer; however, it has also been used definitively to treat as a boost with external beam, for postoperative adjuvant therapy and for definitive treatment of isolated recurrent disease [27, 28]. Furthermore, almost all cases of definitive treatment with EBBT are resigned to treatment of non-small cell cancer histology with the rare exception of tumors such as adenoid cystic or carcinoid tumors. For the purposes of this discussion, we will be referring to non-small cell lung cancer (NSCLC) exclusively.

4.2 Definitive: EBBT Monotherapy

Endobronchial brachytherapy (EBBT) alone as a treatment for NSCLC has been reported in a number of series as shown in Table 1. Selection criteria for definitive EBBT treatment should be strict and include early-stage disease (Tis/T1), small (<1.0 cm) tumors, and node-negative, nonmetastatic, and radiographically occult lesions. These patients should be evaluated for resection and must either not be surgical candidates or refuse resection as surgery remains the standard of care. Furthermore, adequate nodal staging with imaging such as PET-CT and pathologic assessment with mediastinoscopy is warranted unless contraindicated prior to definitive EBBT. Factors that have been associated with a lower incidence of nodal metastasis include tumor size <1.0 cm and squamous cell cancer histology and therefore are characteristics that lend well to definitive local therapy alone [27, 28].

Marsiglia et al. treated 34 inoperable patients definitively with EBBT alone that had predominant squamous cell histology with an average tumor size of 1.0 × 0.5 × 0.3 cm [24]. The patients received definitive EBBT to a total dose of 30 Gy in six fractions with a 2-year local control and survival rate of 85 % and 78 %, respectively. The unique aspect of their study was individualized prescription dosing and adherence to techniques eliminating catheter contact with the bronchial mucosa. Accordingly, they achieved no treatment-related late toxicity of hemoptysis or bronchial necrosis. Their one case of fatal hemoptysis was attributed to a transbronchial biopsy in a patient with no evidence of tumor or

Table 1 HDR endobronchial brachytherapy treatment as sole modality in NSCLC

Study	N	Size	Dose (Gy at 1 cm)	Fractions	Response	Survival	Complications
Gollins [29, 30]	37 (84 % SCC)	<2.0 cm	15 or 20	1	Not reported	2-yr OS 49.4 % 5-yr OS 14.1 %	13.5 % fatal hemoptysis
Tauelle [31]	22 (84 % SCC)	"Small" endobronchial tumors	8–10	3–4	96 % endoscopic CR	1-yr OS 71 % 2-yr OS 46 %	7 % massive hemoptysis 4 % necrosis
Marsiglia [24]	34 (97 % SCC)	Average size 1.0×0.5×0.3 cm	5[a]	6	2-yr LC 85 %	2-yr OS 78 %	1 case of fatal hemoptysis
Hennequin [32]	106 (95 % SCC)	1.9 cm mean length	5 or 7	6	81 % endoscopic CR 2-yr LC 60 %	3-yr OS 47 % 5-yr OS 24 %	2 % fatal hemoptysis 3 % fatal necrosis
Aumont-Le Guilcher [33]	226 (96 % SCC)	Tis = 27 % T1 = 68 %	4–7	4–6	93.6 % endoscopic CR	2-yr OS 57 % 5-yr OS 29 %	5 % fatal hemoptysis 4 % necrosis

SCC squamous cell carcinoma of lung, *CR* complete response, *LC* local control, *EBBT* endobronchial brachytherapy, *Endoscopic CR* macroscopic negative findings on repeat bronchoscopy at 3 months, *2-yr OS* 2-year overall survival, *3-yr OS* 3-year overall survival, *5-yr OS* 5-year overall survival, *CR* complete response, *LC* local control
[a]Prescribed at 0.5–1.0 cm

bronchial necrosis. They concluded that EBBT was a treatment option in nonoperable patients with early, small NSCLC [24].

Hennequin et al. treated 106 patients not suitable for surgery or further EBRT with definitive HDR-EBBT to total doses between 30 and 42 Gy in six fractions, prescribed to a 1.0 cm depth [32]. They noted a 59.4 % complete histologic response at 3 months and a 3-year overall survival (OS) of 47.4 %. A total of five fatal events attributed to treatment (two hemoptyses and three bronchial necroses) occurred. Predictors of local failure included tumors greater than 2.0 cm and/or occlusion of >25 % of the bronchial lumen. They concluded that HDR-EBBT can be considered a curative modality for early-stage endobronchial NSCLC [32].

More recently, Aumont-Le Guilcher et al. published a series of 226 inoperable patients with Tis, T1, and T2 NSCLC treated definitively with HDR-EBBT to total doses ranging from 24 to 35 Gy in 4–6 fractions [33]. They noted a complete endoscopic response rate of 93.6 % at 3 months with median overall survival of 28.6 months. Also noted was a 5 % incidence of fatal hemoptysis, and they concluded that HDR-

EBBT was a safe and effective treatment for inoperable endobronchial carcinoma [33].

In summary, EBBT as sole definitive treatment for early-stage endobronchial NSCLC is not standard of care, but may be utilized in certain situations where other more conventional options such as surgery and stereotactic body radiotherapy cannot be utilized. Patient selection is quite important with most reported series having a predilection for squamous cell histology, radiographic occult cancers, no evidence of nodal metastasis on staging, and small (<1–2 cm) lesions. The reported series in the literature vary significantly in dosing regimens. The American Brachytherapy Society recommends either a total dose of 22.5 Gy in three fractions or 25 Gy in five fractions prescribed to a 1 cm depth for well-selected patients [34].

4.3 Definitive: External Beam Radiotherapy (EBRT) + EBBT

Endobronchial brachytherapy has been combined with external beam radiotherapy in a number of reports as outlined in Table 2 [35–43].

Table 2 Select studies of combined EBRT/EBBT for definitive treatment of NSCLC

Study	N	Stage	EBRT (Gy)	HDR-EBBT (at 1 cm depth)	Response	Median overall survival (months)	Hemoptysis (%)
Aygun [35]	67	I–IIIB	50–60	3–5×5 Gy	LC 36–75 %	13	15
Nori [36]	17 (group 1)	IIIB	50	3×5 Gy	LC 88 %	17.7	0
Huber [37]	56	IIIA–IV	50+10 boost	2×4.8 Gy	NR	40 weeks	18.9
Anacak [38]	30	III	60	3×5 Gy	CR 53.3 %	11	10.5
Langendijk [39]	47	I–IIIB	30–60	2×7.5 Gy	NR	7.0	15
Gejerman [40]	33	III–IV	37.5	3×5 Gy	BR 54 %	5.2	0
Ozkok [41]	43 (group A)	III	60	3×5 Gy	CR 67 %	11	5
Rochet [42]	35	I–III	50	3×5 Gy	CR 57 %	39.1	9

NSCLC non-small cell lung cancer, *EBRT* external beam radiotherapy, *HDR-EBBT* high-dose rate endobronchial brachytherapy, *LC* local control, *NR* not reported, *CR* complete response, *BR* bronchoscopic response, *Hemoptysis* reported massive or fatal hemoptysis

Endobronchial brachytherapy as a boost to EBRT in advanced non-small cell lung cancer patients may improve local control in select patients, particularly with squamous cell histology. Huber et al. conducted a randomized prospective trial with 98 nonoperable advanced-stage non-small cell lung cancer patients randomized to 60 Gy of external beam radiotherapy with or without a 4.8 Gy HDR-EBBT boost 1 week before and 3 weeks after completion of EBRT. With a median follow-up of 2.5 years, there was no statistically significant difference in overall survival or toxicity; however, there was a trend toward a local control benefit, especially in patients with squamous cell histology with EBBT [37].

Several studies have shown durable palliation of symptoms when adding EBBT to definitive external beam therapy in locally advanced non-small cell lung cancer patients. Langendijk et al. conducted a randomized prospective trial of 95 newly diagnosed stage I–IIIB NSCLC patients having proximal tumors with an endobronchial component treated definitively with EBRT +/− EBBT [39]. They showed no difference in survival or toxicity, but did reveal a statistically significant improvement in relief of dyspnea longer than 3 months, in re-expansion of atelectactic lung (57 % vs. 35 %), and improvement in inspiratory vital capacity with the addition of EBBT. They concluded that addition of EBBT to definitive radiotherapy improves symptomatic

dyspnea without added toxicity [39]. Anacak et al. similarly published a phase II prospective study of 30 newly diagnosed stage III NSCLC patients treated with EBRT to a total dose of 60 Gy with an HDR-EBBT boost of 15 Gy in three fractions showing symptomatic relief of cough, hemoptysis, chest pain, and dyspnea [38]. Gejerman et al. also showed overall symptomatic improvement of 72 % in 33 NSCLC patients treated with EBRT + EBBT boost [40].

HDR-EBBT as an adjunct/boost to external beam radiation in the nonoperative definitive management of locally advanced NSCLC has not translated into a survival benefit [35–43]. Furthermore, studies of EBRT + EBBT do not include concurrent chemotherapy as part of the treatment regimen which is the current standard of care. Accordingly, definitive treatment of locally advanced NSCLC remains chemoradiation with EBBT reserved for palliation of symptoms.

4.4   Definitive: Postoperative EBBT

Definitive adjuvant HDR-EBBT in the postoperative setting for close or positive margins has also been described. Skowronek et al. described a heterogeneous group of 34 patients with positive margins or bronchial stump recurrence treated definitively with HDR-EBBT. They reported a

73.5 % complete response rate and a median over-all survival of 18.8 months. Such therapy, however, is not considered a standard of care. Further options to also be considered include further surgery, external beam radiation, and chemotherapy [44].

4.5 Palliation

Despite definitive treatment, many patients with NSCLC and lung metastasis alike present with symptomatic airway obstruction. EBBT is best known for its use as a palliative modality. Although most series describe palliation of primary lung malignancy, EBBT has been effective in palliation of metastatic disease as well [45]. Endobronchial brachytherapy's characteristics of rapid dose falloff make it ideal for palliation of endobronchial lesions, as normal tissue is spared excess radiation dose thereby minimizing side effects. Symptoms from endobronchial obstruction such as cough, hemoptysis, dyspnea, and lung collapse are palliated effectively with EBBT; however, symptoms of chest pain and dysphagia may not be as effectively palliated with EBBT as they are often caused by bulky extrinsic lung masses rather than endobronchial disease [46]. When considering palliation of lung malignancy, external beam radiotherapy has been found to provide effective symptom relief [47]. Yet, there still remains a subset of patients that may benefit from EBBT such as those patients with prior history of EBRT or poor pulmonary reserve precluding EBRT. Multidisciplinary treatment teams including thoracic surgeons, internists, pulmonologists, and medical and radiation oncologists must choose which patients to select for EBBT based on acuity of symptoms, size/location of disease, life expectancy, performance status, potential toxicity, and prior/future treatments.

Endobronchial brachytherapy has been found to be effective in providing prompt and durable symptom control. Symptom relief can be obtained as early as 24–48 h after EBBT [48], and many studies have shown duration of relief for approximately 6–12 months [29, 49, 50]. Accordingly, with this enhanced duration of symptom relief, many series have shown a decreased need for further EBRT and/or bronchoscopic interventions [29, 50]. Overall symptom relief after brachytherapy is approximately 70–90 % [27, 51]. Mallick et al. have shown increased quality of life (QOL) with EBBT [52]. Hemoptysis, dyspnea, cough, and atelectasis show 67–100 %, 33–100 %, 46–88 %, and 20–83 % improvement after EBBT, respectively, based on standardized symptom scoring in a number of series as detailed in Table 3 [29, 31, 36, 41, 45, 46, 49, 53–61].

Endobronchial brachytherapy may be safely utilized in combination with multiple therapies such as Nd:YAG laser photocoagulation, photodynamic therapy, stenting, or EBRT [62]. Patients with symptomatic lung lesions are a difficult challenge to provide adequate palliation, and multimodality approaches have been shown to be beneficial [62]. Laser photocoagulation has shown to be safe and effective in combination with EBBT [50, 63, 64]. Photodynamic therapy has been used in combination with EBBT with no increased toxicity and enhanced duration of benefit indicating a synergistic effect [65, 66]. Most often EBBT is used in conjunction with EBRT, and this has also proven safe in a number of series when conventional EBBT dose and fractionations are used [27, 36, 41, 67]. Multimodality aggressive airway management with multiple combined treatment modalities has been shown to be beneficial, and EBBT is safely utilized in conjunction with other modalities [62].

When treating in a palliative fashion, toxicity of treatment must be minimized. With EBBT, acute toxicity including pleuritic chest pain, pneumothorax, bronchospasm, and bronchitis are infrequent [36, 51, 67]. Late toxicity includes bronchial stenosis, pneumonitis, dysphagia, odynophagia, bronchial necrosis, fistula, and hemoptysis. Bronchial necrosis, fistula, and hemoptysis are devastating toxicities of treatment. The true incidence of massive or fatal hemoptysis after EBBT is unclear. Reports cite rates between 0 and 32 %, but more modern series with acceptable dosing and fractionation schedules have rates closer to 5–10 % [29, 36, 49, 50, 53, 67, 68]. However, the true incidence of iatrogenic hemoptysis is clouded by the high inci-

Table 3 Palliative HDR endobronchial brachytherapy treatment

Study	N	EBBT dose per fraction (Gy) at 1 cm	Fractions	Prior or concurrent EBBT	Percentage of palliation in patients with presenting symptoms			
					Hemoptysis	Dyspnea	Cough	Atelectasis
Burt [46]	50	15–20	1	98 %	86	64	50	46
Bedwinek [53]	38	6	3	100 %	80	71	80	64
Speiser [54]	295	7.5–10	3	41 %	99	86	85	–
Nori [36]	32	5	3	100 %	100	100	86	44
Pisch [55]	39	10	1–2	85 %	93	–	80	20
Chang [49]	76	7	3	78 %	95	87	79	–
Gollins [29]	406	10–20	1	20 %	88	60	62	46
Kohek [56]	79	5	1–5	68 %	86	67	70	70
Tredaniel [57]	51	7	2	63 %	85	55	85	–
Ofiara [58]	30	8	3	100 %	79	33	46	43
Taulelle [31]	131	8–10	3–4	62 %	74	54	54	–
Quantrill [45]	37	10–20	1	11 %	67	42	50	–
Escobar-Sacristan [59]	81	5[a]	4	63 %	96	75	88	–
Kubaszewska [60]	270	8–10[a]	1–4	86 %	92	76	77	73
Ozkok [41]	158	5–7.5	2–3	100 %	100	77	58	–
Guarnechelli [61]	52	5–7.5	1–3	100 %	94	–	64	–

[a]0.5–1.0 cm depth

dence of recurrent disease in patients who develop post-EBBT hemoptysis. When accounting for this, published rates of hemoptysis are lower at around 5 % [68, 69]. Factors associated with increased risk of hemoptysis include dosing, fraction size, performance status, proximity to mediastinal vessels, history of chemotherapy (concurrent and/or sequential), and prior EBRT [53, 69].

Overall, EBBT is a well-tolerated and safe treatment for the palliation of airway obstruction in select patients with endobronchial disease. It is effective in palliating symptoms of dyspnea, hemoptysis, cough, and atelectasis with long-lasting duration of relief [29, 49, 50]. The risk of causing massive/fatal hemoptysis must be considered, and particular attention should be paid to past and ongoing treatments to mitigate this risk and therefore dose/fractionate accordingly. Common treatment regimens for palliation include 4–7.5 Gy/fraction for 2–4 fractions. Table 4 reviews the American Brachytherapy Society's dosing recommendations [34]. Dosing should be adjusted depending on prior treatment history and concurrent chemotherapy administration should be avoided.

4.6   EBBT and Benign Disease

Although endobronchial brachytherapy (EBBT) is a modality used almost exclusively for malignant disease, there remains a select group of refractory benign conditions in which EBBT may be considered as a treatment option. These benign conditions include airway stenosis secondary to hyperplastic granulation tissue post-lung transplantation, post-intubation tracheomalacia, bronchomalacia from various inflammatory causes, and benign complex tracheobronchial stenosis due to tuberculosis [70–80]. The literature on brachytherapy for benign disease should be interpreted with some caution, as there are limited patient numbers and the groups are heterogeneous in terms of HDR-EBBT dosing. In all benign disease, the risk of acute and late radiation toxicity and risk of long-term oncogenesis must be weighed against the potential therapeutic benefit. Accordingly, most if not all of the literature supporting EBBT in benign disease occurs after many attempts at conservative management have failed.

Table 4 ABS dosing recommendations for HDR and LDR endobronchial brachytherapy based on intent of treatment

	HDR dosing[a]	LDR dosing
Palliative intent alone	6 Gy × 4 fractions 7.5 Gy × 3 fractions 10 Gy × 2 fractions	30 Gy to a 1 cm depth
Palliative intent combined with EBRT (30 Gy in 10–12 fractions)	4 Gy × 4 fractions 5 Gy × 3 fractions 7.5 Gy × 2 fractions	20–25 Gy to a 1 cm depth
Definitive intent alone	5 Gy × 5 fractions 7.5 Gy × 3 fractions	Not reported
Definitive intent combined with EBRT (60 Gy in 30 fractions)	5 Gy × 3 fractions 7.5 Gy × 3 fractions	Not reported

[a]Level of evidence: category 2; 1 cm prescribed depth, fractions given every 1–2 weeks, reduce dose if sequential/concurrent chemotherapy is administered

Radiobiologically, hyperplastic granulation and tracheobronchial malacia as insults from disruptive inflammation can be therapeutically targeted by radiotherapy. Radiation is thought to interrupt macrophage migration within the first 48–72 h after an inflammatory response mounts [73, 78]. This causes downstream alteration in the inflammatory microenvironment and cytokine production which is theoretically responsible for the benign stenosis in question [73, 78]. Tendulkar et al. reported the successful treatment of eight patients with benign airway obstruction due to granulation tissue treated with HDR-EBBT within 48–72 h of bronchoscopic debridement [79]. This indicates that for HDR-EBBT to be effective in benign disease, first the obstruction must be debrided followed by prompt HDR-EBBT within 48 h for adequate disruption of the pathogenic inflammatory response.

There are several published reports of the use of EBBT in the treatment of hyperplastic granulation tissue causing airway obstruction in the setting of lung transplantation. Bronchial stenosis due to hyperplastic granulation tissue at the anastomotic site is a common complication occurring in approximately 7–15 % of patients' post-lung transplant [73]. This complication is usually managed conservatively; however, when refractory, EBBT has been shown to be an option in select cases [72, 73, 75, 76].

Kennedy et al. reported two cases of symptomatic airway obstruction from anastomotic stenosis and malacia post-lung transplantation. Both patients failed stenting, laser ablation, and

dilation attempts. They performed HDR-EBBT delivering 1–2 fractions of 3 Gy/fraction to a 1.0 cm depth. At 6 and 7 months, they reported successful resolution of symptomatic obstruction and stenosis on repeat bronchoscopy with no toxicity of treatment [73].

Halkos et al. reported four cases of refractory anastomotic airway obstruction posttransplantation treated with HDR-EBBT after stenting and laser or electrocautery debridement. A dose of 3 Gy/fraction in 2–4 fractions was prescribed to a 1 cm depth with a treated length approximately 0.5 cm proximal and distal to the area at risk determined by thoracic surgery at time of bronchoscopy [72]. In their report, two patients had a significant response, one patient had a partial response, and no patient experienced toxicity from EBBT [72].

Similarly, Madu et al. reported HDR-EBBT treatment of four post-lung transplant patients with benign bronchial obstruction due to hyperplastic granulation tissue and one patient with tracheal stenosis/obstruction due to prolonged intubation [75]. They reported success in symptomatic relief, increase in posttreatment FEV1, and significant decreased quantity of interventional bronchoscopic procedures post-brachytherapy. They prescribed total doses ranging between 10 and 21 Gy in 5–7Gy treatment fractions. One patient did experience nonfatal radiation-induced bronchitis [75].

Meyer et al. described the largest series to date of 12 post-lung transplant patients with benign airway obstruction with mean follow-up of 34.1 months [76]. HDR-EBBT was delivered in 1–4 fractions of 3 Gy/fraction to a prescribed depth of 0.5–1.0 cm and treatment length 0.5 cm proximal and distal to the area at risk. They reported symptomatic improvement in dyspnea, improved quality of life, and a decreased number of bronchoscopic interventions as well as a statistically significant ($p < 0.02$) improvement in mean FEV1 in all patients after HDR-EBBT with no brachytherapy-related complications [76].

Nonmalignant airway obstruction due to hyperplastic granulation tissue and bronchomalacia is not restricted to only the post-lung transplant setting. Kramer et al. reported a case of a 19-year-old male with airway obstruction due to hyperplastic granulation tissue after airway trauma, prolonged intubation, and stent placement [74]. After failure of other measures, they successfully used HDR-EBBT with a single application of 10 Gy prescribed to a 1 cm depth with long-lasting airway patency [74]. The largest series of HDR-EBBT for benign disease was published in 2012 by Allen and colleagues [70]. They published a series of 29 patients with hyperplastic granulation tissue of the trachea caused mostly by prolonged intubation and mechanical ventilation. Patients were treated with a single fraction of HDR-EBBT to a dose of 10 Gy prescribed to a 1 cm depth with 66 % achieving resolution of granulation with median follow-up of 36 months [70]. Similarly, Rahman et al. published a series of 28 patients with refractory airway obstruction due to prolonged mechanical ventilation treated with a single HDR-EBBT fraction to a dose of 10 Gy [77]. Post-brachytherapy, all patients had a decreased need for interventional bronchoscopic procedures with no associated treatment-related toxicity.

In summary, limited reported series have shown a potential role for HDR-EBBT in the treatment of benign airway obstruction caused by hyperplastic granulation tissue post-lung transplantation, post-intubation tracheomalacia, and bronchomalacia from various inflammatory conditions when other measures have failed. These reports should be interpreted with some caution as they have limited patient numbers and are heterogeneous in terms of HDR-EBBT dos-

ing. The potential risk of HDR-EBBT-induced oncogenesis must also be addressed when considering HDR-EBBT in the treatment of these benign conditions.

5 Conclusions

HDR endobronchial brachytherapy can be a useful treatment modality for lung cancer and is commonly used in the palliative setting for endobronchial malignant airway obstruction and in select circumstances for definitive management. In the hands of an experienced bronchoscopist and radiation oncologist, it is well tolerated and can be performed on an outpatient basis. The published reports of EBBT are heterogeneous in terms of dosing and fractionation and vary depending on the extent of prior treatment (prior external beam radiation/chemotherapy), patient performance status, extent of disease, and intent of treatment. In general, HDR brachytherapy is performed every 1–2 weeks and usually prescribed to a 1 cm depth with 1–2 cm margin on gross disease. Review of the literature shows a trend to increased toxicity (hemoptysis in particular) with increasing dose/ fraction. Administration of sequential/concurrent chemotherapy may also increase the risk. Accordingly, the American Brachytherapy Society has published recommended dose and fractionation schedules as described in Table 4 [81].

6 Interstitial Brachytherapy

6.1 Background

LDR interstitial lung brachytherapy has been utilized in the treatment of lung cancer. The experience of Nori and Hilaris from Memorial Sloan Kettering of iodine-125 (I-125) brachytherapy implantation in lung cancer patients has been extensively reported in the past [14, 82–84]. In general, it was used in unresectable patients or in patients with close/positive margins placed along the chest wall/pleural surface or for paraspinal tumors [85]. The outcomes in patients where such invasive brachytherapy techniques have been used have not materialized into improved survival; however, they have paved the way for further applications.

One such patient population where permanent lung brachytherapy has shown a potential beneficial impact is in high-risk resectable stage I non-small cell lung cancer patients. High-risk resectable patients are defined as patients that cannot tolerate an anatomic lobectomy due to physiologic, functional, and/or comorbid status but can tolerate a sublobar resection such as a wedge resection. High-risk resectable patients include, but are not limited to, patients with marginal cardiopulmonary reserve ($FEV1 \leq 50$ % of predicted, $DLCO \leq 50$ % of predicted), increased age, pulmonary hypertension, left ventricular dysfunction, elevated $pCO2$, and increased Modified Research Council Dyspnea scale [86]. Multiple surgical series of such high-risk patients that were treated with wedge resection have shown a significantly worse local failure rate in the order of 15–20 % when compared with lobectomy historical controls which have local failure rates well under 10 % [87–89]. A randomized trial from the Lung Cancer Study Group confirmed an increased local failure rate in patients with T1N0 non-small cell lung cancer randomized to lobectomy vs. sublobar resection with no impact on overall survival [90].

In order to potentially improve local control in the setting of sublobar resection for these high-risk resectable patients, radionuclide impregnated sutures can be placed at the time of surgery along the sublobar resection staple line.

Iodine-125 is the most commonly utilized isotope in this application. Other isotopes that can also be used are cesium-131 (Cs-131), palladium-103 (Pd-103), and iridium-192 (Ir-192). Table 5 summarizes some potential isotopes with isotope characteristics and commonly prescribed doses.

7   125-I Technique

7.1   Impregnated Mesh

The I-125 mesh technique has been described in prior publications [91, 92]. Iodine-125 seeds are ordered from a supplier and arrive embedded in a polyglycolic suture attached to a curved needle on one end. There are ten seeds per suture at 1 cm spacing. The number of seeds and rows of I-125 suture that are implanted is dependent on the activity of the sources and the desired prescribed total dose. Table 6 is an in house reference table developed at Allegheny General Hospital that aids in defining the seed spacing based on various seed activities to give a desired total dose of 100–120 Gy to a 0.5 cm planar depth.

With a sterile technique, a template is drawn onto the mesh with row spacing defined by the lookup table. The I-125 suture is then sewn onto the mesh and secured to each end of the mesh with staples by the radiation oncologist (Fig. 5). The impregnated mesh (Fig. 6) is then delivered intraoperatively to the thoracic surgeon and placed along the sublobar resection staple line. Figure 7 depicts the wedge resec-

Table 5 Isotope characteristics and commonly prescribed doses for lung brachytherapy

Isotope	Average energy (kev)	Half-life (days)	Brachytherapy technique	Prescribed total dose	Prescription depth (cm)
Iodine-125	28	60	LDR mesh	100–140 Gy	0.5
Cesium-131	30	9.7	LDR mesh	80 Gy	0.5
Palladium-103	20	17	LDR mesh	100–125 Gy	0.5
Iridium-192	380	74	HDR remote afterloading	24.5 Gy (3.5 Gy twice daily in seven fractions) (103)	1.0

LDR low-dose rate, *HDR* high-dose rate

Table 6 Lookup table for I-125 mesh technique

Treatment area of 4.0 cm × 9.0 cm

120 Gy activity/ seed (mCi)	100 Gy activity/seed (mCi)	Number of rows	Row spacing (cm)
0.37	0.31	6	0.8
0.44	0.37	5	1.0
0.63	0.53	4	1.3
0.74	0.62	4	1.5

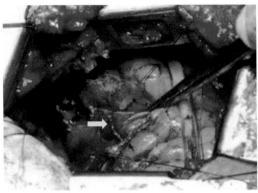

Fig. 7 Intra-operative view of the resection bed and wedge resection staple line (*arrow*)

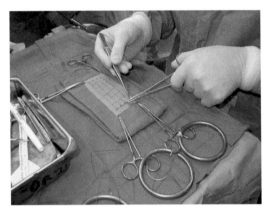

Fig. 5 The I-125 suture is sown onto the mesh by the radiation oncologist

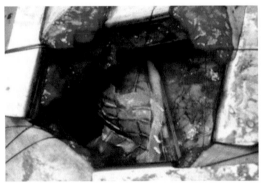

Fig. 8 Intra-operative view of the resection bed with the I-125 mesh implant placed over the wedge resection staple line

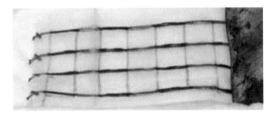

Fig. 6 The I-125 mesh implant

tion staple line and Fig. 8 shows the same staple line with I-125 implant placement. In general, the goal is to place the implant on the staple line with a 2 cm lateral margin on either side. The implant can be sutured into place with 2-0 or 3-0 silk or polyglycolic suture. When reinflating the lung, the implant should constantly be visualized to ensure there is no migration away from the staple line. Premade radioactive Cs-131 and I-125 mesh implants are also available and can be ordered directly from the vendor.

7.2 Double-Suture Technique

Iodine-125 seeds embedded in polyglactin 910 suture (Oncura, Princeton, NJ) in strands of ten seeds are sutured at a 0.5 cm distance on both sides of the visualized resection margin [93]. A common seed activity is between 0.7 and 0.8 mCi/seed with prescribed total dose of 125–140 Gy to a 1 cm depth along the central axis or resection margin [86].

8 Dosimetry

CT-based implant dosimetry occurs between 3 and 6 weeks postoperatively. A non-contrast chest CT simulation is performed using 0.3 cm slice

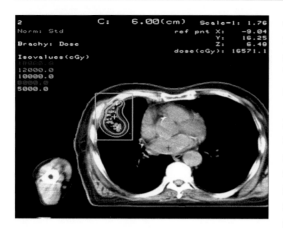

Fig. 9 CT based dosimetry of an I-125 implant with iso-dose lines (*gold line* represents the prescibed dose of 120 Gy)

thickness through the lungs. The clinical tumor volume equals the resection margin or sublobar staple line. The radioactive seeds are digitized into the treatment planning system and dose is calculated based on AAPM TG 43 [26]. Figure 9 is indicative of such a brachytherapy CT plan.

9   Outcomes

Numerous centers have reported their institutional experience regarding lung brachytherapy in this clinical scenario [86, 93–96]. Table 7 shows a summary of reported series showing a benefit with lung brachytherapy when compared to historical controls. These series utilized permanent low-dose rate (LDR) techniques with the exception of one that utilized a remote afterloading high-dose rate (HDR) technique [95].

A series from Allegheny General Hospital in Pittsburgh reported on 145 patients with high-risk stage I NSCLC that underwent sublobar resection and placement of I-125 mesh brachytherapy intraoperatively along the sublobar resection staple line [94]. The median prescribed total dose was 120 Gy with a median total number of seeds implanted of 40. The median total implant activity was 20.2 mCi (range, 11.1–29.7). Postoperative CT scans of the chest revealed no seed migration. They reported a local failure rate

of 4.1 % which compares favorably with local failure rates of 15–20 % in sublobar resection alone in historical control series [87, 90, 93, 94]. Three- and 5-year overall survivals were 65 % and 35 %, respectively.

Lee et al. reported their experience on 33 T1-2N0M0 patients with NSCLC that were not candidates for lobectomy [93]. The double-suture technique was utilized using I-125 prescribed to a total dose of 125–140 Gy. At a median follow-up of 51 months, there were two recurrences at the resection margin with a 5-year survival of 47 % [93]. The authors concluded that limited resection and brachytherapy is associated with "a relatively low incidence of local recurrence and may prolong survival" [93].

Parashar et al. published their institutional retrospective experience using wedge resection and Cs-131 brachytherapy (either mesh- or double-suture technique) and compared it to patients treated with wedge resection alone and stereotactic body radiotherapy [96]. The use of brachytherapy was based on the thoracic surgeon's assessment of whether margins would be close/positive. Fifty-two patients underwent wedge resection followed by Cs-131 brachytherapy application and at a median follow-up of 14 months in the brachytherapy group; local control was 96.2 % [96].

In light of these multiple single institution series showing a potential local control benefit, a randomized phase III trial from the American College of Surgeons Oncology Group (ACOSOG) was conducted [86]. This study randomized 224, high-risk operable stage I non-small cell lung cancer patients with lesions 3 cm or less to sublobar resection alone versus sublobar resection plus I-125 lung brachytherapy (using either the mesh- or double-suture techniques). Local recurrence was defined as failure at the staple line (local progression), failure within the involved lobe, and/or failure in the ipsilateral hilar lymph nodes. At a median follow-up of 4.38 years, there was no difference in local progression, local recurrence, or survival between the two arms. The 3-year overall survival was 71 % in each arm. Brachytherapy was not associated with

Table 7 Various series of sublobar resection and brachytherapy

	N	T stage	Type of surgery	Isotope	Brachytherapy technique	Prescribed dose (Gy)	Median follow-up (months)	Local recurrence	5-year overall survival
Colonias et al. [94]	145	T1-2	WR/Seg	I-125	LDR mesh	Median 120	38.3	4.1 %	35 %
Lee et al. [93]	33	T1-2	WR/Seg	I-125	LDR double suture	125–140	51	6.1 %	47 %
Parashar et al. [96]	52	T1-2	WR	Cs-131	LDR mesh	80	14	3.8 %	100 %
McKenna et al. [95]	48	T1-4 N0-2	WR	Ir-192	HDR remote afterloading	24.5	13.5 (mean)	6.25 %	–
ACOSOG Z4032 brachytherapy arm [86]	108	T1-2 (T3: 1 patient)	WR/Seg	I-125	LDR mesh or double suture	100	4.38 years	7.7 % (in both arms)	55.6 %

WR wedge resection, *Seg* segmentectomy

increased perioperative pulmonary adverse events and at 3 months did not affect pulmonary function [97]. Furthermore, there was no difference in quality of life measures or dyspnea score between the two arms [98].

Even though the ACOSOG Z4032 trial was an overall negative brachytherapy study, the authors concluded that certain situations may still exist to warrant the use of brachytherapy to improve local control. These scenarios revolve around margin status or as the authors state in patients with "potentially compromised margins" and include positive cytology at the staple line, margins of less than 1 cm, margin to tumor ratio <1, tumor size >2 cm, and wedge resection (vs. segmentectomy) [86]. Although subset analysis revealed no statistically significant benefit with brachytherapy in these settings, further study of such "compromised margin" patients with a larger sample size may be warranted.

10   Other Potential Indications

Mutyala et al. reported on a series of 59 patients with various thoracic malignancies (including non-small cell lung cancer, sarcoma, giant cell tumor, and carcinoid) treated with primary surgery with the use of I-125 mesh brachytherapy as an adjunct if the patient was at risk of close or positive margins [99]. The prescribed dose of the implants ranged between 100 and 150 Gy to a 0.5 cm depth for radiation naïve patients and 50–70 Gy for patients having received prior radiation [99]. At a median follow-up of 17 months, 1- and 2-year local control was 80.1 % and 67.4 %, respectively [99]. The authors concluded that brachytherapy is associated with low toxicity and should be further studied in incompletely resected patients.

11   Brachytherapy in Esophageal Cancer

11.1   Incidence/Epidemiology

The American Cancer Society estimates 16,900 cases of esophageal cancer will be diagnosed in

the United States in 2015. It will account for an estimated 15,590 cancer-related deaths in the United States in 2015 [1]. Worldwide, esophageal cancer accounted for over 482,000 cases and over 406,000 cancer-related deaths in 2008 [100].

Squamous cell carcinoma and adenocarcinoma of the esophagus account for the overwhelming majority of esophageal cancers. Historically, squamous cell carcinoma was the predominant type of esophageal cancer. The incidence of squamous cell carcinoma in the United States has been declining. The incidence of adenocarcinoma, however, has increased dramatically, now accounting for over 60 % of esophageal cancers. Worldwide, squamous cell carcinoma remains more common. Men are affected much more commonly than women. Squamous cell carcinoma of the esophagus is more common in African-American men, while adenocarcinoma of the esophagus is more common in Caucasian men [101].

The main risk factors for the development of squamous cell carcinoma of the esophagus are tobacco and alcohol use. Lower socioeconomic status is also associated with the development of squamous cell carcinoma of the esophagus. The main risk factor for the development of adenocarcinoma of the esophagus is the presence of Barrett's esophagus with intestinal metaplasia, a consequence of gastroesophageal reflux disease. Additionally, obesity and tobacco use are associated with adenocarcinoma of the esophagus.

11.2   Diagnosis and Staging

The majority of patients with esophageal cancer are symptomatic. Dysphagia and weight loss are common. Typically, diagnosis is established with upper endoscopy and biopsies. Surveillance endoscopy may identify early-stage esophageal cancer in the asymptomatic patient with Barrett's esophagus. A barium esophagram may also help diagnose esophageal cancer.

Staging of esophageal cancer is dependent on the tumor-node-metastasis classification. Squamous cell carcinoma and adenocarcinoma of the esophagus are considered separately [102]. Tumor status relates to the depth of tumor involvement of the esophageal wall, while nodal status relates to the number of regional lymph nodes. Metastasis relates to the presence of distant disease.

CT and PET scans are routinely obtained, primarily to rule out distant disease. CT and PET scan are inadequate in regard to accurate evaluation of the tumor involvement of the esophageal wall and periesophageal lymphadenopathy. Endoscopic ultrasound provides a much better assessment of local tumor extent and periesophageal nodal involvement. Laparoscopy, thoracoscopy, and bronchoscopy are adjunct staging modalities that may be considered in specific cases, based on imaging and tumor location.

11.3 Survival

Survival correlates with stage of disease in patients with localized, potentially resectable disease. Infrequently, patients with cancer limited to the mucosa or submucosa may be identified. These patients represent the best chance for long-term survival and possible cure.

Unfortunately, the majority of patients present with locally advanced or metastatic disease. Long-term survival is poor in patients with locally advanced disease, with cure rates of approximately 15 %, following multimodality therapy. Long-term survival is highly unlikely in patients with metastatic disease.

12 Treatment Overview

For patients with early-stage disease, limited to the mucosa (T1aN0), endoscopic mucosal resection may be curative. Pathologic review of the lesion is critical. Involvement of the submucosa (T1bN0) generally mandates esophageal resection, due to potential lymphatic spread into the rich submucosal lymphatic network. Patients with involvement of the muscularis propria (T2N0) may be considered for esophagectomy as the initial treatment strategy.

For medically operable patients with locally advanced, potentially resectable disease (typi-

cally T2 or greater or patients with nodal disease), neoadjuvant (induction) chemoradiotherapy or chemotherapy is offered, followed by restaging and possible resection. Induction chemoradiation followed by resection demonstrates improved survival over surgery alone in multiple reports [103–105].

In the medically inoperable patient or in the patient with squamous cell carcinoma of the proximal esophagus, definitive chemoradiation may be considered. Resection may not be possible due to local involvement or proximal extent of tumor in patients with squamous cell carcinoma of the upper third of the esophagus.

For patients with resectable tumors of the mid-thoracic esophagus, total esophagectomy with cervical anastomosis is required. For patients with resectable tumors of the distal esophagus or gastroesophageal junction, esophagectomy with intrathoracic anastomosis or total esophagectomy with cervical anastomosis can be performed. Reconstruction can be accomplished with creation of a gastric conduit or a colonic interposition.

Various surgical approaches can be utilized, including a three-field approach with cervical, thoracic, and abdominal exposure, a trans-hiatal approach (cervical and abdominal exposure), or an Ivor-Lewis approach (abdominal and thoracic exposure). Minimally invasive techniques can be incorporated into any of these approaches, during the abdominal and/or thoracic portions of the procedure.

In addition to esophageal resection and restoration of gastrointestinal continuity, the procedure may include a concomitant gastric drainage procedure (botulinus toxin injection of the pylorus, pyloromyotomy, or pyloroplasty) and insertion of a jejunal feeding tube.

In patients with metastatic disease (stage IV) and patients who are not candidates for surgery or systemic therapy, palliation of esophageal cancer can be considered. This may involve endoluminal therapies, including dilation, stenting, cryotherapy, and photodynamic therapy, and high-dose rate brachytherapy can be considered in the management of malignant stricture, obstruction from tumor, or bleeding.

13 Esophageal Brachytherapy

13.1 Overview

Esophageal brachytherapy can be performed using high-dose rate or low-dose rate techniques. Remote afterloading HDR has the advantage of being an outpatient procedure and limits radiation exposure to health-care workers. Studies comparing LDR with HDR have shown equivalent outcomes in terms of palliation of dysphagia [106] and locoregional control and survival [107]. The most commonly used radioisotope for esophageal HDR is iridium-192. Californium-252, a neutron-emitting isotope, can also be utilized and dose is specified in Gy-equivalent [108].

13.2 Indications

High-dose rate esophageal brachytherapy is used in the palliation of symptoms caused by endoluminal disease, most commonly dysphagia. Other less common uses are in the definitive setting as a boost combined with external beam radiation or as sole therapy in superficial cancers. The American Brachytherapy Society has published consensus guidelines for esophageal brachytherapy [109]. Good candidates for brachytherapy include patients with tumors <10 cm in length and confined to the esophageal wall, thoracic location, and patients without regional nodal involvement [109–111]. Patients with cervical esophageal tumors and/or fistulas should not undergo brachytherapy as these conditions are associated with significant toxicity [109, 112]. Likewise, concurrent chemotherapy is associated with increased treatment-related toxicity including fistula formation [109, 113] and esophageal stricture/ulcer formation [114, 115]. The ABS does not recommend concurrent chemotherapy and brachytherapy [109]. Furthermore, patients with tumor extending into the gastroesophageal junction and proximal stomach are not optimal candidates for brachytherapy as target coverage may not be optimal [109].

13.3 HDR Technique

The technique for endoluminal HDR esophageal brachytherapy requires an esophagogastroduodenoscopy (EGD) with placement of a brachytherapy catheter. At the time of EGD, the distance of the endoluminal lesion from the incisors and length of the lesion should be recorded. The brachytherapy catheter is then placed beyond the lesion, and the scope is removed, while fluoroscopy is performed to make sure that the brachytherapy catheter remains in place. The catheter should be placed at least 3–4 cm past the lesion to insure treating the usual margin of 1–2 cm proximal and distal to the visible mucosal disease. A metallic clip can also be placed submucosally at the proximal edge of the lesion so that the lesion can be readily identified at the time of CT simulation during target delineation and for treatment planning [116]. Once the patient recovers from anesthesia, he or she is transported to the radiation oncology department for CT simulation with a similar process for simulation, planning, and treatment as stated in the endobronchial brachytherapy section of this chapter.

13.4 Definitive Therapy: Superficial Cancer

The standard definitive treatment for esophageal cancer depends on the stage and extent of disease along with the patient's comorbidities, performance status, and their preference. To properly stage these patients, endoluminal ultrasound is required to evaluate the depth of invasion of the primary tumor and to evaluate for regional nodal metastasis. For early mucosal disease, local measures such as mucosal resections are warranted [117–119]. In the event that such interventions cannot be performed, brachytherapy with or without external beam radiation can be used [120, 121]. External beam radiation combined with brachytherapy is recommended when there is significant risk of nodal involvement.

Pasquier et al. reported on 66 patients with superficial (Tis or T1) esophageal cancers that were not surgical candidates or refused surgery

[121]. These patients received external beam radiation and HDR brachytherapy without chemotherapy. The most common treatment regimen was external beam radiation to a total dose of 60 Gy combined with an HDR boost of 14 Gy in two fractions, prescribed to a 0.5 cm depth. The median survival was 3.8 years with a 6 % rate of severe toxicity (primarily esophageal stenosis). The authors concluded that this regimen was tolerable and an option for inoperable patients with superficial esophageal cancer [121].

Ishikawa et al. reported on 59 patients with submucosal esophageal cancer that were treated with external beam radiation therapy. Thirty-six had an esophageal brachytherapy boost using LDR cesium-37 until 1997 and then HDR iridium-192. Brachytherapy was performed after external beam was complete and chemotherapy was not given. Overall locoregional control was 75 % at 5 years. Five-year cause-specific survival was better in the patients that received a brachytherapy boost (86 % vs. 62 %; $p = 0.04$) [120]. The authors concluded that external beam radiation followed by brachytherapy was superior to external beam alone.

13.5 Definitive Therapy: Advanced Disease

In more advanced disease (T2 disease or greater or nodal involvement), the standard therapy is esophagectomy vs. induction chemoradiation then resection vs. definitive chemoradiation [104, 105, 122]. Brachytherapy can be added to external beam radiation as a boost modality in advanced disease but may be associated with significant toxicity and is not considered standard therapy in the United States. Reports from two randomized studies that compared external beam radiation alone with external beam radiation combined with esophageal brachytherapy showed better survival and local control as well as increased toxicity in the combined treatment arm [123, 124]. Numerous other series have been published using brachytherapy in the definitive setting with conflicting results [108, 113,

125–127]. Many of these studies did not utilize concurrent chemotherapy which remains the standard of care.

Muijs et al. reported on 62 patients with esophageal cancer treated with external beam radiation to a total dose of 60 Gy combined with an LDR or HDR boost [126]. About one-third of these patients had nodal disease and almost half had T3–4 disease. Patients received a 12 Gy boost in two fractions with either LDR (cesium-134) or HDR (iridium-192). No patient received chemotherapy. There was a 16 % rate of grade III toxicity including esophageal ulceration, stricture, radiation pneumonitis, fistula, and bleeding. The authors concluded that due to complications, the addition of brachytherapy was not recommended [126].

The Radiation Therapy Oncology Group (RTOG) performed a phase I/II study (RTOG 9207) utilizing concurrent cisplatin/5-FU chemotherapy with external beam radiation combined with HDR brachytherapy in esophageal cancer patients [113]. HDR brachytherapy was initially performed in three fractions of 5 Gy/fraction prescribed to a 1 cm depth from mid-source on weeks 8, 9, and 10 but due to toxicity was reduced to only two fractions. Low-dose rate brachytherapy was also allowed but had poor accrual. The study reported a 12 % incidence of treatment-related fistula within 7 months of therapy and a 10 % incidence of treatment-related death [113].

13.6 Palliation

Numerous series have reported their experience on the effective use of brachytherapy in the palliative setting with most reporting on dysphagia [109, 116, 128–131]. In the palliative setting, the ABS recommends HDR total doses of 15–20 Gy in 2–4 fractions prescribed to a 1 cm depth in weekly fractions (LDR dose of 25–40 Gy at 0.4–1 Gy/h) [109]. Brachytherapy can also be combined with palliative external beam radiation. In this setting the ABS recommends a lower HDR dose of 10–14 Gy in 1–2 weekly fractions (LDR dose of 20–25 Gy at 0.4–1 Gy/h) [109].

Fabrini et al. reported their single institution experience of 104 patients that received brachytherapy as part of their treatment regimen [116]. The report included definitively and palliatively treated patients. The HDR dosing regimen for the palliative patients was 15 Gy in 3 weekly fractions. The authors reported an 84.6 % rate of improvement of dysphagia and a median dysphagia-free interval of 17.5 months. Lymph node involvement was a predictor for overall survival and dysphagia. Three patients developed esophagotracheal fistulas [116].

Rupinski et al. reported on 93 patients with dysphagia due to malignant esophageal disease randomized to argon plasma coagulation laser (APC) alone vs. APC combined with brachytherapy vs. APC combined with photodynamic therapy (PDT) [130]. There was no survival difference between the three treatment arms. The two combined treatment arms had better palliation of dysphagia than the APC alone group. There was no significant difference in palliation of dysphagia between the two combined groups. The patients in the HDR + APC group, however, had fewer complications and better quality of life than the PDT + APC patients [130].

Palliative esophageal brachytherapy can also be combined with self-expanding metal stent (SEMS) placement [128]. Amdal et al. reported a study of 41 patients with malignant esophageal dysphagia randomized to SEMS + brachytherapy vs. brachytherapy alone. Both arms received 8 Gy in three fractions. There was improved dysphagia relief at 3-week follow-up in the combined treatment arm, but at 7 weeks, dysphagia relief was similar between the two arms. Four patients in the combined arm experienced complications requiring a prolonged hospitalization (two had aspiration pneumonia, one aspiration pneumonia and bleeding, and one stent migration) with no reported fistulas or perforations [128]. Based on this study, combining SEMS with brachytherapy can be performed but may be associated with increased risks when compared to brachytherapy alone due to risk of stent migration and other complications. An alternative to SEMS placement may be APC combined with brachytherapy [130]. Esophageal dilatation can also be performed but

should not be performed on the day of brachytherapy as there may be an association with fistula formation [113].

Conclusions

HDR brachytherapy is primarily used in the palliative setting with common dosing schedules of 15–20 Gy in 2–4 fractions as monotherapy or 10–14 Gy in 1–2 fractions when combined with external beam radiation [109]. In the definitive setting, brachytherapy is not considered standard therapy. In early disease, surgical resection is usually performed and in more advanced disease, various regimens can be performed including chemoradiation or trimodality therapy (depending on the extent of disease). In the event that surgery and chemotherapy cannot be performed, external beam radiation with or without brachytherapy can be considered. The ABS recommends 45–50 Gy of external beam radiation followed by either HDR to a total dose of 10 Gy in 2 weekly fractions or LDR to a total dose of 20 Gy at 0.4–1 Gy/h (2–3 weeks after completion of external beam radiation) with a 2–3-week interval between chemotherapy and brachytherapy. Concurrent chemotherapy is not recommended due to risk of severe toxicity including fistula formation.

References

1. American Cancer Society (2015) Cancer facts & figures 2015. American Cancer Society, Atlanta
2. Brambilla E, Travis WD (2014) Lung cancer. In: Stewart BW, Wild CP (eds) World cancer report. World Health Organization, Lyon
3. Alberg AJ, Samet JM (2003) Epidemiology of lung cancer. Chest 123(1 Suppl):21S
4. Goldstraw P, Crowley J, Chansky K et al (2007) The IASLC Lung Cancer Staging Project: proposals for the revision of the TNM stage groupings in the forthcoming (seventh) edition of the TNM Classification of malignant tumours. J Thorac Oncol 2(8):694
5. Arriagada R, Bergman B, Dunant A et al (2004) Cisplatin-based adjuvant chemotherapy in patients with completely resected non-small-cell lung cancer. N Engl J Med 350:351
6. Pignon JP, Tribodet H, Scagliotti GV et al (2008) Lung adjuvant cisplatin evaluation: a pooled analysis

by the LACE Collaborative Group. J Clin Oncol 26:3552

7. Strauss GM, Herndon JE 2nd, Maddaus MA et al (2008) Adjuvant paclitaxel plus carboplatin compared with observation in stage IB non-small-cell lung cancer: CALGB 9633 with the Cancer and Leukemia Group B, Radiation Therapy Oncology Group, and North Central Cancer Treatment Group Study Groups. J Clin Oncol 26:5043

8. Yankauer S (1922) Two cases of lung tumour treated bronchoscopically. NY Med J 21:741–742

9. Kernan JD, Cracovaner AJ (1929) Carcinoma of the lung. Arch Surg 18:315–325

10. Kernan JD (1933) Carcinoma of the lung and bronchus treatment with radon implantations and diathermy. Arch Otolaryngol 17(4):457–475

11. Pool JL (1961) Bronchoscopy in the treatment of lung cancer. Trans Am Bronchoesoph Assoc 41: 128–136

12. Graham EA, Singer JJ (1933) Successful removal of an entire lung for carcinoma of the bronchus. JAMA 18(101):1371–1374

13. Henschke UK (1959) Interstitial implantation in the treatment of primary bronchogenic carcinoma. Am J Roentgenol Radium Ther Nucl Med 79:981–987

14. Hilaris B, Martini N (1988) The current state of intraoperative interstitial brachytherapy in lung cancer. Int J Radiat Oncol Biol Phys 15:1347–1354

15. Hilaris B, Liskow A, Bains M et al (1979) A new endobronchial implanter. Memorial Sloan Kettering Clin Bull 9(1):21–23

16. Mittal B, Matuschak C, Culpepper J (1984) Endobronchial interstitial brachytherapy using a bronchofiberscope with a flexible injector system. Radiology 152:219–220

17. Mittal B, Parsons J, Webster J et al (1986) Transbronchial radioactive implantation using a flexible injector system: an improved technique for endobronchial brachytherapy. Radiother Oncol 5:11–13

18. Mendiondo OA, Dillon M, Beach LJ (1983) Endobronchial brachytherapy in the treatment of recurrent bronchogenic carcinoma. Int J Radiat Oncol Biol Phys 9(4):579–582

19. Seagren S, Harrell J, Horn R (1985) High dose rate intraluminal irradiation in recurrent endobronchial carcinoma. Chest 88:810–814

20. Speiser B, Spratling L (1990) Intermediate dose rate remote afterloading brachytherapy for intraluminal control of bronchogenic carcinoma. Int J Radiat Oncol Biol Phys 18(6):1443–1448

21. Gaspar L (1998) Brachytherapy in lung cancer. J Surg Oncol 67:60–70

22. Lo TCM, Girshovich L, Healey GA et al (1995) Low dose rate versus high dose rate intraluminal brachytherapy for malignant endobronchial tumors. Radiother Oncol 35(3):193–197

23. Lo TC, Beamis JF, Villanueva AG et al (2001) Intraluminal brachytherapy for malignant endobronchial tumors: an update on low-dose rate versus high-dose rate radiation therapy. Clin Lung Cancer 3(1):65–68

24. Marsiglia H, Baldeyrou P, Lartigau E et al (2000) High-dose-rate brachytherapy as sole modality for early-stage endobronchial carcinoma. Int J Radiat Oncol Biol Phys 47(3):665–672

25. Van Limbergen E, Pötter R (2002) Chapter 26. Bronchus cancer. In: GEC ESTRO handbook of brachytherapy, 1st edn. ESTRO, Leuven: ACCO; pp 545–560

26. Rivard M, Coursey BM, DeWerd LA et al (2004) Update of AAPM TG no. 43 report: a revised AAPM protocol for brachytherapy dose calculations. Med Phys 31(3):633–674

27. Gerbaulet A, Pötter R, Mazeron JJ, Meertens H, Van Limbergen E. The GEC ESTRO handbook of brachytherapy. Copyright 2002 by The Authors and ESTRO Printed by ACCO, Leuven

28. Joslin CAF, Flynn A, Hall EJ (2001) Principles and practice of brachytherapy using remote afterloading systems, 1st edn. Oxford University Press Inc, New York

29. Gollins SW, Burt PA, Barber PV et al (1994) High dose rate intraluminal radiotherapy for carcinoma of the bronchus: outcome of treatment of 406 patients. Radiother Oncol 33:31–40

30. Gollins SW, Burt PA, Barber PV et al (1996) Long-term survival and symptom palliation in small primary bronchial carcinomas following treatment with intraluminal radiotherapy alone. Clin Oncol (R Coll Radiol) 8(4):239–246

31. Taulelle M, Chauvet B, Vincent P et al (1998) High dose rate endobronchial brachytherapy: results and complications in 189 patients. Eur Respir J 11: 162–168

32. Hennequin C, Bleichner O, Tredaniel J et al (2007) Long-term results of endobronchial brachytherapy: a curative treatment? Int J Radiat Oncol Biol Phys 67(2):425–430

33. Aumount-Le Guilcher M, Prevost B et al (2011) High-dose-rate brachytherapy for non–small cell lung carcinoma: a retrospective study of 226 patients. Int J Radiat Oncol Biol Phys 79(4):1112–1116

34. Nag S, Kelly JF, Horton JL et al (2001) Brachytherapy for carcinoma of the lung. Oncology (Williston Park) 15(3):371–381

35. Aygun C, Weiner S, Scariato A et al (1992) Treatment of non-small cell lung cancer with external beam radiotherapy and high dose rate brachytherapy. Int J Radiat Oncol Biol Phys 23:127–132

36. Nori D, Allison R, Kaplan B et al (1993) High dose rate intraluminal irradiation in bronchogenic carcinoma* technique and results. Chest 104:1006–1011

37. Huber RM, Fischer R, Hautmann H et al (1997) Does additional brachytherapy improve the effect of external irradiation? A prospective, randomized study in central lung tumors. Int J Radiat Oncol Biol Phys 38:533–540

38. Anacak Y, Mogulkoc N, Ozkok S et al (2001) High dose rate endobronchial brachytherapy in

combination with external beam radiotherapy for stage III non-small cell lung cancer. Lung Cancer 34:253–259

39. Langendijk H, Jong J, Tjwa M et al (2001) External irradiation versus external irradiation plus endobronchial brachytherapy in inoperable non-small cell lung cancer: a prospective randomized study. Radiother Oncol 58:257–268

40. Gejerman G, Mullokandov EA, Bagiella E et al (2002) Endobronchial brachytherapy and external-beam radiotherapy in patients with endobronchial obstruction and extrabronchial extension. Brachytherapy 1:204–210

41. Ozkok S, Karakoyun-Celik O, Goksel T et al (2008) High dose rate endobronchial brachytherapy in the management of lung cancer: response and toxicity evaluation in 158 patients. Lung Cancer 62: 326–333

42. Rochet N, Hauswald H, Stoiber EM et al (2013) Primary radiotherapy with endobronchial high-dose-rate brachytherapy boost for inoperable lung cancer: long-term results. Tumori 99(2):183–190

43. Cotter GW, Herbert DE, Ellingwood KE et al (1991) Inoperable endobronchial obstructing lung carcinoma treated with combined endobronchial and external beam irradiation. South Med J 84(5): 562–565

44. Skowronek J, Piorunek T, Kanikowski M et al (2013) Definitive high-dose-rate endobronchial brachytherapy of bronchial stump for lung cancer after surgery. Brachytherapy 12(6):560–566

45. Quantrill SJ, Burt PA, Barber PV et al (2000) Treatment of endobronchial metastases with intraluminal radiotherapy. Respir Med 94:369–372

46. Burt PA, O'Driscoll BR, Notley HM et al (1990) Intraluminal irradiation for the palliation of lung cancer with the high dose rate micro-Selectron. Thorax 45:765–768

47. Reveiz L, Rueda JR, Cardona AF. Palliative endobronchial brachytherapy for non-small cell lung cancer (Review). The Cochrane Library. 2012; (12):CD004284.

48. Delclos MR, Komaki R, Morice RC et al (1996) Endobronchial brachytherapy with high-dose-rate remote afterloading for recurrent endobronchial lesions. Radiology 201:279–282

49. Chang LL, Horvath J, Peyton W et al (1994) High dose rate afterloading intraluminal brachytherapy in malignant airway obstruction of lung cancer. Int J Radiat Oncol Biol Phys 28(3):589–596

50. Chella A, Ambrogi MC, Ribechini A et al (2000) Combined Nd-YAG laser: HDR brachytherapy versus Nd-YAG laser only in malignant central airway involvement: a prospective randomized study. Lung Cancer 27:169–175

51. Ung YC, Yu E, Falkson C et al (2006) The role of high-dose-rate brachytherapy in the palliation of symptoms in patients with non-small-cell lung cancer: a systematic review. Brachytherapy 5:189–202

52. Mallick I, Sharma SC, Behera D (2007) Endobronchial brachytherapy for symptom palliation in non-small cell lung cancer- analysis of symptom response, endoscopic improvement and quality of life. Lung Cancer 55:313–318

53. Bedwinek J, Petty A, Bruton C et al (1991) The use of high dose rate endobronchial brachytherapy to palliate symptomatic endobronchial recurrence of previously irradiated bronchogenic carcinoma. Int J Radiat Oncol Biol Phys 22:23–30

54. Speiser BL, Spratling L (1993) Remote afterloading brachytherapy for the local control of endobronchial carcinoma. Int J Radiat Oncol Biol Phys 25: 579–587

55. Pisch J, Villamena PC, Harvey JC et al (1993) High dose-rate endobronchial irradiation in malignant airway obstruction. Chest 104:721–725

56. Kohek PH, Pakisch B, Glanzer H (1994) Intraluminal irradiation in the treatment of malignant airway obstruction. Eur J Surg Oncol 20:674–680

57. Tredaniel J, Hennequin C, Zalcman G et al (1994) Prolonged survival after high-dose rate endobronchial radiation for malignant airway obstruction. Chest 105:767–772

58. Ofiara L, Roman T, Schwartzman K et al (1997) Local determinants of response to endobronchial high-dose rate brachytherapy in bronchogenic carcinoma. Chest 112:946–953

59. Escobar-Sacristan JA, Granda-Orive JI, Jimenez GT et al (2004) Endobronchial brachytherapy in the treatment of malignant lung tumours. Eur Respir J 24:348–352

60. Kubaszewsk M, Skowronek J, Chichel A et al (2008) The use of high dose rate endobronchial brachytherapy to palliate symptomatic recurrence of previously irradiated lung cancer. Neoplasma 55(3):239–245

61. Guarnaschelli JN, Jose BO (2010) Palliative high-dose–rate endobronchial brachytherapy for recurrent carcinoma: the University of Louisville experience. J Palliat Med 12(8):981–989

62. Santos RS, Raftopoulos Y, Keenan RJ et al (2004) Bronchoscopic palliation of primary lung cancer. Surg Endosc 18:931–936

63. Miller JL, Phillips TW (1990) Neodymium:YAG laser and brachytherapy in the management of inoperable bronchogenic carcinoma. Ann Thorac Surg 50:190–196

64. Shea JM, Allen RP, Tharratt RS et al (1993) Survival of patients undergoing Nd:YAG laser therapy compared with Nd:YAG laser therapy and brachytherapy for malignant airway disease. Chest 103:1028–1031

65. Freitag L, Ernst A, Thomas M et al (2004) Sequential photodynamic therapy (PDT) and high dose brachytherapy for endobronchial tumour control in patients with limited bronchogenic carcinoma. Thorax 59:790–793

66. Weinberg BD, Allison RR, Sibata C et al (2010) Results of combined photodynamic therapy (PDT)

and high dose rate brachytherapy (HDR) in treatment of obstructive endobronchial non-small cell lung cancer (NSCLC). Photodiagnosis Photodyn Ther 7:50–58

67. Gauwitz M, Ellerbroek N, Komaki R et al (1991) High dose endobronchial irradiation in recurrent bronchogenic carcinoma. Int J Radiat Oncol Biol Phys 23:397–400

68. Kelly JF, Delclos MR, Morice RC et al (2000) High-dose-rate endobronchial brachytherapy effectively palliates symptoms due to airway tumors: the 10-year M.D. Anderson Cancer Center experience. Int J Radiat Oncol Biol Phys 48(3):697–702

69. Hennequin C, Tredaniel J, Chevret S et al (1998) Predictive factors for late toxicity after endobronchial brachytherapy: a multivariate analysis. Int J Radiat Biol Phys 42(1):21–27

70. Allen AM, Abdelrahman N, Silvern D et al (2012) Endobronchial brachytherapy provides excellent long-term control of recurrent granulation tissue after tracheal stenosis. Brachytherapy 11(4):322–326, Epub 2012 Feb 28

71. Brenner B, Kramer MR, Katz A et al (2003) High dose rate brachytherapy for nonmalignant airway obstruction* New treatment option. Chest 124:1605–1610

72. Halkos ME, Godette KD, Lawrence C et al (2003) High dose rate brachytherapy in the management of lung transplant airway stenosis. Ann Thorac Surg 76:381–384

73. Kennedy AS, Sonnett JR, Orens JB et al (2000) High dose rate brachytherapy to prevent recurrent benign hyperplasia in lung transplant bronchi: theoretical and clinical considerations. J Heart Lung Transplant 19:155–159

74. Kramer MR, Katz A, Yarmolovsky A et al (2001) Successful use of high dose rate brachytherapy for non-malignant bronchial obstruction. Thorax 56:415–416

75. Madu CN, Machuzak MS, Sterman DH et al (2006) High-dose-rate (Hdr) brachytherapy for the treatment of benign obstructive endobronchial granulation tissue. Int J Radiat Oncol Biol Phys 66(5):1450–1456

76. Meyer A, Warszawski-Baumann A, Baumann R et al (2012) HDR brachytherapy: an option for preventing nonmalignant obstruction in patients after lung transplantation. Strahlenther Onkol 188:1085–1090

77. Rahman NA, Fruchter O, Shitrit D et al (2010) Flexible bronchoscopic management of benign tracheal stenosis: long term follow-up of 115 patients. J Cardiothorac Surg 5:2

78. Serber W, Dzeda MF, Hoppe RT (1998) Radiation treatment of benign disease. In: Perez CA, Brady LW (eds) Principles and practice of radiation oncology. Lippincott-Raven Publishers, Philadelphia, pp 2170–2172

79. Tendulkar RD, Fleming PA, Reddy CA et al (2008) High-dose-rate endobronchial brachytherapy for recurrent airway obstruction from hyperplastic granulation tissue. Int J Radiat Oncol Biol Phys 70(3):701–706

80. Tscheikuna J, Disayabutr S, Kakanaporn C et al (2013) High dose rate endobronchial brachytherapy (HDR-EB) in recurrent benign complex tracheobronchial stenosis: experience in two cases. J Med Assoc Thai 96(Suppl 2):S252–S256

81. Nag S, Abitbol AA, Anderson LL et al (1993) Consensus guidelines for high-dose-rate remote brachytherapy in cervical, endometrial, and endobronchial tumors. Int J Radiat Oncol Biol Phys 27:1241–1244

82. Hilaris BS (1994) Lung brachytherapy: an overview and current indications. Curr Perspect Thorac Oncol 4:45–53

83. Hilaris BS, Martini N (1979) Interstitial brachytherapy in cancer of the lung: a 20 year experience. Int J Radiat Oncol Biol Phys 5:1951–1956

84. Hilaris BS, Nori D, Martini N (1987) Intraoperative radiotherapy in stage I and II lung cancer. Semin Surg Oncol 3:22–32

85. Armstrong JG, Fass DE, Bains M et al (1991) Paraspinal tumors: techniques and results of brachytherapy. Int J Radiat Oncol Biol Phys 20:787–790

86. Fernando HC, Landreneau R, Mandrekar S et al (2014) Impact of brachytherapy on local recurrence rates after sublobar resection: results from ACOSOG Z4032 (Alliance), a phase III randomized trial for high-risk operable non-small cell lung cancer. J Clin Oncol 32:2456–2462

87. Landreneau RJ, Sugarbaker DJ, Mack MJ et al (1997) Wedge resection versus lobectomy for stage I (T1-T2 N0 M0) non-small cell lung cancer. J Thorac Cardiovasc Surg 113:691–700

88. Martini N, Bains MS, Burt ME et al (1995) Incidence of local recurrence and second primary tumors in resected stage I lung cancer. J Thorac Cardiovasc Surg 109:120–129

89. Miller JI, Hatcher CR (1987) Limited resection of bronchogenic carcinoma in the patient with marked impairment of pulmonary function. Ann Thorac Surg 44:340–343

90. Ginsberg RJ, Rubinstein LV (1995) Lobectomy versus limited resection for T1 N0 non-small cell cancer by the Lung Cancer Study Group. Ann Thorac Surg 60:615–623

91. Chen A, Galloway M, Landreneau R et al (1999) Intraoperative 125I brachytherapy for high-risk stage I non-small cell lung carcinoma. Int J Radiat Oncol Biol Phys 44(5):1057–1063

92. D'Amato TA, Galloway M, Szydlowski G et al (1998) Intraoperative brachytherapy following thoracoscopic wedge resection of stage I lung cancer. Chest 114(4):1112–1115

93. Lee W, Daly BD, DiPetrillo TA et al (2003) Limited resection for non-small cell lung cancer: observed local control with implantation of I-125 brachytherapy seeds. Ann Thorac Surg 75:237–242

94. Colonias A, Betler J, Trombetta M et al (2011) Mature follow-up for high-risk stage I non-small cell lung carcinoma treated with sublobar resection and intraoperative 125-I brachytherapy. Int J Radiat Oncol Biol Phys 79(1):105–109

95. McKenna RJ, Mahtabifard A, McKenna R et al (2008) Wedge resection and brachytherapy for lung cancer in patients with poor pulmonary function. Ann Thorac Surg 85(2):S733–S736

96. Parashar B, Port J, Arora S et al (2015) Analysis of stereotactic radiation vs. wedge resection vs. wedge resection plus Cesium-131 brachytherapy in early stage lung cancer. Brachytherapy 2015. pii: S1538-4721(15)00455-9. doi:10.1016/j.brachy.2015.04.001

97. Fernando HC, Landreneau R, Mandrekar S et al (2011) The impact of adjuvant brachytherapy with sublobar resection on pulmonary function and dyspnea in high-risk patients with operable disease: preliminary results from the American College of Surgeons Oncology Group Z4032 trial. J Thorac Cardiovasc Surg 142(3):554–562

98. Fernando HC, Landreneau R, Mandrekar S et al (2015) Analysis of longitudinal quality-of-life data in high-risk operable patients with lung cancer: Results from ACOSOG Z4032 (Alliance) multicenter randomized trial. J Thorac Cardiovasc Surg 149:718–726

99. Mutyala S, Stewart A, Khan A et al (2010) Permanent Iodine-125 interstitial planar seed brachytherapy for close or positive margins for thoracic malignancies. Int J Radiat Oncol Biol Phys 76(4):1114–1120

100. Jemal A, Bray F, Center MM et al (2011) Global cancer statistics. CA Cancer J Clin 61:69

101. Baquet CR, Commiskey P, Mack K et al (2005) Esophageal cancer epidemiology in blacks and whites: racial and gender disparities in incidence, mortality, survival rates and histology. J Natl Med Assoc 97:1471

102. Edge SB, Byrd DR, Compton CC et al (eds) (2010) American Joint Committee on cancer staging manual, 7th edn. Springer, New York

103. Tepper J, Krasna MJ, Niedzwiecki D et al (2008) Phase III trial of trimodality therapy with cisplatin, fluorouracil, radiotherapy, and surgery compared with surgery alone for esophageal cancer: CALGB 9781. J Clin Oncol 26:1086

104. Van Hagen P, Hulshof MC, van Lanschot JJ et al (2012) Preoperative chemoradiotherapy for esophageal or junctional cancer. N Engl J Med 366(22):2074–2084

105. Walsh TN, Noonan N, Hollywood D et al (1996) A comparison of multimodal therapy and surgery for esophageal adenocarcinoma. N Engl J Med 335:462

106. Harvey JC, Fleischman EH, Bellotti JE et al (1993) Intracavitary radiation in the treatment of advanced esophageal carcinoma: a comparison of high dose rate vs. low dose rate brachytherapy. J Surg Oncol 52:101–104

107. Tamaki T, Ishikawa H, Takahashi T et al (2012) Comparison of efficacy and safety of low-dose-rate vs. high-dose-rate intraluminal brachytherapy boost in patients with superficial esophageal cancer. Brachytherapy 11:130–136

108. Liu H, Wang Q, Wan X et al (2014) Californium-252 neutron brachytherapy combined with external beam radiotherapy for esophageal cancer: long-term treatment results. Brachytherapy 13:514–521

109. Gaspar LE, Nag S, Herskovic A et al (1997) American brachytherapy society consensus guidelines for brachytherapy of esophageal cancer. Int J Radiat Oncol Biol Phys 38(1):127–132

110. Hareyama M, Nishio M, Kagami Y et al (1992) Intracavitary brachytherapy combined with external beam irradiation for squamous cell carcinoma of the thoracic esophagus. Int J Radiat Oncol Biol Phys 24:235–240

111. Hishikawa Y, Kurisu K, Taniguchi M et al (1991) High-dose-rate intraluminal brachytherapy for esophageal cancer: 10 years' experience in Hyogo College of Medicine. Radiother Oncol 21:107–114

112. Gaspar LE, Kocha WI, Barnett R et al (1993) Cancer of the esophagus: brachytherapy, external beam radiation and chemotherapy. Cancer J 6:196–200

113. Gaspar LE, Winter K, Kocha WI et al (2000) A phase I/II study of external beam radiation, brachytherapy and concurrent chemotherapy for patients with localized carcinoma of the esophagus (RTOG 9207): final report. Cancer 88(5):988–995

114. Sharma V, Agarwal J, Dinshaw K et al (2000) Late esophageal toxicity using a combination of external beam radiation, intraluminal brachytherapy and 5-fluorouracil infusion in carcinoma of the esophagus. Dis Esophagus 13:219–225

115. Yorozu A, Dotiya T, Oki Y (1999) High-dose-rate brachytherapy boost following concurrent chemoradiotherapy for esophageal carcinoma. Int J Radiat Oncol Biol Phys 45:271–275

116. Fabrini MG, Perrone F, DeLiguoro M et al (2010) A single-institutional brachytherapy experience in the management of esophageal cancer. Brachytherapy 9(2):185–191

117. Lin J (2013) T1 esophageal cancer; request an endoscopic mucosal resection (EMR) for in-depth review. J Thorac Dis 5(3):353–356

118. Manner H, May A, Pech O et al (2008) Early Barrett's carcinoma with "low-risk" submucosal invasion: long-term results of endoscopic resection with a curative intent. Am J Gastroenterol 103:2589–2597

119. Manner H, Pech O, Heldmann Y et al (2013) Efficacy, safety, and long-term results of endoscopic treatment for early stage adenocarcinoma of the esophagus with low-risk sm1 invasion. Clin Gastroenterol Hepatol 11:630–635

120. Ishikawa H, Nonaka T, Sakurai H et al (2010) Usefulness of intraluminal brachytherapy combined with external beam radiation therapy for submucosal

esophageal cancer: long-term follow-up results. Int J Radiat Oncol Biol Phys 76(2):452–459

121. Pasquier D, Mirabel X, Adenis A et al (2006) External beam radiation therapy followed by high-dose-rate brachytherapy for inoperable superficial esophageal carcinoma. Int J Radiat Oncol Biol Phys 65(5):1456–1461

122. Cooper JS, Guo MD, Herskovic A et al (1999) Chemoradiothcrapy of locally advanced esophageal cancer: long-term follow-up of a prospective randomized trial (RTOG 85–01). Radiation Therapy Oncology Group. JAMA 281(17):1623–1627

123. Sur RK, Singh DP, Sharma SC et al (1992) Radiation therapy of esophageal cancer: role of high dose rate brachytherapy. Int J Radiat Oncol Biol Phys 22:1043–1046

124. Yin WB (1990) Brachytherapy of carcinoma of the esophagus in China, 1970–1974 and 1982–1984. In: Martinez AA, Orton CG, Moulds RF (eds) Brachytherapy: HDR and LDR. Nucletron Corp, Columbia, pp 52–56

125. Kumar S, Dimri K, Khurana R et al (2007) A randomized trial of radiotherapy compared with cisplatin chemo-radiotherapy in patients with unresectable squamous cell cancer of the esophagus. Radiother Oncol 83:139–147

126. Muijs CT, Beukema JC, Mul VE et al (2012) External beam radiotherapy combined with intraluminal brachytherapy in esophageal carcinoma. Radiother Oncol 102:303–308

127. Vuong T, Szego P, David M et al (2005) The safety and usefulness of high-dose-rate endoluminal brachytherapy as a boost in the treatment of patients with esophageal cancer with external beam radiation with or without chemotherapy. Int J Radiat Oncol Biol Phys 63(3):758–764

128. Amdal CD, Jacobsen AB, Sandstad B et al (2013) Palliative brachytherapy with or without primary stent placement in patients with oesophageal cancer, a randomized phase III trial. Radiother Oncol 107(3):428–433

129. Grazziotin Reisner R, Reisner ML, Ferreira MA et al (2015) Measuring relief of dysphagia in locally advanced esophageal carcinoma patients submitted to high-dose-rate brachytherapy. Brachytherapy 14(1): 84–90

130. Rupinski M, Zagorowicz E, Regula J et al (2011) Randomized comparison of three palliative regimens including brachytherapy, photodynamic therapy, and APC in patients with malignant dysphagia (CONSORT 1a)(Revides II). Am J Gastroenterol 106(9):1612–1620

131. Skowronek J, Piotrowski T, Zwierzchowski G (2004) Palliative treatment by high-dose-rate intraluminal brachytherapy in patients with advanced esophageal cancer. Brachytherapy 3(2):87–94

Image-Guided High-Dose Rate Brachytherapy in the Treatment of Liver Cancer

Nikolaos Tselis, Konrad Mohnike, and Jens Ricke

Abstract

High-dose rate brachytherapy for primary and secondary liver malignancies is an innovative radio-oncological modality enjoying rapid acceptance and adoption in the field of interventional oncology. It is a safe and effective treatment most useful in the salvage situation in patients with large hepatic tumors or an intermediate number of lesions unsuitable for thermal ablation or stereotactic external radiotherapy. In this chapter the radiobiological and technical aspects of CT-guided brachytherapy for the treatment of liver cancers are discussed. Clinical toxicity and efficacy outcomes after this technique are described including a comprehensive data review.

1 Introduction

According to estimations of the World Health Organization, liver cancer presents the fifth most common cancer type among men and the seventh among women accounting for approximately 746,000 deaths worldwide in 2012 [1]. Against

N. Tselis, MD, PhD (✉)
Department of Radiation Oncology
and Interdisciplinary Oncology,
Sana Klinikum, Offenbach, Germany
e-mail: nikolaos.tselis@klinikum-offenbach.de

K. Mohnike, MD • J. Ricke, MD
Department of Radiology and Nuclear Medicine,
Otto-von-Guericke-University Magdeburg,
Magdeburg, Germany
e-mail: jens.ricke@med.ovgu.de

this background, primary hepatocellular carcinoma (HCC) is increasing in incidence and it is now the sixth most common malignancy [2]. Because of its high fatality rate with the mortality to incidence ratio being almost united [3, 4], treatment improvements are widely sought after with complete surgical resection remaining the gold standard for the cure of primary hepatic malignancies [5]. Similarly, it is widely accepted in colorectal cancer that surgical treatment of liver metastases is associated with a significant chance of cure [6]. In addition, emerging data suggest benefits of therapeutic hepatic metastasectomy also for other primary sites, such as breast cancer [7]. Unfortunately, many patients with malignant hepatic tumors are not candidates for resection due to the extent of their underlying liver disease or the burden of tumor present in the liver. Although recent

© Springer International Publishing Switzerland 2016
P. Montemaggi et al. (eds.), *Brachytherapy: An International Perspective*, Medical Radiology,
DOI 10.1007/978-3-319-26791-3_13

advances in patient selection and surgical technique have resulted in low mortality after liver resection [8], the mortality rate for extended hepatectomy is up to 5 % with a morbidity rate of 50 % [9]. For those patients, hyperthermal techniques such as radiofrequency ablation (RFA) and laser-induced thermotherapy have been reported to be alternative local treatment choices [10–17]. However, one of the major challenges with these percutaneous approaches is residual cancer tissue after incomplete treatment of larger tumors or lesions with proximity to voluminous vascular structures. Factors impairing the therapeutic ratio are tumor size, with an accepted upper size limit of 3–4 cm for optimal treatment [18–20], and the heat-sink effect, hampering effective cytoreduction in perivascular lesions [19, 21–23]. In fact, the likelihood of recurrence increases rapidly beyond a threshold of 3-cm lesion diameter [24, 25] with tumor location next to the liver hilum being an additional contraindication because of the risk of bile duct injury. These limitations of hyperthermal techniques and the need for nonsurgical local therapies were the primary motivation that led to the implementation of computed tomography (CT)-guided interstitial (IRT) high-dose rate (HDR) brachytherapy (BRT) in the treatment of hepatic tumors. It enables the conformal administration of very large radiation doses to a circumscribed volume, allowing not only precisely predictable energy deposition but complete tumor sterilization regardless of tissue inhomogeneity, thermal conductivity, or tumor perfusion. It has proven safe and effective in the treatment of primary and secondary liver malignancies with no known restriction concerning the location or maximum lesion size for successful radioablation [21–23, 26–36].

2 Treatment Procedure

2.1 Implantation Techniques

Interstitial catheter implantation is usually performed under local or general anesthesia with various catheter placement patterns being described. Extensive experience exists for the technique of CT-guided implantation [21, 23, 28, 35]; however, MRI-based approaches have also been reported in the literature [37–39].

For CT-guided implantation, two similar approaches have been described with one incorporating the Seldinger catheter replacement technique [22] and one without this interventional radiology procedure step [34]. In both experiences the clinical workflow includes the creation of virtual volumes prior to implantation for treatment preplanning in order to estimate the number and alignment of catheters required to be placed percutaneously. After completion of the virtual preplanning, a fluoroscopy CT scan is used to aid in positioning of the catheters. After puncture of the hepatic lesion with a coaxial needle, a very stiff angiography guide wire is introduced. The needle is then exchanged over the wire against an angiography sheath of 6-F diameter. Sheaths with hydrophilic coating are favorable because they cause less pain during insertion through the liver capsule (e.g., Radifocus, Terumo; Tokyo, Japan). After removal of the guide wire, a BRT catheter can be placed in the sheath. Closure of the puncture tracts at the end of the entire procedure including irradiation is achieved by filling the puncture tract with Gelfoam during sheath removal. Similar to the Seldinger-based technique described by Ricke et al. [22], the procedure without catheter replacement employs also CT guidance in appropriate patient position [34]. Round-tip plastic catheters of 6-F diameter and 200-mm length (OncoSmart ProGuide Round Needle: Nucletron B.V., Veenendaal, The Netherlands) are implanted directly into the hepatic lesion through skin incision using a rigid tungsten alloy obturator (Fig. 1). In general, number, geometrical alignment, and distance between the catheters are dependent on the size, shape, and location of the hepatic lesion. Practically, one catheter is inserted per 1–2-cm tumor diameter.

In MRI-based implantation [22], catheter placement is also performed percutaneously including a preplanning step based on three-dimensional (3D) image volumes acquired by pre-interventional MRI sequences. The number, distribution, and distance between the catheters are determined by preplanning which calculates the peripheral catheter arrangement with arbitrary optimization for target coverage. Catheter implantation with control of maximum insertion depth and positional verification of the implanted catheters is performed by interactive MRI scanning employing again the catheter replacement technique (Fig. 2).

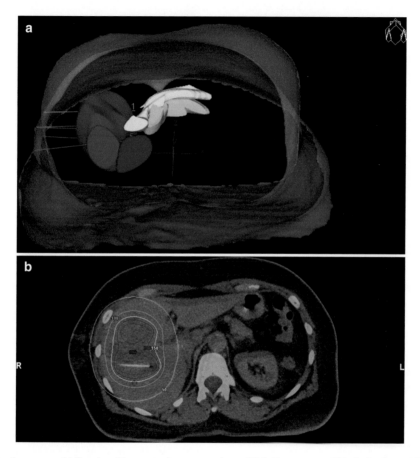

Fig. 1 Fifty-three-year-old female with a metachronous liver metastasis from breast cancer. The patient received single-fractionated IRT BRT after failure of multiple systemic chemotherapies. The HDR BRT was delivered in a single fraction of 15.0 Gy. (**a**) 3D implant reconstruction for CT-based treatment planning showing the irregularly shaped liver tumor (red volume) with the five implanted catheters. The volumetrically calculated lesion size was 261.8 cm³. (**b**) Axial CT/MRI image fusion illustrating the dose distribution of the implant based on a 3D registration of the post-implant CT data set with a pre-interventional contrast-enhanced MRI data set. The color gradation represents: *red* = 300 %, isodose = 45.0 Gy; *blue* = 200 %, isodose = 30.0 Gy; *yellow* = 150 %, isodose = 22.5 Gy; *orange* = 100 %, isodose = 15.0 Gy; and *green* = 50 %, isodose = 7.5 Gy. One of the five implanted catheters is identifiable by radiopaque markers along its axis. Intended minimal tumor dose per fraction is the reference dose of 15.0 Gy, specified as the 100 % – isodose. The central part of the tumor is covered at least by the 300 % – isodose and receives total doses clearly above 45 Gy within a single treatment fraction. (**c**) Pre-interventional T2 MRI imaging showing the extensive liver metastasis. (**d**) T2 MRI imaging at 3 weeks after BRT showing early response of the hepatic metastasis expressed as partial remission with discrete perilesional edema

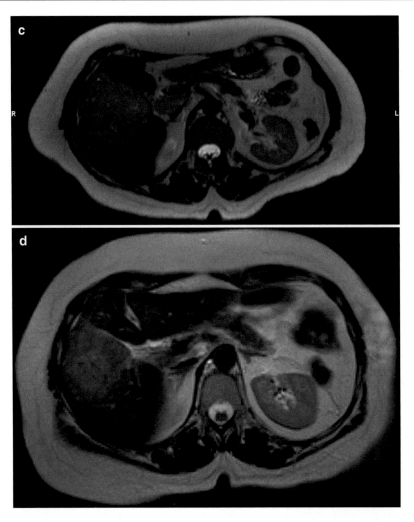

Fig. 1 (continued)

2.2 Imaging for Treatment Planning

After completion of the catheter implantation procedure, an adequate image series is acquired for the process of anatomy-oriented treatment planning. Treatment planning after CT-guided implantation is most commonly performed using CT imaging [21, 23, 26, 35]. In addition, MRI-based treatment planning (with or without MRI-guided implantation) has also been implemented in clinical practice [37–39]. In both cases a breath-hold contrast-enhanced image acquisition with slice thickness of ≤0.5 cm is recommended to ensure accurate anatomy delineation and reproducible catheter reconstruction as part of 3D treatment planning [39, 40]. For a more accurate delineation of the target volume, MRI and CT co-registration can be considered. Alternatively, only MRI can be used where both T1- and T2-weighted images should be considered for an optimal visualization of anatomy and catheter position [37]. Irrespective of the imaging modality for interventional guidance or treatment planning, HDR irradiation is performed using a remote afterloading system. A typical HDR afterloading system features a

192-iridium (^{192}Ir) source of a maximum 10 Ci. The duration of the irradiation ranges from 20 to 40 min depending on the size of the target, the accuracy of the catheter array inserted, and the respective age of the ^{192}Ir source.

2.3 Anatomy Definition

Even though the concepts of target volumes and organs at risk (OAR) were formalized by ICRU Report 50 [41], BRT practitioners have reported different target and treatment philosophies in the literature [23, 35, 38, 42, 43]. In order to develop consistency in target and volume definition for liver BRT, the following may be considered for treatment planning independent of the acquired imaging modality:

(a) In image-guided IRT BRT, the implanted catheters are positioned and fixed inside the target volume. Hence, organ motion is not a limiting factor and the clinical target volume (CTV) and planning target volume (PTV) are theoretically not different. Therefore, CTV = PTV with CTV being defined as the gross tumor volume as outlined in contrast-enhanced CT/MRI.

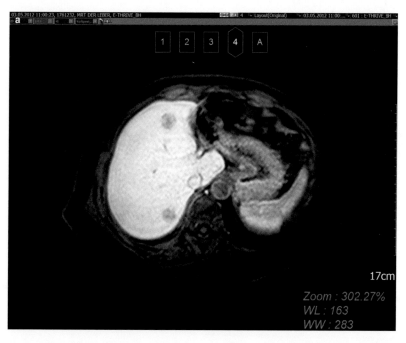

Fig. 2 Sixty-two-year-old female with synchronous liver metastases from colorectal cancer. The patient received single-fractionated IRT BRT after failure of multiple systemic chemotherapies including FOLFOX, FOLFIRI, and irinotecan/Erbitux. The HDR BRT was delivered in single fractions per tumor between 19.4 and 22.8 Gy covering in total five metastases in the right liver lobe in two treatment sessions at an interval of 2 weeks. The left liver lobe was aplastic. (**a**) Pre-interventional contrast-enhanced T1 MRI imaging showing three of the five lesions. (**b**) 3D implant reconstruction for MRI-based treatment planning showing three of the five metastases with the implanted catheters and the isodose lines. The volumetrically calculated lesion size was between 2.1 and 9.9 cm³. The respective color gradation scale for the isodose lines is explained on the left. The tumor volume is delineated in red. Intended minimal tumor dose per fraction is the reference dose of 20.0 Gy, specified as the 100 % – isodose. (**c**) Contrast-enhanced T1 MRI imaging at 12 weeks after BRT shows a sharply defined scar at the place of the former metastases. The patient developed limited and sequential progression with new metastases at different time points during follow-up in the liver and lung, all of them ablated with either HDR BRT or radiofrequency ablation. Thirty-six months after the first BRT and 48 months after initial diagnosis, the patient is still alive and doing well

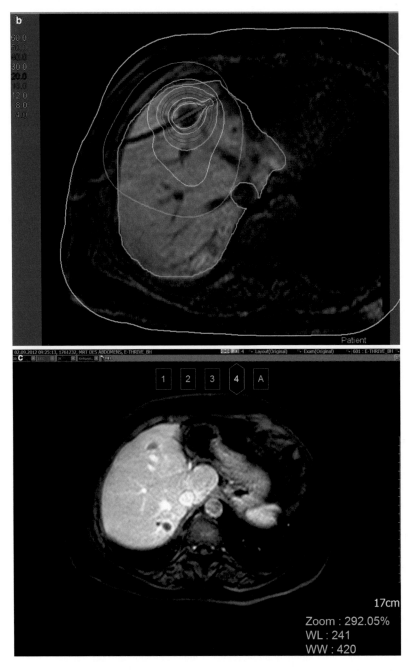

Fig. 2 (continued)

(b) The dominant organ at risk (OAR) is the liver itself. Further OARs to be considered at the time of 3D treatment planning include the stomach and the duodenum and in patients with direct tumor contact, the biliary tree bifurcation.

2.4 Dose Prescription

Initial studies of intraoperative BRT for liver cancers suggested that tumor enclosing isodoses of 15–30 Gy should be used irrespective of the tumor histology [44, 45]. However, advanced

CT-guided HDR BRT has provided more accurate data on what dose levels are necessary to achieve durable tumor control in various tumor types. In a prospective randomized trial of 73 patients with 199 colorectal liver metastases, minimal dose levels enclosing the PTV of 15, 20, and 25 Gy were tested [31]. A dose dependency for local tumor control was shown with no local recurrences observed if the minimum dose to the target (D_{100}) exceeded 23 Gy. In another prospective trial evaluating the effect of CT-guided HDR BRT in HCC, a minimal dose of 15 Gy was prescribed, with local control after 1 year of >90 % [30]. There is also evidence that breast cancer metastases may be treated successfully with a 15 Gy – covering isodose – whereas other tumor subtypes such as colorectal carcinoma likely require a minimum dose >18 Gy [27, 36, 46]. In spite of the high sensitivity of the minimum dose (D_{100}) to small delineation inaccuracies in the PTV, there is also literature referring to planned dose as the achieved D_{90}-values for the PTV [34, 35]. In this methodology the dose distribution is normalized to the calculated mean dose value on the PTV surface to be 100 % and the reference dose specified at the 100 % isodose surface. Those values are more stable regarding delineation inaccuracies and resolution of the calculation grid or the number of sample points than the minimum peripheral dose values. However, no consensus on the required methodology for dose prescription in HDR liver BRT exists. The foregoing notwithstanding in large tumors (>8 cm) excessive irradiation time and unpredictable risks can hamper the delivery of >20 Gy in a single fraction. This problem may be overcome by treating large tumor volumes in multiple sessions. As a rule of thumb, liver tumors more than 8 cm in diameter should be treated in two or more implants or with fractionated single-implant BRT schemes. In addition, to prevent loss of local tumor control by continuous growth of micrometastases after single-fraction irradiation of colorectal liver metastases and HCC, a dose of at least 15.4 Gy at a distance of 0.21 cm to the gross tumor margin has been recommended [47].

For the protection of OARs, a maximum dose exposure of 5 Gy to not more than two-thirds of the liver is recommended [22, 35, 48] with the 12-week threshold dose for hepatocyte function being estimated at approximately 14 Gy for 500 cm^3, approximately 16 Gy for 100 cm^3, and approximately 18 Gy for 10 cm^3 of irradiated liver volume [48]. With regard to stomach and duodenum, a threshold dose $D_{0.1\,cm^3}$ of 11 Gy for general gastric toxicity and 15.5 Gy for gastric ulceration has been found [49]. A gastric prophylaxis (pantoprazol 1×40 mg/day for 3 months and magaldrate H_2O) should be prescribed if the gastric or duodenal mucosa is calculated to receive more than 10 Gy per 1 cm^3 of organ wall. In addition, the maximum dose to the organ wall should be <14 Gy/1 cm^3. In patients with tumor in direct contact with the biliary tree bifurcation, a clinically relevant stenosis of the bile duct is rarely seen, and steroid prophylaxis to reduce the risk of radiation-induced edema and subsequent bile duct obstruction is therefore not generally recommended. However, in studies of intraoperative and CT-guided HDR BRT, doses of 20 Gy have been prescribed to the hepatic bifurcation without evident complications [22, 26, 35, 44, 50]. For verification of treatment delivery in the case of multifractionated implants, repeat CT scans may be obtained before each treatment fraction for fusion with the initial treatment planning image set. With this procedure, the position of every catheter can be verified in comparison to the initial 3D treatment plan [35].

3 Radiobiological and Physical Considerations

Radiobiological research demonstrates that the probabilities of acute and late radiation reactions vary between normal tissues and tumors and between different radiotherapy (RT) dose-fractionation schedules. More precisely, radiation-induced cell death has been modeled according to the linear-quadratic (LQ) model which postulates that multiple radio-induced lesions interact in the cell to trigger cell killing with the α/β ratio, a means of expressing the sensitivity of a particular tissue to altered fraction size, being used to estimate the impact of a given schedule on tumor control and toxicity [51]. For RT of the liver, a clear dose-response relationship has been reported with the delivery of higher doses, resulting in improved clinical outcomes [52]. However, there is an increasing risk of radiation-induced liver disease (RILD) when the whole organ is exposed to even moderate doses with an estimated TD5/5 of 30 Gy for the whole liver [53], while one-third to two-thirds of the organ tolerates doses of 35 Gy to 50 Gy, respectively [54]. Notwithstanding, according to the LQ model, escalated biologically effective doses through high-dose fractions are needed to enhance hepatic tumor cell death [55, 56]. Not least for this reason, total liver external beam radiotherapy (EBRT) plays a very limited role in the treatment of intrahepatic tumors, whereas focal liver irradiation by hypofractionated stereotactic body radiation therapy (SBRT) is becoming more widely used [57–59]. Nevertheless, the rapid clinical implementation of SBRT must not allow us to overlook the fact that the development of SBRT is based on the principles of HDR BRT, aiming to reduce the volume of normal tissue exposed to therapeutic doses while allowing for biologic dose escalation through larger fractional dose delivery for hepatic lesions predominantly less than 4 cm [57, 59–62]. Compared to SBRT, HDR BRT enables the superior partitioning of radiation between tumor and healthy organs by generating unlimited radiation source positions and source dwell times using image-based treatment planning with anatomy-oriented dose optimization [40, 63]. It surpasses the intrinsic capability of SBRT to perform simultaneous intratumoral dose boosting while providing greater dose heterogeneity with higher average doses and a more rapid dose falloff due to the inverse-square law [64, 65]. This can be illustrated by the following example as a case in point: If a BRT catheter is positioned under image guidance in an assumed metastatic liver lesion of 4-cm extension, a dose of 20 Gy is typically prescribed enclosing the PTV. For the inner sphere of a 3.6-cm diameter within the 4-cm tumor, the dose will be > 25 Gy, and for the 3.2-cm sphere, far more than 30 Gy will be delivered. This dose enhancement in most parts of the target volume is beneficial in light of the proven dose-response relationship for metastatic lesions from 15 to 25 Gy [31]. Accordingly, estimations based on the LQ model confirm that approximately 20 Gy might be sufficient for a tumor nodule with a radiosensitivity of $\alpha \approx 0.3$ Gy^{-1} and $\alpha/\beta \approx 10$ Gy [66]. However, the control dose increases toward 40 Gy for less sensitive tumor cell populations with $\alpha \approx 0.1$ Gy^{-1} and $\alpha/\beta \approx 10$ Gy [66]. This is particularly relevant assuming that radioresistant clonogenic tumor cells are considered to reside in central hypoxic tumor parts [67]. The dose escalation within this volume is inherently improved with HDR BRT since the dose gradient from the enclosing radioablative 20-Gy isodose to the periphery is steeper than for any EBRT technique, and considerably less liver tissue is exposed to doses above tolerance. Assuming a TD5/5 of conventionally fractionated 30 Gy for the whole liver [53], a single HDR dose of 10 Gy is biologically equivalent for $\alpha/\beta \approx 2$ Gy [68]. In our example, however, the prescribed reference dose declines from 20 to 10 Gy in a short distance from 2.0 to 2.8 cm (the dose is halved along 0.8 cm assuming the inverse-square law dependency). A 0.8-cm shell of liver tissue around the tumor of 4 cm is exposed to a potentially harmful dose, > 10 Gy, which, however, has only a limited volume of ≈ 60 cm^3. This is much smaller than the volume required to be irradiated with EBRT because of the dose falloff. In addition, for small volumes of liver tissue irradiated with associated steep dose gradients, there is a greater volume of spared liver that may regenerate in response to small-volume irradiation injury, likely increasing the overall tolerance of the liver to radiation. This volume effect has been confirmed in studies of HDR BRT for small liver volumes [49, 68, 69].

Next to temporary HDR BRT, permanent LDR BRT has also been described for the treatment of liver malignancies [42, 43, 70, 71]. In comparison to LDR, however, 3D HDR dosimetry is "high density" because of a vast array of HDR dwell positions (with variable dwell times) as permanent seeds in LDR liver implants. The prospective nature of HDR dosimetry ensures excellent target coverage without dosimetric changes caused by source migration and tissue deformity which can occur with seed implantation.

4   Clinical Data

A large amount of data is available on local tumor control (LC) after CT-guided HDR BRT with consistent and reproducible 1-year LC rates reported for patients with primary (81–96 %) and metastatic liver tumors (73–100 %) [21–23, 26–33, 35, 36, 46, 66, 72–75] (Table 1). Furthermore, a growing body of literature corroborates CT-guided HDR BRT as a safe and effective modality for the radioablation of especially larger tumors. Collettini et al. [26] reported on 35 lesions ranging from 5 to 12 cm (mean 7.1 cm) in 35 patients with unresectable HCC. Treatment consisted of single-fraction CT-guided ^{192}Ir HDR BRT of 15–25 Gy with a mean treatment dose of 15.8 Gy. Local control was 96 % at 12 months

Table 1 Literature results of CT-guided interstitial HDR brachytherapy for primary and metastatic liver malignancies

Author	n	Tumor entity	HDR dose	Tumor size	Results	Toxicity
Schnapauff et al. [32]	15	Primary	Median 20 Gy (15–20)	Median 61 cm³ (2.1–257)	Median LC 10 months	3.7 % major complications
Mohnike et al. [30]	83	Primary	Median 15 Gy (12–25)	Median 3.4 cm (1–15)	1-year LC 95 %	7.2 % major complications
Collettini et al. [26]	35	Primary	Median 15 Gy (15–20)	Mean 7.1 cm (5–12)	1-year LC 96 %	No toxicity reported
Denecke et al. [75]	12	Primary	Minimal 15–20 Gy	Mean 3.6 cm	10 % LR at 3 years	1 major complication
Collettini et al. [74]	98	Primary	Mean minimum 16.51 Gy	Mean 5 cm (1.8–12)	Mean LC 21.1 months	1 major complication
Collettini et al. [72]	7	Metastases	Median 15 Gy	Median 3.19 cm (1.3–12)	100 % LC at median 15.4 months	No complications
Geisel et al. [29]	8	Metastases	Median 20 Gy	Median 4.6 cm (1.4–6.8)	100 % LC at median 6.1 months	1 perihepatic hematoma
Collettini et al. [73]	80	Metastases	Median 19.1 Gy (15–20)	Mean 2.85 cm (0.8–10.7)	3-year LC 68.4 %	No major complications
Ricke et al. [31]	73	Metastases	Median 20 Gy (15–25)	Median 3.1 cm (1–13.5)	Mean LC 34 months	2.5 % major complications
Wieners et al. [36]	41	Metastases	Median 18.5 Gy (12–25)	Mean 83.3 cm³ (4.5–392)	1-year LC 93.5 %	1.4 % major complications
						8.6 % minor complications
Ricke et al. [23]	37	Primary/ metastases	Median 18 Gy (10–20)	Median 4.8 cm (2.5–11)	9-month LC 87 %	41 % minor complications
Ricke et al. [22]	20	Primary/ metastases	Median 17 Gy (12–25)	Mean 87 cm³ (7–367)	9-month LC 80 %	10 % major complications
						40 % minor complications
Tselis et al. [35]	41	Primary/ metastases	Median 20 Gy (7–32)	Median 84 cm³ (38–1348)	1-year Lc primary 81 %	5 % major complications
					1-year LC metastases 73 %	15.2 % minor complications

CT computed tomography, *HDR* right dose rate, *BRT* brachytherapy, *LC* local control, *LR* local recurrence with an overall survival (OS) of mean 15.4 months. Wieners et al. [36] reported on 115 unresectable breast cancer metastases of median 4.6 cm (1.5–11 cm) in 41 patients. Treatment consisted of single-fraction CT-guided ^{192}Ir HDR BRT of median 18.5 Gy (12–25 Gy) yielding an LC and OS rate of 93.5 and 79 % at 12 months, respectively. Tselis et al. [35] generated an LC rate of 79 % at 12 months for liver metastases and 88 % for primary hepatic tumors in 41 patients treated with median 20 Gy in twice daily fractions of median 7.0 Gy. The median tumor volume was 99 cm^3 with an overall LC rate of 80 % at 1 year. In analogy to tumor control, the rate of complications is also consistent in many published series on CT-guided HDR BRT for unresectable liver tumors [21, 26, 30–32, 36]. Mohnike et al. [30] performed 124 BRT sessions in 83 patients with 140 HCC lesions. The authors reported 7.2 % complications requiring intervention with one case of treatment-related death. Wieners et al. [36], however, only documented 1.4 % toxicity necessitating intervention (symptomatic post-interventional hemorrhage) and 8.6 % complications which were self-limiting. Tselis et al. [35] encountered seven (16.5 %) minor and two (4.7 %) major adverse events with no biliary toxicity, confirming that fractionated HDR BRT can be applied at the liver hilum without destroying the integrity of ducts and vessels.

Local control alone as a clinical endpoint does not necessarily reflect the full potential of HDR BRT in the management of cancer patients with liver-confined metastases. In situations of local or even systemic progression, CT-guided HDR BRT may be repeated in most cases. Two prospective trials assessing survival of patients undergoing multiple treatments against control are available, one of which is a randomized trial on colorectal liver metastases and one representing a matched-pair analyses in advanced HCC [30, 31]. In both trials, increased patient survival was significantly correlated with extensive or repeated CT-guided BRT. In the HCC trial [30], survival after BRT was doubled from 18 to 37 months with BRT, and in the colorectal study [31], survival was highest in patients receiving repeated BRT of evolving new metastases at any location with a larger

benefit than further chemotherapy in a selected salvage population.

Permanent IRT BRT techniques have also been used in the liver. Numerous studies employed intraoperative implantation of iodine-125 (^{125}I) seeds for LDR irradiation of unresectable microscopic or gross residual disease [43, 71, 76]. Nag et al. [71] treated 64 patients with incomplete resection of intrahepatic malignancies by intraoperative ^{125}I LDR BRT with a median minimum peripheral dose of 160 Gy. The median implant volume was 16 cm^3. The overall LC rate was 44 % and 22 % at 12 and 36 months, respectively, with an overall recurrence rate of 75 %. The authors reported 9 % treatment-related complications with one case of liver abscess and one case of wound abscess. In contrast to LDR BRT as an adjunctive modality after incomplete resection of liver tumors, very few studies have employed ^{125}I implants for patients with liver malignancies who were not suitable for surgery. Lin et al. [42] treated 23 patients with 65 inoperable HCC lesions by MRI-guided ^{125}I LDR BRT. The minimum dose was 144 Gy with a total mean dose of 173 Gy. The overall response rate was 84.5 %. The authors did not observe any clinically relevant complications during intervention and concluded that MRI-guided LDR BRT is both technically feasible and effective.

Stereotactic body radiation therapy has emerged as a noninvasive technique to facilitate dose escalation for the RT of extracranial tumors. Doses in hypofractionated treatment schemes range from 21 Gy in three fractions up to 60 Gy in 3–6 fractions with local control rates from 55 to 100 % at 24 months [57–60, 77–83]. Similarly, different schedules have been reported for single-fraction approaches with doses from 14 to 30 Gy yielding control rates up to 86 % at 24 months [57, 83–86]. The median lesion volumes in the largest reported SBRT studies range from 2.7 to 75.2 ml [57, 58, 60, 77, 78, 80, 82–84]. In HDR BRT series, the median lesion volumes are in the range of 61–99 cm^3 with median tumor diameters of 31–71 mm ([22, 23, 26–36, 46, 66, 72–75]). With this in mind, CT-guided IRT HDR BRT is an effective alternative for patients who are not candidates for SBRT due to extended tumor size or central tumor location.

In conclusion, image-guided IRT HDR BRT is a safe, effective treatment that is generally well tolerated. It has been most useful in salvage situations in patients with large hepatic tumors or an intermediate number of lesions unsuitable for thermal ablation or SBRT. In contrast to thermal ablation, the technique is well suited to lesions larger than 5 cm or in tumors close to or invading large vessels. Hence, the technique is a valuable adjunct in the large toolbox of interventional and irradiation techniques for the treatment of primary and metastatic liver cancers. In contrast to other locoregional therapies, a higher accuracy of dose delivery reliably leads to extensive cell kill through biologic dose escalation. It is not affected by any organ motion either intra- or inter-fractionally since they can be corrected with interactive online dosimetry during the implantation procedure or modified during real-time anatomy-based 3D treatment planning before dose delivery. Therefore, it may be the least likely to entail unexpected pitfalls such as the uncertainty of dose distribution caused by the interplay effect when segmented or spotted beams are used in EBRT techniques [87]. The next evolutionary step for CT-guided HDR BRT will be related to improvements of image guidance for the interventional oncologist by switching to MRI.

References

1. Ferlay J, Soerjomataram I, Dikshit R et al (2015) Cancer incidence and mortality worldwide: sources, methods and major patterns in GLOBOCAN 2012. Int J Cancer 136(5):E359–E386. doi:10.1002/ijc.29210
2. Torre LA, Bray F, Siegel RL et al (2015) Global cancer statistics, 2012. CA Cancer J Clin 65(2):87–108. doi:10.3322/caac.21262
3. El-Serag HB (2002) Hepatocellular carcinoma: an epidemiologic view. J Clin Gastroenterol 35(5 Suppl 2):S72–S78
4. Yang JD, Roberts LR (2010) Hepatocellular carcinoma: a global view. Nat Rev Gastroenterol Hepatol 7(8):448–458. doi:10.1038/nrgastro.2010.100
5. Akoad ME, Pomfret EA (2015) Surgical resection and liver transplantation for hepatocellular carcinoma. Clin Liver Dis 19(2):381–399. doi:10.1016/j.cld.2015.01.007
6. Poultsides GA, Schulick RD, Pawlik TM (2010) Hepatic resection for colorectal metastases: the impact of surgical margin status on outcome. HPB (Oxford) 12(1):43–49. doi:10.1111/j.1477-2574.2009.00121.x
7. Charalampoudis P, Mantas D, Sotiropoulos GC et al (2015) Surgery for liver metastases from breast cancer. Future Oncol 11(10):1519–1530. doi:10.2217/fon.15.43
8. Belghiti J, Hiramatsu K, Benoist S et al (2000) Seven hundred forty-seven hepatectomies in the 1990s: an update to evaluate the actual risk of liver resection. J Am Coll Surg 191(1):38–46
9. Yu D, Chen W, Jiang C et al (2013) Risk assessment in patients undergoing liver resection. Hepatobiliary Pancreat Dis Int 12(5):473–479
10. Buscarini E, Savoia A, Brambilla G et al (2005) Radiofrequency thermal ablation of liver tumors. Eur Radiol 15(5):884–894. doi:10.1007/s00330-005-2652-x
11. Chen M, Li J, Zheng Y et al (2006) A prospective randomized trial comparing percutaneous local ablative therapy and partial hepatectomy for small hepatocellular carcinoma. Ann Surg 243(3):321–328. doi:10.1097/01.sla.0000201480.65519.b8
12. Goldberg SN, Grassi CJ, Cardella JF et al (2009) Image-guided tumor ablation: standardization of terminology and reporting criteria. J Vasc Interv Radiol 20(7 Suppl):S377–S390. doi:10.1016/j.jvir.2009.04.011
13. Livraghi T, Solbiati L, Meloni F et al (2003) Percutaneous radiofrequency ablation of liver metastases in potential candidates for resection: the "test-of-time approach". Cancer 97(12):3027–3035. doi:10.1002/cncr.11426
14. Mack MG, Straub R, Eichler K et al (2004) Breast cancer metastases in liver: laser-induced interstitial thermotherapy--local tumor control rate and survival data. Radiology 233(2):400–409. doi:10.1148/radiol.2332030454
15. Nikfarjam M, Muralidharan V, Christophi C (2006) Altered growth patterns of colorectal liver metastases after thermal ablation. Surgery 139(1):73–81. doi:10.1016/j.surg.2005.07.030
16. Vogl TJ, Straub R, Eichler K et al (2004) Colorectal carcinoma metastases in liver: laser-induced interstitial thermotherapy--local tumor control rate and survival data. Radiology 230(2):450–458. doi:10.1148/radiol.2302020646
17. Vogl TJ, Straub R, Zangos S et al (2004) MR-guided laser-induced thermotherapy (LITT) of liver tumours: experimental and clinical data. Int J Hyperthermia 20(7):713–724
18. Crocetti L, de Baere T, Lencioni R (2010) Quality improvement guidelines for radiofrequency ablation of liver tumours. Cardiovasc Intervent Radiol 33(1):11–17. doi:10.1007/s00270-009-9736-y
19. Paulet E, Aubé C, Pessaux P et al (2008) Factors limiting complete tumor ablation by radiofrequency ablation. Cardiovasc Intervent Radiol 31(1):107–115. doi:10.1007/s00270-007-9208-1

20. Yin X, Xie X, Lu M et al (2009) Percutaneous thermal ablation of medium and large hepatocellular carcinoma: long-term outcome and prognostic factors. Cancer 115(9):1914–1923. doi:10.1002/cncr.24196

21. Pech M, Wieners G, Kryza R et al (2008) CT-guided brachytherapy (CTGB) versus interstitial laser ablation (ILT) of colorectal liver metastases: an intraindividual matched-pair analysis. Strahlenther Onkol 184(6):302–306. doi:10.1007/s00066-008-1815-5

22. Ricke J, Wust P, Wieners G et al (2004) Liver malignancies: CT-guided interstitial brachytherapy in patients with unfavorable lesions for thermal ablation. J Vasc Interv Radiol 15(11):1279–1286. doi:10.1097/01.RVI.0000141343.43441.06

23. Ricke J, Wust P, Stohlmann A et al (2004) CT-guided interstitial brachytherapy of liver malignancies alone or in combination with thermal ablation: phase I-II results of a novel technique. Int J Radiat Oncol Biol Phys 58(5):1496–1505. doi:10.1016/j.ijrobp.2003.09.024

24. Curley SA (2008) Radiofrequency ablation versus resection for resectable colorectal liver metastases: time for a randomized trial? Ann Surg Oncol 15(1):11–13. doi:10.1245/s10434-007-9668-1

25. Stang A, Fischbach R, Teichmann W et al (2009) A systematic review on the clinical benefit and role of radiofrequency ablation as treatment of colorectal liver metastases. Eur J Cancer 45(10):1748–1756. doi:10.1016/j.ejca.2009.03.012

26. Collettini F, Schnapauff D, Poellinger A et al (2012) Hepatocellular carcinoma: computed-tomography-guided high-dose-rate brachytherapy (CT-HDRBT) ablation of large (5–7 cm) and very large (7 cm) tumours. Eur Radiol 22(5):1101–1109. doi:10.1007/s00330-011-2352-7

27. Collettini F, Golenia M, Schnapauff D et al (2012) Percutaneous computed tomography-guided high-dose-rate brachytherapy ablation of breast cancer liver metastases: initial experience with 80 lesions. J Vasc Interv Radiol 23(5):618–626. doi:10.1016/j.jvir.2012.01.079

28. Collettini F, Singh A, Schnapauff D et al (2013) Computed-tomography-guided high-dose-rate brachytherapy (CT-HDRBT) ablation of metastases adjacent to the liver hilum. Eur J Radiol 82(10):e509–e514. doi:10.1016/j.ejrad.2013.04.046

29. Geisel D, Denecke T, Collettini F et al (2012) Treatment of hepatic metastases from gastric or gastroesophageal adenocarcinoma with computed tomography-guided high-dose-rate brachytherapy (CT-HDRBT). Anticancer Res 32(12):5453–5458

30. Mohnike K, Wieners G, Schwartz F et al (2010) Computed tomography-guided high-dose-rate brachytherapy in hepatocellular carcinoma: safety, efficacy, and effect on survival. Int J Radiat Oncol Biol Phys 78(1):172–179. doi:10.1016/j.ijrobp.2009.07.1700

31. Ricke J, Mohnike K, Pech M et al (2010) Local response and impact on survival after local ablation of liver metastases from colorectal carcinoma by computed tomography-guided high-dose-rate brachytherapy. Int J Radiat Oncol Biol Phys 78(2):479–485. doi:10.1016/j.ijrobp.2009.09.026

32. Schnapauff D, Denecke T, Grieser C et al (2011) Computed tomography-guided interstitial HDR brachytherapy (CT-HDRBT) of the liver in patients with irresectable intrahepatic cholangiocarcinoma. Cardiovasc Intervent Radiol. doi:10.1007/s00270-011-0249-0

33. Schnapauff D, Collettini F, Hartwig K et al (2015) CT-guided brachytherapy as salvage therapy for intrahepatic recurrence of HCC after surgical resection. Anticancer Res 35(1):319–323

34. Tselis N, Chatzikonstantinou G, Kolotas C et al (2012) Hypofractionated accelerated computed tomography-guided interstitial high-dose-rate brachytherapy for liver malignancies. Brachytherapy. doi:10.1016/j.brachy.2012.02.006

35. Tselis N, Chatzikonstantinou G, Kolotas C et al (2013) Computed tomography-guided interstitial high dose rate brachytherapy for centrally located liver tumours: a single institution study. Eur Radiol 23(8):2264–2270. doi:10.1007/s00330-013-2816-z

36. Wieners G, Mohnike K, Peters N et al (2011) Treatment of hepatic metastases of breast cancer with CT-guided interstitial brachytherapy – a phase II-study. Radiother Oncol 100(2):314–319. doi:10.1016/j.radonc.2011.03.005

37. Ricke J, Thormann M, Ludewig M et al (2010) MR-guided liver tumor ablation employing open high-field 1.0T MRI for image-guided brachytherapy. Eur Radiol 20(8):1985–1993. doi:10.1007/s00330-010-1751-5

38. Wonneberger U, Fischbach F, Bunke J et al (2012) MRI-guided brachytherapy in the liver. In: Kahn T, Busse H (eds) Interventional magnetic resonance imaging. Springer, Berlin/Heidelberg, pp 381–387

39. Wybranski C, Eberhardt B, Fischbach K et al (2015) Accuracy of applicator tip reconstruction in MRI-guided interstitial (192)Ir-high-dose-rate brachytherapy of liver tumors. Radiother Oncol. doi:10.1016/j.radonc.2015.01.018

40. Tsalpatouros A, Baltas D, Kolotas C et al (1997) CT-based software for 3-D localization and reconstruction in stepping source brachytherapy. IEEE Trans Inf Technol Biomed 1(4):229–242

41. Purdy JA (2004) Current ICRU definitions of volumes: limitations and future directions. Semin Radiat Oncol 14(1):27–40. doi:10.1053/j.semradonc.2003.12.002

42. Lin Z, Lin J, Lin C et al (2012) 1.5T conventional MR-guided iodine-125 interstitial implants for hepatocellular carcinoma: feasibility and preliminary clinical experience. Eur J Radiol 81(7):1420–1425. doi:10.1016/j.ejrad.2011.03.043

43. Martinez-Monge R, Nag S, Nieroda CA et al (1999) Iodine-125 brachytherapy in the treatment of colorectal adenocarcinoma metastatic to the liver. Cancer 85(6):1218–1225

44. Donath D, Nori D, Turnbull A et al (1990) Brachytherapy in the treatment of solitary colorectal metastases to the liver. J Surg Oncol 44(1):55–61

45. Thomas DS, Nauta RJ, Rodgers JE et al (1993) Intraoperative high-dose rate interstitial irradiation of hepatic metastases from colorectal carcinoma. Results of a phase I-II trial. Cancer 71(6):1977–1981

46. Wieners G, Pech M, Rudzinska M et al (2006) CT-guided interstitial brachytherapy in the local treatment of extrahepatic, extrapulmonary secondary malignancies. Eur Radiol 16(11):2586–2593. doi:10.1007/s00330-006-0241-2

47. Seidensticker M, Wust P, Rühl R et al (2010) Safety margin in irradiation of colorectal liver metastases: assessment of the control dose of micrometastases. Radiat Oncol 5:24. doi:10.1186/1748-717X-5-24

48. Wybranski C, Seidensticker M, Mohnike K et al (2009) In vivo assessment of dose volume and dose gradient effects on the tolerance dose of small liver volumes after single-fraction high-dose-rate 192Ir irradiation. Radiat Res 172(5):598–606. doi:10.1667/RR1773.1

49. Streitparth F, Pech M, Böhmig M et al (2006) In vivo assessment of the gastric mucosal tolerance dose after single fraction, small volume irradiation of liver malignancies by computed tomography-guided, high-dose-rate brachytherapy. Int J Radiat Oncol Biol Phys 65(5):1479–1486. doi:10.1016/j.ijrobp.2006.02.052

50. Dritschilo A, Harter KW, Thomas D et al (1988) Intraoperative radiation therapy of hepatic metastases: technical aspects and report of a pilot study. Int J Radiat Oncol Biol Phys 14(5):1007–1011

51. Franken NAP, Oei AL, Kok HP et al (2013) Cell survival and radiosensitisation: modulation of the linear and quadratic parameters of the LQ model (Review). Int J Oncol 42(5):1501–1515. doi:10.3892/ijo.2013.1857

52. Park HC, Seong J, Han KH et al (2002) Dose-response relationship in local radiotherapy for hepatocellular carcinoma. Int J Radiat Oncol Biol Phys 54(1):150–155

53. Guha C, Kavanagh BD (2011) Hepatic radiation toxicity: avoidance and amelioration. Semin Radiat Oncol 21(4):256–263. doi:10.1016/j.semradonc.2011.05.003

54. Lawrence TS, Robertson JM, Anscher MS et al (1995) Hepatic toxicity resulting from cancer treatment. Int J Radiat Oncol Biol Phys 31(5):1237–1248. doi:10.1016/0360-3016(94)00418-K

55. Brenner DJ (2008) The linear-quadratic model is an appropriate methodology for determining isoeffective doses at large doses per fraction. Semin Radiat Oncol 18(4):234–239. doi:10.1016/j.semradonc.2008.04.004

56. Milano MT, Constine LS, Okunieff P (2008) Normal tissue toxicity after small field hypofractionated stereotactic body radiation. Radiat Oncol 3:36. doi:10.1186/1748-717X-3-36

57. Chang DT, Swaminath A, Kozak M et al (2011) Stereotactic body radiotherapy for colorectal liver metastases: a pooled analysis. Cancer 117(17):4060–4069. doi:10.1002/cncr.25997

58. Dewas S, Mirabel X, Kramar A et al (2012) Radiothérapie stéréotaxique hépatique par CyberKnife(®): l'expérience lilloise (Stereotactic body radiation therapy for liver primary and metastases: the Lille experience). Cancer Radiother 16(1):58–69. doi:10.1016/j.canrad.2011.06.005

59. Rule W, Timmerman R, Tong L et al (2011) Phase I dose-escalation study of stereotactic body radiotherapy in patients with hepatic metastases. Ann Surg Oncol 18(4):1081–1087. doi:10.1245/s10434-010-1405-5

60. Seo YS, Kim M, Yoo SY et al (2010) Preliminary result of stereotactic body radiotherapy as a local salvage treatment for inoperable hepatocellular carcinoma. J Surg Oncol 102(3):209–214. doi:10.1002/jso.21593

61. Timmerman RD, Kavanagh BD, Cho LC et al (2007) Stereotactic body radiation therapy in multiple organ sites. J Clin Oncol 25(8):947–952. doi:10.1200/JCO.2006.09.7469

62. van der Pool AEM, Méndez Romero A, Wunderink W et al (2010) Stereotactic body radiation therapy for colorectal liver metastases. Br J Surg 97(3):377–382. doi:10.1002/bjs.6895

63. Kolotas C, Baltas D, Zamboglou N (1999) CT-Based interstitial HDR brachytherapy. Strahlenther Onkol 175(9):419–427

64. Kamrava M, Loh C, Banerjee R et al (2013) Dosimetric comparison of image-guided high-dose-rate interstitial liver brachytherapy vs liver stereotactic body radiation therapy. Brachytherapy 12:S18. doi:10.1016/j.brachy.2013.01.024

65. Li D, Kang J, Golas BJ et al (2014) Minimally invasive local therapies for liver cancer. Cancer Biol Med 11(4):217–236. doi:10.7497/j.issn.2095-3941.2014.04.001

66. Ricke J, Wust P (2011) Computed tomography-guided brachytherapy for liver cancer. Semin Radiat Oncol 21(4):287–293. doi:10.1016/j.semradonc.2011.05.005

67. Ruggieri R, Naccarato S, Nahum AE (2010) Severe hypofractionation: non-homogeneous tumour dose delivery can counteract tumour hypoxia. Acta Oncol 49(8):1304–1314. doi:10.3109/0284186X.2010.486796

68. Rühl R, Lüdemann L, Czarnecka A et al (2010) Radiobiological restrictions and tolerance doses of repeated single-fraction hdr-irradiation of intersecting small liver volumes for recurrent hepatic metastases. Radiat Oncol 5:44. doi:10.1186/1748-717X-5-44

69. Ricke J, Seidensticker M, Lüdemann L et al (2005) In vivo assessment of the tolerance dose of small liver volumes after single-fraction HDR irradiation. Int J Radiat Oncol Biol Phys 62(3):776–784. doi:10.1016/j.ijrobp.2004.11.022

70. Lin Z, Chen J, Deng X (2012) Treatment of hepatocellular carcinoma adjacent to large blood vessels using 1.5T MRI-guided percutaneous radiofrequency ablation combined with iodine-125 radioactive seed implantation. Eur J Radiol 81(11):3079–3083. doi:10.1016/j.ejrad.2012.05.007

71. Nag S, DeHaan M, Scruggs G et al (2006) Long-term follow-up of patients of intrahepatic malignancies treated with iodine-125 brachytherapy. Int J Radiat Oncol Biol Phys 64(3):736–744. doi:10.1016/j.ijrobp.2005.08.029

72. Collettini F, Poellinger A, Schnapauff D et al (2011) CT-guided high-dose-rate brachytherapy of metachronous ovarian cancer metastasis to the liver: initial experience. Anticancer Res 31(8):2597–2602

73. Collettini F, Lutter A, Schnapauff D et al (2014) Unresectable colorectal liver metastases: percutaneous ablation using CT-guided high-dose-rate brachytherapy (CT-HDBRT). Rofo 186(6):606–612. doi:10.1055/s-0033-1355887

74. Collettini F, Schreiber N, Schnapauff D et al (2015) CT-gesteuerte Hochdosis-Brachytherapie beim inoperablen hepatozellulären Karzinom (CT-guided high-dose-rate brachytherapy of unresectable hepatocellular carcinoma). Strahlenther Onkol 191(5):405–412. doi:10.1007/s00066-014-0781-3

75. Denecke T, Stelter L, Schnapauff D et al (2015) CT-guided interstitial brachytherapy of hepatocellular carcinoma before liver transplantation: an equivalent alternative to transarterial chemoembolization? Eur Radiol. doi:10.1007/s00330-015-3660-0

76. Armstrong JG, Anderson LL, Harrison LB (1994) Treatment of liver metastases from colorectal cancer with radioactive implants. Cancer 73(7):1800–1804

77. Andolino DL, Johnson CS, Maluccio M et al (2011) Stereotactic body radiotherapy for primary hepatocellular carcinoma. Int J Radiat Oncol Biol Phys 81(4):e447–e453. doi:10.1016/j.ijrobp.2011.04.011

78. Katz AW, Carey-Sampson M, Muhs AG et al (2007) Hypofractionated stereotactic body radiation therapy (SBRT) for limited hepatic metastases. Int J Radiat Oncol Biol Phys 67(3):793–798. doi:10.1016/j.ijrobp.2006.10.025

79. Kwon JH, Bae SH, Kim JY et al (2010) Long-term effect of stereotactic body radiation therapy for primary hepatocellular carcinoma ineligible for local ablation therapy or surgical resection. Stereotactic radiotherapy for liver cancer. BMC Cancer 10:475. doi:10.1186/1471-2407-10-475

80. Lee MT, Kim JJ, Dinniwell R et al (2009) Phase I study of individualized stereotactic body radiotherapy of liver metastases. J Clin Oncol 27(10):1585–1591. doi:10.1200/JCO.2008.20.0600

81. Rusthoven KE, Kavanagh BD, Cardenes H et al (2009) Multi-institutional phase I/II trial of stereotactic body radiation therapy for liver metastases. J Clin Oncol 27(10):1572–1578. doi:10.1200/JCO.2008.19.6329

82. Tse RV, Hawkins M, Lockwood G et al (2008) Phase I study of individualized stereotactic body radiotherapy for hepatocellular carcinoma and intrahepatic cholangiocarcinoma. J Clin Oncol 26(4):657–664. doi:10.1200/JCO.2007.14.3529

83. Wulf J, Guckenberger M, Haedinger U et al (2006) Stereotactic radiotherapy of primary liver cancer and hepatic metastases. Acta Oncol 45(7):838–847. doi:10.1080/02841860600904821

84. Goodman KA, Wiegner EA, Maturen KE et al (2010) Dose-escalation study of single-fraction stereotactic body radiotherapy for liver malignancies. Int J Radiat Oncol Biol Phys 78(2):486–493. doi:10.1016/j.ijrobp.2009.08.020

85. Herfarth KK, Debus J, Wannenmacher M (2004) Stereotactic radiation therapy of liver metastases: update of the initial phase-I/II trial. Front Radiat Ther Oncol 38:100–105

86. Stintzing S, Hoffmann R, Heinemann V et al (2010) Radiosurgery of liver tumors: value of robotic radiosurgical device to treat liver tumors. Ann Surg Oncol 17(11):2877–2883. doi:10.1245/s10434-010-1187-9

87. Abbas H, Chang B, Chen ZJ (2014) Motion management in gastrointestinal cancers. J Gastrointest Oncol 5(3):223–235. doi:10.3978/j.issn.2078-6891.2014.028

Gynecologic Brachytherapy: Endometrial Cancer

John A. Vargo, Akila N. Viswanathan,
Beth A. Erickson, and Sushil Beriwal

Abstract

The management of endometrial cancer generally involves surgical extirpation of tumor as a primary therapeutic endeavor. Following surgery, and in some cases in lieu of surgery (in medically inoperable patients), brachytherapy is frequently required as part of the definitive treatment scheme. We present management guidelines and techniques in this chapter to aid in the therapeutic management of these patients.

1   Introduction

In the United States, endometrial cancer represents the most common gynecologic cancer and the 4th most common cancer in females, with an estimated 49,560 new cases in 2013 [1]. In keeping with the change in the 1988 FIGO staging from a clinical to surgical staging system, the primary treatment for endometrial cancer is surgical staging including hysterectomy and bilateral salpingo-oophorectomy with or without pelvic and/or para-aortic nodal dissection. Adjuvant brachytherapy has a key role in decreasing vaginal failures following surgical staging [2]. Endometrial cancer is most common in patients of advancing age with multiple medical comorbidities including obesity, cardiovascular disease, diabetes, and others. For patients who are unfit for surgical staging, definitive radiation therapy, including brachytherapy, remains a viable alternative for medically inoperable patients. Additionally, while the majority of endometrial cancer patients present with early-stage disease, some have locally advanced disease extending to the cervix and parametria. For these locally advanced disease patients, initial surgical staging with simple hysterectomy may potentially transect disease; however a radical hysterectomy is difficult in this population due to

J.A. Vargo, MD • S. Beriwal, MD (✉)
Department of Radiation Oncology, University of Pittsburgh, Pittsburgh, PA, USA
e-mail: vargoja2@upmc.edu

A.N. Viswanathan, MD, MPH
Department of Radiation Oncology, Brigham and Women's Hospital and Dana-Farber Cancer Institute, Harvard Medical School, Boston, MA, USA

B.A. Erickson, MD, FACR, FASTRO
Department of Radiation Oncology, Medical College of Wisconsin, Milwaukee, WI, USA
e-mail: berickson@mcw.edu

© Springer International Publishing Switzerland 2016
P. Montemaggi et al. (eds.), *Brachytherapy: An International Perspective*, Medical Radiology,
DOI 10.1007/978-3-319-26791-3_14

their advanced age and associated medical comorbidities. Neoadjuvant radiotherapy, including external beam and brachytherapy, has been used to downstage disease, affording a less extensive subsequent hysterectomy for these locally advanced patients. Finally, for patients suffering a vaginal recurrence following initial surgical staging alone, radiotherapy, including external beam and brachytherapy, remains the preferred treatment modality offering long-term salvage in up to 50 % of patients with an isolated vaginal recurrence [3, 4]. The combination of external beam radiotherapy and brachytherapy has a clear role throughout the management of endometrial cancer, much of which is explored in detail in this chapter. Brachytherapy for vaginal recurrence of endometrial cancer is detailed in the following chapter.

2   Postoperative Vaginal Cuff Brachytherapy: Indications

While the majority of patients with early-stage endometrial cancers are cured with surgical staging, 10–15 % of all surgically staged patients and up to 35 % of high-risk subsets will suffer pelvic relapse [5]. Randomized trials, including GOG-99 and PORTEC-1, have shown that adjuvant pelvic radiotherapy improved pelvic control without improving overall survival [6, 7]. Given that 75 % of pelvic relapses are isolated vaginal recurrences, PORTEC 2 was designed to address the question of whether vaginal brachytherapy alone could rival outcomes with external beam while decreasing treatment-related morbidity [8]. With no significant differences in vaginal (1.8 versus 1.6 %) or locoregional

(5.1 versus 2.1 %) recurrences comparing vaginal brachytherapy to pelvic external beam radiotherapy, PORTEC 2 established vaginal brachytherapy as an important non-inferior treatment strategy for high- to intermediate-risk early-stage endometrial cancers [8]. Postoperative vaginal brachytherapy is tailored to the findings at surgical staging and the projected risk of vaginal recurrence according to a number of well-defined histopathologic risk factors: stage, depth of myometrial invasion, grade, histology, lymphovascular space invasion, tumor size, and lower uterine segment involvement. Age is also a risk factor that is carefully considered. Balancing these tumor and patient-related risks factors with medical comorbidities, such as ulcerative colitis and other conditions that may predispose patients to treatment induced morbidity, remains important in selecting patients for adjuvant brachytherapy. Table 1 summarizes the National Comprehensive Cancer Network (NCCN) guidelines for adjuvant therapy following surgical staging in FIGO stage I endometrial cancer, which are endorsed by the American Brachytherapy Society as indications for vaginal brachytherapy [9]. A comprehensive summary of indications for postoperative vaginal cuff brachytherapy is found in the comprehensive executive summary evidence-based guideline from the American Society for Radiation Oncology [10].

3   Postoperative Vaginal Cuff Brachytherapy: Technique

HDR vaginal cuff brachytherapy is performed using a number of commercially available cylindrical vaginal applicators. The most appropriate

Table 1 Summary of indications for brachytherapy following surgical staging for FIGO stage I endometrial cancer

	Grade 1	Grade 2	Grade 3
Stage IA without risk factors	Observation[a]	Observation[a]	Observation or vaginal brachytherapy
Stage IA with risk factors	Observation or vaginal brachytherapy	Observation or vaginal brachytherapy	Observation or vaginal brachytherapy and/or EBRT
Stage IB without risk factors	Observation or vaginal brachytherapy	Observation or vaginal brachytherapy	Vaginal brachytherapy and/or EBRT
Stage IB with risk factors	Vaginal brachytherapy and/or EBRT	Observation or vaginal brachytherapy and/or EBRT	EBRT ± vaginal brachytherapy ± chemotherapy

[a]Part of ASTRO Choosing Wisely campaign, recommending "Don't recommend radiation following hysterectomy for endometrial cancer patients with low-risk disease." Potential risk factors include age >60, lymphovascular space invasion, tumor size, and lower uterine (cervical/glandular) segment involvement

applicator is selected based on the pre-application assessment. The pre-application assessment begins with a gynecologic examination to define vaginal anatomy and to ensure appropriate healing of the vaginal cuff with documentation of cuff integrity, the absence of small bowel herniation through the vaginal apex, and the absence of disease recurrence. Brachytherapy should be started as soon as adequate healing is documented which is usually 4–8 weeks postoperatively and ideally not to exceed a maximum of 12-weeks postoperatively [11]. Based on the gynecologic examination, the largest diameter cylinder is selected that the patient can comfortably tolerate. This allows for maximal vaginal distention, minimizing air pockets and decreasing vaginal surface dose. Figure 1 highlights the difference in vaginal surface dose with decreasing cylinder diameter. The total number of cylinder segments is defined by the vaginal length; typically one dome and two segments are used,

aiming for the cylinder not to extend outside of the vaginal introitus unless the target includes the distal vagina. Most commonly for adjuvant vaginal cuff brachytherapy, a single-channel applicator is employed [12]. A multichannel applicator may allow for differential loading to more conformally shape the dose distribution. This can allow higher dose to areas of residual disease and lower doses to areas of subclinical disease. This represents a reasonable method of delivering vaginal brachytherapy, but the potential dosimetric benefits of a multichannel cylinder versus a single-channel cylinder have yet to be proven clinically significant [13, 14]. In addition, realization of the potential for delivering excessive mucosal doses with a multichannel versus a single-channel applicator must be made. Other applicators for vaginal brachytherapy include ovoids, ring, or custom mold applicators, which may improve vaginal mucosal dose in comparison to a cylinder by decreasing air pockets,

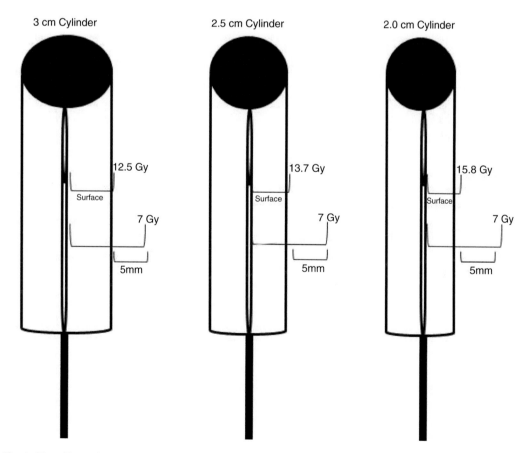

Fig. 1 The effects of vaginal cylinder size on vaginal surface dose. All representative doses are for a single fraction with a prescription dose of 7 Gy to 0.5 cm depth

especially for patients with "dog-ear" vaginal anatomy [15, 16].

Patients are instructed to empty their bladder prior to the procedure [17]. A bladder catheter is not routinely inserted unless the patient is unable to maintain bladder continence for the duration of the procedure. Rarely bowel may lie in close proximity to the vaginal cuff and the bladder can be filled during treatment to displace the bowel and significantly decrease bowel dose [18]. Following a detailed explanation of the proposed application, the patient is placed in the dorsal lithotomy position, while the selected cylinder is measured, assembled, and coated generously with a lubricant (consider use of lidocaine jelly to reduce discomfort). By gently dilating the vagina with a fingertip and then advancing the applicator forward and dorsally, away from the urethra, the applicator is advanced into the vaginal cuff. Once at the cuff, confirmation that it is in contact with the vaginal apex is made by exerting gentle cephalad pressure while monitoring the patient for discomfort. After returning the applicator to a more neutral position, a perineal bar or other external immobilization devices are secured, a radiopaque marker wire is placed in the central channel, and the patient's legs are positioned in a more natural supine position supported on pillows. Once in the legs down position, the applicator should again be checked for its contiguity with the vaginal apex by exerting gentle pressure and releasing to a neutral position and again securing the applicator with the immobilization device.

Two important potential sources for error at the first vaginal brachytherapy insertion are lack of approximation of the applicator with the vaginal apex and selection of the wrong size or shape of applicator. There are a number of different techniques for confirming that the applicator is in contact with the vaginal apex. Two orthogonal radiographs (AP and lateral) can be taken to confirm appropriate placement relative to a radiopaque fiducial marker placed at the time of gynecologic examination or matching the applicator length with the pre-insertion vaginal length. CT evaluation is, however, preferred to allow three-dimensional dosimetric evaluation. Another potential error is to insert the wrong diameter cylinder at repeat fractions. At the time of the first and subsequent insertions, vaginal cylinder diameter should always be measured and confirmed with the measurement of prior insertions. As a second safety confirmation, the cylinder diameter can be measured on the orthogonal films or CT images to document that the appropriate diameter cylinder was placed. A CT simulation is performed for the first fraction of vaginal cuff brachytherapy with a non-contrast-enhanced CT from the mid-pelvis to below the ischial tuberosities using a 0.25 cm slice thickness. CT-based planning offers a number of clinical advantages (see Fig. 2): 3-dimensional (3D) confirmation of appropriate applicator placement and cuff integrity (see Fig. 2a), assessment of dose relative to the thickness of the rectovaginal septum and apical vaginal tissue (see Fig. 2b–c), and assessment of air pockets created between the vaginal mucosa and the applicator (see Fig. 2d) [19]. As the clinical significance of interfraction changes in 3D planning is small for most patients, we do not routinely advocate 3-D planning with each fraction, but rather confirmation of applicator placement on orthogonal films or CT scan imaging with subsequent insertions [20]. On the planning CT, the clinical target volume and critical organs (the bladder, rectum, and small bowel) can be contoured. The clinical target volume typically includes the proximal 3–5 cm of vagina, except for patients with type II histology (clear cell carcinoma and uterine papillary serous carcinoma) or extensive lymphovascular space invasion where treating the entire length of the vagina should be considered for treatment [2]. However, many of these patients with type II histology or extensive lymphovascular space invasion have other risk factors that would favor treatment with a combination of external beam radiotherapy and brachytherapy, wherein the entire vagina could be treated with the external beam fields and brachytherapy would be used to boost just the proximal vagina to minimize the morbidity of treating the entire vagina with brachytherapy. The plan is optimized using points in the apex, curvature of the cylinder dome, and the lateral vaginal mucosa as detailed in the American Brachytherapy Society guidelines [2].

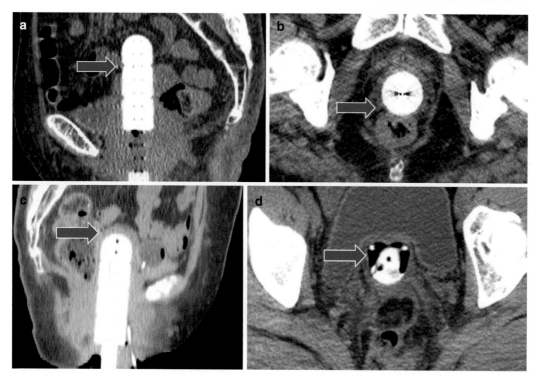

Fig. 2 Benefits of image-based brachytherapy for vaginal cuff brachytherapy. (**a**) Inadvertent perforation of the vaginal apex with vaginal cylinder placement (highlighted by *arrow*) which is easily recognizable on the CT-image completed for image-based planning. (**b**) A thinned submillimeter rectovaginal septum (highlighted by *arrow*) for which a higher dose to the rectum would be administered using two-dimensional planning; however, with image-based planning, the rectal dose was reduced by 14 % over a standard two-dimensional plan. (**c**) Thickened vaginal apex measuring 0.82 cm (highlighted by the *arrow*) for which image-based planning increased the $D_{90\%}$ to the CTV as compared to a standard two-dimension plan. (**d**) Air pockets between the vaginal mucosa and cylinder surface (highlighted by the *arrow*) which can be accounted for in image-based planning

A variety of dose fractionation schemas are employed [12]. For brachytherapy alone, as used in the PORTEC 2, a dose of 7 Gy times 3 fractions specified at a depth of 0.5 cm is a frequently used fractionation schedule [8]. Others have favored using more protracted fractionation schemas including 6 Gy times 5 fractions (M.D. Anderson) or 4 Gy times 6 fractions (Dana-Farber/Brigham and Women's) prescribed to the cylinder surface in an attempt to decrease the vaginal surface dose and subsequent late vaginal morbidity including fibrosis, telangiectasia, dryness, shortening, and narrowing [21]. The American Brachytherapy Society consensus guidelines mention a number of dose fractionation schemes and however purposely do not endorse any one schema over another as there is little agreement when it comes to dose fractionation schemes [2, 12]. A random-ized study by Sorbe et al. showed that vaginal recurrence rates were similar between 2.5 and 5 Gy times 6 fractions prescribed to 0.5 cm depth, with less vaginal shortening with the 2.5 Gy per fraction schema [22]. The ongoing PORTEC 4 is currently comparing 15Gy to 21Gy over 3 fractions prescribed to a 0.5 cm depth to prospectively define if lowering the dose per fraction can maintain excellent tumor control while decreasing the long-term risks of vaginal morbidity. For a brachytherapy boost following external beam, doses such as 6 Gy times 2–3 fractions prescribed to the cylinder surface based on risk factors with external beam radiotherapy doses of 45–50.4 Gy are reasonable and concordant with dose fractionation schemas used in contemporary cooperative group trials such as (RTOG 0921 and 0418). As detailed in Fig. 1, it is important to consider the increasing vaginal surface dose with decreasing cylinder size. For patients with a narrow vagina necessitating a 2.0–2.5 cm cylinder, consideration of decreasing the brachytherapy dose per fraction is warranted. For HDR brachytherapy, daily fractionation is not recommended, and multiple fractions per week are favored using at most an every-other-day application.

4 Postoperative Vaginal Cuff Brachytherapy: Alternate Techniques

While recent international patterns of care have shown 85 % utilize HDR brachytherapy techniques, viable alternatives include LDR and PDR brachytherapy techniques [23]. LDR brachytherapy commonly requires the patient to remain in the hospital, with some component of analgesia, immobilization precautions (deep vein thrombosis prophylaxis), bladder catheter placement, antidiarrheals (to prevent bowel movements), and special precautions to maintain applicator placement. The treatment duration varies according to the dose and dose rate chosen. Historical doses include approximately 60 Gy LDR to the vaginal surface at a dose rate of 60–100 cGy/h for adjuvant vaginal brachytherapy alone and a combined external beam radiotherapy and LDR equivalent of 70 Gy to the vaginal surface when brachytherapy is used as a boost following external beam radiotherapy.

5 Postoperative Vaginal Cuff Brachytherapy: Quality and Reporting Standards

A detailed, signed prescription including the treatment site, prescription point(s), total dose, dose per fraction, number of fractions, where the dose is specified, and radioisotope is imperative. It is recommended that both the dose to 0.5 cm and the vaginal surface be documented. While no specific validated volumetric constraints for CT-based planning in vaginal cuff brachytherapy are currently available, we recommend that the dose to rectum and bladder±bowel (depending on proximity) is recorded usually as D_{2cc}. There are several AAPM task group publications that serve as invaluable resources for brachytherapy quality assurance [24–27].

6 Postoperative Vaginal Cuff Brachytherapy: Results

Two important randomized trials place the comparative effectiveness of adjuvant brachytherapy following surgical staging for endometrial cancer in the context of observation and pelvic external beam radiotherapy. Sorbe et al. completed a multi-institutional trial which compared surgical staging to surgical staging plus adjuvant brachytherapy alone in low-risk (FIGO grades 1–2, with ≤50 % myometrial invasion) endometrioid endometrial cancers [28]. At a mean follow-up of 68 months, adjuvant brachytherapy alone leads to a non-significant (60 %) decrease in vaginal failures (3.1 versus 1.2 %, $p=0.114$) with no grade 3+ complications in either arm, suggesting that brachytherapy reduces the rates of vaginal recurrence without significantly increasing complications; however in subgroups with a low rate of recurrence following surgical staging (FIGO stages 1A–1B, grades 1–2, without risk factors), there is likely limited benefit to adding brachytherapy over close observation following surgical staging [28]. Similarly in PORTEC 2, vaginal brachytherapy alone was compared to pelvic external beam radiotherapy in a prospective phase III setting showing no significant difference in vaginal recurrence (1.8 versus 1.6 %, $p=0.74$), locoregional relapse (5.1 versus 2.1 %, $p=0.17$), disease-free survival (83 versus 78 %, $p=0.74$), or overall survival (85 versus 80 %, $p=0.57$); however brachytherapy resulted in significantly lower gastrointestinal toxicity (grades 1–2 13 % versus 54 %) [8]. These results from PORTEC 2 highlight that brachytherapy can maintain improvements in pelvic control while decreasing toxicity relative to pelvic external beam radiotherapy for intermediate-risk patients [8]. Table 2 summarizes additional results for select series using HDR brachytherapy with >100 included patients [8, 28–34]. Despite differences in patient selection, technique, and follow-up across the studies, Table 2 consistently highlights that vaginal brachytherapy alone results in low rates of vaginal

Table 2 Results for adjuvant vaginal brachytherapy alone following surgical staging for endometrial cancer

Study	n	Treatment	Vaginal recurrence	5-year overall survival	Grade 3+ complications
Swedish Randomized [28]	319	3–8 Gy × 3–6 at 0.5 cm	1.2 %	96 %	0 %
PORTEC 2 [8]	213	7 Gy × 3 at 0.5 cm	1.8 %	85 %	2.3 %
Orebro Medical Center, Sweden [29]	404	4.5–9 Gy × 4–6 at 1 cm	0.7 %	92 %	NR
Royal Prince Alfred, Australia [30]	141	8.5 Gy × 4 at surface	1.4 %	91 %	0 %
University of Goettingen [31]	122	7 Gy × 3 at surface	1.6 %	94 %	0 %
University of Arizona [32]	102	5 Gy × 3 at 0.5 cm	1.0 %	84 %	0 %
Swedish Medical Center [33]	164	7 Gy × 3 at 0.5 cm	1.2 %	87 %	0 %
Memorial Sloan Kettering [34]	382	7 Gy × 3 at 0.5 cm	0.8 %	93 %	1 %

failure to ≤2 % and is associated with an exceedingly low risk of severe grade 3+ complications ≤2 % [8, 28–34]. The potential added benefits of a brachytherapy boost following pelvic external beam radiotherapy remain less well established [35]. However, numerous series have similarly documented low rates of recurrence and toxicity with the combination of external beam radiotherapy and vaginal brachytherapy boost [36, 37]. A randomized Norwegian trial attempted to evaluate the additional benefit of pelvic external beam radiotherapy to surgical staging and low-dose-rate vaginal brachytherapy to 60 Gy at the vaginal surface [38]. Randomizing 540 stage I patients, pelvic external beam radiotherapy reduced the rates of vaginal/pelvic failure (5 % versus 20 %) and improved death from cancer (18 versus 28 %) only in patients with deeply invasive (>50 % myometrial invasion) and grade 3 tumors, highlighting that the combination of external beam radiotherapy plus brachytherapy may be best reserved for high-risk patients [38]. Careful attention to bladder and rectal doses in patients receiving combined external beam and brachytherapy is required to minimize late morbidity which has been observed in some historical series.

7 Postoperative Vaginal Cuff Brachytherapy: Complications and Management

Acute side effects of vaginal cuff brachytherapy typically include vaginitis and rarely mild cystitis or proctitis. Rare irritation of the small bowel, with associated diarrhea, can occur in patients with small bowel gravitating to the pelvic floor. These side effects are commonly self-limited and resolve without intervention. The predominant complications of concern following vaginal brachytherapy are vaginal dryness, vaginal telangiectasia leading to bleeding, and vaginal fibrosis leading to narrowing and shortening of the vagina which potentially compromise sexual function and quality of life [39]. In PORTEC 2, while brachytherapy decreased the rates of gastrointestinal toxicity as compared to pelvic external beam radiotherapy (grade 1–2 gastrointestinal toxicity 13 % versus 54 %, grade 3 gastrointestinal toxicity <1 % versus 2 %), rates of vaginal atrophy were slightly increased with vaginal brachytherapy (grade 3 vaginal atrophy 2 % versus <1 %) [8]. With long-term follow-up, patient-reported quality of life analysis from PORTEC-2 highlighted that vaginal brachytherapy improved social functioning and decreased bowel symptoms including diarrhea and fecal leakage, but did not improve sexual function as compared to pelvic external beam radiotherapy [40]. To mitigate risks of late vaginal dysfunction, a vaginal dilator is commonly recommended following radiation which helps to maintain patency of the vagina by disrupting the formation of adhesions and fibrous tissue, typically advocating for use at minimum two to three times per week beginning within 1 month following the completion of brachytherapy [41–43]. Ongoing studies are currently looking at modifications such as vibrator use, which may help to further reduce vaginal brachytherapy morbidity and improve long-term patient quality of life.

8   Definitive Brachytherapy for Medically Inoperable Endometrial Cancer: Indications

Despite improvements in surgical technique, including minimally invasive laparoscopic and robotic techniques, an ever aging population of patients with significant comorbidities leads to 4–9 % of endometrial cancer patients to be considered medically inoperable [44–47]. The combination of advancing age and a multitude of medical comorbidities (obesity, diabetes, cardiovascular disease, etc.) places this cohort of endometrial cancer patients at a higher risk of death from intercurrent disease (approximately threefold greater risk of death from causes other than endometrial cancer) or from surgery than from their cancer [48]. Nonetheless, definitive radiotherapy, either via brachytherapy alone or a combination of external beam radiotherapy plus brachytherapy, remains an important treatment aimed at controlling disease and maintaining quality of life.

9   Definitive Brachytherapy for Medically Inoperable Endometrial Cancer: Technique

HDR brachytherapy for medically inoperable endometrial cancer can be completed either as monotherapy or as a boost following external beam irradiation. The optimal technique depends on the patients' performance status and the staging imaging if technically feasible. Staging imaging should include pelvic MRI whenever feasible. Additionally for patients with high-grade disease, a CT of the chest, abdomen, and pelvis or whole body PET/CT to assess for regional nodal involvement or distant metastases should be considered. Pelvic MRI can reveal tumor size as well as the presence and depth of myometrial invasion and the presence of cervical extension superior to CT or ultrasound [49–51]. This information is critical in defining the role and type of brachytherapy in

addition to the need for external beam irradiation. For patients with FIGO grade 1–2 endometrioid endometrial carcinoma, with <50 % myometrial invasion and low-volume disease (≤2 cm), brachytherapy alone can be used, while for patients with high-grade disease, deep myometrial invasion, or large-volume disease, a combination of external beam irradiation followed by a brachytherapy boost is generally recommended as these patients are a higher risk for extrauterine extension (most notably pelvic node involvement) which will be inadequately covered with brachytherapy alone. Additionally, this pre-brachytherapy assessment helps to define the optimal brachytherapy applicator and dose. The most common applicators include an intracavitary tandem and cylinder or a dual-tandem or Y applicator, a triple-tandem applicator, or a modified Heyman packing. At the exam under anesthesia, the uterine sound length is measured to define the tandem length required and the vaginal vault size assessed for optimal vaginal applicator selection. Typically the largest size that can be accommodated is selected. For institutions favoring an intracavitary applicator, a maximum uterine width >4–5 cm by pre-brachytherapy imaging helps to select for patients in which the full thickness of the uterus may be under-dosed with a single-tandem-cylinder applicator (see Fig. 3a). For these patients with a maximum uterine width >5 cm, a dual-tandem Y applicator (see Fig. 3b) or triple-tandem applicator may more optimally cover the full thickness of the uterus [44, 52]. Applicator selection should be defined based on the individual patient anatomy; a dual-tandem Y applicator may help improve lateral coverage over a single-tandem applicator while a triple-tandem may increase coverage both laterally and in an anterior/posterior direction [44, 52]. However the inherent challenges in inserting two or three tandems and the associated prolonged immobilization and anesthesia requirements may make them suboptimal for some medically inoperable patients (such as those with baseline coagulopathy or baseline orthopnea from underlying congestive heart failure, sleep apnea, or other similar comorbidities). There is also increased

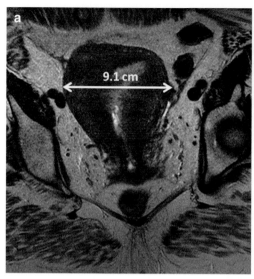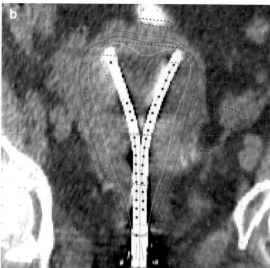

Fig. 3 Uterine width limitations of single-tandem brachytherapy ameliorated with a Rotte Y applicator. (**a**) Pre-brachytherapy MRI showing a maximal uterine width measuring 9.1 cm which would be inadequately covered with a single-tandem applicator. (**b**) Image-based brachytherapy plan for the same patient treated with a Rotte Y applicator to improve lateral coverage. For panel **b**: GTV (*green dotted line*), CTV (*red dotted line*), 150 % isodose line (*yellow solid line*), 100 % isodose line (*red solid line*), and 80 % isodose line (*green solid line*)

risk of perforation with multiple tandems. Others have favored using modified Hyman packing (Norman Simon's applicators) which consist of capsules of varying sizes (usually between 0.4 and 0.8 cm selected based on pre-brachytherapy assessment for packing within the uterine fundus) mounted on long flexible tubing [53, 54]. The modified Heyman packing also requires insertion under anesthesia for insertion of multiple capsules (5–18 capsules) and prolonged immobilization which, as the dual and triple tandems, is challenging in these medically inoperable endometrial cancer patients. This sometimes makes the single-tandem and vaginal cylinder applicator the most reasonable choice.

The brachytherapy procedure begins with some component of analgesia, such as IV conscious sedation, spinal or epidural anesthesia, a paracervical block, or oral pain medication, depending on the applicator type and patient tolerance both to pain and considering the risks associated with increasing depth of analgesia. In some patients a combination of IV sedation and a paracervical block can be helpful in achieving improved comfort while lowering the associated

risks. Patients should always be evaluated for anesthesia risk prior to the procedure. The patient is placed in the dorsal lithotomy position with a bladder catheter inserted to empty the bladder. Using downward traction as needed, the tandem is inserted through a previously placed Smit sleeve, with subsequent vaginal dome segments threaded onto the tandem to optimally fill the vagina without undue discomfort, ranging in size from 2.0 to 4.0 cm. For patients whose placement is difficult or those requiring a dual- or triple-tandem applicator, ultrasound can be used for image guidance during applicator placement. Following applicator placement, if possible, image-based planning should follow to allow for confirmation of appropriate applicator placement relative to the 3-dimensional anatomy and to maximize dose to the target while minimizing dose to critical organs [55]. Others have published their experience using image-based planning for modified Heyman packing [54]. The American Brachytherapy Society guidelines for medically inoperable endometrial cancer are currently being updated and underscore the importance of imaging and volumetric rather than just point-based planning. Additional information regarding the technique for point-based planning as outlined in the 2000 American Brachytherapy Society guidelines will be reviewed in the alternate technique section below [56]. Here the technique description will focus on the preferred technique of image-based planning. Following applicator insertion, a T2-weighted MRI (or non-contrast-enhanced pelvic CT in patients with a contraindication to MRI or with a uterine length >8 cm for which the availability of a MRI-compatible tandem is limited) is obtained with the applicator in place and with each subsequent fraction. The GTV is the entire endometrial cavity (in patients with no identifiable gross tumor at the time of brachytherapy) plus any gross tumor visualized at the time of brachytherapy. The CTV is defined to include the GTV plus the entire uterus, cervix, and upper 1–2 cm of the vagina. When HDR brachytherapy is integrated with pelvic external beam radiotherapy (usually to 45 Gy at 1.8 Gy per fraction), brachytherapy doses range from 4 to 5.5 Gy times 4–5 fractions based on response to external beam, extent of disease, and normal tissue proximity aiming for the CTV to receive a dose sufficient for microscopic disease between 45 and 60 Gy EQD_{2Gy}, whereas the GTV receives a boost to an EQD_{2Gy} of at least 80–90 Gy. Fewer HDR fractions are also reasonable if the organs at risk are in close proximity to the uterus and/or the uterine wall is thin. Brachytherapy planning is completed first by optimizing to point W (2 cm inferior from the tandem tip along the tandem and then lateral to the mid-uterine width or approximately 2 cm) and then using manual optimization to achieve a CTV $D_{90\%} \geq 100$ % while maintaining a rectal D_{2cc} $EQD_{2Gy} \leq 70$ Gy, sigmoid $D_{2cc} \leq 70$ Gy, and bladder $D_{2cc} \leq 80$ Gy [57]. Other recommended dose fractionation schemas for HDR brachytherapy following external beam radiotherapy (45 Gy at 1.8 Gy per fraction) as outlined in the American Brachytherapy Society guidelines are 8.5 Gy times 2 fractions, 6.3 Gy times 3 fractions, and 5.2 times 4 fractions [56]. For brachytherapy alone, 8.5 Gy times 4 fractions, 7.3 Gy times 5 fractions, 6.4 Gy times 6 fractions, or others are

possible options for fractionation schemas [56]. Recognizing that medically inoperable patients are at a threefold higher risk of death from intercurrent disease, a higher priority is placed on critical organ constraints than CTV coverage [48]. These patients cannot afford to have a complication as the intervention for the complication could be life threatening. HDR brachytherapy with a tandem-cylinder applicator is completed on an outpatient basis, using at maximum every-other-day fractionation. If there is concern about the sedation required for applicator insertion, it is possible to hospitalize the patient and deliver two to three fractions for each insertion of the applicator. The risks of bed rest must be balanced with the risks of multiple sedations.

For patient requiring a dual- or triple-tandem applicator, MRI-compatible applicators are not yet commercial available; thus CT-based planning is used. Due to the difficulty in applicator placement, these applications are completed on an inpatient basis. The applicator is placed under anesthesia in the operating room with full relaxation to allow for uterine dilation. For a Y applicator, the two curved tandems are selected to the measured uterine length and then gently advanced toward the opposite uterine cornu under ultrasound guidance. The two tandems are subsequently fixed together and vaginal packing is inserted to keep the applicator in place and displace the rectum and bladder. Following applicator placement, the labia can be sutured to prevent applicator extrusion from the vagina. Confirmation of placement and image-based planning is completed using a non-contrast-enhanced pelvic CT with the applicator in place. Contrast can be inserted into the rectum and sigmoid as well as the bladder to better define these critical organs. For patients receiving a combination of external beam radiotherapy plus brachytherapy, a dose 4–5 Gy times 5 fractions delivery twice daily with a minimum inter-fraction interval of 6 h is used, while for those receiving brachytherapy alone, 7–7.5 Gy times 5 fractions delivered twice daily with a minimum inter-fraction interval of 6 h is used with a similar optimization and planning technique as described above for a single-tandem-cylinder application. Similarly, the American Brachytherapy Society guidelines recommend a dose per fraction of 7.3 Gy when 5 fractions are used for brachytherapy alone and 5.2 Gy per fraction for up to 4 fractions following external beam radiation therapy, among other possible acceptable options [56].

10 Definitive Brachytherapy for Medically Inoperable Endometrial Cancer: Alternate Techniques

Brachytherapy planning can be either image based (preferably) relative to cross-sectional imaging or point based relative to fixed geometry or localization radiographs (Ap and lateral or stereoshift radiographs). Relying on point-based planning increases the risk of complications over image-based planning in a medically inoperable population vulnerable to serious complications [58]. Integration of image-based planning allows for dose painting such that the high dose is confined to the defined areas of disease, which is not feasible with point-based planning [55, 58]. The intended target volume for point-based planning includes the uterus, cervix, and proximal 3–5 cm of vagina, with recommendations to aim for the prescription isodose line to include the entire uterine serosa and vaginal wall (to 0.5 cm depth). The dose is specified to a point defined as 2 cm from the central axis at the midpoint along the uterine applicator. The prescription at the vaginal level can be adjusted depending on the cylinder diameter to meet the 0.5 cm prescription depth or a surface dose prescription. Traditional International Commission of Radiation Units (ICRU) points for rectum and bladder are used to record critical organ doses. Assessment of dose to the sigmoid is also critical in this population where the sigmoid is often close to the uterus. This technique of attempting to cover the entire uterus is technically challenging and often not feasible when considering normal tissue constraints; therefore point-based planning should be avoided in favor of image-based planning in the modern brachytherapy era [59].

11 Definitive Brachytherapy for Medically Inoperable Endometrial Cancer: Quality and Reporting Standards

A detailed, signed prescription including the treatment site, prescription point, total dose, dose per fraction, fractionation, and radioisotope is again imperative. Prescribed dose is recorded as $D_{90\%}$ for the contoured CTV, aiming for a $D_{90\%} \geq 100\%$ when image-based planning is incorporated. We recommend that the critical organ doses be carried across brachytherapy fractions and incorporate any external beam radiotherapy dose, using an EQD_{2Gy} calculator, aiming for the rectal D_{2cc} EQD_{2Gy} ≤ 70 Gy, sigmoid D_{2cc} ≤ 70 Gy, and bladder D_{2cc} ≤ 80 Gy. There are several American Association of Physicists in Medicine (AAPM) task group publications that serve as invaluable resources for brachytherapy quality assurance [24–27].

12 Definitive Brachytherapy for Medically Inoperable Endometrial Cancer: Results

The importance of brachytherapy utilization for inoperable endometrial cancer was highlighted in a recent Surveillance, Epidemiology, and End Results (SEER) analysis from 2004 to 2010, which showed that despite only 5 % brachytherapy utilization, inoperable endometrial cancer patients treated with brachytherapy had significantly improved overall survival with a 3-year overall survival of 45–59 % (depending on age) compared to 21–23 % for external beam radiotherapy alone ($p < 0.001$) [60]. However, owing to the uncommon nature of medically inoperable endometrial cancer, the body of literature supporting definitive brachytherapy for endometrial cancer is confined to retrospective cohort studies, the largest of which is from Vienna. Reporting on their institutional experience for 280 inoperable endometrial cancer patients (84 % stage I) predominately treated with HDR brachytherapy alone, at a median follow-up of 49 months, the 5-year disease-specific survival and local control rates were 76 and 75 % with a 5-year probability of grade 3 late complications of 5.2 % [61]. Similarly in a multi-institutional collaboration including 74 patients from five large US academic cancer institutions, the median progression-free survival was 44 months and overall survival was 47 months with a hazard ratio for risks of death from causes other than endometrial cancer of 3.4 (95 % CI 1.4–9.4, $p=0.003$) again highlighting the burden of comorbidity and competing risks of mortality in this cohort of endometrial cancer patients [48]. More recently, image-based brachytherapy has been integrated in the management of medically inoperable patients which has translated into high local control rates 91–92 % and no grade 3+ complications across two international series; further follow-up will help to better define if these high rates of local control and low rates of complication relative to older two-dimensional series are maintained [54, 55].

13 Definitive Brachytherapy for Medically Inoperable Endometrial Cancer: Complications and Management

In the largest series using definitive brachytherapy for endometrial cancer from the Vienna group, overall rates of complications were low with only 12.5 % of patients experiencing any acute side effects (9.1 % were grade I involving the rectum, bladder, or vagina which resolved without interventions) and 21 % of patients experiencing any late complication (5.2 % of which were grade 3–4 complications, the majority of which were small bowel complications with a 3.5 % grade 3–4 bowel complications) [61]. These severe late small bowel complications often require surgical intervention in a challenging subset of patients. Image-based planning may help to reduce this risk of bowel complications over two-dimensional planning by accounting for small bowel and sigmoid dose [58]. Moreover, one treatment-related death in the Vienna series was due to an unrecognized perforation during the application resulting in small bowel necrosis and peritonitis [61]. This highlights the impor-

tance of careful applicator placement as the postmenopausal uterine wall is often thin and recognition of applicator perforation prior to treatment. It also highlights one of the important advantages of image-based planning over conventional two-dimensional point-based planning.

14 Preoperative Brachytherapy for Locally Advanced Disease: Indications

Locally advanced endometrial cancer extending to the cervix at presentation is an uncommon and challenging presentation. Two potential plans of care thus exist:

1. Radical hysterectomy (if feasible) followed by tailored adjuvant therapy
2. Neoadjuvant radiochemotherapy (including a combination of external beam radiotherapy plus brachytherapy) to downstage disease followed by extrafascial hysterectomy

15 Preoperative Brachytherapy for Locally Advanced Disease: Techniques

Preoperative brachytherapy for locally advanced endometrial cancer is not covered in the previous guideline publications from the American Brachytherapy Society; thus the presented technique reflects the current practice. For patients with disease clinically extending to the cervix/parametria, these clinical findings are confirmed with additional pre-brachytherapy imaging including a pelvic MRI and PET/CT. If extension to the cervix/parametria is confirmed, preoperative external beam radiotherapy (with concurrent weekly cisplatin) is planned with the volume of treatment to include the pelvis only up to the common iliac nodal regions for patients whose PET/CT is negative for nodal disease. For patients with nodal disease, the pelvis plus para-aortic nodes +/− a simultaneous integrated boost to the positive nodes is recommended [62]. In the 4th or 5th week of chemoradiotherapy, patients undergo a repeat exam under anesthesia to assess response and an MR-compatible Smit sleeve is placed followed by 3–4 fractions of image-based HDR brachytherapy. The sound length of the uterus at the time of exam under anesthesia helps to define the required tandem length and the extent of disease defines the applicator selection. Brachytherapy is completed using either a tandem-ring (preferred applicator), tandem-cylinder (used at our institutions primarily when a tandem length of 8 cm or greater is required), or template-based interstitial applicator. HDR brachytherapy is completed as an outpatient, with at maximum every-other-day fractionation. A bladder catheter is placed prior to beginning the procedure with either oral analgesia or conscious sedation incorporated. The patient is placed in the dorsal lithotomy position, and the tandem is inserted with ultrasound guidance used on an as-needed basis based on the difficulty of insertion. Then, either the ring or subsequent dome segments are assembled accordingly with rectal retraction or vaginal packing per institutional practice. The patient is returned to a more comfortable supine position with placement of an external stabilizing device such as a perineal bar. HDR brachytherapy is completed using image-based planning with each fraction, with T2-weight pelvic MRI as the preferred image-based planning modality. CT-based brachytherapy

planning is used for patients with a contraindication to MRI or for those requiring non-MRI-compatible applicators (based on institutional availability). The CTV includes the gross tumor volume plus the entire uterus and cervix (see Fig. 4). Fractionation schedules vary between 5 and 5.5 Gy times three to four fractions, aiming for a cumulative EQD_{2Gy} of 60–70 Gy modulated based on response and extent of disease. The plan is first optimized to point A, with subsequent manual optimization aiming for a CTV $D_{90\%} \geq 100$ % while maintaining a rectal D_{2cc} $EQD_{2Gy} \leq 65$ Gy, sigmoid $D_{2cc} \leq 65$ Gy, and bladder $D_{2cc} \leq 70$ Gy (see Fig. 4). Restaging CT imaging is performed 4–5 weeks following completion of chemoradiotherapy followed by extrafascial hysterectomy at a 4–8-week-interval post-completion of neoadjuvant brachytherapy.

16 Preoperative Brachytherapy for Locally Advanced Disease: Alternate Techniques

An alternative technique would be to use LDR as described in the older University of Kentucky experience [63, 64]. Preoperative brachytherapy using LDR would include all the above steps for

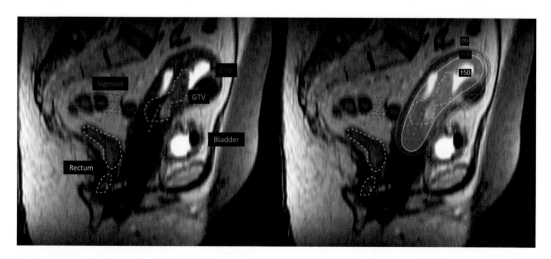

Fig. 4 MRI-based planning for preoperative brachytherapy in locally advanced endometrial cancer clinical extending to the cervix. The GTV at the time of brachytherapy is outlined in green. The CTV is outlined in *red*, which incorporates the GTV plus the entire uterus and cervix. The isodose cloud highlights MRI-based planning where the *yellow* cloud represents the 150 % isodose, *red* represents to 100 % isodose, and *green* represents the 80 % isodose

applicator placement; however additional consideration of prolonged immobilization and radiation exposure would apply. This older technique described traditional point-based planning to point A while limiting the maximum point dose to the rectum and bladder of 80 % of the prescription dose using the ICRU points previously described for gynecologic cancer planning.

17 Preoperative Brachytherapy for Locally Advanced Disease: Quality and Reporting Standards

A detailed, signed prescription including the treatment site, prescription point, total dose, dose per fraction, fractionation, and radioisotope is again imperative. Prescribed dose is recorded as $D_{90 \%}$ for the contoured CTV, aiming for a $D_{90 \%}$ ≥ 100 % when image-based planning is incorporated. We recommend that the critical organ doses be carried across brachytherapy fractions and incorporate any external beam radiotherapy dose, using an EQD_{2Gy} calculator, aiming for the EQD_{2Gy} rectal $D_{2cc} \leq 65$ Gy, sigmoid $D_{2cc} \leq 65$ Gy, and bladder $D_{2cc} \leq 70$ Gy. There are several AAPM task group publications that serve as invaluable resources for brachytherapy quality assurance [24–27].

18 Preoperative Brachytherapy for Locally Advanced Disease: Results

Larger series from the 2-dimensional non-image-based era showed the potential value of a neoadjuvant radiotherapy approach to a total dose of 60–65 Gy with a combination of external beam radiotherapy and LDR brachytherapy using a tandem and cylinder applicator evincing an 88 % 5-year overall survival with only 5 % vaginal failure [63, 64]. These results have been more recently validated in the image-based HDR brachytherapy era, with a similar 3 % vaginal failure and 100 % 3-year survival [62].

19 Preoperative Brachytherapy for Locally Advanced Disease: Complications and Management

One potential concern of a preoperative approach is the potential for increasing surgical complications following neoadjuvant therapy. A recent detailed analysis of surgical complications following neoadjuvant chemoradiation therapy and extrafascial hysterectomy showed acceptable low rates of postoperative ileus and vaginal cuff dehiscence of 10 and 3 %, respectively [65]. This suggests that neoadjuvant therapy does not increase complications over upfront surgical staging followed by tailored adjuvant therapy.

References

1. Siegel R, Naishadham D, Jemal A (2013) Cancer statistics, 2013. CA Cancer J Clin 63:11–30
2. Small W, Beriwal S, Demanes DJ et al (2012) American brachytherapy society consensus guidelines for adjuvant vaginal cuff brachytherapy after hysterectomy. Brachytherapy 11:58–67
3. Creutzberg CL, Van Putten WL, Koper PC et al (2003) Survival after relapse in patients with endometrial cancer: results from a randomized trial. Gynecol Oncol 89:201–209
4. Jhingran A, Burke TW, Eifel PJ (2003) Definitive radiotherapy for patients with isolated vaginal recurrence of endometrial carcinoma after hysterectomy. Int J Radiat Oncol Biol Phys 56:1366–1372
5. Morrow CP, Bundy BN, Kurman RJ et al (1991) Relationship between surgical-pathological risk factors and outcome in clinical stage I and II carcinoma of the endometrium: a Gynecologic Oncology Group Study. Gynecol Oncol 40:55–65
6. Keys HM, Roberts JA, Brunetto VL et al (2004) A phase III trial of surgery with or without adjunctive external pelvic radiation therapy in intermediate risk endometrial adenocarcinoma: a Gynecologic Oncology Group Study. Gynecol Oncol 92:744–751
7. Nout RA, Van de Poll-Franse LV, Lybeert ML et al (2011) Long-term outcome and quality of life of patients with endometrial carcinoma treated with or without pelvic radiotherapy in the post-operative radiation in endometrial carcinoma 1 (PORTEC-1) trial. J Clin Oncol 29:1692–1700
8. Nout RA, Smit VT, Putter H et al (2010) Vaginal brachytherapy versus pelvic external beam radiotherapy for patients with endometrial cancer of high-intermediate risk (PORTEC-2): an open-label, non-inferiority, randomized trial. Lancet 375:816–823

9. NCCN clinical practice guidelines in oncology (NCCN Guidelines®) uterine neoplasms version 1 2015 (Nov 2014). Available at www.nccn.org

10. Klopp A, Smith BD, Alektiar K et al (2014) The role of postoperative radiation therapy for endometrial cancer: executive summary of an American Society for Radiation Oncology evidence-based guideline. Pract Radiat Oncol 4:137–144

11. Cattaneo R, Hanna RK, Jacobsen G et al (2014) Interval between hysterectomy and start of radiation treatment is predictive of recurrence in patients with endometrial carcinoma. Int J Radiat Oncol Biol Phys 88:866–871

12. Small W, Erickson B, Kwakwa F (2005) American Brachytherapy Society survey regarding practice patterns of postoperative irradiation for endometrial cancer: current status of vaginal brachytherapy. Int J Radiat Oncol Biol Phys 63:1502–1507

13. Demanes DJ, Rege S, Rodriguez RR et al (1999) The use and advantages of a multichannel vaginal cylinder in high-dose-rate brachytherapy. Int J Radiat Oncol Biol Phys 44:211–219

14. Peng J, Sinha R, Patel R, Lebovic G (2011) A comparison of 3D dose planning regimens for vaginal cuff brachytherapy using a flexible inflatable multichannel gynecologic applicator. Brachytherapy 10:S67

15. El Khoury C, Dumas I, Tailleur A et al (2015) Adjuvant brachytherapy for endometrial cancer: advantaged of the vaginal mold technique. Brachytherapy 14:51–55

16. Tuncell N, Toy A, Demiral AN, Cetingoz R et al (2009) Dosimetric comparison of ring and ovoid applicators. J Buon 14:451–454

17. Stewart AJ, Cormack RA, Lee H et al (2008) Prospective clinical trial of bladder filling and tree-dimensional dosimetry in high-dose-rate vaginal cuff brachytherapy. Int J Radiat Oncol Biol Phys 72:843–848

18. Hung J, Shen S, De Los Santos JF et al (2012) Image-based 3D treatment planning for vaginal cylinder brachytherapy: dosimetric effects of bladder filling on organs at risk. Int J Radiat Oncol Biol Phys 83:980–985

19. Kim H, Kim H, Houser C et al (2012) Is there any advantage to three-dimensional planning for vaginal cuff brachytherapy? Brachytherapy 11:398–401

20. Zhou J, Prisiandaro J, Lee C et al (2014) Single or multi-channel vaginal cuff high-dose-rate brachytherapy: is replanning necessary prior to each fraction? Pract Radiat Oncol 4:20–26

21. Townamchai K, Lee L, Viswanathan AN (2012) A novel low dose fractionation regimen for adjuvant vaginal brachytherapy in early stage endometrial cancer. Gynecol Oncol 127:351–355

22. Sorbe B, Staumtis A, Karlsson L (2005) Intravaginal high-dose brachytherapy for stage I endometrial cancer: a randomized study of two dose-per-fraction levels. Int J Radiat Oncol Biol Phys 62:1385–1389

23. Viswanathan AN, Creutzberg CL, Craighead P et al (2012) International brachytherapy practice patterns: a survey of the Gynecologic Cancer Intergroup (GCIG). Int J Radiat Oncol Biol Phys 82:250–255

24. Fraass B, Doppke M, Hunt M et al (1998) American Association of Physicists in Medicine Radiation Therapy Committee Task Group 53: quality assurance for clinical radiotherapy treatment planning. Med Phys 25:1773–1829

25. Glasgow GP, Bourland JD, Grigsby PW et al (1993) Remote afterloading technology: a report of AAPM Task Group No. 41. American Institute of Physics, New York

26. Kubo HD, Glasgow GP, Pethel TD et al (1998) High dose-rate brachytherapy treatment delivery: a report of the AAPM Radiation Therapy Committee Task Group No. 59. Med Phys 25:375–403

27. Nath R, Anderson LL, Meli JA et al (1997) Code of practice for brachytherapy physics: report of the AAPM Radiation Therapy Committee Task Group No. 56. Med Phys 24:1557–1598

28. Sorbe B, Nordstrom B, Maenpaa J et al (2009) Intravaginal brachytherapy in FIGO stage I low-risk endometrial cancer: a controlled randomized study. Int J Gynecol Cancer 19:873–878

29. Sorbe BG, Smeds AC (1990) Postoperative vaginal irradiation with high dose rate afterloading technique in endometrial carcinoma stage I. Int J Radiat Oncol Biol 18:305–314

30. MacLeod C, Fowler A, Duval P et al (1998) High-dose-rate brachytherapy alone post-hysterectomy for endometrial cancer. Int J Radiat Oncol Biol 42:1033–1039

31. Weiss E, Hirnle P, Arnold-Bofinger H et al (1998) Adjuvant vaginal high-dose-rate afterloading alone in endometrial carcinoma: patterns of relapse and side effects following low-dose therapy. Gynecol Oncol 71:72–76

32. Anderson JM, Stea B, Hallum AV et al (2000) High-dose-rate postoperative vaginal cuff irradiation alone for stage IB and IC endometrial cancer. Int J Radiat Oncol Biol Phys 46:417–425

33. Horowitz NS, Peters WA, Smith MR et al (2002) Adjuvant high dose rate vaginal brachytherapy as treatment of stage I and II endometrial carcinoma. Obstet Gynecol 99:235–240

34. Alektiar KM, Venkatraman E, Chi DS, Barakat RR (2005) Intravaginal brachytherapy alone for intermediate-risk endometrial cancer. Int J Radiat Oncol Biol Phys 62:111–117

35. Greven KM, D'Agostino RB, Lanciano RM et al (1998) Is there a role for a brachytherapy vaginal cuff boost in the adjuvant management of patients with uterine-confined endometrial cancer? Int J Radiat Oncol Biol Phys 42:101–104

36. Kucera H, Vavra N, Weghaupt K (1990) Benefit of external irradiation in pathologic stage I endometrial carcinoma: a prospective clinical trial of 605 patients who received post-operative vaginal irradiation and additional pelvic irradiation in the presence of unfavorable prognostic factors. Gynecol Oncol 38:99–104

37. Lybeert ML, van Putten WL, Ribot JG et al (1989) Endometrial carcinoma: high dose rate brachytherapy in combination with external irradiation: a multivariate analysis of relapse. Radiother Oncol 16:245–252

38. Aalders J, Abeler V, Kolstad P et al (1980) Postoperative external irradiation and prognostic parameters in stage I endometrial carcinoma: clinical and histopathologic study of 540 patients. Obstet Gynecol 56:419–427

39. Bruner DW, Lanciano R, Keegan M et al (1993) Vaginal stenosis and sexual function following intracavitary radiation for the treatment of cervical and endometrial carcinoma. Int J Radiat Oncol Biol Phys 27:825–830

40. Nout RA, Putter H, Jurgenliemk-Schultz IM et al (2009) Quality of life after pelvic radiotherapy or vaginal brachytherapy for endometrial cancer: first results of the randomized PORTEC-2 trial. J Clin Oncol 27:3547–3556

41. Decruze SB, Guthrie D, Magnani R (1999) Prevention of vaginal stenosis in patients following vaginal brachytherapy. Clin Oncol (R Coll Radiol) 11:46–48

42. Friedman LC, Abdallah R, Schluchter M et al (2011) Adherence to vaginal dilation following high doe rate brachytherapy for endometrial cancer. Int J Radiat Oncol Biol Phys 80:751–757

43. Lancaster L (2004) Preventing vaginal stenosis after brachytherapy for gynecological cancer: an overview of Australian practices. Eur J Oncol Nurs 8:30–39

44. Coon D, Beriwal S, Heron DE et al (2008) High-dose-rate Rotte "Y" applicator brachytherapy for definitive treatment of medically inoperable endometrial cancer: 10-year results. Int J Radiat Oncol Biol Phys 71: 779–783

45. Fishman DA, Roberts KB, Chambers JT et al (1996) Radiation therapy as exclusive treatment for medically inoperable patients with stage I and II endometrioid carcinoma with endometrium. Gynecol Oncol 61: 189–196

46. Nguyen TV, Petereit DG (1998) High-dose-rate brachytherapy for medically inoperable stage I endometrial cancer. Gynecol Oncol 71:196–203

47. Rouanet P, Dubois JB, Gely S, Pourquier H (1993) Exclusive radiation therapy in endometrial carcinoma. Int J Radiat Oncol Biol Phys 26:223–228

48. Podzielinski I, Randall ME, Breheny PJ et al (2012) Primary radiation therapy for medically inoperable patients with clinical stage I and II endometrial carcinoma. Gynecol Oncol 124:36–41

49. Cunha TM, Felix A, Cabral I (2001) Preoperative assessment of deep myometrial and cervical invasion in endometrial carcinoma: comparison of magnetic resonance imaging and gross visual inspection. Int J Gynecol Cancer 11:130–136

50. Frei KA, Kinkel K, Bonel HM et al (2000) Prediction of deep myometrial invasion in patients with endometrial cancer: clinical utility of contrast-enhanced MR imaging a meta-analysis and Bayesian analysis. Radiology 216:444–449

51. Kinkel K, Kaji Y, Yu KK et al (1999) Radiologic staging in patients with endometrial cancer: a meta-analysis. Radiology 212:711–718

52. Johnson SB, Zhou J, Jolly S et al (2014) The dosimetric impact of single, dual, and triple tandem applicators in the treatment of intact uterine cancer. Brachytherapy 13:268–274

53. Herbolsheimer M, Sauer O, Rotte K (1992) Primary irradiation of endometrial cancer: technical aspects, individual treatment planning, and first results in a modified Heyman Packing with high dose rate after loading. Endocurieth Hypertherm Oncol 8:11–18

54. Weitmann HD, Pötter R, Waldhause C et al (2005) Pilot study in the treatment of endometrial carcinoma with 3D image-based high-dose-rate brachytherapy using modified Heyman packing: clinical experience and dose-volume histogram analysis. Int J Radiat Oncol Biol Phys 62:468–478

55. Gill BS, Kim H, Houser C et al (2014) Image-based three-dimensional conformal brachytherapy for medically inoperable endometrial carcinoma. Brachytherapy 13:542–547

56. Nag S, Erickson B, Parikh S et al (2000) The American Brachytherapy Society recommendations for high-dose-rate brachytherapy for carcinoma of the endometrium. Int J Radiat Oncol Biol Phys 48:779–790

57. Stitt J (1991) Dose specification for inoperable endometrial carcinoma: the Madison system. Brachytherapy J 2:32–34

58. Beriwal S, Kim H, Heron DE, Selvaraj R (2006) Comparison of 2D vs 3D dosimetry for Rotte Y applicator high dose rate brachytherapy for medically inoperable endometrial cancer. Technol Cancer Res Treat 5:521–527

59. Mock U, Knocke TH, Fellner C et al (1998) Analysis of different application systems and CT-controlled treatment planning variants in the treatment of primary endometrial carcinomas: is brachytherapy treatment of the entire uterus technically possible? Strahlenther Onkol 174:320–328

60. Patel S, Tenapel M, Button A et al (2014) Impact on survival of brachytherapy in inoperable endometrial cancer: the (SEER) experience from 2004–2010. Int J Radiat Oncol Biol Phys 90:S111–S112

61. Knocke TH, Kucera H, Weidinger B et al (1997) Primary treatment of endometrial carcinoma with high-dose-rate brachytherapy: results of 12 years of experience with 280 patients. Int J Radiat Oncol Biol Phys 37:359–365

62. Vargo JA, Boisen MM, Comerci JT et al (2014) Neoadjuvant radiotherapy with or without chemotherapy followed by extrafascial hysterectomy for locally advanced endometrial cancer clinically extending to the cervix or parametria. Gynecol Oncol 135:190–195

63. Higgins RV, van Nagell JR, Horn EJ et al (1991) Preoperative radiation therapy followed by extrafascial hysterectomy in patients with stage II endometrial carcinoma. Cancer 68:1261–1264

64. Maruyama Y, Yoneda J, Coffey C et al (1992) Tandem-vaginal cylinder applicator for radiation therapy of uterine adenocarcinoma. Radiother Oncol 25:140–141

65. Boisen MM, Vargo JA, Beriwal S et al (2015) Surgical outcomes of patients undergoing extrafascial hysterectomy following neoadjuvant high-dose-rate brachytherapy for locally advanced endometrial cancer clinically extending to the cervix and parametria. Gynecol Oncol 137(Suppl 1):1–210

Gynecologic Brachytherapy: Cervical Cancer

John A. Vargo, Akila N. Viswanathan,
Beth A. Erickson, and Sushil Beriwal

Abstract

Cervical cancer is the 3rd most common malignancy in the world. Despite national trends of declining utilization, brachytherapy plays an integral role in the curative management of all locally-advanced and medically inoperable early-stage cervical cancer. Herein we review the practice implementation of brachytherapy critical to curing patients of cervical cancer, especially modern image-based high-dose rate brachytherapy.

1 Introduction

Over 275, 000 women die of cervical cancer per year worldwide, with cervical cancer representing the 3rd most common cancer in women [1, 2]. Brachytherapy is an integral part of cervical cancer management which has consistently been shown to improve overall survival [3–6]. Despite the consistent survival improvement associated with brachytherapy utilization, in the context of modern radiation therapy such as intensity-modulated radiation therapy and stereotactic body radiation therapy, brachytherapy utilization has decreased which has led to a survival decrement [5, 6].

2 Indications

Surgery is generally considered the preferred curative treatment for early-stage IA cervical cancer because of the opportunity for fertility and ovarian preservation in premenopausal women, decreased risk of second cancers, and decreased overall treatment time. However for medically inoperable patients with International Federation of Gynecology and Obstetrics (FIGO) stage IA1–IB1 cervical cancer, definitive radiation therapy is the preferred alternative to surgery. Radical

J.A. Vargo, MD • S. Beriwal, MD (✉)
Department of Radiation Oncology, University of Pittsburgh, Pittsburgh, PA, USA
e-mail: vargoja2@upmc.edu

A.N. Viswanathan, MD, MPH
Department of Radiation Oncology, Brigham and Women's Hospital and Dana-Farber Cancer Institute, Boston, MA, USA

B.A. Erickson, MD, FACR, FASTRO
Department of Radiation Oncology, Medical College of Wisconsin, Milwaukee, WI, USA
e-mail: berickson@mcw.edu

© Springer International Publishing Switzerland 2016
P. Montemaggi et al. (eds.), *Brachytherapy: An International Perspective*, Medical Radiology,
DOI 10.1007/978-3-319-26791-3_15

hysterectomy (± adjuvant external beam radiotherapy) and definitive radiation therapy result in equivalent cancer-specific and overall survival for patients with clinical stage IB–IIA cervical cancer, with increased acute and late toxicity in those patients requiring radical hysterectomy plus adjuvant radiotherapy [7]. Intravaginal brachytherapy may selectively be integrated with adjuvant external beam radiotherapy for intermediate- and high-risk patients following surgery, especially when only a simple hysterectomy has been performed inadvertently or when vaginal margins are close or positive. For all patients with clinical node-positive or locally advanced cervical cancers (stages IB2–IVA), concurrent cisplatin-based chemoradiotherapy with the addition of brachytherapy is the accepted standard.

3   Technique

Comprehensive staging and disease assessment is critical; thus a thorough gynecologic examination and cross-sectional imaging are essential to guide the plan of care based on the clinical stage. Pelvic MRI with water-based vaginal gel to enhance vaginal contrast is a more sensitive test for parametrial, uterine, and vaginal extension and tumor size measurements than CT [8, 9]. PET/CT provides a valuable assessment of nodal spread and distant metastases [10, 11]. Except for the rare situation of medically inoperable stage IA1 cervical cancer without lymphovascular space invasion, where the risk of extra-cervical spread is low and brachytherapy alone is indicated, external beam radiotherapy is integrated with weekly cisplatin 40 mg/m^2 (for FIGO IB2-IVA and node-positive patients) before brachytherapy. Prolongation of total treatment duration, including external beam and brachytherapy, beyond 8 weeks results in a 0.1–1 % decreases in local control and survival per day [12–15]. Thus, a detailed pelvic exam is performed in the 4th or 5th week of external beam radiotherapy to assess response to external beam and to prepare for the optimal timing of brachytherapy to minimize overall treatment time. This response-based evaluation will also help to make the final determination of the most appropriate

brachytherapy application: intracavitary, hybrid intracavitary-interstitial, or interstitial.

For most patients, brachytherapy is completed using an intracavitary technique with either a tandem-and-ring or tandem-and-ovoid applicator. A tandem-and-ring applicator has the advantages of easier placement and fixed reproducible geometry. However, in comparison to tandem and ovoids, it can increase dose to the vaginal surface, has less lateral throw-off of dose, and is sometimes not suitable for patients with a narrow vagina [16]. Compared to intracavitary applicators, a hybrid intracavitary-interstitial applicator offers the ability to increase lateral coverage in patients with residual bulky central or medial parametrial disease, to increase dose to asymmetric cervical tumors, or to decrease dose to critical organs while maintaining adequate coverage of the target volume [17–19]. While a hybrid intracavitary-interstitial applicator can improve lateral coverage, the range of improvement over an intracavitary application is usually at maximum 1 cm; thus template-based interstitial brachytherapy is the treatment of choice for patients with residual disease extending to the lateral parametria and distal half of the vagina, bladder, or rectum or for patients where the endocervical canal cannot be located because of distorted anatomy [16].

For intracavitary brachytherapy, dilation of the endocervical canal for tandem insertion is required. This can either be completed under general anesthesia followed by Smit sleeve placement at the first fraction, with subsequent applications performed on an outpatient basis with oral analgesia or conscious sedation or with serial dilations under general anesthesia or conscious sedation for each fraction. Brachytherapy is usually held should the absolute neutrophil count fall below 500 cells/μl and concurrent brachytherapy on the same day as chemotherapy is avoided to minimize increasing the risk of normal tissue complications. The patient is placed in the dorsal lithotomy position and a bladder catheter is placed. For difficult applications where ultrasound guidance is used (see Fig. 1), the bladder may be filled with saline to increase visualization of the uterus and cervix. Prior to the procedure, the patient is given instructions for a low-residue diet to minimize rectal distention. Rectosigmoid and bladder contrast are not necessary with MR-based brachytherapy planning, but are helpful with CT-based planning. A sterile speculum is inserted into the vagina to visualize the cervix. The tandem is inserted with the angle matching the direction of uterine flexion (with the length of the tandem based on uterine sound measurements and prior MRI imaging). Then the largest size ring or ovoids the patient can accommodate are placed followed by a rectal retractor or appropriate vaginal packing. The placement of an external stabilization device such as a perineal bar or base plate and clamp is then performed. Applicator placement geometry can be confirmed on fluoroscopy or orthogonal films or CT or MR scout films after the patient is returned to a more neutral supine position with thighs together, before the CT or MR scans are obtained in the event that applicator repositioning is needed.

Three-dimensional image-based planning offers a number of distinct clinical advantages over traditional two-dimensional point-based planning: confirmation of applicator placement including recognition of inadvertent perforation (see Fig. 1), improved tumor coverage (see Fig. 2), and decreased dose to critical organs (see Fig. 2) [20]. MRI-based planning offers superior soft tissue contrast and remains the standard for GTV and CTV definition [21]. The benefits of MRI over CT-based planning were highlighted by a prospective international comparison between CT- and MRI-based brachytherapy which showed that CT-based brachytherapy significantly overestimates the tumor width especially in the context of disease extending to the parametria [22]. More recently, a consensus contouring atlas by gynecologic brachytherapy experts was created comparing MRI- and CT-based planning, again highlighting that, for patients with a good treatment response and no parametrial involvement, CT- and MRI-based contouring were similar; however there was greater variation for cases with parametrial or sidewall extension especially those with a good response favoring MRI-based planning [23]. If MRI-based planning with each fraction is not possible, alternative methods include MRI with the first fraction and subsequent serial CT-based planning [24–26], CT-based planning [22, 27], or ultrasound-based planning [28, 29].

Guidelines for target and organ-at-risk contouring are outlined in the GEC-ESTRO and ABS working group consensus statements [16, 30–34]. The high-risk CTV (HR-CTV) includes the entire cervix (defined as 1 cm superior to the insertion of the uterine arteries, to the point of uterine widening, or a total length of approximately 3 cm) plus any residual tumor extension at the time of brachytherapy. The intermediate-risk CTV (IR-CTV) includes the HR-CTV plus the tumor extension at the time of diagnosis. The optimization process begins with

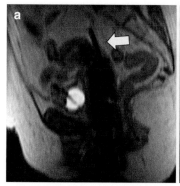 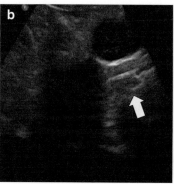 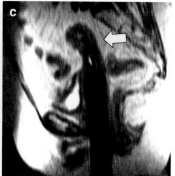

Fig. 1 Inadvertent uterine perforation recognized by image-based planning and ameliorated by ultrasound image-guided application. (**a**) Inadvertent perforation of the tandem through the posterior wall of the uterus. (**b**) Ultrasound-based image-guided replacement of the tandem. (**c**) Subsequent MRI-based planning confirming appropriate tandem placement

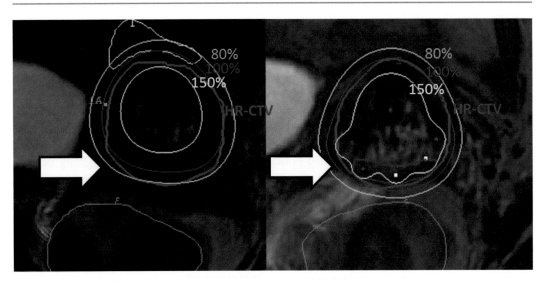

Fig. 2 Image-based brachytherapy benefits. Highlighted by the *arrows* is the HR-CTV volume extending posterior beyond the 100 % isodose line with significant unnecessary dose to the bladder neck, which is improved with posteriorly placed interstitial needles using a hybrid intracavitary-interstitial applicator and image-based manual optimization

a digitization of the source track, aided with a CT- or MR-compatible marker placed prior to image acquisition. Dwell positions and times are manually optimized for each fraction aiming for a HR-CTV $D_{90\%}$ ≥80–90 Gy while limiting the equivalent dose at 2 Gy per fraction ($EQD_{2\,Gy}$) to $D_{2\,cc}$ of the rectum/sigmoid and bladder ≤70 Gy and 80 Gy. Based on prospective studies from Korea and Vienna, if these organ-at-risk constraints are met, the risk of grade 2+ late toxicities should be <5 % [35–37]. For patients with a good response, the target HR-CTV $D_{90\%}$ $EQD_{2\,Gy}$ is 80–85 Gy, while for patients with a poor response, bulky tumors, or a histology of adenocarcinoma, dose escalation to an aimed $EQD_{2\,Gy}$ of 85–90 Gy may improve outcomes based on published dose response data [38, 39]. Fractionation patterns commonly used in the United States for intracavitary brachytherapy as outlined in the ABS guidelines are detailed in Table 1.

For hybrid intracavitary-interstitial applications, the decision to insert needles may be based on clinical examination or an MRI obtained after external beam indicating significant residual disease. Alternatively, intracavitary brachytherapy can be completed for the

Table 1 Regimens frequently used in the United States for intracavitary brachytherapy as outlined in the American Brachytherapy Society consensus guidelines

HDR brachytheraphy dose (after 1.8 Gy × 25 fractions of EBRT)	$EQD_{2\,Gy}$ (α/β of 10)
7 Gy × 4 fractions	84.0 Gy
6 Gy × 5 fractions	84.3 Gy
5 Gy × 6 fractions	81.8 Gy
5.5 Gy × 5 fractions	79.8 Gy

Gy gray, *$EQD_{2\,Gy}$* equivalent dose at 2 Gy per fraction, *HDR* high dose rate, *EBRT* external beam radiotherapy

first fraction; should HR-CTV $D_{90\%}$ ≥100 % coverage or critical organ dosimetry be suboptimal, then for subsequent fractions the planning MRI for the first fraction can be used to select interstitial needle location and depth for subsequent fractions [19]. Similar to the intracavitary technique, MRI-based planning is used to confirm applicator and interstitial needle placement. Planning is similar to that described above for intracavitary brachytherapy, with subsequent additive manual optimization to supplement missing coverage with the needles while respecting the previously described constraints for the rectum, bladder, and sigmoid [18, 34]. To avoid increasing mucosal dose at the needle region, on average only approximately 10 % of the total dwell time is linked to the needles [18, 34].

For interstitial applications, needle placement is typically performed under general or spinal anesthesia, with an epidural anesthesia catheter placed preoperatively in order to augment postoperative pain control. A tandem should be placed whenever feasible, as tandem placement is critical to maintaining adequate HR-CTV dose and central dose inhomogeneity [40]. To provide countertraction for needle insertion, a series of sutures can be placed in the cervix. Ideally needles should be placed with 1 cm spacing aiming to cover the gross disease plus an additional 1 cm margin; the spacing and geometry are often best maintained through the use of a perineal template. Perineal templates include the Syed-Neblett template or a MUPIT applicator or institutional customized variations [41, 42]. Titanium or plastic needles may help to reduce CT artifact and facilitate MRI-based planning [43]. Image guidance (either via transabdominal or transrectal ultrasound, CT, or MRI) helps to reduce the likelihood of inadvertent needle placement in the bowel, rectum, or bladder [44–47]. Needles placed within the bladder, rectum, or sigmoid should either be removed or not loaded unless there is direct extension of disease to these adjacent organs [48]. Antibiotic prophylaxis is administered to all patients after needle insertion. Following needle placement, the applicator may be sutured to the perineum to minimize interfraction displacement, and the needles are attached to the template with an adhesive bond if necessary. The patient is maintained on standard medical precautions for patients requiring prolonged immobilization including deep vein thrombosis prophylaxis, bladder catheter placement, analgesia with an epidural catheter if feasible, and antidiarrheal medications to prevent a bowel movement during the implant duration. CT- or MRI-based planning has also shown superiority over film-based planning [16]. Upon leaving the recovery room, a pelvic CT or MRI is completed for image-based planning with needle adjustment as needed under epidural analgesia [49–51]. Prior to image acquisition for CT-based planning, dilute contrast (30–70 cc) is placed into the bladder and 20–40 cc is inserted into the rectum. The CTV definition again follows the GEC-ESTRO and ABS guidelines as previously described [16, 30–34]. The goal of planning is to achieve a HR-CTV $D_{90\%} \geq 75$–85 Gy while limiting the $EQD_{2\,Gy}$ to $D_{2\,cc}$ of the rectum/sigmoid and bladder ≤ 70 Gy and 80 Gy, respectively. Fractionation schedules as outlined in the ABS guidelines include 3–3.5 Gy times 9 fractions, 4.25 Gy times 7 fractions, or 4.5–5 Gy times 5 fractions. The plan is manually optimized aiming for a CTV $D_{90\%}$ of approximately 75–85 Gy based on the extent of disease, critical organ doses, histology, and response to external beam radiotherapy.

4 Alternate Techniques

An alternative technique is to use low-dose-rate (LDR) or pulse-dose-rate brachytherapy (PDR). PDR brachytherapy uses a remote afterloading ^{192}IR source with a source strength of approximately 1 Ci (as compared to the 10 Ci ^{192}IR source used in HDR brachytherapy) to approximate the 0.4–0.6 Gy/h dose rate of LDR with the added benefit of optimization of source stepping and dwell times [31]. The lower dose rate of LDR or PDR as compared to HDR may reduce toxicity by enhancing sublethal damage repair; however this potential radiobiological advantage over HDR comes at the cost of increased applicator movement during treatment [52]. Cervical cancer brachytherapy using LDR or PDR would include all the above steps for applicator placement and immobilization precautions (with the added precaution of radiation exposure precautions for LDR). Typically for intracavitary applications, LDR or PDR brachytherapy is completed in two applications one within 4–6 weeks after the initiation of external beam radiotherapy and a second 1–2 weeks later, again maintaining a total treatment time of <8 weeks. The target contouring, aimed HR-CTV $D_{90\%}$, critical organ $D_{2\,cc}$, and manual optimization process remain similar to those described above.

5   Quality and Reporting Standards

There are several American Association of Physicists in Medicine (AAPM) task group publications that serve as invaluable resources for brachytherapy quality assurance; additionally the American Society for Radiation Oncology (ASTRO) has recently published an executive summary [53–57]. As outlined in the ABS guidelines for intracavitary brachytherapy, recommended documentation includes the type of applicator, prescription (including dose per fraction, total dose, and designated target volume), dose to point A or other prescription points, total reference air kerma, loading patterns, HR-CTV $D_{90\%}$ $D_{100\%}$ $V_{100\%}$, critical organ $D_{0.1\,cc}$ and $D_{2\,cc}$, vaginal mucosa dose, and isodose distributions [16].

6   Results

While the integration of concurrent chemotherapy translated into a significant improvement in overall survival across multiple prospective randomized trials, outcomes especially for locally advanced cervical cancer can still be improved [58]. However, more recently a number of publications have shown the value of image-based brachytherapy as the latest major improvement in cervical cancer [27, 39, 59–67]. Table 2 summarizes the outcomes of published international experiences for modern image-based brachytherapy with local control rates ranging from 79 to 100 % and grade 3+ complications from 0 to 14 %. When compared to conventional 2-dimensional brachytherapy, 3-dimensional image-based brachytherapy significantly improves local control and decreases the risk of significant morbidity. This was best highlighted in a recently published French prospective multi-institutional trial enrolling >700 cervical cancer patients across 20 centers, which compared 2-dimensional LDR or PDR brachytherapy to modern 3-dimensional (mainly CT-based) image-based PDR brachytherapy [59]. Three-dimensional image-based brachytherapy

significantly improved local control across subgroups (79–100 % versus 74–92 %, $p=0.003$) with a strong trend toward improved disease-free survival (60–90 % versus 55–87 %, $p=0.086$) while more than halving the risk of toxicity (3–9 % versus 13–23 %, $p=0.002$) as compared to conventional 2-dimensional film-based brachytherapy [59]. This prospective data is further validated by three-large international retrospective comparisons also showing a significant reduction in toxicity and improved local control and survival with image-based brachytherapy when compared to two-dimensional film-based brachytherapy [63, 65, 66]. Combined, these series set the standard for modern brachytherapy in cervical cancer with local control consistently >80–90 % (even in locally advanced disease) with the risk of grade 3+ toxicity <5–10 % (see Table 2).

7   Complications and Management

Increased adoption of image-based brachytherapy will help to reduce the risk of severe complications by more than half that are seen with two-dimensional film-based brachytherapy; however up to 5–10 % will still experience severe grade 3+ complications [59, 63, 65, 66]. The most severe complication is rectovaginal or vesicovaginal fistulae formation, which causes significant physical, social, and psychological distress due to persistent leakage of flatus, stool, or urine and associated bleeding, pain, and increased risk of infection. Management typically includes imaging (with contrast-enhanced pelvic MRI with water-based vaginal gel representing the preferred modality) and exam under anesthesia to confirm the presence of a fistula and rule out recurrent disease [68]. While it is important to confirm disease recurrence in the setting of fistulae as this often directs management, it must be recognized that mucosal changes are common following chemoradiation therapy and indiscriminate biopsies are a significant precipitant of fistula formation and are often low yield [69, 70]. Once a fistula is

Table 2 Summary of results for modern image-based brachytherapy in cervical cancer

	Local control (Actuarial)	Grade 3+ late toxicity (Actuarial)	Overall survival (Actuarial)
STIC (2-year) [59]	79–100 %	3–9 %	74–96 %
Vienna (3-year) [65]	95 %	8 %[a]	68 %
Leiden (3-year) [66]	93 %	7 %[a]	86 %
Aarhus (3-year) [63]	91 %	7 %	79 %
Milwaukee (2 year) [62]	100 %	11 %[a]	93 %
Thailand (2-year) [67]	98 %	4 %[a]	94 %
Paris (4-year) [60]	91 %	0 %	94 %
Australia (5-year) [64]	87–88 %	1–5 %	60 %
Korea (3-year) [61]	97 %	1 %	NR
Pittsburgh (3-year) [39]	92 %	3 %	77 %
Addenbrooke (3-year) [27]	96 %	14 %	82 %

NR not reported
[a]Crude toxicity rate as actuarial estimate was not reported

confirmed, fecal or urinary diversion is warranted, with the type of diversion individualized based on patient performance status, disease status, extent of prior radiotherapy, bowel health, and other factors. In the absence of recurrent disease, hyperbaric oxygen may promote fistula healing. Less commonly complex surgical repair may be attempted especially for vesicovaginal fistulae; however the success rate is significantly reduced in a previously irradiated field ranging from 40 to 100 % and must be balanced with increasing risks of surgical complications [71, 72]. More commonly patients may experience chronic rectal bleeding (daily or episodic, not uncommonly associated with incontinence or diarrhea) as a result of radiation proctopathy. In the era of 2-dimensional brachytherapy, the incidence of mild to severe rectal bleeding ranged from 5 to 30 % [73]. A retrospective cohort study comparing image-based brachytherapy to conventional film-based planning highlighted the opportunity for image-based planning to reduce the risk of rectal bleeding, where severe rectal bleeding was documented in 2 % of patients treated with CT-based brachytherapy as compared to 13 % of those treated with conventional 2-dimensional brachytherapy planning, $p = 0.02$ [61]. For patients experiencing mild to moderate bleeding, conservative management with corticosteroid, sucralfate, or mesalamine enemas is effective in >70–80 % of patients [73–78].

Should bleeding persist or increase in severity, endoscopic evaluation with intrarectal thermal or photocoagulation is the most effective means of reducing moderate to severe bleeding [79, 80]. Vaginal stenosis remains a significant source of morbidity with most patients (upwards of 90 %) experiencing mild to moderate vaginal morbidity most commonly manifested as vaginal stenosis or dryness [81]. Dilator use remains an important part of mitigating risks of vaginal stenosis.

References

1. Jemal A, Bray F, Center MM et al (2011) Global cancer statistics. CA Cancer J Clin 61:69–90
2. Parkin DM, Bray F, Ferlay J, Pisani P (2005) Global cancer statistics, 2002. CA Cancer J Clin 55:74–108
3. Lanciano RM, Won M, Coia LR, Hanks GE (1991) Pretreatment and treatment factors associated with improved outcomes in squamous cell carcinoma of the uterine cervix: a final report of the 1973 and 1978 patterns of care studies. Int J Radiat Oncol Biol Phys 20:667–676
4. Montana GS, Hanlon AL, Brickner TJ et al (1995) Carcinoma of the cervix: patterns of care studies: reviews of 1978, 1983, and 1988–1989 surveys. Int J Radiat Oncol Biol Phys 32:1481–1486
5. Han K, Milosevic M, Fyles A, Pintilie M, Viswanathan AN (2013) Trends in the utilization of brachytherapy in cervical cancer in the United States. Int J Radiat Oncol Biol Phys 87:111–119
6. Gill BS, Lin JF, Krivak TC et al (2014) National cancer data base analysis of radiation therapy consolidation modality for cervical cancer: the impact

of new technological advancements. Int J Radiat Oncol Biol Phys 90:1083–1090

7. Landoni F, Maneo A, Colombo A et al (1997) Randomized study of radical surgery versus radiotherapy for stage Ib-IIa cervical cancer. Lancet 350:535–540

8. Hricak H, Gatsonis C, Coakley FV et al (2007) Early invasive cervical: CT and MRI imaging in preoperative evaluation – ACRIN/GOG comparative study of diagnostic performance and interobserver variability. Radiology 245:491–498

9. Mitchell DG, Snyder B, Coakley F et al (2006) Early invasive cervical cancer: tumor delineation by magnetic resonance imaging, computed tomography, and clinical examination, verified by pathologic results, in the ACRIN 6651/GOG 183 Intergroup Study. J Clin Oncol 24:5687–5694

10. Kidd EA, Sigel BA, Dehdashti F et al (2010) Lymph node staging by positron emission tomography in cervical cancer: relationship to prognosis. J Clin Oncol 28:2108–2113

11. Tsai CS, Lai CH, Chang TC et al (2010) A prospective randomized trial to study the impact of pretreatment FDG-PET for cervical cancer patients with MRI-detected positive pelvic but negative para-aortic lymphadenopathy. Int J Radiat Oncol Biol Phys 76:477–484

12. Grinsky T, Rey A, Roche B et al (1993) Overall treatment time in advanced cervical carcinomas: a critical parameter in treatment outcome. Int J Radiat Oncol Biol Phys 27:1051–1056

13. Lanciano RM, Pajak TF, Matrz K et al (1993) The influence of treatment time on outcome for squamous cell cancer of the uterine cervix treated with radiation: a patterns-of-care study. Int J Radiat Oncol Biol Phys 25:391–397

14. Perez CA, Grigsby PW, Castro-Vita H et al (1995) Carcinoma of the uterine cervix: impact of prolongation of overall treatment time and timing of brachytherapy on outcome of radiation therapy. Int J Radiat Oncol Biol Phys 32:1275–1288

15. Petereit DG, Sarkaria JN, Chappell R et al (1995) The adverse effect of treatment prolongation in cervical carcinoma. Int J Radiat Oncol Biol Phys 32:1301–1307

16. Viswanathan AN, Thomadsen B, American Brachytherapy Society Cervical Cancer Recommendations Committee, American Brachytherapy Society (2012) American brachytherapy society guidelines for locally advanced carcinoma of the cervix: part I general principles. Brachytherapy 11:33–46

17. Dimopoulos JC, Kirisits C, Petric P et al (2006) The Vienna applicator for combined intracavitary and interstitial brachytherapy of cervical cancer: clinical feasibility and preliminary results. Int J Radiat Oncol Biol Phys 66:83–90

18. Kirisits C, Lang S, Dimopoulos J et al (2006) The Vienna applicator for combined intracavitary and interstitial brachytherapy of cervical cancer: design, application, treatment planning, and dosimteric results. Int J Radiat Oncol Biol Phys 65:624–630

19. Nomden CN, de Leeuw AA, Moerland MA et al (2012) Clinical use of the Utrecht applicator for combined intracavitary/interstitial brachytherapy treatment in locally advanced cervical cancer. Int J Radiat Oncol Biol Phys 82:1424–1430

20. Vargo JA, Beriwal S (2014) Image-based brachytherapy for cervical cancer. World J Clin Oncol 5:921–930

21. Dimopoulos JC, Schard G, Berger D et al (2006) Systematic evaluation of MRI findings in different stages of treatment of cervical cancer: potential of MRI on delineation of target, pathoanatomic structures, and organs at risk. Int J Radiat Oncol Biol Phys 64:1380–1388

22. Viswanathan AN, Dimopoulos J, Kirisits C et al (2007) Computed tomography versus magnetic resonance imaging-based contouring in cervical cancer brachytherapy: results of a prospective trial and preliminary guidelines for standardized contours. Int J Radiat Oncol Biol Phys 68:491–498

23. Viswanathan AN, Erickson B, Gaffney DK et al (2014) Comparison and consensus guidelines for delineation of clinical target volume for CT- and MR-based brachytherapy in locally advanced cervical cancer. Int J Radiat Oncol Biol Phys 90:320–328

24. Beriwal S, Kim H, Coon D et al (2009) Single magnetic resonance imaging vs magnetic resonance imaging/computed tomography planning in cervical cancer brachytherapy. Clin Oncol (R Coll Radiol) 21:483–487

25. Beriwal S, Kannan N, Kim H et al (2011) Three-dimensional high dose rate intracavitary image-guided brachytherapy for the treatment of cervical cancer using a hybrid magnetic resonance imaging/computed tomography approach: feasibility and early results. Clin Oncol (R Coll Radiol) 23:685–690

26. Nesvacil N, Pötter R, Sturdza A et al (2013) Adaptive image guided brachytherapy for cervical cancer: a combined MRI-/CT-planning technique with MRI only at first fraction. Radiother Oncol 107:75–81

27. Tan LT, Coles CE, Hart C et al (2009) Clinical impact of computed tomography-based image-guided brachytherapy for cervix cancer using the tandem-ring applicator – the Addenbrooke's experience. Clin Oncol (R Coll Radiol) 21:175–182

28. Mahantshetty U, Khanna N, Swamidas J et al (2012) Trans-abdominal ultrasound (US) and magnetic resonance imaging (MRI) correlation for conformal intracavitary brachytherapy in carcinoma of the uterine cervix. Radiother Oncol 102:130–134

29. Van Dyk S, Narayan K, Fisher R et al (2009) Conformal brachytherapy planning for cervical cancer using transabdominal ultrasound. Int J Radiat Oncol Biol Phys 75:64–70

30. Haie-Meder C, Pötter R, Van Limbergen E et al (2005) Recommendations from gynecological (GYN) GEC-ESTRO working group (I): concepts and terms

in 3D image based treatment planning in cervix cancer brachytherapy with emphasis on MRI assessment of GTV and CTV. Radiother Oncol 74:235–245

31. Lee LJ, Das IJ, Higgins SA et al (2012) American brachytherapy society consensus guidelines for locally advanced carcinoma of the cervix: Part III low-dose-rate and pulsed-dose-rate brachytherapy. Brachytherapy 11:53–57

32. Nag S, Cardenes H, Chang S et al (2004) Proposed guidelines for image-based intracavitary brachytherapy for cervical carcinoma: report from image-guided brachytherapy working group. Int J Radiat Oncol Biol Phys 60:1160–1172

33. Pötter R, Haie-Meder C, Van Limbergen E et al (2006) Recommendations from gynecological (GYN) GEC-ESTRO working group (II): concepts and terms in 3D image based treatment planning in cervix cancer brachytherapy-3D dose volumes parameters and aspects of 3D image-based anatomy, radiation physics, radiobiology. Radiother Oncol 78:67–77

34. Viswanathan AN, Beriwal S, De Los Santos JF et al (2012) American brachytherapy society consensus guidelines for locally advanced carcinoma of the cervix: part II high-dose-rate brachytherapy. Brachytherapy 11:47–52

35. Georg P, Kirisits C, Goldner G et al (2009) Correlation of dose-volume parameters, endoscopic and clinical rectal side effects in cervix cancer patients treated with definitive radiotherapy including MRI-based brachytherapy. Radiother Oncol 91:173–180

36. Georg P, Pötter R, Georg D et al (2012) Dose effect relationship for late side effects of the rectum and urinary bladder in magnetic resonance image-guided adaptive cervix cancer brachytherapy. Int J Radiat Oncol Biol Phys 82:653–657

37. Koom WS, Sohn DK, Kim JY et al (2007) Computed tomography-based high-dose-rate intracavitary brachytherapy for uterine cervical cancer: preliminary demonstration of correlation between dose-volume parameters and rectal mucosal changes observed by flexible sigmoidoscopy. Int J Radiat Oncol Biol Phys 68:1446–1454

38. Dimopoulos JC, Lang S, Kirisits C et al (2009) Dose-volume histogram parameters and local tumor control in magnetic resonance image-guided cervical cancer brachytherapy. Int J Radiat Oncol Biol Phys 75: 56–63

39. Gill BS, Kim H, Houser CJ et al (2015) MRI-guided high dose rate intracavitary brachytherapy for treatment of cervical cancer: the University of Pittsburgh experience. Int J Radiat Oncol Biol Phys 91(3):540–547

40. Viswanathan A, Cormack R, Rawal B et al (2009) Increasing brachytherapy dose predicts survival for interstitial and tandem-based radiation for stage IIIB cervical cancer. Int J Gynecol Cancer 19:1402–1406

41. Martinez A, Cox RS, Edmundson GK (1984) A multiple-site perineal applicator (MUPIT) for treatment of prostatic, anorectal, and gynecologic malignancies. Int J Radiat Oncol Biol Phys 10:297–305

42. Syed A, Putjawala AA, Neblett D et al (1986) Transperineal interstitial intracavitary "Syed-Neblett" applicator in the treatment of carcinoma of the uterine cervix. Endocuriether hypertherm Oncol 2:1–13

43. Popowski Y, Hiltbrand E, Joliat D et al (2004) Open magnetic resonance imaging using titanium-zirconium needles: improved accuracy for interstitial brachytherapy implants? Int J Radiat Oncol Biol Phys 47:759–765

44. Fokdal L, Tanderup K, Nielsen SK et al (2011) Image and laparoscopic guided interstitial brachytherapy for locally advanced primary or recurrent gynaecological cancer using the adaptive GEC ESTRO target concept. Radiother Oncol 100:473–479

45. Lee LJ, Damato AL, Viswanathan AN (2013) Clinical outcomes of high-dose-rate interstitial gynecologic brachytherapy using real-time CT guidance. Brachytherapy 12:303–310

46. Stock RG, Chan K, Terk M et al (1997) A new technique for performing Syed-Neblett template interstitial implants for gynecologic malignancies using transrectal-ultrasound guidance. Int J Radiat Oncol Biol Phys 37:819–825

47. Viswanathan AN, Szymonifka J, Tempany-Afdhal CM et al (2013) A prospective trial of real-time magnetic resonance-guided catheter placement in interstitial gynecologic brachytherapy. Brachytherapy 12:240–247

48. Shah AP, Strauss JB, Gielda BT et al (2010) Toxicity associated with bowel or bladder puncture during gynecologic interstitial brachytherapy. Int J Radiat Oncol Biol Phys 77:171–179

49. Eisbruch A, Johnston CM, Martel MK et al (1998) Customized gynecologic interstitial implants: CT-based planning, dose evaluation, and optimization aided by laparotomy. Int J Radiat Oncol Biol Phys 40:1087–1093

50. Erickson B, Albano K, Gillin M (1996) CT-guided interstitial implantation of gynecologic malignancies. Int J Radiat Oncol Biol Phys 36:699–709

51. Erickson B, Albano K, Gillin M (1996) Magnetic resonance imaging following interstitial implantation of pelvic malignancies. Radiat Oncol Invest 2: 298–300

52. Brenner DJ, Hall EJ (1991) Conditions for the equivalence of continuous to pulsed low dose rate brachytherapy. Int J Radiat Oncol Biol Phys 20: 181–190

53. Fraass B, Doppke M, Hunt G et al (1998) American Association of Physicists in Medicine Radiation Therapy Committee Task Group 53: quality assurance for clinical radiotherapy treatment planning. Med Phys 25:1773–1829

54. Glasgow GP, Bourland JD, Grigsby PW et al (1993) Remote afterloading technology: a report of AAPM Task Group No. 41. American Institute of Physics, New York

55. Kubo HD, Glasgow GP, Pethel TD et al (1998) High dose-rate brachytherapy treatment delivery: a report of the AAPM Radiation Therapy Committee Task Group No. 59. Med Phys 25:375–403

56. Nath R, Anderson LL, Meli JA et al (1997) Code of practice for brachytherapy physics: report of the AAPM Radiation Therapy Committee Task Group No. 56. Med Phys 24:1557–1598

57. Thomadsen BR, Erickson BA, Eifel PJ et al (2014) A review of safety, quality management, and practice guidelines for high-dose-rate brachytherapy: executive summary. Pract Radiat Oncol 4:65–70

58. Chemoradiotherapy for Cervical Cancer Meta-Analysis Collaboration (2008) Reducing uncertainties about the effects of chemoradiotherapy for cervical cancer: a systematic review and meta-analysis of individual patient data from 18 randomized trials. J Clin Oncol 26:5802–5812

59. Charra-Brunaud C, Harter V, Delannes M et al (2012) Impact of 3D image-based PDR brachytherapy on outcome of patients treated for cervix carcinoma in France: results of the French STIC prospective study. Radiother Oncol 103:305–313

60. Haie-Meder C, Chargari C, Rey A et al (2009) DVH parameters and outcome for patients with early-stage cervical cancer treated with preoperative MRI-based low dose rate brachytherapy followed by surgery. Radiother Oncol 93:316–321

61. Kang HC, Shin KH, Park SY et al (2010) 3D CT-based high-dose-rate brachytherapy for cervical cancer: clinical impact on late rectal bleeding and local control. Radiother Oncol 97:507–513

62. Kharofa J, Morrow N, Kelly T et al (2014) 3-T MRI-based adaptive brachytherapy for cervix cancer: treatment technique and initial clinical outcomes. Brachytherapy 13:319–325

63. Lindegaard JC, Fokdal LU, Nielsen SK et al (2013) MRI-guided adaptive radiotherapy in locally advanced cervical cancer from a Nordic perspective. Acta Oncol 52:1510–1519

64. Narayan K, van Dyk S, Bernshaw D et al (2009) Comparative study of LDR (Manchester system) and HDR image-guided conformal brachytherapy of cervical cancer: patterns of failure, late complications, and survival. Int J Radiat Oncol Biol Phys 74:1529–1535

65. Pötter R, Georg P, Dimopoulos JC et al (2011) Clinical outcome of protocol based image (MRI) guided adaptive brachytherapy combined with 3D conformal radiotherapy with or without chemotherapy in patients with locally advanced cervical cancer. Radiother Oncol 100:116–123

66. Rijkmans EC, Nout RA, Rutten IH et al (2014) Improved survival of patients with cervical cancer treated with image-guided brachytherapy compared with conventional brachytherapy. Gynecol Oncol 135:231–238

67. Tharavichitkul E, Chakrabandhu S, Wanwilairat S et al (2013) Intermediate-term results of image-guided brachytherapy and high-technology external beam radiotherapy in cervical cancer: Chiang Mai University experience. Gynecol Oncol 130:81–85

68. Narayanan P, Nobbenhuis M, Reynolds KM et al (2009) Fistulas in malignant gynecologic disease: etiology, imaging, and management. Radiographics 29:1073–1083

69. Anderson JR, Spence RA, Parks TG et al (1984) Rectovaginal fistulae following radiation treatment for cervical carcinoma. Ulster Med J 53:84–87

70. Feddock J, Randall M, Kudrimoti M et al (2014) Impact of post-radiation biopsies on development of fistulae in patients with cervical cancer. Gynecol Oncol 133:263–267

71. Angioli R, Penalver M, Muzi L et al (2003) Guidelines of how to manage vesicovaginal fistula. Crit Rev Oncol Hematol 48:295–304

72. Jao SW, Beart RW, Gunderson LL (1986) Surgical treatment of radiation injuries of the colon and rectum. Am J Surg 151:272–277

73. Chun M, Kang S, Kil HJ et al (2004) Rectal bleeding and its management after irradiation for uterine cervical cancer. Int J Radiat Oncol Biol Phys 58:98–105

74. Colwell JC, Goldberg M (2000) A review of radiation proctitis in the treatment of prostate cancer. J Wound Ostomy Continence Nurs 27:179–187

75. Kochhar R, Patel F, Dhar A et al (1991) Radiation-induced proctosigmoiditis: prospective, randomized, double-blind controlled trial of oral sulfasalazine plus rectal steroids versus rectal sucralfate. Dig Dis Sci 36:103–107

76. Kochhar R, Sriram PV, Sharma SC et al (1999) Natural history of late radiation proctosigmoiditis treated with topical sucralfate suspension. Dig Dis Sci 44:973–978

77. Shipley WU, Zietman AL, Hanks GE et al (1994) Treatment related sequelae following external beam radiation for prostate cancer: a review with an update in patients with stages T1 and T2 tumor. J Urol 152:1799–1805

78. Teshima T, Hanks GE, Hanlon AL et al (1997) Rectal bleeding after conformal 3D treatment of prostate cancer: time to occurrence, response to treatment and duration of morbidity. Int J Radiat Oncol Biol Phys 39:77–83

79. Jensen DM, Machicado GA, Cheng S et al (1997) Randomized prospective study of endoscopic bipolar electrocoagulation and heater probe treatment of chronic rectal bleeding from radiation telangiectasia. Gastrointest Endosc 45:20–25

80. Viggiano TR, Zighelboim J, Ahlquist DA et al (1993) Endoscopic Nd: YAG laser coagulation of bleeding from radiation proctopathy. Gastrointest Endosc 39:513–517

81. Kirchheiner K, Nout RA, Tanderup K et al (2014) Manifestation pattern of early-late vaginal morbidity after definitive radiation (chemo) therapy and image-guided adaptive brachytherapy for locally advanced cervical cancer: an analysis from the EMBRACE study. Int J Radiat Oncol Biol Phys 89:88–95

Gynecologic Brachytherapy: Vaginal Cancer

John A. Vargo, Akila N. Viswanathan,
Beth A. Erickson, and Sushil Beriwal

Abstract

Primary vaginal cancer is the rarest of gynecologic malignancies by anatomic site. Despite the rarity, vaginal cancer requires special consideration in treatment and frequently requires brachytherapy for local control and cure.

1   Introduction

Primary vaginal cancer is a rare malignancy representing <2 % of all gynecologic cancers; more commonly vaginal cancers represent extension from cervical or vulvar cancer, metastases, or recurrences from endometrial, cervical, vulvar, or other primary sites. The majority (80–90 %) of primary vaginal cancers are squamous cell histology, followed by adenocarcinoma (including clear-cell adenocarcinoma linked to diethylstilbestrol exposure in utero), melanoma, and sarcomas, respectively. Human papillomavirus (HPV, most commonly the HPV-16 serotype) is an oncogenic driver in 50–75 % of primary vaginal cancer, with HPV-positive vaginal cancers carrying an improved prognosis [1, 2]. Except for highly select stage I patients, oncologic organ preserving surgery is not feasible. Thus definitive radiotherapy is the preferred local treatment modality, with brachytherapy considered an integral part of definitive radiotherapy for primary and recurrent vaginal cancers [3–5].

J.A. Vargo, MD • S. Beriwal, MD (✉)
Department of Radiation Oncology,
University of Pittsburgh, Pittsburgh, PA, USA
e-mail: vargoja2@upmc.edu; beriwals@upmc.edu

A.N. Viswanathan, MD, MPH
Department of Radiation Oncology, Brigham and
Women's Hospital and Dana-Farber Cancer Institute,
Harvard Medical School, Boston, MA, USA

B.A. Erickson, MD, FACR, FASTRO
Department of Radiation Oncology,
Medical College of Wisconsin, Milwaukee, WI, USA
e-mail: berickson@mcw.edu

2   Indications

For patients with FIGO stage I disease, brachytherapy alone or in combination with external beam radiotherapy or surgical resection represents potentially reasonable plans of care [6].

© Springer International Publishing Switzerland 2016
P. Montemaggi et al. (eds.), *Brachytherapy: An International Perspective*, Medical Radiology,
DOI 10.1007/978-3-319-26791-3_16

Otherwise for patients with FIGO stage II–IVA primary vaginal cancer or vaginal recurrences of other gynecological primaries, brachytherapy is commonly used to boost sites of gross disease following concurrent pelvic chemoradiotherapy to address the at-risk intervening lymphatics, paravaginal tissue, and regional lymph nodes [5–7].

3   Technique

The key first step in vaginal brachytherapy includes a pre-therapy gynecologic exam and staging imaging commonly including a CT of the chest, abdomen, and pelvis or full-body PET/CT, plus a pelvic MRI with water-based vaginal gel [8, 9]. The selection of intracavitary versus interstitial brachytherapy depends on the location, extent, and thickness of disease assessed both on pre- and post-external beam radiotherapy, wherein an exam and staging pelvic MRI with water-based vaginal gel are extremely helpful in guiding subsequent brachytherapy planning. Fiducial markers can be placed at the time of exam to mark gross disease. For patients with superficial lesions (≤0.5 cm in thickness on gynecologic exam following external beam radiotherapy), especially those in the proximal or mid-vagina, intracavitary brachytherapy is commonly completed using a single-channel vaginal cylinder or other intravaginal applicators. The technique for intracavitary vaginal brachytherapy has been extensively detailed in the endometrial cancer section including applicator placement and planning for patients following hysterectomy. For patients with an intact uterus, an intrauterine tandem is commonly used to improve vaginal forniceal coverage. For intracavitary brachytherapy in patients with disease limited to a single-wall or distal vaginal cancer, some institutions advocate for a shielded single-channel vaginal cylinder to minimize dose to uninvolved vagina and critical organs (most notably urethra and rectum); however this technique is challenged by applicator availability, applicator weight, and non-compatibility with

image-based planning [10]. Others have advocated for the use of a multichannel intravaginal cylinder (see Fig. 1), which may allow for improved dose modulation over a single-channel intravaginal cylinder especially in vaginal cancers limited to a single vaginal wall in the middle or distal vagina [11–13].

Image-based planning for vaginal cancer is currently the preferred technique [14–18]. Following intracavitary applicator placement, image-based planning using either a T2-weighted pelvic MRI or non-contrast-enhanced pelvic CT is completed with each fraction. The CTV is based on a combination of both the pre- and post-external beam radiotherapy extent of disease [17]. The HR-CTV includes the post-external beam radiotherapy GTV to the residual disease thickness and the circumference of vagina at the level of residual disease to the vaginal surface (see Fig. 1). The IR-CTV includes the regional of initial tumor extension plus the remaining vagina to account for potential microscopic submucosal spread through intervening lymphatics [17]. Based on patterns of failure predominately in the HR-CTV volume, others are exploring the hypothesis that the 45–50.4 Gy of external beam radiotherapy may be sufficient to address this microscopic disease by modifying the IR-CTV from the entire vagina to the length of initially involved vagina in an attempt to reduce vaginal morbidity [14, 17]. The HDR dose and fractionation is modulated based on the extent of disease, response to external beam radiotherapy, location within the vagina, and dose of external beam radiation therapy. Following 45–50.4 Gy of external beam radiation therapy with concurrent weekly cisplatin chemotherapy [19], fractionation schedules as outlined in the American Brachytherapy Society guidelines include 4–5.5 Gy times 5 fractions, 3 Gy times 9–10 fractions, or 7 Gy times 3 fractions, though other fractionations are feasible while respecting organs-at-risk dose limits [20]. The plan is optimized using points in the apex, curvature of the cylinder dome, and the lateral vaginal mucosa. The plan is then manually optimized to cover the contoured HR-CTV aiming for a $D_{90\%}$ EQD_{2Gy} of 75 Gy with a range of 70–80 Gy as described in

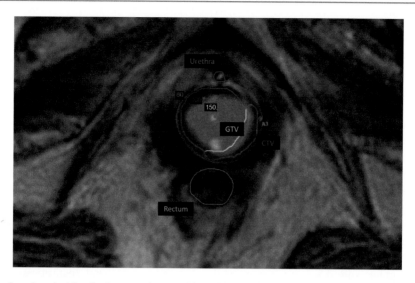

Fig. 1 Image-based vaginal brachytherapy using a multi-channel intravaginal cylinder with MRI-based planning. The GTV at the time of brachytherapy is outlined in green. The CTV is outlined in *red*, which incorporates the entire circumference of the vagina at the level of disease to the surface of the vaginal cylinder and the thickness of the GTV at the time of brachytherapy. The isodose cloud highlights that the multichannel cylinder and image-based planning allow the dose to be extended laterally to increase coverage of the GTV at the time of brachytherapy, the *yellow* cloud represents the 150 % isodose, *red* represents the 100 % isodose, and *green* represents the 80 % isodose

the American Brachytherapy Society guidelines [20], while maintaining the rectal $D_{2\,cc}$ <70 Gy, sigmoid $D_{2\,cc}$ <70 Gy, bladder $D_{2\,cc}$ <80 Gy, and urethral maximum dose <100 % of the prescription dose [21, 22]. No vaginal dose constraint is implemented, though it should be recognized that the estimated tolerance of the distal vagina (~80 Gy) is significantly less than the proximal vagina (~120 Gy).

Interstitial brachytherapy is recommended for patients with disease thickness beyond the range of a cylinder following external beam radiotherapy and is used at some institutions for distal vaginal cancers confined to a single wall to limit dose to the uninvolved vagina and surrounding critical organs [20]. Interstitial needle placement is typically completed under general or spinal anesthesia. Additionally, epidural anesthesia augments pain control postoperatively and allows for applicator adjustment based on imaging. For patients with apical lesions, a perineal template with a vaginal cylinder is recommended to guide needle placement. For distal vaginal lesions, either a free-hand or template-based technique can be used. Ideally needles should be placed with 1 cm spacing aiming to cover the gross disease plus an additional 1 cm margin. While traditionally steel needles were used for interstitial brachytherapy, titanium or plastic needles may help to reduce CT artifact and facilitate MRI-based planning [23]. Laparoscopic guidance (especially for apical lesions in close proximity to small bowel) or image guidance (either via ultrasound, CT, or MRI depending on expertise and availability) helps to reduce the likelihood of inadvertent needle placement in the bowel, rectum, or bladder [24–28]. Additionally, needle placement within the urethra or rectovaginal septum should be avoided, unless one is intentionally attempting to place a hydrogel spacer in between the rectum and vaginal wall or there is tumor extending to these locations [29]. Following needle placement, the applicator may be sutured to the labia to minimize interfraction displacement. The patients are maintained on standard medical precautions for patients requiring prolonged immobilization including deep vein thrombosis prophylaxis, Foley catheter placement, analgesia with an epidural catheter if feasible, and antidiarrheal medications.

Following postoperative recovery, pelvic CT or MRI depending on image-based planning preference is taken with needle adjustment as needed. To improve organ-at-risk delineation for CT-based planning, diluted contrast 50–70 cc is placed into the bladder with 20–40 cc of rectal contrast. Needles inadvertently placed in the bladder or rectum do not necessarily need to be removed; however, loading in these locations must be avoided and antibiotic prophylaxis should be given [30]. CTV delineation includes the pretreatment vaginal circumference length and the gross disease at the time of brachytherapy. Optimization points are placed within the outer portion of the CTV volume, aiming for between 100 and 200 points with 0.5–1 cm spacing, and then the plan is manually optimized aiming for a CTV $D_{90\%}$ between 70 and 80 Gy modified based on the extent of disease, location within the vagina, and response to external beam radiotherapy. Interstitial HDR brachytherapy is delivered on an inpatient basis delivered twice daily with a minimum interaction interval of 6 h [18, 20].

4   Alternate Techniques

An alternative technique would be to use low-dose rate brachytherapy as described in a number of older institutional series [31–41]. Vaginal brachytherapy using LDR would include all the above steps for applicator placement and immobilization precautions (with the added precaution of radiation exposure precautions). Depending on external beam radiotherapy dose, extent of disease, and response to external beam radiation therapy, LDR would be administered at a dose rate of 35–70 cGy/h with a prescription dose between 25 and 40 Gy aiming for a total dose of 70–85 Gy.

5   Quality and Reporting Standards

A detailed, signed prescription including the treatment site, prescription point, total dose, dose per fraction, fractionation, and radioiso-

tope is imperative. Prescribed dose is recorded as $D_{90\%}$ for the contoured CTV, aiming for a $D_{90\%} \geq 100\%$. We recommend that the critical organ doses be carried across brachytherapy fractions and incorporate any external beam radiotherapy dose, using an $EQD_{2\,Gy}$ calculator, aiming for the rectal $D_{2\,cc} \leq 70$ Gy, sigmoid $D_{2\,cc} \leq 70$ Gy, and bladder $D_{2\,cc} \leq 80$ Gy. There are several AAPM task group publications that serve as invaluable resources for brachytherapy quality assurance [42–45].

6   Results

A number of recent institutional series have documented high rates of local control (92–96 %) and low rates of toxicity (2–23 %) when incorporating image-based brachytherapy for primary vaginal cancer [14, 16–18]; however, the majority of outcome data for brachytherapy in vaginal cancer comes from series examining the role of definitive radiation therapy as a salvage modality for patients with vaginal recurrence of endometrial cancer. Table 1 highlights the results of numerous institutional series using a combination of external beam radiation therapy and LDR brachytherapy for vaginal recurrence of endometrial cancer highlighting that definitive radiation therapy, including brachytherapy, salvages approximately 50 % of patients with vaginal recurrence of endometrial cancer with published 5-year overall sur-

Table 1 Summary of clinical outcomes for two-dimensional LDR brachytherapy plus external beam radiotherapy salvage for vaginal recurrence of endometrial cancer

	n	Local control (%)	5-year overall survival (%)
Jhingran et al. [34]	91	75	43
Currant et al. [35]	47	48	31
Lin et al. [36]	50	74	53
Sears et al. [37]	45	54	44
Hoekstra et al. [38]	26	84	44
Wylie et al. [39]	58	65	53
Jereczek et al. [40]	73	48	25
Morgan et al. [41]	34	85	68

vivals ranging from 25 to 68 % and local control of 48–85 % [34–41]. Table 2 summarizes the results for HDR brachytherapy for vaginal recurrence of endometrial cancer, highlighting the importance of image-based planning where the rates of local control are similar across the point-based and image-based series ranging from 74 to 100 % [46–48]; however, grade 3+ toxicity in series incorporating image-based planning ranges from 0 to 5 % compared to 5–50 % for series using two-dimensional point-based planning [15, 16].

7 Complications and Management

As highlighted in Table 2, the major toxicity following definitive radiation therapy for vaginal cancer, including vagina brachytherapy, is vaginal stenosis or other toxicity such as ulceration, for which the use of modern radiation planning techniques including image-based brachytherapy can help to reduce such toxicity. Similar to the description in the cervix brachy-

therapy section, a vaginal dilator is recommended to maintain patency of the vagina by disrupting the formation of adhesions and fibrous tissue. For patients who develop vaginal ulceration, initial management with hydrogen peroxide douching (1/10 dilution with water) intravaginally one to two times per day for 2–4 weeks can aid healing. While rare, patients who suffer persistent vaginal ulceration or necrosis, hyperbaric oxygen therapy should be considered as small series have shown high rates of resolution both for vaginal ulceration and vaginal ulceration in association with rectovaginal fistula [49, 50]. Additionally, Trental (400 mg tid) can also aid in healing necrotic vaginal tissue. Chronic toxicities and management for rectal and bladder injury are reviewed extensively in the cervical cancer brachytherapy section. A comprehensive discussion of the management of complication following pelvic radiation therapy is beyond the scope of this text, and for additional information the reader is directed to a recently published dedicated review of complication following pelvic radiotherapy including brachytherapy [51].

Table 2 Summary of clinical outcomes for HDR brachytherapy (including image-based planning) plus external beam radiotherapy salvage for vaginal recurrence of endometrial cancer

	n	Technique	CR (%)	LC	Vaginal toxicity (%)	Bladder toxicity (%)	Gastrointestinal toxicity (%)
Petignat et al. [46]	22	4-field EBRT 2D HDRB	100	100 %, 5 years	50	0	18
Pai et al. [47]	20	4-field EBRT 2D HDRB	90	74 %, 10 years	0	5	5
Sorb et al. [48]	40	4-field EBRT 2D HDRB	92	75 %, 5 years	19[a]	3	11
Image-based HDR							
Vargo et al. [15]	41	IMRT 3D-based HDRB	93 %	95 %, 3 years	5	0	4
Lee et al. [16]	31[b]	4-field EBRT 3D-based HDRB	NR	94 %, 2 years	3	0	0

IMRT intensity modulated radiotherapy, *3D* three-dimensional, *2D* two-dimensional, *HDRB* high-dose rate brachytherapy, *NR* not recorded, *GI* gastrointestinal
[a]19 % grade 2–3 vaginal toxicity
[b]Results for the 31 patients not receiving prior radiotherapy, local failure from this series in re-irradiation cohort was 39 % with a 23 % rate of grade 3 complications

References

1. Alemany L, Saunier M, Tinoco L et al (2014) Large contribution of human papillomavirus in vaginal neoplastic lesions: a worldwide study in 597 samples. Eur J Cancer 50:2846–2854

2. Brunner AH, Grimm C, Polterauer S et al (2011) The prognostic role of human papillomavirus in patients with vaginal cancer. Int J Gynecol Cancer 21:923–929

3. Stock RG, Mychalczak B, Armstrong JG et al (1992) The importance of brachytherapy technique in the management of primary carcinoma of the vagina. Int J Radiat Oncol Biol Phys 24:747–753

4. Rajagopalan MS, Xu KM, Lin J et al (2015) Patterns of care and brachytherapy boost utilization for vaginal cancer in the United States. Pract Radiat Oncol 5:56–61

5. Rajagopalan MS, Xu KM, Lin JF et al (2014) Adoption and impact of concurrent chemoradiation therapy for vaginal cancer: a National Cancer Data Base (NCDB) study. Gynecol Oncol 135:495–502

6. Frank SJ, Jhingran A, Levenback C et al (2005) Definitive radiation therapy for squamous cell carcinoma of the vagina. Int J Radiat Oncol Biol Phys 62:138–147

7. Yeh AM, Marcus RB, Amdur RJ, Morgan LS, Million RR (2000) Patterns of failure in carcinoma of the vagina treated with definitive radiotherapy alone: what is the appropriate field volume? Int J Cancer 96:S109–S116

8. Taylor MB, Dugar N, Davidson SE et al (2007) Magnetic resonance imaging of primary vaginal carcinoma. Clin Radiol 62:549–555

9. Lamoreaux WT, Grigsby PW, Dehdashti F et al (2005) FDG-PET evaluation of vaginal carcinoma. Int J Radiat Oncol Biol Phys 62:733–737

10. Waterman FM, Holcomb DE (1994) Dose distributions produced by a shielded vaginal cylinder using high-activity iridium-192 source. Med Phys 21:101–106

11. Kim H, Rajagopalan MS, Houser C et al (2014) Dosimetric comparison of multichannel with one single-channel vaginal cylinder for vaginal cancer treatments with high-dose-rate brachytherapy. Brachytherapy 13:263–267

12. Park SJ, Chung M, Demanes DJ et al (2013) Dosimetric comparison of 3-dimensional planning techniques using an intravaginal multichannel balloon applicator for high-dose-rate gynecologic brachytherapy. Int J Radiat Oncol Biol Phys 87:840–846

13. Tanderup K, Lindegaard JC (2004) Multichannel intracavitary vaginal brachytherapy using three-dimensional optimization of source geometry. Radiother Oncol 70:81–85

14. Vargo JA, Kim H, Houser CJ et al (2015) Image-based multichannel vaginal cylinder brachytherapy for vaginal cancer. Brachytherapy 14:9–15

15. Vargo JA, Kim H, Houser CJ et al (2014) Definitive salvage for vaginal recurrence of endometrial cancer: The impact of modern intensity-modulated-radiotherapy with image-based HDR brachytherapy and the interplay of the PORTEC 1 risk stratification. Radiother Oncol 113:126–131

16. Lee LJ, Damato AL, Viswanathan AN (2013) Clinical outcomes following 3D image-guided brachytherapy for vaginal recurrence of endometrial cancer. Gynecol Oncol 131:586–592

17. Dimopoulos JC, Schmid MP, Fidarova E et al (2012) Treatment of locally advanced vaginal cancer with radiochemotherapy and magnetic resonance image-guided adaptive brachytherapy: dose-volume parameters and first clinical results. Int J Radiat Oncol Biol Phys 82:1880–1888

18. Beriwal S, Rwigema JC, Higgins E et al (2012) Three-dimensional image-based high-dose-rate interstitial brachytherapy for vaginal cancer. Brachytherapy 11:176–180

19. Miyamoto DT, Viswanathan AN (2013) Concurrent chemoradiation for vaginal cancer. PLoS One 8, e65048

20. Beriwal S, Demanes DJ, Erickson B et al (2012) American Brachytherapy Society consensus guidelines for interstitial brachytherapy for vaginal cancer. Brachytherapy 11:68–75

21. Georg P, Pötter R, Georg D et al (2012) Dose effect relationship for late side effects of the rectum and urinary bladder in magnetic resonance image-guided adaptive cervix cancer brachytherapy. Int J Radiat Oncol Biol Phys 82:653–657

22. Rajagopalan MS, Kannan N, Kim H et al (2013) Urethral dosimetry and toxicity with high-dose-rate interstitial brachytherapy for vaginal cancer. Brachytherapy 12:248–253

23. Popowski Y, Hiltbrand E, Joliat D et al (2004) Open magnetic resonance imaging using titanium-zirconium needles: improved accuracy for interstitial brachytherapy implants? Int J Radiat Oncol Biol Phys 47:759–765

24. Choi JC, Ingenito AC, Nanda RK et al (1999) Potential decreased morbidity of interstitial brachytherapy for gynecologic malignancies using laparoscopy: a pilot study. Gynecol Oncol 73:210–215

25. Corn BW, Lanciano RM, Rosenblum N et al (1995) Improved treatment planning for Syed-Neblett template using endorectal-coil magnetic resonance and intraoperative (laparotomy/laparoscopy) guidance: a new integrated technique for hysterectomized women with vaginal tumors. Gynecol Oncol 56:255–261

26. Fokdal L, Tanderup K, Nielsen SK et al (2011) Image and laparoscopic guided interstitial brachytherapy for locally advanced primary or recurrence gynaecological cancer using the adaptive GEC ESTRO target concept. Radiother Oncol 100:473–479

27. Viswanathan AN, Cormack R, Holloway CL et al (2006) Magnetic resonance-guided interstitial therapy for vaginal recurrence of endometrial cancer. Int J Radiat Oncol Biol Phys 66:91–99

28. Stock RG, Chan K, Terk M et al (1997) A new technique for performing Syed-Neblett template interstitial implants for gynecologic malignancies using transrectal-ultrasound guidance. Int J Radiat Oncol Biol Phys 37:819–825

29. Viswanathan AN, Damato AL, Nguyen PL (2013) Novel use of hydrogel spacer permits reirradiation in otherwise incurable recurrent gynecologic cancers. J Clin Oncol 31:e446–e447

30. Shah AP, Strauss JB, Gielda BT et al (2010) Toxicity associated with bowel or bladder puncture during gynecologic interstitial brachytherapy. Int J Radiat Oncol Biol Phys 77:171–179

31. Perez CA, Grigsby PW, Garipagaoglu M et al (1999) Factors affecting long-term outcome of irradiation in carcinoma of the vagina. Int J Radiat Oncol Biol Phys 44:37–45

32. Chyle V, Zagars GK, Wheeler JA, Wharton JT, Delclos L (1996) Definitive radiotherapy for carcinoma of the vagina: outcomes and prognostic factors. Int J Radiat Oncol Biol Phys 35:891–905

33. Kucera H, Vavra N (1991) Radiation management of primary carcinoma of the vagina: clinical and histopathological variables associated with survival. Gynecol Oncol 40:12–16

34. Jhingran A, Burke TW, Eifel PJ (2003) Definitive radiotherapy for patients with isolated vaginal recurrence of endometrial carcinoma after hysterectomy. Int J Radiat Oncol Biol Phys 56:1366–1372

35. Curran WJ, Whittington R, Peters AJ et al (1988) Vaginal recurrences of endometrial carcinoma: the prognostic value of staging by a primary vaginal carcinoma system. Int J Radiat Oncol Biol Phys 15:803–808

36. Lin LL, Grigsby PW, Powell MA et al (2005) Definitive radiotherapy in the management of isolated vaginal recurrences of endometrial cancer. Int J Radiat Oncol Biol Phys 63:500–504

37. Sears JD, Greven K, Hoen HM et al (1994) Prognostic factors and treatment outcome for patients with locally recurrent endometrial carcinoma. Cancer 74:1303–1308

38. Hoekstra CJ, Koper PC, van Putten WL (1993) Recurrent endometrial adenocarcinoma after surgery alone: prognostic factors and treatment. Radiother Oncol 27:164–166

39. Wylie J, Irwin C, Pintilie M et al (2000) Results of radical radiotherapy for recurrent endometrial cancer. Gynecol Oncol 77:66–72

40. Jereczek-Fossa B, Badzio A, Jassem J (2000) Recurrent endometrial cancer after surgery alone: results of salvage radiotherapy. Int J Radiat Oncol Biol Phys 48:405–413

41. Morgan J, Reddy S, Sarin P et al (1993) Isolated vaginal recurrences of endometrial carcinoma. Radiology 189:609–613

42. Nath R, Anderson LL, Meli JA et al (1997) Code of practice for brachytherapy physics: report of the AAPM Radiation Therapy Committee Task Group No. 56. Med Phys 24:1557–1598

43. Glasgow GP, Bourland JD, Grigsby PW et al (1993) Remote afterloading technology: a report of AAPM Task Group No. 41. American Institute of Physics, New York

44. Fraass B, Doppke M, Hunt M et al (1998) American Association of Physicists in Medicine Radiation Therapy Committee Task Group 53: quality assurance for clinical radiotherapy treatment planning. Med Phys 25:1773–1829

45. Kubo HD, Glasgow GP, Pethel TD et al (1998) High dose-rate brachytherapy treatment delivery: report of the AAPM Radiation Therapy Committee Task Group No. 59. Med Phys 25:375–403

46. Petignat P, Jolicoeur M, Alobaid A et al (2006) Salvage treatment with high-dose-rate brachytherapy for isolated vaginal endometrial cancer recurrence. Gynecol Oncol 101:445–449

47. Pai HH, Souhami L, Clark BG et al (1997) Isolated vaginal recurrences in endometrial carcinoma: treatment results using high-dose-rate intracavitary brachytherapy and external beam radiotherapy. Gynecol Oncol 66:300–307

48. Sorbe B, Söderström K (2013) Treatment of vaginal recurrences in endometrial carcinoma by high-dose-rate brachytherapy. Anticancer Res 33:241–247

49. Williams JA, Clarke D, Dennis WA et al (1992) The treatment of pelvic soft tissue radiation necrosis with hyperbaric oxygen. Am J Obstet Gynecol 167:412–415

50. Safra T, Gutman G, Fishlev G et al (2008) Improved quality of life with hyperbaric oxygen therapy in patients with persistent pelvic radiation-induced toxicity. Clin Oncol (R Coll Radiol) 20:284–287

51. Viswanathan AN, Lee LJ, Eswara JR et al (2014) Complications of pelvic radiation in patients treated for gynecologic malignancies. Cancer 120:3870–3883

Gynecologic Brachytherapy: Image Guidance in Gynecologic Brachytherapy

Patrizia Guerrieri and Bryan C. Coopey

Abstract

This chapter is a practical guide for image-guided high-dose-rate (HDR) brachytherapy in gynecologic cancers treated definitively with radiation therapy. It will focus predominantly on the use of intracavitary brachytherapy with either ring and tandem or tandem and ovoid devices since this is the most frequent scenario, but it will also give a brief example of an interstitial implant. It is intended as a practical "checklist," especially useful for someone who wants to implement his/her practice with a focus in gynecologic oncology. The theoretical background and techniques are discussed extensively elsewhere in this book.

1 Introduction

Image-guided brachytherapy is defined by the use of imaging to define the gross tumor volume (GTV) of brachytherapy, which is usually the residual tumor at time of the implant, as well as the areas at risk for microscopic involvement known as the high-risk CTV (HR-CTV).

Clinical examination is an important step for evaluation of the areas that should be addressed by brachytherapy at the time of the implant. As well, images from different diagnostic studies should be reviewed and the imaging importance should not be underestimated. According to the aim of the chapter as a practical guide for correct planning of gynecological brachytherapy, and in view of the fact that clinical tumor evaluation at diagnosis and its modification during treatment are part of the definition of HR-CTV as defined by the GEC-ESTRO-ABS guidelines, we will begin from the point where the patient is first seen by the radiation oncologist. We will describe the role and use of imaging (especially MRI) to guide the contouring of the brachytherapy target and of the organs at risk (OARs).

Finally, we will discuss dosimetric planning of the implant basing our discussion on dose prescription and constraints as recommended by the ABS-GEC-ESTRO guidelines.

P. Guerrieri, MD, MS (✉)
Department of Radiation Oncology, Allegheny Health Network, Temple University of College of Medicine, Pittsburgh Campus, Pittsburgh, PA, USA
e-mail: pguerrie@wpahs.org

B.C. Coopey, MS
Department of Radiation Oncology, Allegheny Health Network, Pittsburgh, PA, USA

© Springer International Publishing Switzerland 2016
P. Montemaggi et al. (eds.), *Brachytherapy: An International Perspective*, Medical Radiology,
DOI 10.1007/978-3-319-26791-3_17

2   Clinical Algorithm

1. *Initial evaluation*
   Pelvic examination:
   (a) Inspection, including bimanual and recto-vaginal palpation
       (i) Tumor dimensions
       (ii) Vaginal involvement +/−
       (iii) Parametrial involvement +/−
       (iv) Vaginal size and pliability
   Imaging data
   Pelvic MRI (*T1 with contrast and T2-weighted images*) to evaluate:
   (i) Circumferential extension
   (ii) Parametrial extension
   (iii) Bladder involvement
   (iv) Rectal involvement
   (v) Vertical extension into the vagina (*clinical assessment may be more reliable*)
   PET/CT
   (i) To evaluate the presence of metastatic disease
   (ii) To evaluate the metabolic activity of primary tumor/lymph nodes
2. *During and at the end of pelvic radiation therapy*
   Pelvic examination: inspection and rectovaginal palpation to evaluate and determine:
   Tumor response to chemoradiation in terms of:
   (i) Residual tumor size
   (ii) Vaginal involvement response
   (iii) Parametrial involvement response
   (iv) Vaginal size and pliability
   (v) Anatomy of the cervix, fornices, and vagina
3. *Prior to first implant*
   Pelvic MRI (T2-weighted images):
   (i) To evaluate and contour shape and size of residual tumor
   (ii) To evaluate circumferential extension: parametrial, bladder, or rectal involvement
   (iii) To evaluate clinical vertical extension into the vagina (*clinical assessment is better in this situation*)
   (iv) For OAR contouring

Pelvic CT
(i) To fuse with MRI images for OAR contouring

4. *Post-implant*
   Pelvic CT
   (i) For OAR dosimetry and constraints
   Pelvic MRI (T2-weighted images):
   (i) To evaluate and contour shape and size of residual tumor
   (ii) To evaluate circumferential extension: parametrial, bladder, or rectal involvement
   (iii) To evaluate clinical vertical extension into the vagina (*clinical assessment is better in this situation*)
   (iv) For OAR contouring
   Integrated image evaluation to determine:
   (i) Does the patient need a parametrial boost?
   (ii) Does the patient need a pelvic lymph node boost?
   (iii) Summation of pelvic dose contribution from different techniques.
5. *Follow-up*
   A protocol must be set to determine when to schedule:
   (i) PET/CT
   (ii) Clinical evaluation
   (iii) Consideration for salvage surgery

3   Cervical Cancer Consultation

Together with the history and physical examination, it is important to review all referring physician's notes, pathology report, and available staging studies. It is recommended to have a full pelvic MRI with and without contrast and consider infusing water-soluble aqueous gel into the vagina to better appreciate the possible involvement of the parametria, rectum, bladder, or vagina. These will be important pieces of information when planning for the implant (Figs. 1, 2, and 3). A PET/CT should also be part of the staging to evaluate the presence or absence of metastatic disease and to plan for the external beam portion of the treatment. Also, it is of importance for the brachytherapy planning, since the possible FDG avid nodes will

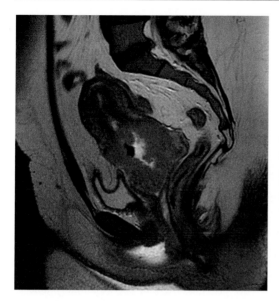

Fig. 1 Sagittal MRI initial presentation of locally advanced cervical cancer (T2 image)

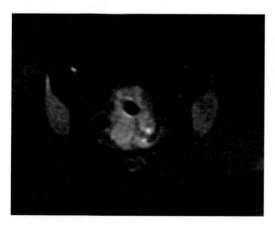

Fig. 2 Initial presentation of locally advanced cervical cancer (axial DWI MRI image)

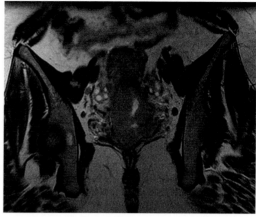

Fig. 3 Initial presentation of locally advanced cervical cancer (coronal T2 MRI image)

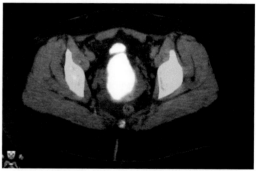

Fig. 4 Initial presentation of locally advanced cervical cancer (PET/CT image of the primary tumor)

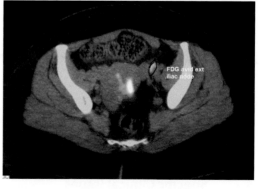

Fig. 5 Initial presentation of locally advanced cervical cancer (PET/CT image of nodal involvement)

be contoured and the necessity for a final boost dose will be evaluated in consideration of the brachytherapy contribution to the composite plan (Figs. 4 and 5). This is particularly important when delivering brachytherapy with HDR as compared to LDR because of the different dose falloffs at the periphery of the implant.

An essential part of the consultation will be the planning of an examination under anesthesia in conjunction with the gynecologic oncologist. Among other things this will allow staging according to the FIGO classification. It will accomplish visualization of bladder and rectal mucosa through cysto-proctoscopy and allow for a better appreciation of parametrial and vaginal involvement. Keeping in mind the initial clinical presentation will help in planning the brachytherapy implant at the time of boost. There is now a tendency to shy away from EUA in favor of MRI and this has some advantages; however, clinical evaluation of the vagina, rectum, or bladder is more accurate when coupling images with clinical data. The EUA and MRI should be thought of as *complimentary* necessities. A further advantage of the EUA is the possibility of placing fiducial markers at the most caudal aspect of the tumor to facilitate external beam planning. However, we should consider that moving toward MRI image-guided brachytherapy could make placement of cervical fiducials for brachytherapy unnecessary and they could possibly be detrimental to MRI image quality.

During EUA and standard pelvic examination, particular attention must be given to the following:

- Size of the cervix/tumor, extension into the parametria: Does the tumor involve the pelvic sidewall?
- The vaginal fornices: Are they involved by tumor?
- Size and pliability of the vagina: Will it accommodate easily a ring and tandem or an ovoid and tandem device?
- Extension into the vagina: Which part of the vagina is involved? Remember that all vaginal walls must be examined turning the speculum 90°, especially when using a metallic speculum!
- Which diameter of the cervix is the largest (in cm), anteroposterior, latero-lateral, or craniocaudal?
- Is there any gross involvement of the bladder or rectum?

4 Specific Clinical Issues

4.1 Extension into the Parametria

Extensive involvement: This situation is unlikely to be managed by a purely endocavitary brachytherapy treatment, since even in case of a good response to concurrent chemoradiation, some gross tumor extension into the parametria might still exist with a consequent need to treat that portion with brachytherapy. That residual disease might be addressed with a pure interstitial implant or with a combination of endocavitary/interstitial implant. Such a combined approach has been made possible by the availability of applicators such as the Vienna or Utrecht that allow the insertion of needles into the proximal part of the parametria through the ring (Vienna) or ovoids (Utrecht).

4.2 Gross Involvement of the Vagina

Unless there is involvement of only the first 2 cm of the proximal vagina, one is unlikely able to manage gross extension into the vagina with classic applicators like a ring and tandem or ovoids and tandem following chemoradiation. Two different clinical scenarios are possible at the time of the implant:

1. *Complete response or nearly complete response of vaginal disease at time of implant*: If the residual tumor is less than 0.5 cm in thickness, one should plan to deliver at least part of the treatment via a vaginal cylinder together with an intrauterine tandem to treat distal microscopic disease. Unfortunately, this technique is based on a single radioactive linear dosimetry, and dose optimization is therefore limited by the size of the cervix, the dose to the vaginal mucosa, and the dose to the rectum and bladder. It is not possible to optimize the shape of the isodoses that, in this case, resemble a cylinder.

2. *Residual vaginal tumor is more than 0.5 cm in thickness or the vagina is very narrow*: The patient may be better served with an interstitial implant via a Syed-Neblett or a MUPIT template that allows treatment of the vagina and the parametria, if necessary, along with the cervix. The same is true in the presence of a narrow vagina that cannot accommodate a standard size ring and tandem. In this situation, mini-colpostats could be a possible valid alternative, but the dosimetry, even if optimized, may not be so favorable, and the

risk of important side effects like rectovaginal fistulas is higher.

We have already anticipated some issues that must be taken into account at the time of the implant, to stress the need to properly plan brachytherapy since the beginning of treatment planning and optimizing ahead the proper integration of treatment different steps. These aspects and issues will be reviewed later.

5   Imaging Considerations

5.1   Pretreatment MRI: What Is It for and How to Use the Findings

MRI is not part of the FIGO staging for cervix cancer, but it is an important part of the overall treatment planning for several reasons:

1. Parametrial extension discovered at MRI will question the feasibility of surgery (calling for an upfront chemoradiation treatment), since parametrial infiltration represents one of the high-risk factors assessed by Peters in the GOG 109 trial [1] and will require treatment with adjuvant concurrent chemoradiation.
2. Clinical vaginal extension can be confirmed or sometimes discovered at MRI. This will once again question the feasibility of immediate surgery because of the high risk of tumor "cut-through." Staging MRI will also establish baseline data for evaluating vaginal tumor response and to discern whether or not there may be a need to address residual vaginal disease at the time of the implant. MRI images may also guide in identifying the caudal extent of the external beam fields.
3. Bladder or rectal involvement on MRI will not change the FIGO staging of the disease in the absence of positive bladder or rectal biopsies, but it might favor the use of an interstitial implant to adequately treat gross tumor extension anteriorly or posteriorly.
4. MRI may identify nodal involvement not otherwise appreciated on CT. Although nodal involvement is not part of the FIGO staging

system, it is an essential part of the TNM and, together with PET and CT, will determine the need to plan IMRT treatment especially for the para-aortic nodes or the use of a simultaneous boost to other involved nodes.

This last point is of importance to brachytherapy, especially if HDR brachytherapy is to be used. Pelvic lymph nodes in proximity of the implant will receive a sizable dose contribution from the implant itself that needs to be taken into account in a composite plan to avoid overdosing OARs and therefore increasing the risk of important side effects. For lymph node treatment in these areas, it is better to plan the boost with ERT after the implant following an accurate evaluation of the composite isodoses (Figs. 1, 2, and 3).

5.2   PET/CT

The role of this critical modality is to identify occult disease that may change the treatment intent and/or to evaluate the metabolic activity of the tumor cells in the primary site and nodal disease. It will also help in designing the external beam as well as the brachytherapy targets. It will finally be part of the evaluation of the final response to treatment (Figs. 4 and 5).

Upon completion of staging, the patient will be ready to start treatment, usually concurrent chemoradiation to the pelvis (+/−para-aortic nodes), with weekly cisplatin. During chemoradiation, a weekly on-treatment visit must be done. This will allow both for early detection and treatment of acute adverse events, as well as for adequate implant timing and proper brachytherapy technique choice.

6   Finalized Brachytherapy Planning During the Course of Concomitant Chemoradiation

Weekly pelvic examinations should begin no later than the third week of treatment to determine the ideal time to initiate brachytherapy during the course of the external beam radiotherapy (ERT), especially if HDR will be used. An earlier brachytherapy start will allow for a shorter overall treatment time, potentially increasing the local control rate. With HDR, only 1 fraction/week should be administered during external beam (not on chemotherapy days). In addition, ERT will be held. An anatomic complete assessment of the vagina and cervix and the tumor size and shape will determine the feasibility of an earlier implant and will help in the choice of the ideal brachytherapy technique. Vaginal accommodation and symmetry, cervix size and distortion along with patency of cervical canal, and forniceal and parametrial infiltration must be attentively determined to select the best technique and device. If desired, a cervical sleeve can be placed by the gynecologic oncologist to facilitate the positioning of the device on an outpatient basis.

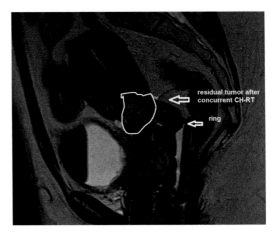

Fig. 6 Locally advanced cervical cancer at first brachytherapy fraction (sagittal T2W MRI image with device in site highlighting of the residual tumor)

7   Finalized Brachytherapy Planning Following Concomitant Chemoradiation

Should the anatomy remain unfavorable for an intercurrent implant during chemoradiation, then the entirety of brachytherapy should be performed upon completion of EBT, keeping in mind that it is imperative that all therapy be completed within 8 weeks of initiation to maximize local control and survival [2, 3]. To meet that timeline, brachytherapy must be started immediately following completion of chemoradiation, using an appropriate fractionation schedule. Several fractionation schedules have been proposed by the American Brachytherapy Society (ABS) [4].

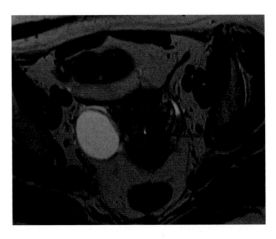

Fig. 7 Locally advanced cervical cancer at first brachytherapy fraction (axial T2 MRI image with device in site. Residual tumor is highlighted)

8   Brachytherapy Schedule

At our institution, we use 5 fractions of 5.5 Gy, two times per week. We use a cervical sleeve that is placed by the gynecologic oncologist, to allow outpatient brachytherapy treatment without subsequent need of general anesthesia in most cases. At the time of sleeve placement, the

patient is further evaluated while under sedation to clinically appreciate the residual tumor. A MRI is performed with the first brachytherapy implant. This MRI is performed on with the applicator in place. To minimize imaging time, only a limited series is performed. We image three orthogonal planes oriented with the applicator. Each plane is acquired with T2 turbo spin echo (TSE) sequence, small field of view (FOV), and 0.3 cm slice thickness with 0.06 cm gap (Figs. 6, 7, and 8).

A CT scan is done for every brachytherapy fraction. The first is fused with the MRI done at

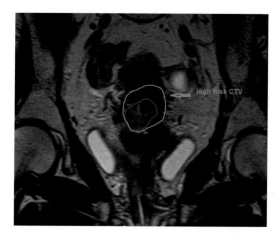

Fig. 8 Locally advanced cervical cancer at first brachytherapy fraction (coronal T2 MRI image with device in site and highlighting of the residual tumor and HR-CTV)

the time of first implant. Evaluation of the following is done on 3D reconstructed images:

1. The position of the tandem within the uterine cavity. The tandem should span the entire cavity length and to fit well into the sleeve when used.
2. The position of the tandem with respect to the pubic symphysis and the sacral promontory. The tandem usually sits1/2 to 2/3 of the way toward the pubic symphysis. It should not be too close to the sacrum to avoid undue irradiation to the bone. The position of the tandem might have an impact on the OAR dose, since a forward position will give more dose to the bladder, while a backward position will contribute preferentially to the dose to the rectum and sigmoid.
3. The geometric relationship of tandem and ring. A tandem that is not centered within the ring usually means that the connection between ring and tandem has been lost.
4. The geometric relationship of tandem and ovoids. Ovoids are positioned immediately below the flange, and the tandem is centered between the ovoids in the coronal and sagittal projections. A loss of symmetry in the coronal plane means more doses to the vaginal wall closer to the tandem, while ovoids not centered with respect to the tandem and

placed distally to the cervix will not effectively contribute to the primary dose.

Errors in the correct positioning of the brachytherapy device are responsible for unwanted areas of very high dosage and a suboptimal implant with consequent increase in side effects and potential decrease in local control.

9 Target Definition in Gynecologic Brachytherapy

In the 3D-CRT era, brachytherapy is shying away from the 2D parameters historically used for dose prescription, e.g., points A and B and maximal point dose to the rectum and bladder. While 2D parameters are still used for dose reporting, they frequently do not accurately reflect the dose to the tumor and the OARs. Some of the traditional Manchester dosimetry points are recorded, but the prescribed dose delivered is a volume isodose.

Three-dimensional volume-based brachytherapy now uses volumes and DVH according to the GEC-ESTRO-ABS guidelines. These define several target volumes that must be taken into account such as high-risk CTV, intermediate-risk CTV, and different sub-volumes of the following OARs, bladder, rectum, sigmoid, and small bowel, with the most useful sub-volumes being the high-risk CTV for dose prescription and the dose to 2 cc of the OARs for dose constraints. They represent the parameters to which one must conform brachytherapy plans. While a full technical discussion of these issues is not part of this chapter (please refer to the previous chapter and to the numerous publications present in the literature), we will illustrate how to use these concepts in clinical practice [5–7].

The high-risk CTV of GYN brachytherapy is related to the extent of GTV at time of brachytherapy. It keeps in mind the tumor extent at diagnosis, to gauge areas at risk of microscopic disease, but has the intent of delivering a high total dose (80–90 Gy) to the residual tumor (high-risk CTV). The dose is comparable to the dose to point A but is prescribed to a volume rather than to a point. This volume includes the whole cervix and the presumed tumor extension as outlined by clinical assessment and the evidence of residual gray zones on T2-weighted MRI images (Figs. 6, 7, and 8) [8].

10 Brachytherapy Procedure

With the sleeve in place, the patient is put in stirrups for the positioning of the brachytherapy device. Usually lorazepam and ibuprofen are enough to keep the discomfort of the procedure under control. A urinary catheter is put in place and the vagina is once again examined to choose the right size of ovoids or ring. There are in fact, several caps that can be chosen to accommodate the vaginal width. The largest one that fits the patient anatomy is chosen to better spare the OARs from unnecessary dose. For ring and tandem combinations, the tandem is chosen on the basis of the natural position of the body of the uterus and ideally spans the entire uterine cavity. The most used tandem angles are usually 60° or 45° and the most used length is 6 or 8 cm. Many HDR tandem and ovoid kits carry either the straight or the curved tandem. Curved tandems are usually chosen, and then a flange is screwed in position according to the length of the intrauterine part of the tandem, so that it will abut the cervical os when positioned.

A rectal retractor is finally positioned along the posterior wall of the vagina to displace the anterior wall of the rectum from the high dosage area. Alternatively, one or two vaginal balloons can be attached to the ring or the ovoids to act as vaginal packing. We find it difficult to do adequate vaginal packing with contrast-soaked gauze in an outpatient setting and prefer the use of balloons or rectal retractors.

The MRI images are registered to the planning CT in the treatment planning software. Since the three orthogonal series are in the same coordinate space, one registration co-registers all series. Thus, contouring that is only performed on the axial CT slices can be viewed on higher-resolution images for the sagittal and coronal reconstruction.

11 Brachytherapy Planning

After fusing the MRI images with the simulation CT, we contour the high-risk CTV using MRI images, while OARs are contoured on CT images to allow for an easier comparison with CT images obtained for the subsequent treatments. The OARs contoured on CT are compared with MRI images and necessary adjustments are done prior to the first brachytherapy plan. Alternatively, an MRI could be done for each single HDR treatment with contouring each time of the target and OARs on the MRI alone [9]. Current treatment planning systems do not calculate dose with heterogeneity corrections. The dose calculation is based on the geometry of the sources and the AAPM Task Group 43 (TG43) formalism. Therefore, CT is not strictly necessary for dosimetry.

Organs at risk (OARs) are contoured in their entirety for DVH purposes, for it has been proven that contouring just the wall of the organ is more subjective and less accurate [10].

The bladder is usually scanned with the urinary catheter open, therefore voiding urine, but it can be scanned with a modest amount of water or saline solution in it to space out possible bowel loops from close proximity to the device. At this time it is possible to develop a rough treatment plan having in mind the dose to point A as a baseline dosimetry. At our institution, we then follow by contouring the cervix and the residual tumor on the fused MRI images and look at the dose to the HR-CTV as well as at the 2 cc OAR volumes. At this point, the prescription isodose is optimized according to the shape of the HR-CTV as delineated on the MRI and as clinically appreciated at the time of the sleeve insertion, and the dose is modulated to meet OAR constraints (Figs. 9, 10, and 11). An appropriate analogy would be to imagine the inflation of a large balloon in the center of a room. The balloon needs to be inflated as large as possible without hitting the walls, floor, or ceiling. The necessary volume of this balloon is the contoured volume of the HR-CTV. The ceiling height and wall distances are the 2 cc OAR dose limits. From one fraction to the next, the ceiling height (bladder proximity and size) may decrease. The balloon can be squeezed in a

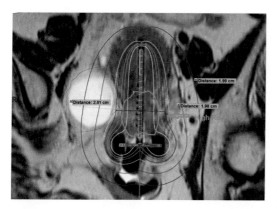

Fig. 9 Locally advanced cervical cancer at first brachytherapy fraction (dosimetric coronal reconstruction of the first treatment on fused T2W MRI image)

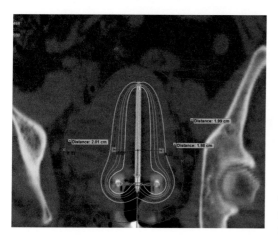

Fig. 10 Locally advanced cervical cancer at first brachytherapy fraction (dosimetric coronal reconstruction of the first treatment on CT image)

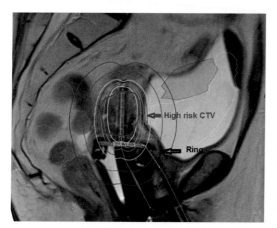

Fig. 11 Locally advanced cervical cancer at first brachytherapy fraction (dosimetric sagittal reconstruction of the first treatment on fused T2 MRI image)

different direction (increasing dwell times in ring or tip of tandem) to keep the same volume but not hit the ceiling. According to GEC-ESTRO-ABS guidelines, the dose of 2 cc for the bladder, rectum, and sigmoid should be kept at less than 80 % of the prescription dose. For the rectum and sigmoid, we tend to stay between 60 and 80 % of the prescribed dose, and we monitor bowel in proximity to the implant. We prefer small bowel D2cc equal to 60 % of the prescribed dose but know that the small bowel loops can shift around between scanning and treatment and between individual treatments; therefore, we review the total D2cc from the entire brachytherapy treatment preferentially over each individual fraction dose. Of course, our priority is to give a meaningful dose to the tumor to maximize local control. Again according to GEC-ESTRO-ABS, the composite dose to the HR-CTV should be between 80 and 90 Gy EQD2, according to primary tumor volume.

In addition to the 2 cc OAR doses, the traditional Manchester calculation points of Pt A and Pt B are calculated on every case. These points can serve as a prescription surrogate to the 3D volume prescription in cases where HR-CTV contouring is not possible. These points also serve as a bridge from the old brachytherapy methods to the new.

Another parameter that is recorded on every case is the source activity (Ci) multiplied by the treatment time in seconds (s). The resulting Ci*s value is fairly constant depending on prescription dose and tandem length. The Ci*s varies little between individual fractions on each patient.

A fractionation schedule of 5.5 Gy × 5 is equivalent to 85–90 Gy EQD2 when combined to 45–50 Gy of pelvic external beam, and we follow the OAR constraints recommended by the GEC-ESTRO-ABS guidelines [7]:

Bladder D2cc	80 Gy EQD2
Rectum D2cc	70–75 Gy EQD2
Sigmoid D2 cc	70–75 Gy EQD2
Small bowel D2cc	60Gy EQD2

We also report the dose to 0.1 cc and value D0.1 cc since it is a representative expression of the maximal dose.

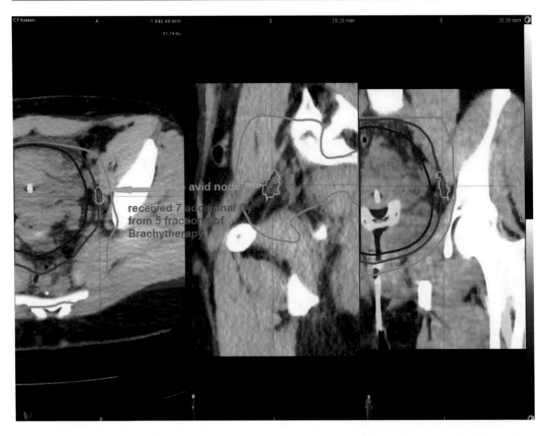

Fig. 12 Locally advanced cervical cancer: dosimetric reconstruction of composite dose from external and intracavitary brachytherapy with highlighting of a small PET positive node

12 Dosimetric Evaluation of the Dose Contribution from External Beam and Brachytherapy

At the end of brachytherapy, especially when there is an initial finding of gross parametrial involvement or evidence of pathologically involved pelvic lymph nodes, it is recommended to evaluate the dose received by the involved parametrium or lymph nodes through combined external and brachytherapy doses. At our institution, we use software to add each fraction's 3D dose to form a composite dose distribution. This composite dose is combined with the 3D dose calculation from the external beam dose. This way we can better evaluate the composite dose to the organs at risk. HDR brachytherapy usually gives a contribution of 6–8 Gy to the distal part of

the parametria, therefore microscopic parametrial disease or a small lymph node might not require additional boost dose (Fig. 12).

13 Interstitial Brachytherapy

Gross residual parametrial or vaginal tumor cannot be treated with a simple endocavitary treatment with ring and tandem or tandem and ovoids in some cases and may require an interstitial implant with a Syed-Neblett or a MUPIT template (Fig. 13); however, the technical explanation of this type of implant goes beyond the scope of this chapter. Suffice it to say that these are more complex implants that can cause a higher risk of significant permanent adverse events and should be therefore carried out in centers with extensive clinical experience.

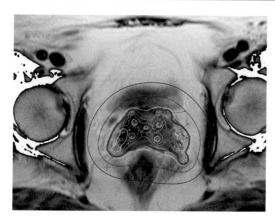

Fig. 13 Locally advanced cervical cancer at first brachytherapy fraction (dosimetric axial reconstruction of the interstitial treatment on fused T2 MRI image)

14   Follow-Up

Follow-up appointments and their timing are important factors that would allow (1) to follow tumor response to treatment, (2) detect important side effects, and (3) assess the need for possible surgical intervention or complication management.

Response to treatment is best evaluated by clinical examination and by a PET/CT at 2–3 months from the end of the treatment. A complete disappearance of the FDG avidity at that point represents a positive prognostic factor [11].

It may take months for the tumor to completely resolve, and sometimes the tumor is replaced by a necrotic process that takes a long time to heal. It is important in this situation to decide timing and opportunity of a biopsy to clarify the issue of tumor necrosis or tumor senescence versus tumor progression or relapse.

Salvage surgery or surgical intervention to symptomatically improve side effects like bowel stenosis and bladder or rectal fistula formation may be necessary, and close collaboration and communication with the surgeon are necessary.

References

1. Peters WA et al (2000) Concurrent chemotherapy and pelvic Radiation Therapy compared with pelvic Radiation Therapy Alone as adjuvant therapy after Radical Surgery in High-Risk Early-Stage cancer of the cervix. J Clin Oncol 18(8):1606–1613
2. Gasinska A, Fowler JF, Lind BK et al (2004) Influence of overall treatment time and radiobiological parameters on biologically effective doses in cervical cancer patients treated with radiation therapy alone. Acta Oncol 43(7):657–666
3. Mandal A, Asthana AK, Aggarwal LM (2007) Clinical significance of cumulative biological effective dose and overall treatment time in the treatment of carcinoma cervix. J Med Phys 32(2):68–72
4. Nag S, Erickson B, Thomadsen B et al (2012) The American Brachytherapy Society recommendations for high-dose-rate brachytherapy for carcinoma of the cervix. American Brachytherapy Society. Brachytherapy 11(1):47–52
5. Haie-Meder C, Pötter R, van Limbergen E (2005) Recommendations from the gynaecological (GYN) GEC-ESTRO working group: concepts and terms in 3D image based 3D treatment planning in cervix cancer brachytherapy with emphasis on MRI assessment of GTV and CTV. Radiother Oncol 74: 235–245
6. Hellebust TP, Kirisits C, Berger D (2010) Recommendations from Gynaecological (GYN) GEC-ESTRO working group: considerations and pitfalls in commissioning and applicator reconstruction in 3D image-based treatment planning of cervix cancer brachytherapy. Radiother Oncol 96:153–160
7. Pötter R, Haie-Meder C, van Limbergen E (2006) Recommendations from gynaecological (GYN) GEC-ESTRO working group (II): concepts and terms in 3D image-based treatment planning in cervix cancer brachytherapy-3D dose–volume parameters and aspects of 3D image-based anatomy, radiation physics, and radiobiology. Radiother Oncol 78:67–77
8. Dimopoulos JCA, Petrow P, Tanderup K et al (2012) Recommendations from Gynaecological (GYN) GEC-ESTRO Working Group (IV): basic principles and parameters for MR imaging within the frame of image based adaptive cervix cancer brachytherapy. Radiother Oncol 103(1):113–122
9. Gill BS, Kim H, Houser CJ et al (2015) MRI-guided high-dose-rate intracavitary brachytherapy for treatment of cervical cancer: the University of Pittsburgh experience. Int J Radiat Oncol Biol Phys 91(3):540–547
10. Yaparpalvi R, Mutyala S, Gorla GR et al (2008) Point vs. volumetric bladder and rectal doses in combined intracavitary-interstitial high-dose-rate brachytherapy: correlation and comparison with published Vienna applicator data. Brachytherapy 7(4):336–342
11. Grigsby PW, Siegel BA, Dehdashti F et al (2003) Post-therapy surveillance monitoring of cervical cancer by FDG-PET. Int J Radiat Oncol Biol Phys 55:907–913

Prostate: Low Dose Rate Brachytherapy

Pei Shuen Lim and Peter Hoskin

Abstract

Brachytherapy has the advantage of delivering a high tumoricidal dose of radiation to the target volume, while giving low doses to the surrounding normal tissues as dose falloff obeys the inverse square law. It therefore offers an elegant means of treating prostate cancer avoiding the anatomical disruption of major surgery or the more widespread radiation effects associated with external beam therapy.

1 Introduction

Prostate cancer is increasing in incidence annually in the USA and Europe with well over one million men diagnosed each year. In the UK it is now the most common cancer in men and accounts for a quarter of all male cancers. The highest incidence worldwide is seen in Australasia with 115 per 100,000 new cases per year. This compares with 98 per 100,000 in the USA and 73 per 100,000 in the UK. Low incidence is seen in Africa and Asia with incidence rates of 31 per 100,000 in Nigeria and Kenya and only 4 per 100,000 in India [1].

In those areas with high incidence, much of the increase can be accounted for by earlier diagnosis using PSA measurements in relatively asymptomatic men together with an aging male population. The majority of these men will present with localized low- to intermediate-risk prostate cancer and be candidates for active surveillance, radical prostatectomy, or brachytherapy. Death from prostate cancer in this group is unlikely whichever treatment is used and therefore with the prospect of many years of life ahead dealing with the legacy of treatment an informed decision is critical.

P.S. Lim, BM, MRCP
Specialist Registrar in Clinical Oncology, Mount Vernon Cancer Centre, Northwood, UK
e-mail: pei.lim@nhs.net

P. Hoskin, MD (✉)
Consultant in Clinical Oncology, Professor, Mount Vernon Cancer Centre and University College Northwood, London, UK
e-mail: peterhoskin@nhs.net

2 Low Dose Rate Prostate Brachytherapy

2.1 Indications and Contraindications

Patients can be considered for LDR brachytherapy if they have localized prostate cancer without

© Springer International Publishing Switzerland 2016
P. Montemaggi et al. (eds.), *Brachytherapy: An International Perspective*, Medical Radiology,
DOI 10.1007/978-3-319-26791-3_18

metastases and a life expectancy of longer than 10 years. Patients can broadly be stratified into different risk groups based on three main prognostic factors: Gleason score, PSA value, and T stage. The American Brachytherapy Society (ABS) recommends using the National Comprehensive Cancer Network guidelines classification [2]:

- Low risk – Gleason score 6 *and* PSA <10 ng/mL *and* T1-T2a tumor
- Medium risk – Gleason score 7 *or* PSA 10–20 ng/mL *or* T2b-T2c tumor
- High risk – Gleason score 8–10 *or* PSA >20 ng/mL *or* T3a tumor

Guidelines by the ESTRO/EAU/EORTC with recommendations on patient selection for LDR brachytherapy are shown in Table 1 [3]. Those predicted to have a poor outcome should be considered for other modalities of treatment or combination treatment.

When selecting patients, it is important to consider the functional outcome as well as the oncological outcome after treatment. A high International Prostate Symptom Score (IPSS) and low flow rate (Qmax) pretreatment are related to an increased risk of catheter use and irritative urinary morbidity post implant [4]. Patients with an IPSS score of more than 20 have been found to have a higher risk of prolonged urethritis and urinary retention [5,6].

A large gland has a higher probability of pubic arch interference where part of the prostate sits behind the bone and physically does not permit a geometrically satisfactory implant. It is recommended that patients with glands larger

than 50–60 cm^3 should undergo a few months of antiandrogen therapy, which normally results in a 30 % volume reduction of the gland.

It is challenging to accomplish optimal seed distribution with acceptable dosimetry in patients with large defects from previous transurethral resection of the prostate (TURP). The risk of incontinence is thought to be higher with patients who have had a TURP [7,8] although this is now challenged [9,10]. If the TURP was performed more than 6 months to a year previously, the urethral cavity may have healed, but care must still be taken to minimize the urethral dose.

Patients on regular anticoagulants and antiplatelet agents should be advised to stop for a few days preimplantation if it is clinically safe to do so. The duration will depend on the half-life of the medication.

Contraindications to LDR brachytherapy as recommended by ABS and ESTRO/EAU/EORTC are summarized in Table 2.

2.2   Equipment Required

- A transrectal ultrasound (TRUS) probe with dedicated prostate brachytherapy software. The ultrasound should ideally be of high resolution, using frequencies between 5 and 12 Mhz with a biplanar system, to allow sagittal and transaxial visualization.
- Stepping unit support system containing a cradle to hold the ultrasound probe and allow three-dimensional movement in the x (left-right), y (anterior-posterior), and z (superior-inferior) axis. The unit can be mounted on the operating table or placed on the ground.

Table 1 ESTRO/EAU/EORTC recommendations for indications on LDR prostate brachytherapy [3]

	Recommended (do well)	Optional (fair)	Investigational (poor outcome)
PSA (ng/mL)	<10	10–20	>20
Gleason score	5–6	7	8–10
Stage	T1c-T2a	T2b-T2c	T3
IPSS	0–8	9–19	>20
Prostate volume (g)	<40	40–60	>60
Qmax (ml/s)	>15	15–10	<10
Residual volume (cm^3)			>200
TURP			+

Table 2 Contraindications to LDR brachytherapy

ABS guidelines [11]		ESTRO/EAU/EORTC guidelines [3]
Absolute	Relative	
Limited life expectancy	High IPSS >20	Life expectancy less than 5 years
Unacceptable operative risks	History of prior pelvic radiotherapy	Metastatic disease
Distant metastases	TURP defects	Recent TURP with persisting large defect
Absence of rectum, precluding the use of TRUS	Large median lobes	Bleeding disorder
Large TURP defects	Prostate gland >60 cm³ at implantation	Prostate gland >50 cm³ at implantation
Ataxic telangiectasia	Inflammatory bowel disease	

- Perineal template that will be fixed onto the stepping system and calibrated to accurately match the grid displayed on the ultrasound image.
- Implantation device and needles. Implantation needles are usually 18 gauge and 20 cm long.
- Locking (stabilization) needles – optional.
- Foley catheter or aerated gel (lubricating gel mixed with air in a syringe to produce tiny bubbles) to visualize the urethra on TRUS.
- Fluoroscopy unit. Some units are able to obtain CT slices to detect areas with cold spots.

2.3   Pretreatment Preparation

1. Patients will require an anesthetic assessment prior to the procedure. Spinal or general anesthetic may be used.
2. Laxatives may be given a few days prior to empty the bowel. An enema is usually given a few hours before the procedure to empty the rectum in order to obtain a good visual field on the TRUS image. If the rectum is still full, a rectal washout may be necessary before starting the procedure.
3. An alpha-blocker may be given a few weeks prior to the procedure if the patient has existing outflow obstructive symptoms.

2.4   Implantation Technique

The introduction of the transperineal approach for Iodine-125 seed implantation using transrectal ultrasound (TRUS) guidance by Holm in 1983 has revolutionized prostate brachytherapy [12]. This method allows direct visualization of needles in the prostate guiding precise seed implantation, which in turn enhances dosimetry, and ultimately translates to improved clinical outcomes. Since then, this technique has been refined and popularized, becoming the standard for prostate brachytherapy [13,14]. The last decade has seen advances in imaging, and the introduction of sophisticated planning software technology has further improved the quality of seed implantation.

2.5   Preimplant Treatment Planning

Before seed implantation, the patient will undergo a prostate volume study. TRUS still remains the standard modality used for the volume study and has been shown to have close approximation with prostatectomy prostate volumes [15]. CT imaging can be used but may overestimate the volume of the prostate [16]. Many newer brachytherapy software systems now allow MRI soft tissue registration with TRUS images, allowing for better soft tissue visualization while contouring the prostate.

The patient is positioned in the lithotomy position as shown in Fig. 1. Hyperextension of the legs can widen the pubic arch for those with a larger gland. The TRUS probe is then inserted into the rectum and fixed onto the cradle of the stepping unit.

The TRUS image of the prostate is positioned centrally within the displayed template grid on

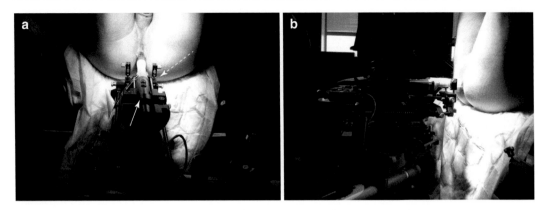

Fig. 1 (**a, b**) Views of a patient setup in lithotomy position with ultrasound probe inserted into the rectum. The probe has been fixed onto the cradle (*full arrow*) of the stepping unit. The *dashed arrow* points to the template holder

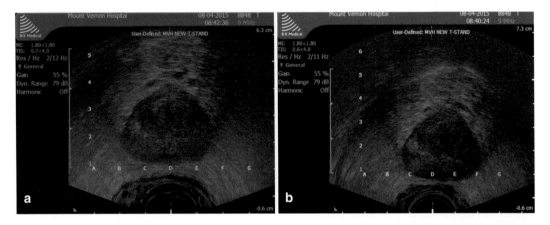

Fig. 2 (**a**) Good TRUS image of the prostate; (**b**) Rotated image

the ultrasound image at its largest transverse slice, usually at the mid-gland. Special attention must be taken to ensure that the TRUS is inserted straight and with little pressure around the probe so that the prostate image is not distorted, angled, or rotated around the probe. A small amount of saline can be injected into the condom over the rectal probe for improved image quality and assistance in positioning the posterior capsule of the prostate. The posterior row of the grid (column D, row 1) should be 0.1–0.2 cm above the posterior prostate capsule to keep the rectal dose below prescription point (Fig. 2).

The urethra should be located in the middle of the grid (column D). A Foley catheter or aerated gel is inserted into the urethra to assist urethral visualization. Insertion of aerated gel (Fig. 3) is preferred as the catheter may pull the urethra anteriorly, compromising the dosimetric outcome once the catheter is removed. The catheter may also distort the prostate leading to inaccurate target volume delineation [17].

Once the clinician is satisfied with the quality and reproducibility of the TRUS setup and image, serial transverse images are taken from the base to the apex as shown in Fig. 4. This should be in no more than 0.5 cm increments; 0.1 cm spacing will improve the 3D reconstruction and also enable more precise definition of base and apex. A sagittal image that displays both the base and apex of the prostate is also obtained to measure the length of the gland. After the images are obtained, data are transferred into the planning computer treatment planning system (TPS). Target volumes and

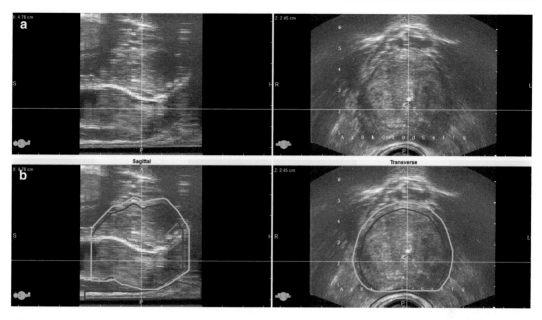

Fig. 3 (**a, b**) Sagittal and transverse view of the prostate on TRUS with aerated gel in the urethra. Inserting a catheter can alter the normal curvature of the urethra, affecting actual dosimetry received by the prostate when the cathe-ter has been removed. *Bottom row*: Same images with target volumes and organs at risk contoured. *Red* prostate, *light blue* prostate with margin, *dark blue* rectum, *green* urethra

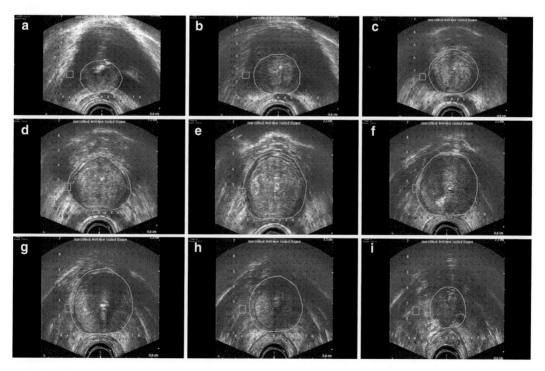

Fig. 4 (**a–i**) TRUS 0.5 cm interval slices obtained at volume study with target volume of the prostate outlined from base (*top left*) to apex (*bottom*)

organ at risk volumes are outlined, followed by the generation of a treatment plan.

2.6 Volume Definition and Dose Parameters

ESTRO/EAU/EORTC volume definitions are as follows in the preimplant setting [18]:

- *Tumor volume definition*
  - *GTV* (gross tumor volume) is contoured on the preimplantation TRUS image in correlation with MRI imaging when available.
  - *CTV* (clinical target volume) is the whole prostate gland with a margin expanded with constrains to the anterior rectal wall (posterior) and bladder neck (cranial):
    - T1-T2 CTV = visible prostate contour + 0.3 cm margin
    - T3 CTV = visible prostate contour + visible extracapsular extension + 0.3 cm margin
  - *PTV* = CTV
- *Organs at risk (OAR)*
  - Prostatic *urethra* – Defined by aerated gel or a small gauge catheter when the surface of the catheter is used to define the urethral surface.
  - *Rectum* – Visualization of the anterior rectal wall is good on TRUS. The outer and inner walls should be outlined.

The preplan dose parameters recommended by ESTRO/EAU/EORTC are summarized in Table 3. The ABS guidelines limit the preplan dose parameters for the dose applied to <1 cc of the rectum to 100 % of the prescription dose (RV 100 < 1 cc) [11]. It is important to aim for a higher preplan D90 as post implant D90 dosimetry is generally lower and targets are often not achieved [19].

2.7 Treatment Planning Techniques

2.7.1 Preplanning

The original approach was to perform a two-step procedure where the volume study is performed during a separate procedure a few days or weeks

Table 3 Dose parameter preplan recommendations by ESTRO/EAU/EORTC for LDR brachytherapy [18]

GTV	GTV >150 %
CTV	V100 ≥ 95 % D90 > 100 % V150 ≤ 50 %
OAR: rectum	Primary: D2cc < 145 Gy Secondary: D0.1 cc (Dmax) < 200 Gy
OAR: prostatic urethra	Primary: D10 < 150 % Secondary: D30 < 130 %

before the implantation. The volume study is undertaken and a dose plan that can be reproduced during the implantation procedure is then created. There are a few benefits to this method. It allows planning of optimal source placement to maximize coverage of the target volume. The exact number of seeds required can be predicted accurately and ordered, or alternatively preloaded needles can be ordered. Pubic arch interference can be assessed and patients with a large gland requiring cytoreduction can be identified.

However, several limitations are associated with this preplanning approach [20]. Reproducibility of TRUS images at implantation to match those obtained at preplanning is extremely challenging due to variation of patient repositioning and TRUS probe setup. The prostate shape or volume may change in between preplanning and implantation with pelvic floor muscle relaxation from anesthesia or the use of antiandrogens. Therefore an implant based on the preplan technique may lead to inaccuracies and poor dose distributions.

2.7.2 Intraoperative Planning

Most units have now moved toward the "intraoperative planning" technique which is a one-step approach where the volume study, treatment planning, and seed implantation are all performed as one procedure to overcome positional uncertainties. This also provides the opportunity to improve the quality of implants by modifying and replanning during the procedure. There are several approaches to intraoperative planning as defined by the American Brachytherapy Society (ABS): intraoperative preplanning, interactive planning, and dynamic dose calculation [21].

Intraoperative Preplanning

This technique brings the planning system into the operating room (OR). As there is no preplan done beforehand, the number of seeds required is determined from a nomogram or table based on the prostate volume deduced from a CT scan or ultrasound. The TRUS images obtained in the OR are transferred real time into the TPS for the treatment plan creation, followed immediately by the implant procedure.

Although operating time is lengthened, dosimetry is generally better with intraoperative preplanning when compared to conventional preplanning. This technique obviates patient repositioning issues but does not account for intraoperative variations in prostate geometry or deviations of the implant needle insertion from the plan [22].

Interactive Planning

Interactive planning allows intraoperative optimization of the treatment plan using real time dose calculation updates from image-based needle position feedback during the implant procedure [21]. The intraoperative preplan method described earlier is used to generate the initial treatment plan. Once the implant needles are inserted into the prostate, the positions are registered by the TPS. The dose is then recalculated based on the imaged needle positions, giving a more accurate dosimetric representation. Seed loading can be modified, individual needle positions can be adjusted, and additional needles can be added to optimize the plan if the dosimetry is found to be suboptimal before the sources are deposited. It has been shown that this method produces better dosimetry for the CTV [23] and has been associated with improved biochemical control [24,25].

Advances in technology with improved ultrasound resolution, automated stepping, and tracking systems allow quicker and more accurate plan modifications [26]. It has also been proposed that the learning curve for new brachytherapists may be reduced as corrections during the procedure can be made. This technique also accommodates intraoperative changes within the prostate and deviations in the inserted implant needle position from the intended position on the

preplan. However, as it uses information based on needle position, it does not account for actual implanted seed location, loose seed migration, or stranded seed retraction from the prostate apex after implantation or the effects of intraoperative prostate edema on final seed placement.

Dynamic Dose Calculation

Dynamic dose calculation refers to optimization of the treatment plan in a 3D setting based on continuous deposited seed position feedback. It is important to note that information is gathered from each individual seed implanted position rather than the needle position as in the interactive planning method. This technique provides the most accurate representation of the dose delivered.

However, it is not yet commercially available as the ability to track individual seeds reliably for dosimetric calculation is limited with current TRUS technology. Several methods are under development including TRUS fusion with fluoroscopy [27,28] and intraoperative C-arm cone beam CT [29].

Robotic systems with promising results are also in development to assist the improvement of seed placement accuracy [30].

2.8 Dosimetry Planning Techniques

There are various seed loading planning techniques used as shown in Fig. 5. The Seattle group initially utilized a *uniform loading* approach with a high number of low-activity seeds evenly distributed at a 1 cm distance throughout the prostate [31] which maintains dose homogeneity despite small variations in seed placement. This however causes underdosing of the periphery due to the "scalloping-in" effect and significant overdosing of the central (urethral) portion of the gland which can approach almost 300 % of the prescribed dose, resulting in increased urinary morbidity [32].

The *peripheral loading* approach has evolved where a lower number of high-activity seeds were implanted only around the periphery of the gland [33]. This technique spares the urethra but at the

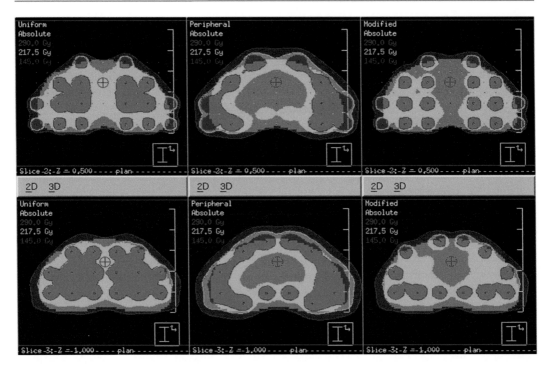

Fig. 5 Dosimetry using the uniform loading approach (*left*), peripheral loading approach (*middle*), and modified approach (*right*)

expense of underdosing the prostate centrally and resulting in undesirable high dose gradients close to the rectum. Slight seed misplacement or migration may also affect dosimetry significantly.

To overcome disadvantages in both techniques, most centers now use a merged approach, *modified uniform* [34] or *modified peripheral loading* [35], depending on the starting reference. Both utilize the concept of increasing the number of seeds at the periphery, especially at the base and apical region of the gland, while reducing central seed density adjacent to the urethra. More sophisticated derivations of this approach may also use seeds of different activity with higher activity seeds around the periphery.

2.9 Implant Procedure

The patient is repositioned in a similar lithotomy position as the volume study if the preplan method is used. The ultrasound setup will then be reproduced as close as possible to that during the volume study. The one-step procedure simply flows continuously from the volume study acquisition to dose plan generation to implantation.

The scrotum is lifted up and taped or suture retracted away from the perineum and the perineal area is disinfected. The perineal template is mounted onto the stepping unit and is checked that it correlates with the template grid displayed on the ultrasound image. Most templates are made with 0.5 cm spacing.

Locking or fixation needles can be used to fix the prostate but are not implemented universally. The prostate is a soft structure that can move and change in shape when needles are inserted. The preplan will contain a needle loading report that indicates for each needle:

- The x and y coordinate
- The number of seeds including special loadings
- Retraction of needle tip from base plane (z coordinate)

Seeds may be ordered loose or stranded. Loose seeds are associated with a higher trend of migration than stranded seeds [36,37]. Seed migration is rare and can occur up to 1-year post-procedure. Seeds may pass through the urine or may migrate to the lung or pelvic lymph nodes. Although there are concerns that stranded seeds are associated with intraprostatic seed movement in the weeks post implantation due to prostate edema, there appears to be little effect on the post implant dosimetry [38]. Increased experience and avoidance of seed placement in periprostatic vessels are associated with a reduction in seed migration [39].

Most needles will implant a fixed number of 2–5 seeds; there may also be special loadings with no seeds in the middle portion of the track. These are normally used adjacent to the urethra to keep the urethral dose low (Fig. 6).

The implantation process is shown in Figs. 7 and 8. It is usually begun from the anterior row first to minimize TRUS interference. The needle is advanced into the prostate guided by the TRUS transverse imaging set at the corresponding retraction plane slice. The needle can be rotated to check that tip of the bevel "flashes" up and down to ensure that it is at the correct depth. The probe is then rotated within the cradle so that the sagittal crystal is focused on the needle to verify its depth. The seeds are then advanced into the intended position along the needle using the stylet, using the final distance from the stylet tip to the needle hub as a reference to the number of seeds in the needle. Special loaded needles will have a longer distance than the total number of seeds in the needle as spacers are used in place of the absent seeds. If the stylet is advanced too deeply or too quickly, the seeds may be pushed beyond the intended position. Once in position, seeds are deposited carefully by holding the stylet stationary and carefully withdrawing the needle over the stylet. If the needle is pulled out too swiftly, the seeds may slip inferiorly due to the suction effect from withdrawal [40].

There are two main methods of seed placement, the preloaded technique and the afterloading technique. With the preloaded technique, seeds are placed into the needle beforehand and deposited immediately into the prostate once the needle is inserted. The needles can be manually preloaded or ordered preloaded based on the needle loading report. With the afterloading technique, the needles are positioned in the prostate first, either all at once or by row. The seeds are then inserted into the needle while it is in the prostate. This generates the desired alignment of a train of seeds and spacers, and the

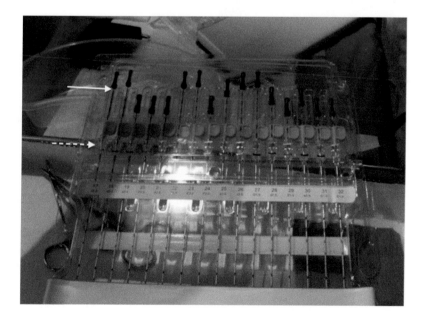

Fig. 6 Tray containing preloaded needles ordered based on the needle implant report. The distance between the stylet tip and needle hub after the seeds are advanced is used as a reference to correlate with the number of seeds contained within the needle

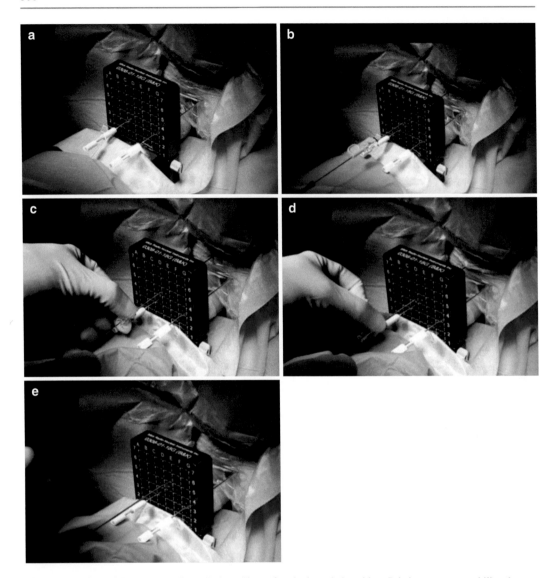

Fig. 7 Insertion of implant needle and deposition of seeds. (**a**) Stabilization needles inserted transperineally via the template into the prostate. (**b**) Preloaded implant needle inserted into the prostate until the tip is visualized on the reference plane on TRUS as shown in (**a**). (**c**) Stylet is slowly pushed in to advance seeds along the needle to the intended position. It is important to stabilize the needle using the nondominant hand (*left* in this picture) to minimize the possibility of pushing the needle further in. (**d**) Needle is withdrawn over the stylet with the stylet held stationary to deposit the seeds. (**e**) Both needle and stylet being removed

train is pushed into the prostate remotely. The needle is retracted until it is just outside of the prostate and is then further retracted by the operator (Fig. 9).

2.9.1 Post Procedure

A fluoroscopic image is taken and an ultrasound scan from base to apex is reviewed to ensure good coverage of the prostate. The number of seeds can be calculated on the fluoroscopic image to ensure all seeds are accounted for before leaving the operating room. A Geiger-Muller counter or scintillation detector is used to survey the operating area for any misplaced seeds.

A cystoscopy may be done if there is concern about loose seeds in the bladder; however, this rarely happens and if so, free seeds will normally pass naturally (Fig. 10).

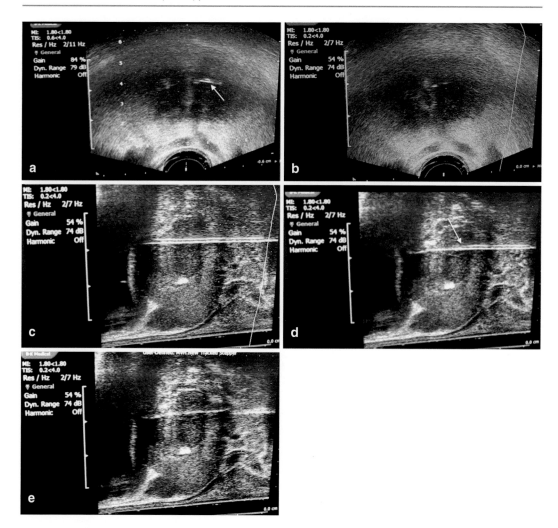

Fig. 8 (a–e) TRUS views showing implant needle insertion and deposition of seeds. (a) Tip of the bevel at reference plane. Two horizontal lines can be seen. When the bevel is rotated, the horizontal line will "flash." (b) Probe is tilted so that the needle image is at midline to visualize the needle in sagittal mode. (c) Needle in sagittal view. (d) Needle being withdrawn over a strand of seeds. (e) Strand of seeds deposited and needle is slowly removed

3 Dosimetry

3.1 Choice of Radioisotopes and Prescription Doses

Permanent seed implants may use Iodine-125, Palladium-103, or Cesium-131. Iodine-125 is the usual isotope used in Europe. The properties and published recommendations for dose prescriptions are summarized in Table 4. The dose is prescribed to a minimum peripheral dose, which is the 100 % isodose.

Iodine-125 dose prescriptions in early literature (pre-TG-43 era) may be reported as 160 Gy, which is equivalent to 144 Gy using TG-43 calculations [41]. Cesium-131 is a fairly new radioisotope introduced recently in 2004, and a prescription dose of 115 Gy is recommended for monotherapy [42]. The ABS guidelines in 2012 have not made any recommendations on the use of Cesium-131 as follow-up data are still immature.

3.2 Post Implant Dosimetry

It is good clinical practice for all implants to undergo evaluation to ensure good quality control of the implant. There is evidence

Fig. 9 Periprostatic vessels (*arrows*). Care should be taken not to insert seeds into this area

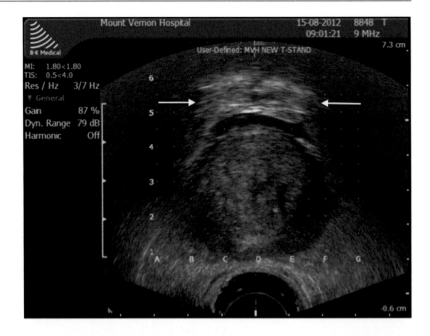

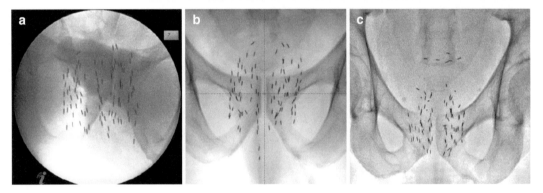

Fig. 10 (**a**) Fluoroscopy at D0 post implant. (**b**) Pelvic radiograph of same patient at D30 showing a strand of seeds migrating inferiorly. (**c**) Pelvic radiograph of another patient with migration of seeds into the bladder

Table 4 Radionuclide properties and prescription doses recommendations for LDR prostate brachytherapy

Radionuclide	Half-life (days)	Initial dose rate (cGy.h⁻¹)	Average energy (keV)	Seed strength mCi	U	Prescription dose (Gy) using AAPM TG-43 formalism Monotherapy (ESTRO) [18]	Monotherapy (ABS) [11]	Combination with EBRT (ABS) [11]
Iodine-125	59.4	7	28.4	0.3–0.6	0.4–0.8	145	140–160	108–110
Palladium-103	17	21	20.7	1.1–2.2	1.4–1.8	125	110–125	90–100
Caesium-131	9.7	30	30.4	2.5–3.9	1.6–2.5	N/A	N/A	N/A

U is the unit for air kerma strength, $1U = 1$ cGy cm² h⁻¹, *EBRT* external beam radiation therapy, Recommended EBRT dose = 41.4–50.4 Gy (1.8 Gy–2 Gy/day)

suggesting that the probability of achieving biochemical control has a strong correlation with the quality of an implant, represented by the D90, the minimum dose delivered to 90 % of the target volume on post implant dosimetric analysis [43,44].

Table 5 Published recommendations from ABS [11,51] and ESTRO/EAU/EORTC [3,18] on post implant dosimetry reporting in LDR prostate brachytherapy

	ABS	ESTRO/EAU/EORTC	
		Primary parameters *Mandatory*	Secondary parameters *May be reported*
Prostate CTV	D_{100}, D_{90}, D_{80} V_{200}, V_{150}, V_{100}, V_{90}, V_{80}	D_{90} V_{100} V_{150}	V_{200} D_{100} Natural dose rate Homogeneity index Conformal index
OAR: rectum	RV_{100}	D_{2cc}	$D_{0.1cc}$ V_{100}
OAR: urethra	UV_{150} UV_5 UV_{30}	D_{10}	$D_{0.1cc}$ D_{30} D_5
Other reporting recommendations	Total volume of prostate Number of days between implantation and post implant imaging study	Volume implanted Number of seeds Number of needles used Total activity implanted Prescribed dose	

ESTRO recommends that volume (V) parameters should always be expressed in absolute values (cc)
OAR organs at risk, *D90* dose covering 90 % of the prostate volume, *V100* volume that has received 100 % of the prescribed dose, *UV* urethral volume, *RV* rectal volume

The timing of post implant imaging will produce different results in post implant dosimetry due to the varying degrees of trauma-related prostatic edema. Imaging performed immediately post implant (day 0) will underestimate the dosimetric parameters by about 10 % as the mean prostatic volume is increased [45]. ABS recommends CT-based post implant dosimetry to be performed within 60 days of the implant with the optimum timing depending on the radionuclide used: 16 ± 4 days for palladium-103 and 30 ± 7 days for iodine-125 [11].

Interobserver and intraobserver variability in CT-based post implant contouring of the prostate due to poor soft tissue visualization contributes to variability in prostate dosimetry [46,47]. CT images may also be degraded due to scatter from the metallic seeds. Despite the fact that MRI improves soft tissue definition, MRI-based post implant contouring of the prostate was also found to have large interobserver variability caused by the lack of uniformity in the interpretation of the prostate CTV [48], despite contouring recommendations from ESTRO mentioned below.

CT imaging still remains the best means of seed localization. On MRI, seeds are seen as sig-

nal voids and are more difficult to individualize. Seeds may appear on more than one CT slice; hence use of a seed sorting software algorithm is recommended. Optimal post implant imaging includes performing both CT and MRI with image fusion to improve the reproducibility of post implant dosimetry [49,50]. However, there are uncertainties on image fusion and these may account for variability up to 16 % for CT and T2 MRI fusion [48].

The ABS and ESTRO have both recommended a set of dose–volume parameters to be reported for post implant evaluation as shown in Table 5.

ESTRO has published recommendations to promote uniformity in contouring the prostate and organs at risk for post implant dosimetry evaluation [18]:

- There are two *prostate CTV* definitions and both should be reported:
  - CTV-P = CTV for prostate, i.e., the prostatic gland capsule on post implant radiological imaging is contoured.
  - CTV-PM = CTV for prostate plus 0.3 cm three-dimensional uniform margin.

- Prostatic *urethra* – Definition is poor both on CT and MRI. It is only accurate when a urinary catheter or aerated gel is inserted during post implant imaging, which may not always be practical. Correlation or fusion of CT or MRI images with TRUS images may be the optimal noninvasive technique for urethral localization. It is recommended that institutional policy should be described if urethral parameters are published.
- *Rectum* – If using CT only, outer rectal wall can be clearly defined. If using MRI, outer and inner walls can be defined. There is controversy as to whether there is a need to outline the inner wall for post implant dosimetry. For dose–volume parameters of D2cc and below, there is no impact, but for larger dose–volume criteria, errors may be introduced from just the outer wall contours [52].

The penile bulb and neurovascular bundles can only be defined accurately on MRI, but dose parameters to these structures are still under investigation.

4   Results

Outcome is generally measured as biochemical relapse-free survival (bRFS) as the natural history of localized prostate cancer is generally slow. Overall survival is not a common end point as most men with low- and intermediate-risk prostate cancer die of other age-related comor-bidities rather than their prostate cancer [53]. Several definitions of biochemical failure have been used, which may contribute to differences in reported outcomes. At present, the "Phoenix definition," a PSA rise of 2 ng/ml above post-treatment nadir, introduced in 2006, is the widely accepted criterion used [54].

There has been extensive literature published on the results of primary LDR prostate brachytherapy monotherapy to date, and as a result, it is a very well-established treatment option for low-risk disease. For LDR brachytherapy alone, the 10-year bPFS is approximately 80 % for low risk, 60–70 % for intermediate risk, and 30–60 % for high-risk disease.

Large studies with more than 900 patients and long-term results on LDR seed monotherapy are summarized in Table 6. The largest cohort is a multi-institutional study by Zelefsky describing outcomes of 2693 patients with T1-T2 disease treated with permanent brachytherapy only without androgen deprivation. 1831 were treated with I-125 implants and 893 were treated with Pd-103 implants. No difference in outcomes was found between the different isotopes. The 8-year PSA relapse-free survival using the Phoenix definition of relapse was 74, 61, and 39 % for the low-risk, intermediate-risk, and high-risk group stratified using the National Comprehensive Cancer Network (NCCN) risk criteria [55].

LDR seed brachytherapy can be used in conjunction with external beam radiotherapy (EBRT) in the intermediate- and high-risk settings to dose escalate. Long-term outcomes are

Table 6 Summary of representative results on LDR seed brachytherapy monotherapy from selected large patient cohorts

Author	Number of patients	Median follow-up (years)	Total follow-up (years)	Recurrence definition	bNED (%)		
					Low risk	Int risk	High Risk
Zelefsky et al. [55]	2693	5.3	8	ASTRO	82	70	48
				Phoenix	74	61	39
Henry et al. [56]	1298	4.9	10	ASTRO	86	77	61
				Phoenix	72	73	58
Hinnen et al. [57]	921	5.75	10	Phoenix	88	61	30

bNED biochemical no evidence of disease, *ASTRO definition* 3 successive rises in PSA after posttreatment nadir achieved [58], *Phoenix definition* absolute posttreatment nadir plus 2 ng/mL [54] shown in Table 7. A recent randomized controlled trial from Canada has been reported in abstract demonstrating the superiority of this approach over external beam radiotherapy to 74 Gy alone [62].

Outcomes for prostate LDR brachytherapy are comparable to other radical treatment modalities, and one large comparative analysis has reported superior bRFS outcomes for LDR brachytherapy compared to radical prostatectomy or EBRT in the low-risk and intermediate-risk setting. Patients in the high-risk group performed better with combined treatment using brachytherapy and EBRT [63].

There is a dose–response relationship between the post implant quality, represented by the post implant D90 and clinical efficacy. Stock first introduced this concept in 1998 when he demonstrated improved bRFS rates with higher D90 values. In this series, the bRFS at 4 years was 92 % for patients with D90 >140 Gy versus 68 % for those with D90 <140 Gy [44]. Zelefsky demonstrated significantly higher 8-year bRFS rates when the D90 was >130 Gy at 93 % versus 76 % when the D90 was <130 Gy [55]. Several other series have also confirmed this association [43,64].

Approximately 30 % of patients experience the PSA "bounce phenomenon," where there is a temporary rise in PSA after an initial fall [65,66]. This is usually seen 12–24 months posttreatment with average rises of <2 ng/ml. The bounce is benign and should not be a trigger for salvage therapy. If a prostate biopsy is undertaken before 30 months following an implant due to a rising PSA, the biopsy result may not be interpretable [67].

The time taken for the PSA to achieve its nadir value is slow and can take up to 6 years [68]. The nadir value has been found to be a prognostic indicator of long-term biochemical outcome. Zelefsky has shown that the 8-year bRFS outcome using the Phoenix definition was 88 %, 69 %, 57 %, and 41 %, respectively, for patients with a 3-year PSA nadir value of 0–0.49, 0.5–0.99, 1.0–1.99, and >2. For patients who maintained bRFS at 8 years, the median PSA nadir level was 0.1 ng/ml [55].

4.1 "Salvage Brachytherapy"

LDR brachytherapy has also been used for salvage after local recurrence following previous radiation therapy. It is feasible but few mature results are available to make firm recommendations. It should be performed at an experienced center in prostate brachytherapy, undertaking prospective data collection.

4.2 Post Implantation Care

- Perineal bruising after implant is common and perineal ice packs may be advised.
- Post implant prophylactic antibiotics are recommended for one week.
- Obstructive and irritative urinary symptoms are very common and can last for a few

Table 7 Summary of representative results on LDR seed brachytherapy combined with EBRT

Author	Number of patients	Median follow-up (years)	Total follow-up (years)	Recurrence definition	bNED (%)		
					Low risk	Int risk	High risk
Sylvester et al. [8]	223	9.43	15	Modified ASTRO	85.8	80.3	67.8
Dattoli et al. [59]	321	10.5	16	Phoenix	–	89	74
Merrick et al. [60]	284	7.8	12	PSA > 0.4 above nadir	–	–	89
				Phoenix	–	–	88.4
Critz and Levinson [61]	1469	6	10	PSA > 0.2	93	80	61

Modified ASTRO definition 2 successive rises in PSA at time of last follow-up months. Prophylactic postoperative alpha-blockers can improve urinary morbidity [69]. Prophylactic anti-inflammatory drugs can also be prescribed to improve dysuria.

- Urine needs to be passed via a sieve while in hospital extended in some recommendations to 3 days after the implant to "catch" any loose seeds passing via the urethra. If a seed is found, then a spoon or forceps is used to pick it and dispose of in a sanitary system. If it is in the lavatory, it can be flushed away. At some institutions, this is not a requirement.
- Sexual intercourse may be resumed, but some practitioners recommend condom use for the first few ejaculations, although the likelihood of ejaculation of a seed is very low.
- The range of radiation outside the patient is very low and there is little radiation risk to others [70]. It is however still recommended that children and pregnant women should avoid close contact (less than one meter) for one half-life of the radionuclide.
- The patient should be given written information about the implanted sources, strength of radiation, date of implantation, and contact numbers. A "wallet card" should also be given to the patient.
- Cremation may cause contamination and release radioactive material into the atmosphere and is not recommended for 2 years post implantation.

Further information regarding radiation safety for permanent prostate implants can be found in more detail in the ICRP 98 document [71].

5   Complications

The main complications from permanent seed implants are from urinary, bowel, and sexual dysfunction.

The majority of patients who develop complications develop urethritis with increased urinary frequency and obstructive and irritative symptoms which start a few days post implant and may persist up to 6–9 months after. The symptoms for 90 % of men resolve at 1 year once most of the

total dose is delivered [72]. For Iodine-125, 75 % is delivered by 4 months and 97 % by 8 months.

Acute urinary retention happens in 5–10 % of patients. It should be managed conservatively in the first instance with alpha-blockers and intermittent self-catheterization or continuous drainage with a Foley catheter. The probability of developing acute retention correlates with the pretreatment IPSS score and prostate size and is related to prior use of alpha-blocking drugs, tobacco use, and age [73]. Retention normally resolves within the first year and should be treated conservatively. If a TURP is performed in the first year post-treatment, there is a higher risk of urinary incontinence [74].

Chronic urinary morbidity can occur secondary to excessive irradiation of the bladder neck or prostatic urethra. RTOG grade 3 toxicity is reported in 1–3 % of treated patients [75] and urethral stricture rates are up to 12 % [76]. Long-term incontinence is strongly associated with previous TURP surgery, with up to 20 % incontinence rates in the group who underwent TURP versus 1 % without TURP in one series [8]. Newer evidence is emerging which may support post TURP implantation in selected circumstances.

Chronic radiation proctitis is rare, seen in less than 5 % of patients. It may present 6 months post implant with rectal bleeding, rectal urgency, rectal incontinence, and pain. Rates of rectal fistulas are low, around 0.6 % [77]. The distance between posterior seeds implanted and the anterior rectal wall is correlated with rectal toxicity, and improved technology in implant positioning accuracy has improved rates of toxicity.

Erectile dysfunction rates are generally lower with permanent seed implants compared to other treatment modalities. The rate of erectile dysfunction has a significant correlation with preimplant erectile status. Thirty percent of men potent prior to the implant will develop impotence but 60 % will respond to phosphodiesterase inhibitors [78].

LDR brachytherapy does not seem to be related with an increased risk of radiation-induced secondary malignancy compared to the general population. A systematic review has supported this conclusion, and it is felt that this could be attributed to the high sterilizing doses received by small regions only around the treated area [79].

6   Summary

Low dose rate brachytherapy using the transperineal transrectal ultrasound-guided approach is now well established as an effective treatment for both low- and intermediate-risk prostate cancer. The technique has evolved from the original two-step process to a single-step procedure in which a preimplant volume study is undertaken, plan produced, and seeds inserted during a single event. This also enables interactive planning with tracking and correction of seed placement as the implant is built up. Seeds may be used singly using a Mick® applicator or in a stranded form with no consistent advantage seen for either approach. Post plan dosimetry is important for quality assurance and governance; a D90 of at least 130 Gy using I-125 should be the target. Overall biochemical relapse-free survival rates of around 90 % in low risk and 80 % in intermediate-risk patients are to be expected. The main toxicities are urinary with acute irritative symptoms in the first year and later urethral stricture as the most common events. Rectal changes are less frequent and erectile dysfunction will occur in 30–40 % of men potent prior to the implant.

References

1. UK, C.R. Cancer incidence worldwide map. 2015; Available from: http://www.cancerresearchuk.org/cancer-info/cancerstats/world/incidence/-By
2. Mohler JL (2010) The 2010 NCCN clinical practice guidelines in oncology on prostate cancer. J Natl Compr Canc Netw 8(2):145
3. Ash D et al (2000) ESTRO/EAU/EORTC recommendations on permanent seed implantation for localized prostate cancer. Radiother Oncol 57(3): 315–321
4. Crook J et al (2002) Factors influencing risk of acute urinary retention after TRUS-guided permanent prostate seed implantation. Int J Radiat Oncol Biol Phys 52(2):453–460
5. Gutman S et al (2006) Severity categories of the International Prostate Symptom Score before, and urinary morbidity after, permanent prostate brachytherapy. BJU Int 97(1):62–68
6. Terk MD, Stock RG, Stone NN (1998) Identification of patients at increased risk for prolonged urinary retention following radioactive seed implantation of the prostate. J Urol 160(4):1379–1382
7. Blasko JC, Ragde H, Grimm PD (1991) Transperineal ultrasound-guided implantation of the prostate: morbidity and complications. Scand J Urol Nephrol Suppl 137:113–118
8. Sylvester JE et al (2007) 15-Year biochemical relapse free survival in clinical Stage T1-T3 prostate cancer following combined external beam radiotherapy and brachytherapy; Seattle experience. Int J Radiat Oncol Biol Phys 67(1):57–64
9. Brousil P et al (2015) Modified transurethral resection of the prostate (TURP) for men with moderate lower urinary tract symptoms (LUTS) before brachytherapy is safe and feasible. BJU Int 115(4):580–586
10. Stone NN, Ratnow ER, Stock RG (2000) Prior transurethral resection does not increase morbidity following real-time ultrasound-guided prostate seed implantation. Tech Urol 6(2):123–127
11. Davis BJ et al (2012) American Brachytherapy Society consensus guidelines for transrectal ultrasound-guided permanent prostate brachytherapy. Brachytherapy 11(1):6–19
12. Holm HH et al (1983) Transperineal 125iodine seed implantation in prostatic cancer guided by transrectal ultrasonography. J Urol 130(2):283–286
13. Sylvester J et al (1997) Interstitial implantation techniques in prostate cancer. J Surg Oncol 66(1):65–75
14. Sylvester JE et al (2009) Permanent prostate brachytherapy preplanned technique: the modern Seattle method step-by-step and dosimetric outcomes. Brachytherapy 8(2):197–206
15. Hastak SM, Gammelgaard J, Holm HH (1982) Transrectal ultrasonic volume determination of the prostate--a preoperative and postoperative study. J Urol 127(6):1115–1118
16. Park H et al (2011) A comparison of preplan MRI and preplan CT-based prostate volume with intraoperative ultrasound-based prostate volume in real-time permanent brachytherapy. Radiat Oncol J 29(3):199–205
17. Anderson C et al (2010) I-125 seed planning: an alternative method of urethra definition. Radiother Oncol 94(1):24–29
18. Salembier C et al (2007) Tumour and target volumes in permanent prostate brachytherapy: a supplement to the ESTRO/EAU/EORTC recommendations on prostate brachytherapy. Radiother Oncol 83(1):3–10
19. Al-Qaisieh B et al (2009) Correlation between pre- and postimplant dosimetry for iodine-125 seed implants for localized prostate cancer. Int J Radiat Oncol Biol Phys 75(2):626–630

20. Polo A et al (2010) Review of intraoperative imaging and planning techniques in permanent seed prostate brachytherapy. Radiother Oncol 94(1):12–23
21. Nag S et al (2001) Intraoperative planning and evaluation of permanent prostate brachytherapy: report of the American Brachytherapy Society. Int J Radiat Oncol Biol Phys 51(5):1422–1430
22. Cormack RA, Tempany CM, D'Amico AV (2000) Optimizing target coverage by dosimetric feedback during prostate brachytherapy. Int J Radiat Oncol Biol Phys 48(4):1245–1249
23. Lee EK, Zaider M (2003) Intraoperative dynamic dose optimization in permanent prostate implants. Int J Radiat Oncol Biol Phys 56(3):854–861
24. Matzkin H et al (2013) Comparison between preoperative and real-time intraoperative planning (1)(2)(5)I permanent prostate brachytherapy: long-term clinical biochemical outcome. Radiat Oncol 8:288
25. Shah JN et al (2006) Improved biochemical control and clinical disease-free survival with intraoperative versus preoperative preplanning for transperineal interstitial permanent prostate brachytherapy. Cancer J 12(4):289–297
26. Beaulieu L et al (2007) Bypassing the learning curve in permanent seed implants using state-of-the-art technology. Int J Radiat Oncol Biol Phys 67(1):71–77
27. Kuo N et al (2014) An image-guidance system for dynamic dose calculation in prostate brachytherapy using ultrasound and fluoroscopy. Med Phys 41(9):091712
28. Todor DA et al (2003) Intraoperative dynamic dosimetry for prostate implants. Phys Med Biol 48(9):1153–1171
29. Westendorp H et al (2007) Intraoperative adaptive brachytherapy of iodine-125 prostate implants guided by C-arm cone-beam computed tomography-based dosimetry. Brachytherapy 6(4):231–237
30. Podder TK et al (2014) AAPM and GEC-ESTRO guidelines for image-guided robotic brachytherapy: report of Task Group 192. Med Phys 41(10):101501
31. Blasko JC, Grimm PD, Ragde H (1993) Brachytherapy and organ preservation in the management of carcinoma of the prostate. Semin Radiat Oncol 3(4):240–249
32. Talcott JA et al (2001) Long-term treatment related complications of brachytherapy for early prostate cancer: a survey of patients previously treated. J Urol 166(2):494–499
33. Wallner K et al (1991) An improved method for computerized tomography-planned transperineal 125iodine prostate implants. J Urol 146(1):90–95
34. Merrick GS, Butler WM (2000) Modified uniform seed loading for prostate brachytherapy: rationale, design, and evaluation. Tech Urol 6(2):78–84
35. Raben A et al (2004) Prostate seed implantation using 3D-computer assisted intraoperative planning vs. a standard look-up nomogram: improved target conformality with reduction in urethral and rectal wall dose. Int J Radiat Oncol Biol Phys 60(5):1631–1638
36. Al-Qaisieh B et al (2004) The use of linked seeds eliminates lung embolization following permanent seed implantation for prostate cancer. Int J Radiat Oncol Biol Phys 59(2):397–399
37. Hinnen KA et al (2010) Loose seeds versus stranded seeds in I-125 prostate brachytherapy: differences in clinical outcome. Radiother Oncol 96(1):30–33
38. Usmani N et al (2011) Lack of significant intraprostatic migration of stranded iodine-125 sources in prostate brachytherapy implants. Brachytherapy 10(4):275–285
39. Stone NN, Stock RG (2005) Reduction of pulmonary migration of permanent interstitial sources in patients undergoing prostate brachytherapy. Urology 66(1):119–123
40. Yu Y et al (1999) Permanent prostate seed implant brachytherapy: report of the American Association of Physicists in Medicine Task Group No. 64. Med Phys 26(10):2054–2076
41. Rivard MJ et al (2004) Update of AAPM Task Group No. 43 Report: a revised AAPM protocol for brachytherapy dose calculations. Med Phys 31(3):633–674
42. Bice WS et al (2008) Recommendations for permanent prostate brachytherapy with (131)Cs: a consensus report from the Cesium Advisory Group. Brachytherapy 7(4):290–296
43. Potters L et al (2003) Importance of implant dosimetry for patients undergoing prostate brachytherapy. Urology 62(6):1073–1077
44. Stock RG et al (1998) A dose-response study for I-125 prostate implants. Int J Radiat Oncol Biol Phys 41(1):101–108
45. Waterman FM et al (1998) Edema associated with I-125 or Pd-103 prostate brachytherapy and its impact on post-implant dosimetry: an analysis based on serial CT acquisition. Int J Radiat Oncol Biol Phys 41(5):1069–1077
46. Al-Qaisieh B et al (2002) Impact of prostate volume evaluation by different observers on CT-based post-implant dosimetry. Radiother Oncol 62(3):267–273
47. Dubois DF et al (1998) Intraobserver and interobserver variability of MR imaging- and CT-derived prostate volumes after transperineal interstitial permanent prostate brachytherapy. Radiology 207(3):785–789
48. De Brabandere M et al (2012) Prostate post-implant dosimetry: interobserver variability in seed localisation, contouring and fusion. Radiother Oncol 104(2):192–198
49. Polo A et al (2004) MR and CT image fusion for postimplant analysis in permanent prostate seed implants. Int J Radiat Oncol Biol Phys 60(5):1572–1579
50. Tanaka O et al (2006) Comparison of MRI-based and CT/MRI fusion-based postimplant dosimetric analysis of prostate brachytherapy. Int J Radiat Oncol Biol Phys 66(2):597–602
51. Nag S et al (2000) The American Brachytherapy Society recommendations for permanent prostate

brachytherapy postimplant dosimetric analysis. Int J Radiat Oncol Biol Phys 46(1):221–230

52. Wachter-Gerstner N et al (2003) Bladder and rectum dose defined from MRI based treatment planning for cervix cancer brachytherapy: comparison of dose-volume histograms for organ contours and organ wall, comparison with ICRU rectum and bladder reference point. Radiother Oncol 68(3):269–276

53. Bittner N et al (2008) Primary causes of death after permanent prostate brachytherapy. Int J Radiat Oncol Biol Phys 72(2):433–440

54. Roach M et al (2006) Defining biochemical failure following radiotherapy with or without hormonal therapy in men with clinically localized prostate cancer: recommendations of the RTOG-ASTRO Phoenix Consensus Conference. Int J Radiat Oncol Biol Phys 65(4):965–974

55. Zelefsky MJ et al (2007) Multi-institutional analysis of long-term outcome for stages T1-T2 prostate cancer treated with permanent seed implantation. Int J Radiat Oncol Biol Phys 67(2):327–333

56. Henry AM et al (2010) Outcomes following iodine-125 monotherapy for localized prostate cancer: the results of leeds 10-year single-center brachytherapy experience. Int J Radiat Oncol Biol Phys 76(1):50–56

57. Hinnen KA et al (2010) Long-term biochemical and survival outcome of 921 patients treated with I-125 permanent prostate brachytherapy. Int J Radiat Oncol Biol Phys 76(5):1433–1438

58. American Society for Therapeutic Radiology and Oncology Consensus Panel (1997) Consensus statement: guidelines for PSA following radiation therapy. American Society for Therapeutic Radiology and Oncology Consensus Panel. Int J Radiat Oncol Biol Phys 37(5):1035–1041

59. Dattoli M et al (2010) Long-term outcomes for patients with prostate cancer having intermediate and high-risk disease, treated with combination external beam irradiation and brachytherapy. J Oncol 2010;(2010):471375. doi:10.1155/2010/471375

60. Merrick GS et al (2011) Prostate cancer death is unlikely in high-risk patients following quality permanent interstitial brachytherapy. BJU Int 107(2):226–232

61. Critz FA, Levinson K (2004) 10-year disease-free survival rates after simultaneous irradiation for prostate cancer with a focus on calculation methodology. J Urol 172(6 Pt 1):2232–2238

62. Morris WJ, Pai HH et al (2015) ASCENDE-RT*: A multicenter, randomized trial of dose-escalated external beam radiation therapy (EBRT-B) versus low-dose-rate brachytherapy (LDR-B) for men with unfavorable-risk localized prostate cancer. J Clin Oncol 33 (Suppl 7; abstr 3)

63. Grimm P et al (2012) Comparative analysis of prostate-specific antigen free survival outcomes for patients with low, intermediate and high risk prostate cancer treatment by radical therapy. Results from the Prostate Cancer Results Study Group. BJU Int 109(Suppl 1):22–29

64. Papagikos MA et al (2005) Dosimetric quantifiers for low-dose-rate prostate brachytherapy: is V(100) superior to D(90)? Brachytherapy 4(4):252–258

65. Patel C et al (2004) PSA bounce predicts early success in patients with permanent iodine-125 prostate implant. Urology 63(1):110–113

66. Toledano A et al (2006) PSA bounce after permanent implant prostate brachytherapy may mimic a biochemical failure: a study of 295 patients with a minimum 3-year followup. Brachytherapy 5(2): 122–126

67. Reed D et al (2003) Clinical correlates to PSA spikes and positive repeat biopsies after prostate brachytherapy. Urology 62(4):683–688

68. Grimm PD et al (2001) 10-year biochemical (prostate-specific antigen) control of prostate cancer with (125) I brachytherapy. Int J Radiat Oncol Biol Phys 51(1):31–40

69. Elshaikh MA et al (2005) Prophylactic tamsulosin (Flomax) in patients undergoing prostate 125I brachytherapy for prostate carcinoma: final report of a double-blind placebo-controlled randomized study. Int J Radiat Oncol Biol Phys 62(1):164–169

70. Michalski J et al (2003) Radiation exposure to family and household members after prostate brachytherapy. Int J Radiat Oncol Biol Phys 56(3):764–768

71. International Commission on Radiological, Physics (2005) Radiation safety aspects of brachytherapy for prostate cancer using permanently implanted sources. A report of ICRP Publication 98. Ann ICRP 35(3):iii–vi, 3–50

72. Merrick GS et al (2000) Temporal resolution of urinary morbidity following prostate brachytherapy. Int J Radiat Oncol Biol Phys 47(1):121–128

73. Neill M et al (2007) The nature and extent of urinary morbidity in relation to prostate brachytherapy urethral dosimetry. Brachytherapy 6(3):173–179

74. Merrick GS et al (2004) Effect of transurethral resection on urinary quality of life after permanent prostate brachytherapy. Int J Radiat Oncol Biol Phys 58(1):81–88

75. Zelefsky MJ et al (1999) Comparison of the 5-year outcome and morbidity of three-dimensional conformal radiotherapy versus transperineal permanent iodine-125 implantation for early-stage prostatic cancer. J Clin Oncol 17(2):517–522

76. Ragde H et al (1997) Interstitial iodine-125 radiation without adjuvant therapy in the treatment of clinically localized prostate carcinoma. Cancer 80(3):442–453

77. Kishan AU, Kupelian P (2015) Late rectal toxicity after low-dose-rate brachytherapy: incidence, predictors, and management of side effects. Brachytherapy 14(2):148–159

78. Bottomley D et al (2007) Side effects of permanent I125 prostate seed implants in 667 patients treated in Leeds. Radiother Oncol 82(1):46–49

79. Murray L et al (2014) Second primary cancers after radiation for prostate cancer: a systematic review of the clinical data and impact of treatment technique. Radiother Oncol 110(2):213–228

Prostate: High-Dose Rate Brachytherapy in the Treatment of Clinically Organ-Confined Prostate Cancer

Nikolaos Tselis, Dimos Baltas, and Nikolaos Zamboglou

Abstract

High-dose rate brachytherapy for prostate cancer has enjoyed rapid acceptance and is one of the most active areas of clinical research in the field. We present this chapter as a comprehensive technical analysis of rationale, methods, and outcomes including a substantive data review.

1 Introduction

In patients with clinically organ-confined prostate cancer, radical prostatectomy [1, 2], external beam radiotherapy (EBRT) [3–5], permanent low-dose rate (LDR) brachytherapy (BRT) [6–8] and temporary high-dose rate (HDR) BRT [9–18] are established treatment options. In the absence of randomized clinical trials, however, survival and biochemical control (BC) data are difficult to assess, and the optimal therapeutic strategy remains controversial. Against this background, quality of life issues have gained increasing importance in the choice of interventional treatment with BRT gaining momentum due to its potential

advantages of convenience, high effectiveness, and relatively low morbidity. By now, a large body of literature corroborates the efficacy of both permanent and temporary BRT in the treatment of localized prostate cancer. Especially research on HDR BRT is accelerating, reporting technological improvements in ultrasound-based real-time image guidance with one-step intraoperative treatment planning which ensures high standards of implant quality [19]. In fact, the superior dosimetry of HDR temporary afterloading BRT is reflected in the growing number of recent publications reporting excellent clinical results [20–22], thus supporting HDR BRT as an innovative alternative to permanent LDR BRT [23].

2 Background

2.1 Rationale for HDR Brachytherapy

Recent clinical research suggests that radiation dose escalation for localized prostate cancer not

N. Tselis, MD, PhD (✉) • N. Zamboglou, MD, PhD
Department of Radiation Oncology and
Interdisciplinary Oncology, Sana Klinikum,
Offenbach, Germany
e-mail: ntselis@hotmail.com;
nikolaos.zamboglou@hotmail.com

D. Baltas, PhD
Department of Medical Physics and Engineering,
Sana Klinikum, Offenbach, Germany
e-mail: dimos.baltas@uniklinik-freiburg.de

© Springer International Publishing Switzerland 2016
P. Montemaggi et al. (eds.), *Brachytherapy: An International Perspective*, Medical Radiology,
DOI 10.1007/978-3-319-26791-3_19

only improves biochemical disease control [4, 5, 24] but also results in improved local control (LC) and metastasis-free survival (MFS) [5, 25–29]. In this context, patients without regionally advanced or metastatic disease may benefit most from dose-escalated radical radiotherapy (RT), and it is reasonable to assume that further improvements in the therapeutic ratio can be generated by escalating the treatment dose while ameliorating dose conformity. High-dose rate BRT meets this objective optimally by exploiting the radiobiological advantage of large fraction sizes [30–32] while ensuring intraoperative real-time treatment planning and delivery [33] with prospective three-dimensional (3D) dosimetry [34]. High-dose rate treatment planning provides anatomy-based multiparametric dose optimization through modulation of catheter geometry, radiation source positions, and source dwell times [35, 36]. The versatility of intratarget dose modulation inherent to HDR BRT can be controlled and directed to deliver higher doses to gross disease or to selectively reduce the dose to organs at risk (OARs) [20]. In comparison to permanent LDR BRT, HDR dosimetry is "high density" because there are approximately twice as many HDR dwell positions as seeds in the typical LDR implant. The prospective nature of HDR dosimetry ensures excellent target coverage and normal tissue sparing without dosimetric changes caused by source migration and tissue deformity which are common problems associated with permanent LDR seed implants [37–39]. Furthermore, variations in internal anatomy secondary to organ motion, which frequently occur during treatment delivery times in EBRT [40–42], and setup inaccuracies are not an issue with HDR because they can be corrected with interactive online dosimetry during the implantation procedure or modified during real-time anatomy-based treatment planning before dose delivery [20]. Since there is no need to add treatment volume beyond the intended target to account for patient motion or variations in beam delivery, the precise 3D dosimetry of HDR allows the technique to be used in combination with EBRT. This is of particular relevance when it is deemed clinically necessary to extend the treat-ment volume to include areas of possible extra-prostatic extension or the regional lymphatic drainage to a moderate dose while administering an escalated dose to the prostate.

2.2　Radiobiological Considerations

Radiobiological research demonstrates that the probabilities of acute and late radiation reactions vary between normal tissues and tumors and between different RT dose fractionation schedules. The α/β ratio, a means of expressing the sensitivity of a particular tissue to altered fraction size, is used to estimate the impact of a given schedule on tumor control and toxicity while enabling comparisons between different treatment schedules. Tissues and tumors with a low α/β ratio have a higher sensitivity to changes in fraction size than those with a high α/β ratio [30, 43–45]. Recent radiobiological findings support a low α/β ratio, 1.2–3.0 Gy, for prostate adenocarcinoma which is lower than the α/β ratio of acutely and late-reacting normal tissues [31, 46, 47]. For prostate cancer, this implies that a hypofractionated dose regimen is favored for tumor control with a reduction in late sequelae. Hypofractionated HDR BRT with anatomy-based dose optimization is an excellent method for conformal dose escalation in terms of both radiation biology and physics [48]. In order to compare HDR regimes with EBRT treatment schemes, the linear-quadratic formula as described by Fowler et al. [43] is usually used:

$$\mathrm{BED} = D\left(1 + \frac{d}{(\alpha/\beta)}\right)$$

where *BED* is the biologically effective dose as a measure of the biological effect delivered by a particular RT regime, *D* is the total treatment dose, and *d* is the dose per fraction. In addition and in accordance with the linear-quadratic formula, the term equieffective dose, EQDX, has been introduced and is defined as the total absorbed dose delivered by the reference treatment plan (fraction size *X*) that leads to the same biological effect as the treatment plan that is conducted with absorbed dose per fraction d and total absorbed dose D [49]. In this sense, BED in the above equation is the equieffective dose EQD0 ($X=0$ Gy). To understand by intuition, the comparison of RT schedules consisting of different total dose or dose per fraction is better possible by converting each RT schedule into an equivalent schedule in 2.0 Gy fractions which would give the same biological effect, the equieffective dose EQD2:

$$EQD2 = D\frac{(d + \alpha/\beta)}{(2 + \alpha/\beta)}$$

where D is the total treatment dose and d the dose per fraction of the fractionation scheme under investigation. Based on those formulae for calculating equieffective dose, when comparing HDR BRT with definitive conventional EBRT (including dose-escalated IMRT), the clinically delivered dose with HDR BRT regimens is up to 50 % higher compared to conventional EBRT schemes [11, 14, 22, 50–56].

2.3   Patient Selection for HDR Brachytherapy

Based on the assumption that failure to eradicate organ-confined prostate cancer may lead to the development of metastatic disease, the main indication for HDR treatment is histologically proven localized disease in patients considered suitable for radical treatment [57, 58]. In this context, the National Comprehensive Cancer Network (NCCN) [59] defined that low- and intermediate-risk cases are more likely to have disease confined to the prostate region and therefore are logically the best candidates for local treatment. Mature results exist for the application of HDR BRT as a boost modality in combination with EBRT for patients with intermediate- and high-risk disease according to the risk stratification schemes as described by D'Amico et al. [2], Zelefsky et al. [60] or the National Comprehensive Cancer Network (NCCN) [61]. In addition, a growing body of

literature corroborates its safe use as monotherapy with excellent oncological results predominantly for low- and intermediate-risk disease. However, some authors have elected to use HDR monotherapy in high-risk patients based on the idea that it provides a treatment margin greater than radical prostatectomy and the dose to the bladder and rectum remain significantly lower than when treating with definitive dose-escalated EBRT. In the clinical setting of regional lymphadenopathy with or without distant disease spread, HDR BRT may be implemented combined with EBRT in individualized treatment schemes in order to avoid increased toxicity where RT is employed with the goal of increased local disease control.

Pretreatment investigations for HDR BRT should follow the European Association of Urology [62], European Society for Radiotherapy and Oncology (ESTRO) [58], and American Brachytherapy Society (ABS) [57] guidelines. All patients considered for interstitial (IRT) irradiation should have histological confirmation of malignancy, and staging tests for evaluation of disease burden should include digital rectal examination, transrectal ultrasound (TRUS), and, if indicated, computed tomography (CT) and/or magnetic resonance imaging (MRI) and bone scintigraphy. In equivocal cases of regional lymphadenopathy, laparoscopic pelvic lymphadenectomy [63] or positron emission tomography [64, 65] may be considered.

Although functional outcome after IRT BRT is predicted by the baseline urinary function [66], neither larger gland size nor previous transurethral resection of the prostate (TURP) are absolute contraindications for treatment. Transperineal TRUS-guided implantation enables the complete and safe coverage of prostate volumes appreciably greater than 50 cm³ provided the patient has a sufficiently broad pelvic inlet and freedom from lower urinary tract symptoms (LUTS) requiring treatment [34, 57, 67–70]. However, HDR appears to be less likely to cause prolonged exacerbation of urination symptoms than LDR or EBRT because even patients with International Prostate Symptom Score (IPSS) of 20 or higher tend to have a relatively rapid return to pre-treatment baseline urinary function [70]. In addition, temporary implantation with HDR irradiation is safely feasible at >3 months after TURP given a sufficient amount of residual gland volume for image-based 3D treatment planning [20, 71–74]. Nonetheless, HDR BRT may be technically feasible even after extensive TURP in selected cases because it uses a scaffolding of catheters to hold the radiation source, and the dose to OARs be anatomy-based optimised given adequate imaging for treatment planning [74].

Selection criteria for HDR BRT as monotherapy or combined with EBRT are shown in Table 1. Unlike for permanent LDR implants, temporary HDR BRT afterloading catheters can be implanted next to extracapsular lesions or the seminal vesicles or even into the bladder pouch. Therefore, the indication for HDR BRT is by various groups extended to even T4 tumors as part of curative treatment schemes [14, 56, 75, 76]. Previous pelvic EBRT, inflammatory bowel disease, and prior pelvic surgery are not absolute contraindications to prostate BRT, but the anatomy-based dosimetry must include carefully defined normal tissue dose constraints and there must be a very cautious evaluation of the potential risks and benefits [20].

Table 1 Patient selection criteria for HDR BRT in the treatment of prostate cancer

Inclusion criteria
Stages T1–T3b[a]
Any Gleason score
Any PSA level
Exclusion criteria
TURP within 3 months
IPSS > 20
Pubic arch interference
Lithotomy position not possible[b]
Anesthesia not possible
Rectal fistula

[a]T4 tumors included with curative intent in the protocols of selected centers [14, 56, 75, 76]
[b]Relevant for TRUS-guided techniques, not relevant for MRI-guided implantation [77, 78]

3   Treatment Procedure

3.1   Implantation Techniques

Interstitial catheter implantation is usually performed under spinal or general anesthesia with various catheter placement patterns being described. Extensive experience exists for the technique of TRUS-guided implantation [9–11, 17, 48, 79]; however, MRI-based implantation techniques have also been reported in the literature [77, 78].

In case of the TRUS-based technique, implantation is performed transperineally in high lithotomy position using a continuous probe movement technique and a template to aid catheter placement. The clinical workflow includes the creation of virtual volumes prior to implantation for inverse treatment preplanning [36], and for this purpose, transverse ultrasound (US) images of the prostate, urethra, and anterior rectal wall are acquired in real time. Three-dimensional (3D) volumes are reconstructed based on a 0.1 cm image distance. The planning target volume (PTV) encompasses the entire prostate gland and the contour definition for the rectum extends cranially (e.g., 1.0 cm) from the prostatic base and caudally (e.g., 1.0 cm) from the prostatic apex. Urethra contouring encounters the intraprostatic urethra marked by the insertion of a radiopaque three-way Foley catheter and extends caudally (at least 0.5 cm) to include the apical membranous urethra. Bladder contouring encompasses the volume visible on US. Based on the acquired 3D anatomy, appropriate virtual catheter positions are generated, catheter source dwell positions located within the PTV are activated, and radioactive source dwell times are calculated using an intraoperative treatment planning system (Fig. 1). The final evaluation of the anatomy-oriented dose optimization [35] is based on the dose-volume histogram (DVH) of the PTV and the OARs (i.e., intraprostatic urethra, anterior rectal wall, and urinary bladder). If the preplanning dosimetry parameters fulfill the dosimetric protocol, TRUS-guided implantation is performed at the previously determined catheter positions (Fig. 2). In MRI-based implantation, catheter placement is

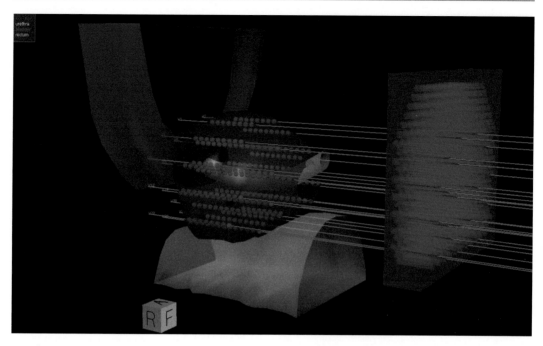

Fig. 1 Three-dimensional reconstruction of the prostate, urethra, rectum, and bladder with ideal template catheter trajectories for TRUS-guided implantation as calculated for preplanning by the real-time treatment planning system SWIFT/Oncentra Prostate (Nucletron – an Elekta Company, B.V., Veenendaal, The Netherlands). The virtual perineal template is displayed on the right side

also performed transperineally with the patient in left lateral decubitus position utilizing a template device. Similar to the workflow of TRUS-guided implantation, the MRI-guided procedure includes a preplanning step based on 3D image volumes acquired by preinterventional MRI sequences of at least 0.3 cm slice thickness. The number, distribution, and distance between the catheters are determined by the preplanning which calculates the peripheral catheter arrangement with arbitrary optimization for target coverage. Catheter implantation with control of maximum insertion depth and positional verification of the implanted catheters is performed by interactive MRI scanning.

3.2 Imaging for Treatment Planning

After completion of the catheter implantation procedure, an adequate image series is acquired for the process of treatment planning. Treatment planning after TRUS-guided implantation is most commonly performed using either TRUS [9–11, 80] or CT imaging [17, 18, 81–83]. In addition, MRI-based treatment planning with or without MRI-guided implantation has also been implemented in clinical practice [77, 78, 84, 85].

3.2.1 Ultrasound-Based Intraoperative Treatment Planning

For US-based intraoperative treatment planning after TRUS-guided implantation, a series of TRUS images are acquired with the patient remaining in lithotomy position. For accurate anatomic delineation and catheter reconstruction, image acquisition in steps of as low as 0.1 cm may be used (Fig. 3a–c). Modern systems allow the continuous movement of the US probe (manually or motorized) without discrete stepping, where US images are automatically grabbed at a predefined interval (0.1–0.5 cm). At this point, attention should be paid when using standoffs for a better coupling of sound-avoiding materials, such as silicone, where geometric shifts are

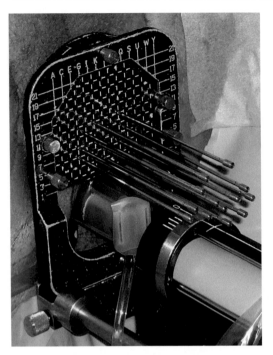

Fig. 2 High-resolution template with implanted interstitial steel catheters (20 cm length, 0.19 cm diameter). The transducer probe for TRUS guidance is attached to a floor-mounted stepping unit and inserted into the rectum. A thin intestinal tube for the discharge of intestinal gases is inserted laterally to the probe and partly visible behind the lower right angle of the template

3.2.2 CT- or MRI-Based Postoperative Treatment Planning

For CT- or MRI-based treatment planning after TRUS-guided implantation, the patient must be transferred after recovery from anesthesia to a CT or MRI scanner, respectively. For accurate anatomy delineation and reproducible catheter reconstruction, an image acquisition with slice thickness of ≤ 0.3 cm is recommended. Considering the craniocaudal scanning extension for adequate inclusion of the OARs, the specifications listed above for the US-based planning procedure should be considered. Since in current clinical practice two-dimensional dose calculation is the standard method (TG 43 formalism without consideration of tissue inhomogeneities and influence of the finite size of the body) [87, 88], it is not necessary to include the patient's body contour for treatment planning purposes. For a more accurate delineation of the prostate, MRI and CT co-registration can be considered [89–91]. Alternatively, only MRI can be used where both T1- and T2-weighted images should be considered for an optimal visualization of anatomy and catheter position [77, 78, 84, 85]. In contrary to the totally TRUS-based clinical workflow, CT- or MRI-based planning bears an additional risk for catheter rearrangement and target volume changes due to transferring of the patient to a CT or MRI scanner which constitutes a deviation of the patient setup [92–94].

Irrespective of the imaging modality for interventional guidance or treatment planning, HDR irradiation is performed using a remote afterloading system. Iridium-192 is the most commonly used isotope with an effective energy of 398 keV, a half-life of 73.81 days, and a half value layer of 3.0 mm of lead [95].

observed due to the differences in sound speed between silicone and soft tissue (981 m/s in silicone versus 1540 m/s in soft tissue) [86]. Alternatively, rotational acquisition can be used whenever this is supported by the intraoperative planning system. The extension of the scanning should be adjusted in such a way that:

- The whole prostate gland is included
- Possible extensions (e.g., seminal vesicles) are covered
- The tip of all catheters is included
- An adequate extension caudally from the prostatic apex to account for delineation of the apical membranous urethra (at least 0.5 cm) is considered
- An adequate extension cranially from the prostatic base and caudally from the prostatic apex for delineation of the rectum or rectal wall (e.g., 1.0 cm) is considered

3.3 Treatment Planning

Postimplantation image-guided treatment planning in temporary HDR prostate BRT encompasses the steps of anatomy definition, localization of the implanted catheters, and dosimetric calculations including dose optimization.

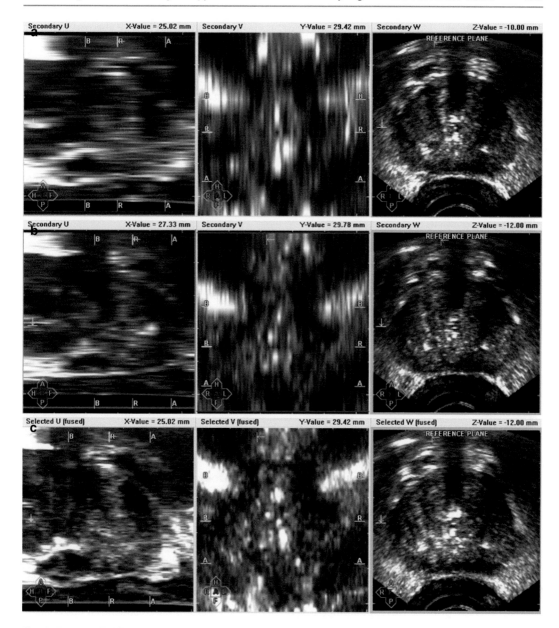

Fig. 3 Impact of different intervals in the ultrasound-based image acquisition using the transversal crystal array and continuous movement with a BK medical ultrasound system (BK medical, Analogic Corporation, USA) and the Oncentra Prostate planning system: (**a**) 0.5 cm interval, (**b**) 0.3 cm interval, and (**c**) 0.1 cm interval. The superior quality of the reconstructed coronal (*left*) and sagittal (*middle*) images is clearly demonstrated

3.3.1   Anatomy Definition

Even though the concepts of target volumes and OARs were formalized by ICRU Report 50 [96, 97], BRT practitioners have reported different target and treatment philosophies in the literature [9, 12, 98–100]. In order to develop consistency in target and volume definition for temporary HDR prostate BRT, the following should be considered for postimplantation treatment planning independent of the acquired imaging modality [58]:

• Clinical target volume (CTV) is defined by:
  – The prostate capsule plus any macroscopic extracapsular disease or seminal vesicle

involvement identified on diagnostic images expanded by 0.3 cm to encompass potential microscopic disease

- Gross tumor volume (GTV) may be defined using information from previous diagnostic imaging. Clinical target subvolumes may include boost volumes to the peripheral zones or other sites defined from imaging where significant tumor volumes are considered.
- Organs at risk should include as a minimum:
  - Rectum: outlining of the outer wall alone is considered adequate for BRT dosimetry as defined for LDR seed techniques.
  - The urethra using the urethral catheter as a landmark on imaging for the urethral contour which should extend from bladder base to 0.5–1.0 cm below the prostatic apex.
- Other OARs may include penile bulb, bladder neck, and the neurovascular bundle.

Consideration should be given to expand the CTV to define a PTV accounting for any uncertainties in the procedure, for example, catheter tracking and image registration.

3.3.2 Catheter Localization and Optimization

The identification of the tip and thereby of the first (most distal) source dwell position for each implanted catheter is essential for the accuracy of the catheter localization process. Due to the partial volume effect of all imaging modalities (US, CT, and MRI), special attention has to be paid. Kim et al. [101] demonstrated that for CT-based HDR prostate BRT planning, a CT slice thickness of maximum 0.3 cm should be used in order to keep the average dose uncertainty acceptable (i.e., 1.0 % or less). The same can be transferred to MRI-based treatment planning [77, 78, 85]. For US-based treatment planning, advanced tools have been developed and are available in dedicated treatment planning systems. In general, the US-based process for catheter tip identification uses the known physical length of the catheter and the measurement of the catheter free length which is the portion from the end of the catheter (outside the

body) to the proximal side of the perineal template [102].

It is widely established in clinical practice that the use of the inverse optimization tools available in modern treatment planning systems for automatically adjusting the dwell times of the source at the different dwell positions of the catheters should be used [103] (Fig. 4a, b). To this end, appropriate dose-volume objectives (objective functions) for the different volumes of interest (PTV, OARs) and their relative importance (penalties or importance factors, Fig. 5) need to be preset. The results of the inverse optimization depend strongly on concrete algorithmic implementation. This is also valid for the influence of the relative importance of the defined dose-volume objectives on the optimization result. Specific sets of parameter values for the specific inverse optimizer and the specific clinically implemented implantation technique can be defined to achieve dose distributions fulfilling, in the best possible way, a specific dosimetric clinical protocol (Fig. 6a–d). These sets can be stored and are available for each new planning process, thus improving efficacy and reproducibility.

3.3.3 Dose Prescription and Dose Fractionation Schemes

In spite of the high sensitivity of the minimum dose (MD) or minimum peripheral dose (MPD) to small delineation inaccuracies in the PTV, in both the ABS consensus guidelines [57] and the ESTRO recommendations [58], the aimed or intended MPD to the PTV is referred to as the prescribed dose for the treatment. In this context, the majority of the relevant literature refers to planned dose to the achieved D_{90}-values for the PTV. Those values are more stable regarding delineation inaccuracies and resolution of the calculation grid or number of sample points than the MD values. In general, it should be distinguished between the aimed or intended dose (prescription) and the realized dose in the planning process. In other words, the aimed D_{90}-value for the PTV (usually at least the aimed dose) should be distinguished from the planned D_{90}-value which is the value that is delivered in the

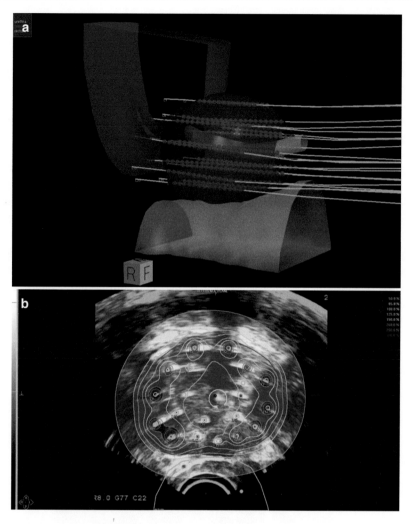

Fig. 4 Intraoperative real-time TRUS-based treatment planning. (**a**) Three-dimensional reconstruction of the prostate, organs at risk (i.e., rectum, urethra, bladder), in situ catheters, and the source dwell positions as calculated using the real-time treatment planning system SWIFT/Oncentra Prostate for the final treatment plan; (**b**) isodose distribution after anatomy-based dose optimization. The isodose color code convention is *dark red* = 300 % {isodose = 28.5 Gy}, *orange* = 200 % {isodose = 19.0 Gy}, *yellow* = 150 % {isodose = 14.25 Gy}, *green* = 125 % {isodose = 11.87 Gy}, *turquoise* = 100 % {isodose = 9.5 Gy}, and *dark blue* = 50 % {isodose = 4.75 Gy}

Name	Type	Class	Dose limit [%]	Dose limit [cGy]	Imp. factor
☑ Normal Tissue	External	External	120.00	1380.00	8.000
☑ Prostate-Low	CTV1	Prostate	100.00	1150.00	20.000
☑ Prostate-Heigh	CTV1	Prostate	150.00	1725.00	5.000
☑ Urethra	OAR	Urethra	120.00	1380.00	10.000
☑ Rectum	OAR	Rectum	75.00	862.50	10.000
Normal Tissue	External	External	120.00	1380.00	8.000

DVHO optimization settings

VOI Settings

Dwell time gradient restr.
0.00   0.15   1.00

ASDPs outside target
☑ Consider ASDPs outside target

Convergence Settings
◉ Standard
○ High Accuracy
Max. Iterations: 1000

Apply and run   OK   Cancel

Fig. 5 An example of graphical user interface for defining the different parameter values for inverse treatment plan optimization. In this case, the HIPO-Optimizer (Pi-Medical Ltd., Athens, Greece) as implemented in Oncentra Prostate individual treatment and represents the individual dose prescription. For example, White et al. [34] reported their dosimetric analysis of 104 consecutive patients (208 temporary HDR implants) treated at the California Endocurietherapy Cancer Center (CET). The authors could demonstrate very high reproducibility of the planned (prescribed) D_{90}-value for the PTV. On average, the planned D_{90}-value was 9.2 % higher than the aimed dose and thus 9.2 % higher than the dose per fraction described by the authors in the two different fractionation schemes which were used (7.25 Gy and 6.0 Gy per fraction). This is the result of the specific implantation and optimization technique used at the CET and has to be taken into consideration when comparing different fractionation schemes. In a similar analysis, the Offenbach group evaluated 120 consecutive HDR monotherapy treatment plans. With an aimed D_{90} for the PTV of 11.5 Gy per fraction, the authors showed that the average planned D_{90} was 102.5 ± 2 % of the aimed value (Fig. 7).

Thus, based on the current Offenbach protocol [9], the planned dose prescription per fraction, expressed as D_{90}, is on average 11.8 Gy, and the total dose achieved in three fractions is on average 35.4 Gy with intended doses of 11.5 Gy and 34.5 Gy, respectively. In comparison, for the CET monotherapy protocol, the corresponding values are on average 7.9 Gy per fraction, and the total dose achieved is 47.4 Gy in six fractions with intended doses of 7.25 Gy and 43.5 Gy, respectively. Independent of the specific aspects concerning the issue of dose prescription, the heterogeneity in clinically implemented dose fractionation schemes makes the establishment of absolute guidelines for total physical prescription doses and normal tissue dose constraints difficult. For illustration, Table 2 lists dose fractionation schedules and normal tissue dose constraints used by various centers. For example, the William Beaumont Hospital monotherapy protocol consists of one implant that delivers four fractions of 9.5 Gy [10]. The current Offenbach

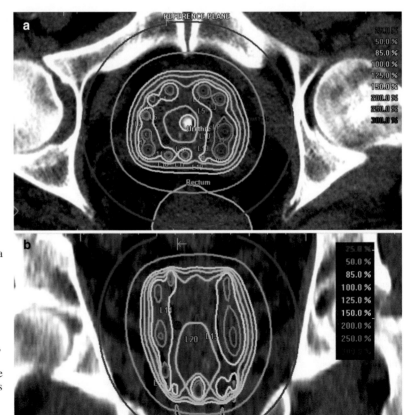

Fig. 6 Results of inverse optimization with Oncentra Prostate RTP using HIPO for a CT-based treatment plan of HDR prostate BRT. The isodose line overlay to (**a**) the central axial plane (reference plane), (**b**) a coronal plane, and (**c**) a representative sagittal plane (**d**) shows the corresponding DVH curves for the PTV, urethra, and rectum. One hundred percent corresponds to the aimed dose prescription

Fig. 6 (continued)

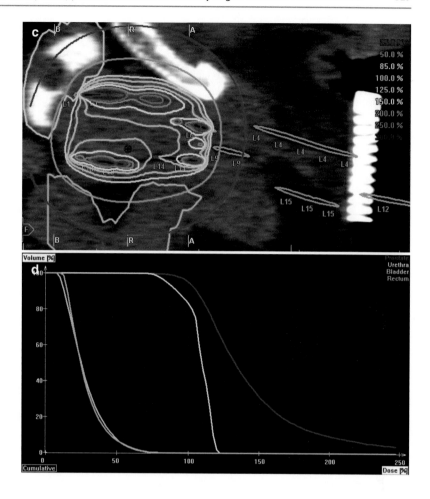

Fig. 7 Mean values and standard deviations for 120 consecutive monotherapy treatment plans with an aimed D_{90} for PTV of 11.5 Gy per fraction for different dose-volume values for PTV and OARs. The values are expressed as percentage of the aimed prescription dose of 11.5 Gy to the 90 % of the PTV

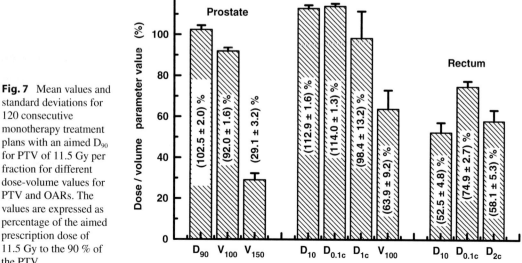

Table 2 Total physical prescription doses and normal tissue HDR dose constraints (as percent of prescribed reference dose or absolute dose value) of various treatment schemes

Treatment protocol	PTV	Rectum	Bladder	Urethra	D_{90}	V_{100}	V_{150}
Demanes et al. 2011 [10][a]							
CET	7.0 Gy × 6 (42 Gy)	$D_{0.1\,cm^3}$ ≤80%	$D_{0.1\,cm^3}$ ≤80%	$D_{0.1\,cm^3}$ ≤110%	>100%	>97%	–
WBH	9.5 Gy × 4 (38 Gy)	$D_{0.1\,cm^3}$ ≤75%	$D_{0.1\,cm^3}$ ≤80%	$D_{0.1\,cm^3}$ ≤120%	>100%	>96%	–
Zamboglou et al. 2012 [9][a]	9.5 Gy × 4 (38 Gy)	$D_{0.1\,cm^3}$ ≤80%	$D_{0.1\,cm^3}$ ≤80%	$D_{0.1\,cm^3}$ ≤120%	≥100%	≥90%	≤35%
	11.5 Gy × 3 (34.5 Gy)	$D_{0.1\,cm^3}$ ≤80%	$D_{0.1\,cm^3}$ ≤80%	$D_{0.1\,cm^3}$ ≤120%	≥100%	≥90%	≤35%
Prada et al. 2012 [144][a]	19 Gy × 1 (19 Gy)	$D_{0.1\,cm^3}$ ≤75%	–	$D_{0.1\,cm^3}$ ≤110%	–	–	–
Hoskin et al. 2007 [82][b]	37.7 Gy EBRT + 2 × 8.5 Gy (17 Gy) BRT	$D_{2.0\,cm^3}$ <6.7 Gy	–	D_{10} <10 Gy	–	–	–
Kotecha et al. 2013 [14][b]	45–50.4 Gy EBRT + 3 × (5.5–7.5 Gy) BRT	$D_{0.1\,cm^3}$ ≤100%	–	$D_{0.1\,cm^3}$ ≤120%	–	≥100%	–
Pistis et al. 2010 [13][b]	60 Gy EBRT + 1 × 9 Gy BRT	$D_{2.0\,cm^3}$ ≤75%	–	$D_{2\%}$ <120%	≥105%	≥98%	≤50%
Morton et al. 2010 [115][b]	1 × 15 Gy BRT + 37.5 Gy EBRT	D_{max}≤80%	D_{max}≤80%	D_{max}≤118%	–	≥95%	≤40%
Agoston et al. 2011 [116][b]	40–61 Gy EBRT + 1 × 8 or 10 Gy BRT	D_{max}≤80%	–	D_{max}≤125%	–	≥95%	–

Abbreviations: D_{10} dose delivered to 10% of the organ, $D_{0.1\,cm^3}$ maximum dose to the most exposed 0.1 cm³ of the organ, $D_{2.0\,cm^3}$ maximum dose to the most exposed 2.0 cm³ of the organ, $D_{2\%}$ maximum dose to the most exposed 2% of the organ, D_{max} maximum dose to the most exposed points of the organ, V_{100}, V_{150} percent of PTV receiving 100% and 150% of the prescription dose, *CET* California Endocurietherapy Cancer Center, *WBH* William Beaumont Hospital
[a] Monotherapy
[b] Combined treatment with supplemental EBRT

monotherapy protocol consists of three implants each delivering one fraction of 11.5 Gy with implants separated by 21 days [9]. At the Catalan Institute of Oncology, combined treatment is delivered with 60 Gy conventionally fractionated EBRT followed by a single-fraction HDR boost of 9 Gy within 21 days [13].

4 Clinical Data

4.1 HDR Boost in Combination with EBRT

In patients with intermediate- and high-risk prostate cancer, dose-escalated RT has been shown to improve both BC and LC [4, 5, 24, 25, 27–29, 104–107]. The combination of EBRT and HDR BRT allows for the safe delivery of escalated biologic equivalent doses to the prostate not achievable in terms of conformality even by image-guided IMRT [3, 108–111]. Two randomized trials have helped to show the superiority of HDR BRT combined with EBRT over EBRT alone in the radical treatment of localized prostate cancer. Sathya et al. [112] assigned 104 patients to conventional EBRT of 66 Gy in 33 fractions or to 35 Gy HDR BRT with supplemental EBRT of 40 Gy in 20 fractions. At a median follow-up of 8.2 years, the authors reported biochemical failure in 17 patients of the combined arm compared with 33 patients in the EBRT alone arm ($p=0.0024$). Overall survival was 94 % in the combined arm versus 92 % in the EBRT arm without statistically significant differences in acute or late genitourinary (GU) and gastrointestinal (GI) toxicity. In an analogous approach, Hoskin et al. [82] randomized 220 patients to either hypofractionated EBRT alone or hypofractionated EBRT combined with HDR BRT. The EBRT group ($n=111$) received 55 Gy in 20 fractions, whereas the combined treatment group ($n=109$) was given 35.75 Gy EBRT in 13 fractions plus a 17-Gy HDR boost applied in two fractions. The mean biochemical failure-free survival in the combined arm was 5.1 vs. 4.3 years in the EBRT-only group ($p=0.03$) without statistically significant differences in higher-grade GU and GI toxicity. The results of these randomized trials are in accordance with the oncological outcomes reported in large retrospective series [13–15]. Kotecha et al. [14] treated 229 patients with an HDR BRT boost followed by EBRT. The boost consisted of three fractions of HDR BRT at 5.5–7.5 Gy per fraction and supplemental EBRT of conventionally fractionated IMRT delivering 45.0–50.4 Gy. The generated $BED_{1.5}$ values ranged from 171 to 226 Gy with a median value of 191.5 Gy. The 7-year biochemical relapse-free survival rates were 95 %, 90 %, and 57 % for low-, intermediate-, and high-risk patients, respectively, with a 7-year BC of 81 % among high-risk patients with $BED_{1.5}$ values >190 Gy. The reported incidence of late Grade 3 GU and GI toxicity was 3.1 % and 0.4 %, respectively. In a scheme consisting of EBRT interdigitated with HDR BRT, Prada et al. [15] reported on 252 high-risk patients treated with 46 Gy EBRT and two fractions of HDR BRT of 10.5–11.5 Gy yielding total combined $BED_{1.5}$ doses ranging from 292 to 366 Gy. The accomplished 5- and 10-year BC rate was 84 % and 78 %, respectively, with 2.7 % late Grade 3 GU and no late GI toxicity.

Although the heterogeneity of clinically implemented treatment schemes makes uniform recommendations concerning the optimal combined treatment protocol challenging, the published oncological results on HDR BRT combined with supplemental EBRT are consistent and reproducible (Table 3). Most authors use BRT fractions ranging from 6 to 10 Gy yielding

total physical HDR doses of 12–20 Gy applied in two to four fractions. The supplemental EBRT doses range from 45 to 54 Gy, generating total $BED_{1.5}$ and EQD2 doses in the range of 171–366 Gy and 74–137 Gy, respectively [12–15, 17, 18, 54, 79, 81, 99, 112–117, 119–121, 123–127]. The reported rates of severe late GU and GI adverse events compare favorably with late toxicity rates in dose-escalated EBRT series [105, 128–130].

4.2 HDR Monotherapy

Although HDR BRT was initially used as a boost modality in conjunction with EBRT because of concerns about the normal tissue toxicity of hypofractionated treatment regimes, dose escalation studies established the safety and efficacy range for HDR in the context of combined EBRT and BRT [17, 131, 132]. These clinical experiences, together with technological advances in real-time image guidance and 3D image-based treatment planning, led to the introduction of HDR monotherapy as a conceptually comprehensible RT approach for organ-confined prostate cancer [132–134]. The rationale for HDR monotherapy was derived from other locally directed treatments such as radical prostatectomy, definitive EBRT, and permanent LDR seed monotherapy considering that image-guided HDR with anatomy-based dose optimization can reliably treat the prostate and simultaneously control the dose to adjacent OARs [20]. There is by now a growing body of literature that corroborates HDR monotherapy as a safe and effective modality for the radical treatment of localized prostate cancer with consistent intermediate- and long-term BC rates reported for all risk groups [9–11, 20, 22, 69, 76, 80, 132, 135–144]. Although direct comparisons are difficult, given the variety of clinically implemented dose fractionation schemes, the oncological outcomes yielded with single- or multiple implant regimes for extreme hypofractionated or multifractionated treatment protocols are uniform (Table 4).

Kukielka et al. [140] reported the oncological outcomes in 77 patients of various risk groups

Table 3 Literature results of HDR BRT as boost modality to EBRT for clinically localized prostate cancer

Study	n	Treatment scheme			Follow-up (years)	Biochemical control[a]
		Total EBRT dose (Gy/fx)	Total HDR dose (Gy/fx)	Total BED/EQD2 (Gy)		
Galalae et al. [81]	144	40/20	18/2	219/94	Median 8.2	74 %/69 % all risk groups at 5years/8 years
Pistis et al. [13]	114	60/20	9/1	203/87	Mean 2.7	97.4 % IR and HR at 4 years
Kotecha et al. [14]	229	45–50.4/25–28	16.5–22.5/3	171–226/74–97	Median 5.1	95 % LR at 7 years, 90 % IR at 7 years, 57 % HR at 7 years (81 % HR with BED > 190 Gy)
Martin et al. [79]	102	45/25	20–28/4	191–251/82–108	Median 2.6	100 % LR/IR at 3 years, 79 % HR at 3 years
Prada et al. [15]	252	46/23	21–23/2	292–366/109–137	Median 6.1	84 %/78 % HR at 5 years/10 years
Åström et al. [113]	214	50/25	20/2	269/116	Median 4	82 % all risk groups at 5 years
Martinez et al. [17]	207	46/23	16.5–23/2–3	184–306/79–131	Mean 4.4	52 % all risk groups for EQD2<93 Gy and 87 % all risk groups for EQD2>93 Gy at 5 years
Noda et al. [114]	59	50/25	15–18/2	191–243/82–104	Median 5.1	100 % LR at 5 years, 92 % IR at 5 years, 72 % HR at 5 years
Hoskin et al. [82]	220	35.75/13	17/2	214/92	Median 2.5	Mean for all risk groups 4.3 years
Morton et al. [115]	123	37.5/15	15/1	265/114	Median 1.2	100 % all risk groups
Agoston et al. [116]	100	40–60/20–30	8/1 or 10/1	144–219/66–94	Median 5.1	85.5 % all risk groups at 5 years with IR 84,2 % at 7 years and HR 81,6 % at 7 years
Hiratsuka et al. [117]	71	41.8 /19 or 45/25	16.5/3 or 22.5/4	176–206/92–110	Median 3.6	93 % at 5 years (ASTRO definition [118])
Pellizzon et al. [119]	209	36–54/20–30	16–24/4	143–237/59–94	Median 5.3	94.2 % all risk groups at 3.3 years with 91.5 % LR, 90.2 % IR, and 88.5 % HR
Phan et al. [120]	309	39.6–50.4/20–28	15-26/3-4	144–218/63–97	Median 4.9	86 % all risk groups at 5 years with 98 % LR, 90 % IR, and 78 % HR (ASTRO definition [164])
Viani et al. [121]	131	45–50/25	16–24/4–6	158–237/67–101	Median 5.2	81 % at 5 years with 87 % IR and 71 % HR

Abbreviations: LR low-risk group, *IR* intermediate-risk group, *HR* high-risk group, *y* years, *BED* biologically effective dose considering an a/β ratio for prostate cancer of 1.5, *EQD2* biologically effective dose administered in 2Gy fractions
[a]Biochemical failure defined by the *Phoenix definition* [122] unless specified otherwise

who were treated with 45 Gy in three single-fraction implants at 15 Gy. The 5-year overall survival was 98.7 % with an actuarial BC rate of 96.7 %. There were no acute Grade 3 or higher toxicities; however, acute Grade 2 GU toxicity was seen in 25 % of patients. One patient experi-

Table 4 Literature results of HDR BRT as monotherapy for localized prostate cancer

Study	n	HDR protocol Gy/fraction	Fractions (implants)	Total	Median f/u (y)	Biochemical control[a]	BED (Gy)	EQD2 (Gy)
Yoshioka et al. [76]	111	6.0 Gy	9 (1 implant)	54 Gy	5.4	93 % IR, 85 % HR at 3 years	270	116
Yoshioka et al. [56]	63	6.5 Gy	7 (1 implant)	45.5 Gy	3.5	96 % IR, 90 % HR at 3 years	243	104
Hoskin et al. [11]	197	8.5–9.0 Gy	4 (1 implant)	34–36 Gy	4.5–5	95 % IR, 87 % HR at 4 years	227–252	97–108
		10.5 Gy	3 (1 implant)	31.5 Gy	3			
		13.0 Gy	2 (1 implant)	26 Gy	0.5			
Rogers et al. [69]	284	6.5 Gy	6 (2 implants)	39 Gy	3	94 % IR at 5 years	208	89
Mark et al. [141]	301	7.5 Gy	6 (2 implants)	45 Gy	8	88 % all risk groups at 8 years	270	117
Prada et al. [144]	40	19.0 Gy	1 (1 implant)	19 Gy	1.6	100 % LR, 88 % IR at 32 months	260	111
Demanes et al. [10]	298	7.0 Gy	6 (2 implants)	42 Gy	5.2	97 % LR/IR at 5 years	238–279	102–119
		9.5 Gy	4 (1 implant)	38 Gy				
Zamboglou et al. [9]	718	9.5 Gy	4 (1 implant)	38 Gy	4.4	95 % LR, 93 % IR 93 % HR at 5 years	279–299	119–128
		9.5 Gy	4 (2 implants)	38 Gy				
		11.5 Gy	3 (3 implants)	34.5 Gy				
Ghadjar et al. [137]	36	9.5 Gy	4 (1 implant)	38	3	100 % LR/IR at 3 years	279	119
Barkati et al. [135]	79	10-11.5 Gy	3 (1 implant)	30–34.5	3.3	85.1 % LR/IR at 5 years	230–299	99–128
Komiya et al. [139]	51	6.5 Gy	7 (1 implant)	45.5	1.4	94 % all risk groups at 17 months	243	104

Abbreviations: LR low-risk group, *IR* intermediate-risk group, *HR* high-risk group, *f/u* follow-up, *y* years, *BED* biologically effective dose considering an a/β ratio for prostate cancer of 1.5, *EQD2* biologically effective dose administered in 2Gy fractions
[a]Biochemical failure defined by the *Phoenix definition* [122]

enced late Grade 3 urethral stenosis with no late Grade 3 GI adverse events detected. Mark et al. [141] reported an actuarial BC rate of 88 % at 8 years in 301 patients of all risk groups treated with two implants at three fractions of 7.5 Gy. Acute urinary retention occurred in 5 % of patients with late Grade 3–4 GU adverse events

in 6 %. Late GI toxicity was Grades 1–2 in 2.3 % and Grades 3–4 in 0.3 % of patients. Similarly, Rogers et al. [69] reported their experience on 284 patients with intermediate-risk prostate cancer treated with two implants to deliver six fractions of 6.5 Gy. The 5-year actuarial BC was 94.4 % with MFS of 99 %. Unlike other reports, there were no Grade 3 urethral strictures with late Grade 1–2 GI toxicity in 4.2 % of patients. All authors included clinical stages ≥ T2b with no exclusions for Gleason score (GS) or pretreatment prostate-specific antigen (PSA) in the series by Mark et al. [141] and Kukielka et al. [140]. These data corroborate the clinical experience of other groups indicating that HDR BRT is applicable for monotherapy over a range of risk groups including intermediate- and selected cases of high-risk disease [9, 11, 76, 139, 145, 146]. Hoskin et al. [11], for example, conducted a dose escalation trial of 197 patients with predominantly intermediate- (52 %) and high-risk (44 %) cases. The implemented monotherapy protocols consisted of 34 Gy in four fractions, 36 Gy in four fractions, 31.5 Gy in three fractions, or 26 Gy in two fractions. The authors reported a 4-year BC rate of 87 % for the high-risk group which included clinical tumor stages ≥ T3 in 21 %, GS ≥ 8 in 10 %, and PSA > 20 ng/ml in 25 % of patients with 92 % of cases receiving temporary ADT. The incidence of acute Grade 3 GU morbidity was 3–7 % with no cases of acute GI toxicity. Late Grade 3 GU toxicity was 3–16 % with late Grade 3 GI toxicity documented in 1 % of patients. Similar results were reported by Zamboglou et al. [9] who treated 718 consecutive patients utilizing three different monotherapy protocols (four fractions of 9.5 Gy in one implant, four fractions of 9.5 Gy in two implants, and three fractions of 11.5 in three implants). The study population included 44.9 % of intermediate- and high-risk patients with clinical tumor stages > T2b in 13 %, GS ≥ 7 in 23 %, and PSA > 11 ng/ml in 7.3 % of all patients. Almost 60 % of high-risk and 27 % of intermediate-risk cases received temporary ADT including all patients with PSA ≥ 20 ng/ml, 93 % of patients with GS ≥ 7b (4 + 3), and more than 90 % of cases staged > T2b. The 5-year BC rate for intermediate- and high-risk patients was 93 % and 93 %, respectively. The authors documented 3.5 % late Grade 3 GU and 1.6 % late Grade 3 GI adverse events with two patients developing Grade 4 urinary incontinence and two patients requiring endoscopic restoration of bowel continuity.

Data on erectile function after HDR monotherapy have been rarely reported using various multidimensional or ordinal scales for assessment. However, potency preservation rates of 75–90 % are documented in the recent literature [9, 69, 139, 143, 144, 147, 148]. Komyia et al. [139] evaluated the quality of life (QOL) in 51 patients of various risk groups who were treated with one implant in seven fractions of 6.5 Gy. Long-term adjuvant ADT was used for high-risk cases. Assessment of QOL included the International Prostate Symptom Score (IPSS) [149] and the International Index of Erectile Function (IIEF) [150] questionnaire. The total IPSS increased significantly at 2 and 4 weeks after BRT but recovered to pretreatment values by 12 weeks in all patients. The erectile function was significantly impaired at 2 and 4 weeks after BRT in patients without ADT; however, it recovered to pretreatment values by 12 weeks with an IIEF score > 21 points. Ghadjar et al. [147] reported on 36 patients with low- and intermediate-risk prostate cancer treated with one implant in four fractions of 9.5 Gy. Fourteen percent of patients received concomitant ADT. At a median follow-up of 6.9 years, 19 % of patients experienced late Grade 3 GU adverse events with no late Grade 2–3 GI toxicities. The crude erectile function preservation rate in patients without ADT was 75 %.

So far, no randomized trial has ever compared LDR and HDR monotherapy, but nonrandomized evaluations have confirmed that both acute and late high-grade toxicities are less frequent after HDR than LDR monotherapy [138, 143]. Martinez et al. [143] performed a comprehensive toxicity comparison between 248 HDR monotherapy and 206 LDR seed patients. The 5-year actuarial BC for monotherapy was 88 % for HDR and 89 % for seeds with no difference in cancer mortality or overall survival. Temporary HDR monotherapy was associated with significantly less Grade 1–2 chronic dysuria (LDR 22 % vs. HDR 15 %) and urinary frequency/urgency (LDR 54 % vs. HDR 43 %). The rate of urethral stricture was equal with 2.5 % for LDR vs. 3 % for HDR. Chronic Grade 3 GU toxicity was low in both groups with about 2 % for HDR, mostly urinary frequency/urgency. The 5-year potency preservation rate was 80 % for HDR and 70 % for permanent LDR BRT.

Overall, the clinical outcome data of HDR monotherapy reflect current radiobiological considerations for optimal tumor control through hypofractionation. The BED values in Table 4 range from 208 to 299 Gy with a median value of 256 Gy, considering an alpha/beta ratio of 1.5 Gy. However, even for an alpha/beta ratio of 3.0 Gy, the BED values would be in the range of 123–167 Gy. In comparison with LDR implants, where attempts are made to attain a BED > 200 Gy by mainly adding EBRT [151, 152], HDR monotherapy generates BED values far higher than 200 Gy by itself. The values for EQD2 in Table 4 range from 89 to 128 Gy for an alpha/beta ratio of 1.5 Gy (77–104 Gy for an alpha/beta ratio of 3.0 Gy) which may be mostly impossible to administer with conventional EBRT. In contrast to clinical data from definitive EBRT, however, the potential advantage of temporary ADT for patients treated with HDR monotherapy remains an issue of ongoing discussion as no corroborative evidence exclusive to this modality exists [20, 153].

The excellent results of HDR prostate BRT have prompted the implementation of stereotactic body radiotherapy (SBRT) for the percutaneous treatment of localized prostate cancer using extreme hypofractionation and utilizing continuous image guidance to automatically track, detect, and correct for intrafraction prostate movement [154–158]. It appears to represent a biologically potent local treatment method, seemingly combining "EBRT-like" noninvasiveness with "HDR BRT-like" biologic potency [159]. However, in a recent dosimetric analysis comparing virtual SBRT with actual HDR monotherapy plans from treated patients, Spratt et al. [160] demonstrated that HDR achieves significantly higher intraprostatic doses while achieving similar urethral doses and lower maximum rectal doses compared with virtual SBRT treatment planning. Although SBRT has the potential to recapitulate HDR dosimetry [161], at present, there are no durable monotherapy outcome data and no direct clinical trials comparing temporary HDR, permanent LDR, or SBRT in the treatment of prostate cancer. In addi-

tion, given the tight "surgical margin" associated with SBRT, it is not recommended for more advanced disease such as extracapsular extension or seminal vesicle involvement [156, 162].

4.3 HDR Monotherapy as Salvage Treatment

The ideal management of patients experiencing a biochemical recurrence (BCR) after radical RT for clinically localized prostate cancer remains a controversial clinical issue [163]. Despite the primary treatment-related variation in the definition of BCR [118, 122], clinical data suggest that up to 70 % of patients with a rising PSA will have local disease as the only demonstrable site of recurrence [164–166]. Therefore, repeat local treatment poses a comprehensible therapeutic approach with different local procedures such as salvage radical prostatectomy, salvage high-intensity focused US, and salvage RT being clinically practiced [167]. For pathologically proven local failure after previous definitive RT, salvage HDR BRT (sHDR BRT) with or without ADT appears to be an effective, well-tolerated treatment option with disease control and toxicity rates which compare favorably to those reported using other nonradiotherapeutic local treatment modalities [165, 168–173]. Lee et al. [168] treated 21 patients (median pre-salvage PSA 3.8ng/ml with median pre-salvage GS 7) after primary EBRT of a median 66.6 Gy with 36 Gy sHDR BRT in six fractions using two TRUS-guided implants separated by 1 week. The reported BC at median 18.7 months of follow-up was 89 % with 86 % Grade 2 and 14 % Grade 3 GU adverse events at 3 months after BRT. Yamada et al. [173] reported the results of a Phase II study of 40 patients (median pre-salvage PSA 3.45ng/ml with 60 % GS 7 and 33 % GS ≥ 8) treated with sHDR BRT after prior definitive EBRT. The protocol prescription dose of 32 Gy was delivered in four fractions of 8 Gy over 30 hours. Twelve patients had neoadjuvant ADT. At a median follow-up of 38 months, the estimated PSA disease-free survival was 70 %. Late Grade 1 and 2 GU toxicities were found in 38 % and 48 %, respectively, with one patient developing Grade 3 urinary incontinence. Late Grade 1 and 2 GI toxicity was noted in 17 % and 8 % of patients, respectively. Three patients developed urethral strictures requiring urethral dilatation. No Grade 4 toxicities were observed. Similarly, Oliai et al. [169] reported on a group of 22 patients who underwent sHDR BRT with or without ADT after primary treatment with EBRT, LDR BRT, or HDR BRT with supplemental EBRT, receiving for salvage 36 Gy HDR BRT in six fractions using two TRUS-guided implants. At a median follow-up of 45 months, the generated BC rate was 75 %. Urethral strictures requiring transurethral resection developed in 32 % of patients and Grade 2 hematuria manifested in 18 % of patients. In the series by Chen et al. [165], which is the largest series of patients treated with sHDR BRT after previous definitive RT, fifty-two patients were analyzed. After pathologic confirmation of locally recurrent disease, patients received 36 Gy HDR BRT in six fractions of 6 Gy. Median follow-up was 59.6 months with an actuarial BC rate of 51 % at 5 years. Acute and late Grade 3 GU adverse events were reported in 2 % and 2 % of patients, respectively. No Grade 2 or higher acute GI adverse events and 4 % late Grade 2 GI toxicity were documented. In summary, sHDR BRT for locally recurrent disease after initial radical treatment appears as a promising RT approach with an acceptable acute and late toxicity profile.

References

1. D'Amico AV, Whittington R, Malkowicz SB et al (2002) Biochemical outcome after radical prostatectomy or external beam radiation therapy for patients with clinically localized prostate carcinoma in the prostate specific antigen era. Cancer 95(2): 281–286. doi:10.1002/cncr.10657
2. D'Amico AV, Whittington R, Malkowicz SB et al (1998) Biochemical outcome after radical prostatectomy, external beam radiation therapy, or interstitial radiation therapy for clinically localized prostate cancer. JAMA 280(11):969–974
3. Kupelian P, Meyer JL (2011) Image-guided, adaptive radiotherapy of prostate cancer: toward new standards of radiotherapy practice. Front Radiat Ther Oncol 43:344–368. doi:10.1159/000322485
4. Kuban D, Tucker S, Dong L et al (2008) Long-term results of the M. D. Anderson randomized dose-escalation trial for prostate cancer. Int J Radiat Oncol Biol Phys 70(1):67–74. doi:10.1016/j.ijrobp.2007.06.054
5. Zelefsky MJ, Yamada Y, Fuks Z et al (2008) Long-term results of conformal radiotherapy for prostate cancer: impact of dose escalation on biochemical tumor control and distant metastases-free survival outcomes. Int J Radiat Oncol Biol Phys 71(4):1028–1033. doi:10.1016/j.ijrobp.2007.11.066
6. Potters L, Morgenstern C, Calugaru E et al (2005) 12-year outcomes following permanent prostate brachytherapy in patients with clinically localized prostate cancer. J Urol 173(5):1562–1566. doi:10.1097/01.ju.0000154633.73092.8e
7. Zelefsky MJ, Kuban DA, Levy LB et al (2007) Multi-institutional analysis of long-term outcome for stages T1-T2 prostate cancer treated with permanent seed implantation. Int J Radiat Oncol Biol Phys 67(2):327–333. doi:10.1016/j.ijrobp.2006.08.056
8. Battermann JJ, Boon TA, Moerland MA (2004) Results of permanent prostate brachytherapy, 13 years of experience at a single institution. Radiother Oncol 71(1):23–28. doi:10.1016/j.radonc.2004.01.020
9. Zamboglou N, Tselis N, Baltas D et al (2012) High-dose-rate interstitial brachytherapy as monotherapy for clinically localized prostate cancer: treatment evolution and mature results. Int J Radiat Oncol Biol Phys. doi:10.1016/j.ijrobp.2012.07.004
10. Demanes DJ, Martinez AA, Ghilezan M et al (2011) High-dose-rate monotherapy: safe and effective brachytherapy for patients with localized prostate cancer. Int J Radiat Oncol Biol Phys 81(5):1286–1292. doi:10.1016/j.ijrobp.2010.10.015
11. Hoskin P, Rojas A, Lowe G et al (2012) High-dose-rate brachytherapy alone for localized prostate cancer in patients at moderate or high risk of biochemical recurrence. Int J Radiat Oncol Biol Phys 82(4):1376–1384. doi:10.1016/j.ijrobp.2011.04.031
12. Galalae RM, Martinez A, Mate T et al (2004) Long-term outcome by risk factors using conformal high-dose-rate brachytherapy (HDR-BT) boost with or without neoadjuvant androgen suppression for localized prostate cancer. Int J Radiat Oncol Biol Phys 58(4):1048–1055. doi:10.1016/j.ijrobp.2003.08.003
13. Pistis F, Guedea F, Pera J et al (2010) External beam radiotherapy plus high-dose-rate brachytherapy for treatment of locally advanced prostate cancer: the initial experience of the Catalan Institute of Oncology. Brachytherapy 9(1):15–22. doi:10.1016/j.brachy.2009.05.001
14. Kotecha R, Yamada Y, Pei X et al (2013) Clinical outcomes of high-dose-rate brachytherapy and external beam radiotherapy in the management of clinically localized prostate cancer. Brachytherapy 12(1):44–49. doi:10.1016/j.brachy.2012.05.003
15. Prada PJ, Mendez L, Fernández J et al (2012) Long-term biochemical results after high-dose-rate

intensity modulated brachytherapy with external beam radiotherapy for high risk prostate cancer. Radiat Oncol 7:31. doi:10.1186/1748-717X-7-31

16. Deutsch I, Zelefsky MJ, Zhang Z et al (2010) Comparison of PSA relapse-free survival in patients treated with ultra-high-dose IMRT versus combination HDR brachytherapy and IMRT. Brachytherapy 9(4):313–318. doi:10.1016/j.brachy.2010.02.196

17. Martinez AA, Gustafson G, Gonzalez J et al (2002) Dose escalation using conformal high-dose-rate brachytherapy improves outcome in unfavorable prostate cancer. Int J Radiat Oncol Biol Phys 53(2):316–327

18. Demanes DJ, Rodriguez RR, Schour L et al (2005) High-dose-rate intensity-modulated brachytherapy with external beam radiotherapy for prostate cancer: California endocurietherapy's 10-year results. Int J Radiat Oncol Biol Phys 61(5):1306–1316. doi:10.1016/j.ijrobp.2004.08.014

19. Milickovic N, Mavroidis P, Tselis N et al (2011) 4-D analysis of influence of patient movement and anatomy alteration on the quality of 3D U/S-based prostate HDR brachytherapy treatment delivery. Med Phys 38(9):4982–4993. doi:10.1118/1.3618735

20. Demanes DJ, Ghilezan MI (2014) High-dose-rate brachytherapy as monotherapy for prostate cancer. Brachytherapy 13(6):529–541. doi:10.1016/j.brachy.2014.03.002

21. Morton GC, Hoskin PJ (2013) Brachytherapy: current status and future strategies – can high dose rate replace low dose rate and external beam radiotherapy? Clin Oncol (R Coll Radiol) 25(8):474–482. doi:10.1016/j.clon.2013.04.009

22. Yoshioka Y, Yoshida K, Yamazaki H et al (2013) The emerging role of high-dose-rate (HDR) brachytherapy as monotherapy for prostate cancer. J Radiat Res 54(5):781–788. doi:10.1093/jrr/rrt027

23. Challapalli A, Jones E, Harvey C et al (2012) High dose rate prostate brachytherapy: an overview of the rationale, experience and emerging applications in the treatment of prostate cancer. Br J Radiol 85 Spec No 1:S18–S27. doi:10.1259/bjr/15403217

24. Kupelian PA, Ciezki J, Reddy CA et al (2008) Effect of increasing radiation doses on local and distant failures in patients with localized prostate cancer. Int J Radiat Oncol Biol Phys 71(1):16–22. doi:10.1016/j.ijrobp.2007.09.020

25. Kim MM, Hoffman KE, Levy LB et al (2012) Prostate cancer-specific mortality after definitive radiation therapy: who dies of disease? Eur J Cancer 48(11):1664–1671. doi:10.1016/j.ejca.2012.01.026

26. Zelefsky MJ, Reuter VE, Fuks Z et al (2008) Influence of local tumor control on distant metastases and cancer related mortality after external beam radiotherapy for prostate cancer. J Urol 179(4):1368–1373. doi:10.1016/j.juro.2007.11.063; discussion 1373

27. Zelefsky MJ, Pei X, Chou JF et al (2011) Dose escalation for prostate cancer radiotherapy: predictors of long-term biochemical tumor control and distant

metastases-free survival outcomes. Eur Urol 60(6):1133–1139. doi:10.1016/j.eururo.2011.08.029

28. Nguyen Q, Levy LB, Lee AK et al (2013) Long-term outcomes for men with high-risk prostate cancer treated definitively with external beam radiotherapy with or without androgen deprivation. Cancer 119(18):3265–3271. doi:10.1002/cncr.28213

29. Pahlajani N, Ruth KJ, Buyyounouski MK et al (2012) Radiotherapy doses of 80 Gy and higher are associated with lower mortality in men with Gleason score 8 to 10 prostate cancer. Int J Radiat Oncol Biol Phys 82(5):1949–1956. doi:10.1016/j.ijrobp.2011.04.005

30. Brenner DJ, Martinez AA, Edmundson GK et al (2002) Direct evidence that prostate tumors show high sensitivity to fractionation (low alpha/beta ratio), similar to late-responding normal tissue. Int J Radiat Oncol Biol Phys 52(1):6–13

31. Nath R, Bice WS, Butler WM et al (2009) AAPM recommendations on dose prescription and reporting methods for permanent interstitial brachytherapy for prostate cancer: report of Task Group 137. Med Phys 36(11):5310–5322

32. Ritter M, Forman J, Kupelian P et al (2009) Hypofractionation for prostate cancer. Cancer J 15(1):1–6. doi:10.1097/PPO.0b013e3181976614

33. Edmundson GK, Yan D, Martinez AA (1995) Intraoperative optimization of needle placement and dwell times for conformal prostate brachytherapy. Int J Radiat Oncol Biol Phys 33(5):1257–1263. doi:10.1016/0360-3016(95)00276-6

34. White EC, Kamrava MR, Demarco J et al (2013) High-dose-rate prostate brachytherapy consistently results in high quality dosimetry. Int J Radiat Oncol Biol Phys 85(2):543–548. doi:10.1016/j.ijrobp.2012.03.035

35. Mavroidis P, Katsilieri Z, Kefala V et al (2010) Radiobiological evaluation of the influence of dwell time modulation restriction in HIPO optimized HDR prostate brachytherapy implants. J Contemp Brachyther 2(3):117–128. doi:10.5114/jcb.2010.16923

36. Karabis A, Giannouli S, Baltas D (2005) HIPO: A hybrid inverse treatment planning optimization algorithm in HDR brachytherapy. Radiother Oncol 76(Suppl 2):29

37. Kono Y, Kubota K, Aruga T et al (2010) Swelling of the prostate gland by permanent brachytherapy may affect seed migration. Jpn J Clin Oncol 40(12):1159–1165. doi:10.1093/jjco/hyq118

38. Knaup C, Mavroidis P, Esquivel C et al (2012) Investigating the dosimetric and tumor control consequences of prostate seed loss and migration. Med Phys 39(6):3291–3298. doi:10.1118/1.4712227

39. Franca CAS, Vieira SL, Carvalho ACP et al (2009) Radioactive seed migration after prostate brachytherapy with iodine-125 using loose seeds versus stranded seeds. Int Braz J Urol 35(5):573–579; discussion 579–580

40. Shah AP, Kupelian PA, Willoughby TR et al (2011) An evaluation of intrafraction motion of the prostate in the prone and supine positions using electromagnetic tracking. Radiother Oncol 99(1):37–43. doi:10.1016/j.radonc.2011.02.012

41. Algan O, Jamgade A, Ali I et al (2012) The dosimetric impact of daily setup error on target volumes and surrounding normal tissue in the treatment of prostate cancer with intensity-modulated radiation therapy. Med Dosim 37(4):406–411. doi:10.1016/j.meddos.2012.03.003

42. Mutanga TF, de Boer HCJ, Rajan V et al (2012) Day-to-day reproducibility of prostate intrafraction motion assessed by multiple kV and MV imaging of implanted markers during treatment. Int J Radiat Oncol Biol Phys 83(1):400–407. doi:10.1016/j.ijrobp.2011.05.049

43. Fowler J, Chappell R, Ritter M (2001) Is alpha/beta for prostate tumors really low? Int J Radiat Oncol Biol Phys 50(4):1021–1031

44. Brenner DJ, Hall EJ (1999) Fractionation and protraction for radiotherapy of prostate carcinoma. Int J Radiat Oncol Biol Phys 43(5):1095–1101

45. Brenner DJ (2004) Fractionation and late rectal toxicity. Int J Radiat Oncol Biol Phys 60(4):1013–1015. doi:10.1016/j.ijrobp.2004.04.014

46. Tucker SL, Thames HD, Michalski JM et al (2011) Estimation of α/β for late rectal toxicity based on RTOG 94-06. Int J Radiat Oncol Biol Phys 81(2):600–605. doi:10.1016/j.ijrobp.2010.11.080

47. Miralbell R, Roberts SA, Zubizarreta E et al (2012) Dose-fractionation sensitivity of prostate cancer deduced from radiotherapy outcomes of 5,969 patients in seven international institutional datasets: α/β = 1.4 (0.9-2.2) Gy. Int J Radiat Oncol Biol Phys 82(1):e17–e24. doi:10.1016/j.ijrobp.2010.10.075

48. Lee WR (2009) Extreme hypofractionation for prostate cancer. Expert Rev Anticancer Ther 9(1):61–65. doi:10.1586/14737140.9.1.61

49. Bentzen SM, Dörr W, Gahbauer R et al (2012) Bioeffect modelling and equieffective dose concepts in radiation oncology--terminology, quantities and units. Radiother Oncol 105(2):266–268. doi:10.1016/j.radonc.2012.10.006

50. Fatyga M, Williamson JF, Dogan N et al (2009) A comparison of HDR brachytherapy and IMRT techniques for dose escalation in prostate cancer: a radiobiological modelling study. Med Phys 36(9):3995–4006

51. Masson S, Persad R, Bahl A (2012) HDR Brachytherapy in the Management of High-Risk Prostate Cancer. Adv Urol 980841. doi:10.1155/2012/980841

52. Bolla M, Poppel HV (2012) Management of prostate cancer. A multidisciplinary approach. Springer, Berlin/New York

53. Hoskin P (2008) High dose rate brachytherapy for prostate cancer. Cancer Radiother 12(6-7):512–514. doi:10.1016/j.canrad.2008.07.012

54. Martinez AA, Gonzalez J, Ye H et al (2011) Dose escalation improves cancer-related events at 10 years for intermediate- and high-risk prostate cancer patients treated with hypofractionated high-dose-rate boost and external beam radiotherapy. Int J Radiat Oncol Biol Phys 79(2):363–370. doi:10.1016/j.ijrobp.2009.10.035

55. Zaorsky NG, Doyle LA, Yamoah K, Andrel JA, Trabulsi EJ, Hurwitz MD, Dicker AP, Den RB. High dose rate brachytherapy boost for prostate cancer: a systematic review.Cancer Treat Rev. 2014;40(3):414–425. doi:10.1016/j.ctrv.2013.10.006

56. Yoshioka Y, Konishi K, Suzuki O et al (2014) Monotherapeutic high-dose-rate brachytherapy for prostate cancer: a dose reduction trial. Radiother Oncol 110(1):114–119. doi:10.1016/j.radonc.2013.10.015

57. Yamada Y, Rogers L, Demanes DJ et al (2012) American Brachytherapy Society consensus guidelines for high-dose-rate prostate brachytherapy. Brachytherapy 11(1):20–32. doi:10.1016/j.brachy.2011.09.008

58. Hoskin PJ, Colombo A, Henry A et al (2013) GEC/ESTRO recommendations on high dose rate afterloading brachytherapy for localised prostate cancer: an update. Radiother Oncol 107(3):325–332. doi:10.1016/j.radonc.2013.05.002

59. Mohler JL, Kantoff PW, Armstrong AJ et al (2013) Prostate cancer, version 1.2014. J Natl Compr Canc Netw 11(12):1471–1479

60. Zelefsky MJ, Leibel SA, Gaudin PB et al (1998) Dose escalation with three-dimensional conformal radiation therapy affects the outcome in prostate cancer. Int J Radiat Oncol Biol Phys 41(3):491–500

61. Mohler J, Bahnson RR, Boston B et al (2010) NCCN clinical practice guidelines in oncology: prostate cancer. J Natl Compr Canc Netw 8(2):162–200

62. Heidenreich A, Bellmunt J, Bolla M et al (2011) EAU guidelines on prostate cancer. Part 1: screening, diagnosis, and treatment of clinically localised disease. Eur Urol 59(1):61–71. doi:10.1016/j.eururo.2010.10.039

63. Touijer K, Fuenzalida RP, Rabbani F et al (2011) Extending the indications and anatomical limits of pelvic lymph node dissection for prostate cancer: Improved staging or increased morbidity? BJU Int 108(3):372–377. doi:10.1111/j.1464-410X.2010.09877

64. Evangelista L, Guttilla A, Zattoni F et al (2013) Utility of choline positron emission tomography/computed tomography for lymph node involvement identification in intermediate- to high-risk prostate cancer: a systematic literature review and meta-analysis. Eur Urol 63(6):1040–1048. doi:10.1016/j.eururo.2012.09.039

65. Maurer T, Eiber M, Krause BJ (2014) Molekulare multimodale Hybridbildgebung des Prostata- und Blasenkarzinoms (Molecular multimodal hybrid imaging in prostate and bladder cancer). Urol A 53(4):469–483. doi:10.1007/s00120-014-3440-5

66. Eid K, Krughoff K, Stoimenova D et al (2013) Validation of the urgency, weak stream, incomplete emptying, and nocturia (UWIN) score compared with the american urological association symptoms score in assessing lower urinary tract symptoms in the clinical setting. Urology 83:181–185. doi:10.1016/j.urology.2013.08.039

67. Le H, Rojas A, Alonzi R et al (2013) The influence of prostate volume on outcome after high-dose-rate brachytherapy alone for localized prostate cancer. Int J Radiat Oncol Biol Phys 87(2):270–274. doi:10.1016/j.ijrobp.2013.05.022

68. Monroe AT, Faricy PO, Jennings SB et al (2008) High-dose-rate brachytherapy for large prostate volumes (≥50cc)—uncompromised dosimetric coverage and acceptable toxicity. Brachytherapy 7(1):7–11. doi:10.1016/j.brachy.2007.10.005

69. Rogers CL, Alder SC, Rogers RL et al (2012) High dose brachytherapy as monotherapy for intermediate risk prostate cancer. J Urol 187(1):109–116. doi:10.1016/j.juro.2011.09.050

70. Yamada Y, Bhatia S, Zaider M et al (2006) Favorable clinical outcomes of three-dimensional computer-optimized high-dose-rate prostate brachytherapy in the management of localized prostate cancer. Brachytherapy 5(3):157–164. doi:10.1016/j.brachy.2006.03.004

71. Ishiyama H, Hirayama T, Jhaveri P et al (2012) Is there an increase in genitourinary toxicity in patients treated with transurethral resection of the prostate and radiotherapy? A systematic review. Am J Clin Oncol. doi:10.1097/COC.0b013e3182546821

72. Luo HL, Fang FM, Chuang YC et al (2009) Previous transurethral resection of the prostate is not a contraindication to high-dose rate brachytherapy for prostate cancer. BJU Int 104(11):1620–1623. doi:10.1111/j.1464-410X.2009.08664.x

73. Luo HL, Fang FM, Kang CH et al (2013) Can high-dose-rate brachytherapy prevent the major genitourinary complication better than external beam radiation alone for patients with previous transurethral resection of prostate? Int Urol Nephrol 45(1):113–119. doi:10.1007/s11255-012-0277-y

74. Peddada AV, Jennings SB, Faricy PO et al (2007) Low morbidity following high dose rate brachytherapy in the setting of prior transurethral prostate resection. J Urol 178(5):1963–1967. doi:10.1016/j.juro.2007.07.028

75. Sakamoto N, Akitake M, Ikoma S et al (2011) Clinical outcome in prostate cancer patients undergoing high-dose-rate brachytherapy with external beam radiotherapy in our institute. Nippon Hinyokika Gakkai Zasshi 102(4):621–627

76. Yoshioka Y, Konishi K, Sumida I et al (2011) Monotherapeutic high-dose-rate brachytherapy for prostate cancer: five-year results of an extreme hypofractionation regimen with 54 Gy in nine fractions. Int J Radiat Oncol Biol Phys 80(2):469–475. doi:10.1016/j.ijrobp.2010.02.013

77. Lakosi F, Antal G, Vandulek C et al (2011) Open MR-guided high-dose-rate (HDR) prostate brachytherapy: feasibility and initial experiences open MR-guided high-dose-rate (HDR) prostate brachytherapy. Pathol Oncol Res 17(2):315–324. doi:10.1007/s12253-010-9319-x

78. Ménard C, Susil RC, Choyke P et al (2004) MRI-guided HDR prostate brachytherapy in standard 1.5T scanner. Int J Radiat Oncol Biol Phys 59(5):1414–1423. doi:10.1016/j.ijrobp.2004.01.016

79. Martin T, Röddiger S, Kurek R et al (2004) 3-D conformal HDR brachytherapy and external beam irradiation combined with temporary androgen deprivation in the treatment of localized prostate cancer. Radiother Oncol 71(1):35–41. doi:10.1016/j.radonc.2003.10.004

80. Ghilezan M, Martinez A, Gustason G et al (2011) High-dose-rate brachytherapy as monotherapy delivered in two fractions within one day for favorable/intermediate-risk prostate cancer: preliminary toxicity data. Int J Radiat Oncol Biol Phys. doi:10.1016/j.ijrobp.2011.05.001

81. Galalae RM, Kovács G, Schultze J et al (2002) Long-term outcome after elective irradiation of the pelvic lymphatics and local dose escalation using high-dose-rate brachytherapy for locally advanced prostate cancer. Int J Radiat Oncol Biol Phys 52(1):81–90

82. Hoskin PJ, Motohashi K, Bownes P et al (2007) High dose rate brachytherapy in combination with external beam radiotherapy in the radical treatment of prostate cancer: initial results of a randomised phase three trial. Radiother Oncol 84(2):114–120. doi:10.1016/j.radonc.2007.04.011

83. Martin T, Kolotas C, Dannenberg T et al (1999) New interstitial HDR brachytherapy technique for prostate cancer: CT based 3D planning after transrectal implantation. Radiother Oncol 52(3):257–260

84. Anderson ES, Margolis DJA, Mesko S et al (2014) Multiparametric MRI identifies and stratifies prostate cancer lesions: implications for targeting intraprostatic targets. Brachytherapy 13(3):292–298. doi:10.1016/j.brachy.2014.01.011

85. Boonsirikamchai P, Choi S, Frank SJ et al (2013) MR imaging of prostate cancer in radiation oncology: what radiologists need to know. Radiographics 33(3):741–761. doi:10.1148/rg.333125041

86. Diamantopoulos S, Milickovic N, Butt S et al (2011) Effect of using different U/S probe Standoff materials in image geometry for interventional procedures: the example of prostate. J Contemp Brachytherapy 3(4):209–219. doi:10.5114/jcb.2011.26472

87. Nath R, Anderson LL, Luxton G et al (1995) Dosimetry of interstitial brachytherapy sources: recommendations of the AAPM Radiation Therapy Committee Task Group No. 43. American Association of Physicists in Medicine. Med Phys 22(2):209–234

88. Perez-Calatayud J, Ballester F, Das RK et al (2012) Dose calculation for photon-emitting brachytherapy sources with average energy higher than 50 keV: report of the AAPM and ESTRO. Med Phys 39(5):2904–2929. doi:10.1118/1.3703892

89. Dinkla AM, Pieters BR, Koedooder K et al (2013) Improved tumour control probability with MRI-based prostate brachytherapy treatment planning. Acta Oncol 52(3):658–665. doi:10.3109/0284186X.2012.744875

90. Tanaka H, Hayashi S, Ohtakara K et al (2011) Usefulness of CT-MRI fusion in radiotherapy

planning for localized prostate cancer. J Radiat Res 52(6):782–788

91. Tzikas A, Karaiskos P, Papanikolaou N et al (2011) Investigating the clinical aspects of using CT vs. CT-MRI images during organ delineation and treatment planning in prostate cancer radiotherapy. Technol Cancer Res Treat 10(3):231–242

92. Holly R, Morton GC, Sankreacha R et al (2011) Use of cone-beam imaging to correct for catheter displacement in high dose-rate prostate brachytherapy. Brachytherapy 10(4):299–305. doi:10.1016/j.brachy.2010.11.007

93. Seppenwoolde Y, Kolkman-Deurloo I, Sipkema D et al (2008) HDR prostate monotherapy: dosimetric effects of implant deformation due to posture change between TRUS- and CT-imaging. Radiother Oncol 86(1):114–119. doi:10.1016/j.radonc.2007.11.004

94. Whitaker M, Hruby G, Lovett A et al (2011) Prostate HDR brachytherapy catheter displacement between planning and treatment delivery. Radiother Oncol 101(3):490–494. doi:10.1016/j.radonc.2011.08.004

95. Baltas D, Zamboglou N, Sakelliou L (2007) The physics of modern brachytherapy for oncology. Series in medical physics and biomedical engineering. Taylor & Francis, Boca Raton

96. Chavaudra J, Bridier A (2001) Définition des volumes en radiothérapie externe: rapports ICRU 50 et 62 (Definition of volumes in external radiotherapy: ICRU reports 50 and 62). Cancer Radiother 5(5):472–478

97. Purdy JA (2004) Current ICRU definitions of volumes: limitations and future directions. Semin Radiat Oncol 14(1):27–40. doi:10.1053/j.semradonc.2003.12.002

98. Borghede G, Hedelin H, Holmäng S et al (1997) Irradiation of localized prostatic carcinoma with a combination of high dose rate iridium-192 brachytherapy and external beam radiotherapy with three target definitions and dose levels inside the prostate gland. Radiother Oncol 44(3):245–250

99. Deger S, Boehmer D, Roigas J et al (2005) High dose rate (HDR) brachytherapy with conformal radiation therapy for localized prostate cancer. Eur Urol 47(4):441–448. doi:10.1016/j.eururo.2004.11.014

100. Hoskin P, Rojas A, Ostler P et al (2014) High-dose-rate brachytherapy alone given as two or one fraction to patients for locally advanced prostate cancer: acute toxicity. Radiother Oncol 110(2):268–271. doi:10.1016/j.radonc.2013.09.025

101. Kim Y, Hsu IJ, Lessard E et al (2004) Dose uncertainty due to computed tomography (CT) slice thickness in CT-based high dose rate brachytherapy of the prostate cancer. Med Phys 31(9):2543–2548

102. Zheng D, Todor DA (2011) A novel method for accurate needle-tip identification in trans-rectal ultrasound-based high-dose-rate prostate brachytherapy. Brachytherapy 10(6):466–473. doi:10.1016/j.brachy.2011.02.214

103. Panettieri V, Smith RL, Mason NJ et al (2014) Comparison of IPSA and HIPO inverse planning

104. Dearnaley DP, Sydes MR, Graham JD et al (2007) Escalated-dose versus standard-dose conformal radiotherapy in prostate cancer: first results from the MRC RT01 randomised controlled trial. Lancet Oncol 8(6):475–487. doi:10.1016/S1470-2045(07)70143-2

105. Peeters STH, Heemsbergen WD, Koper PCM et al (2006) Dose-response in radiotherapy for localized prostate cancer: results of the Dutch multicenter randomized phase III trial comparing 68 Gy of radiotherapy with 78 Gy. J Clin Oncol 24(13):1990–1996. doi:10.1200/JCO.2005.05.2530

106. Pollack A, Zagars GK, Starkschall G (2002) et al; Prostate cancer radiation dose response: results of the M. D. Anderson phase III randomized trial. Int J Radiat Oncol Biol Phys 53(5):1097–1105

107. Zietman AL, Bae K, Slater JD et al (2010) Randomized trial comparing conventional-dose with high-dose conformal radiation therapy in early-stage adenocarcinoma of the prostate: long-term results from proton radiation oncology group/american college of radiology 95-09. J Clin Oncol 28(7):1106–1111. doi:10.1200/JCO.2009.25.8475

108. Hermesse J, Biver S, Jansen N et al (2009) A dosimetric selectivity intercomparison of HDR brachytherapy, IMRT and helical tomotherapy in prostate cancer radiotherapy. Strahlenther Onkol 185(11):736–742. doi:10.1007/s00066-009-2009-5

109. Hermesse J, Biver S, Jansen N et al (2010) Dosimetric comparison of high-dose-rate brachytherapy and intensity-modulated radiation therapy as a boost to the prostate. Int J Radiat Oncol Biol Phys 76(1):269–276. doi:10.1016/j.ijrobp.2009.05.046

110. Hsu IC, Pickett B, Shinohara K et al (2000) Normal tissue dosimetric comparison between HDR prostate implant boost and conformal external beam radiotherapy boost: potential for dose escalation. Int J Radiat Oncol Biol Phys 46(4):851–858

111. Pieters BR, van de Kamer JB, van Herten YRJ et al (2008) Comparison of biologically equivalent dose-volume parameters for the treatment of prostate cancer with concomitant boost IMRT versus IMRT combined with brachytherapy. Radiother Oncol 88(1):46–52. doi:10.1016/j.radonc.2008.02.023

112. Sathya JR, Davis IR, Julian JA et al (2005) Randomized trial comparing iridium implant plus external-beam radiation therapy with external-beam radiation therapy alone in node-negative locally advanced cancer of the prostate. J Clin Oncol 23(6):1192–1199. doi:10.1200/JCO.2005.06.154

113. Aström L, Pedersen D, Mercke C et al (2005) Long-term outcome of high dose rate brachytherapy in radiotherapy of localised prostate cancer. Radiother Oncol 74(2):157–161. doi:10.1016/j.radonc.2004.10.014

114. Noda Y, Sato M, Shirai S et al (2011) Efficacy and safety of high-dose-rate brachytherapy of single implant with two fractions combined with external

optimization algorithms for prostate HDR brachytherapy. J Appl Clin Med Phys 15(6):5055 beam radiotherapy for hormone-naïve localized prostate cancer. Cancers (Basel) 3(3):3585–3600. doi:10.3390/cancers3033585

115. Morton GC, Loblaw DA, Sankreacha R et al (2010) Single-fraction high-dose-rate brachytherapy and hypofractionated external beam radiotherapy for men with intermediate-risk prostate cancer: analysis of short- and medium-term toxicity and quality of life. Int J Radiat Oncol Biol Phys 77(3):811–817. doi:10.1016/j.ijrobp.2009.05.054

116. Agoston P, Major T, Fröhlich G et al (2011) Moderate dose escalation with single-fraction high-dose-rate brachytherapy boost for clinically localized intermediate- and high-risk prostate cancer: 5-year outcome of the first 100 consecutively treated patients. Brachytherapy 10(5):376–384. doi:10.1016/j.brachy.2011.01.003

117. Hiratsuka J, Jo Y, Yoshida K et al (2004) Clinical results of combined treatment conformal high-dose-rate iridium-192 brachytherapy and external beam radiotherapy using staging lymphadenectomy for localized prostate cancer. Int J Radiat Oncol Biol Phys 59(3):684–690. doi:10.1016/j.ijrobp.2003.11.035

118. Consensus statement: guidelines for PSA following radiation therapy. American Society for Therapeutic Radiology and Oncology Consensus Panel (1997) Int J Radiat Oncol Biol Phys 37(5):1035–1041

119. Pellizzon ACA, Salvajoli J, Novaes P et al (2008) The relationship between the biochemical control outcomes and the quality of planning of high-dose rate brachytherapy as a boost to external beam radiotherapy for locally and locally advanced prostate cancer using the RTOG-ASTRO Phoenix definition. Int J Med Sci 5(3):113–120

120. Phan TP, Syed AMN, Puthawala A et al (2007) High dose rate brachytherapy as a boost for the treatment of localized prostate cancer. J Urol 177(1):123–127. doi:10.1016/j.juro.2006.08.109; discussion 127

121. Viani GA, Pellizzon AC, Guimarães FS et al (2009) High dose rate and external beam radiotherapy in locally advanced prostate cancer. Am J Clin Oncol 32(2):187–190. doi:10.1097/COC.0b013e3181841f78

122. Roach M, Hanks G, Thames H et al (2006) Defining biochemical failure following radiotherapy with or without hormonal therapy in men with clinically localized prostate cancer: recommendations of the RTOG-ASTRO Phoenix Consensus Conference. Int J Radiat Oncol Biol Phys 65(4):965–974. doi:10.1016/j.ijrobp.2006.04.029

123. Galalae RM, Martinez A, Nuernberg N et al (2006) Hypofractionated conformal HDR brachytherapy in hormone naïve men with localized prostate cancer. Is escalation to very high biologically equivalent dose beneficial in all prognostic risk groups? Strahlenther Onkol 182(3):135–141. doi:10.1007/s00066-006-1448-5

124. Izard MA, Haddad RL, Fogarty GB et al (2006) Six year experience of external beam radiotherapy,

125. brachytherapy boost with a 1Ci (192) Ir source, and neoadjuvant hormonal manipulation for prostate cancer. Int J Radiat Oncol Biol Phys 66(1):38–47. doi:10.1016/j.ijrobp.2006.04.002

125. Martinez A, Gonzalez J, Spencer W et al (2003) Conformal high dose rate brachytherapy improves biochemical control and cause specific survival in patients with prostate cancer and poor prognostic factors. J Urol 169(3):974–979. doi:10.1097/01.ju.0000052720.62999.a9; discussion 979–980

126. Martinez AA, Demanes DJ, Galalae R et al (2005) Lack of benefit from a short course of androgen deprivation for unfavorable prostate cancer patients treated with an accelerated hypofractionated regime. Int J Radiat Oncol Biol Phys 62(5):1322–1331. doi:10.1016/j.ijrobp.2004.12.053

127. Vargas CE, Martinez AA, Boike TP et al (2006) High-dose irradiation for prostate cancer via a high-dose-rate brachytherapy boost: results of a phase I to II study. Int J Radiat Oncol Biol Phys 66(2):416–423. doi:10.1016/j.ijrobp.2006.04.045

128. de Meerleer G, Vakaet L, Meersschout S et al (2004) Intensity-modulated radiotherapy as primary treatment for prostate cancer: acute toxicity in 114 patients. Int J Radiat Oncol Biol Phys 60(3):777–787. doi:10.1016/j.ijrobp.2004.04.017

129. Liauw SL, Weichselbaum RR, Rash C et al (2009) Biochemical control and toxicity after intensity-modulated radiation therapy for prostate cancer. Technol Cancer Res Treat 8(3):201–206

130. Lips IM, Dehnad H, van Gils CH et al (2008) High-dose intensity-modulated radiotherapy for prostate cancer using daily fiducial marker-based position verification: acute and late toxicity in 331 patients. Radiat Oncol 3:15. doi:10.1186/1748-717X-3-15

131. Martinez AA, Kestin LL, Stromberg JS et al (2000) Interim report of image-guided conformal high-dose-rate brachytherapy for patients with unfavorable prostate cancer: the William Beaumont phase II dose-escalating trial. Int J Radiat Oncol Biol Phys 47(2):343–352

132. Martinez AA, Pataki I, Edmundson G et al (2001) Phase II prospective study of the use of conformal high-dose-rate brachytherapy as monotherapy for the treatment of favorable stage prostate cancer: a feasibility report. Int J Radiat Oncol Biol Phys 49(1):61–69

133. Rodriguez RR, Demanes DJ, Altieri GA (1999) High dose rate brachytherapy in the treatment of prostate cancer. Hematol Oncol Clin North Am 13(3):503–523

134. Yoshioka Y, Nose T, Yoshida K et al (2000) High-dose-rate interstitial brachytherapy as a monotherapy for localized prostate cancer: treatment description and preliminary results of a phase I/II clinical trial. Int J Radiat Oncol Biol Phys 48(3):675–681

135. Barkati M, Williams SG, Foroudi F, Tai KH, Chander S, van Dyk S, See A, Duchesne GM. High-dose-rate brachytherapy as a monotherapy for favorable-risk

prostate cancer: a Phase II trial. Int J Radiat Oncol Biol Phys. 2012;82(5):1889–1896. doi:10.1016/j.ijrobp.2010.09.006

136. Corner C, Rojas AM, Bryant L et al (2008) A phase II study of high-dose-rate afterloading brachytherapy as monotherapy for the treatment of localized prostate cancer. Int J Radiat Oncol Biol Phys 72(2):441–446. doi:10.1016/j.ijrobp.2007.12.026

137. Ghadjar P, Keller T, Rentsch CA et al (2009) Toxicity and early treatment outcomes in low- and intermediate-risk prostate cancer managed by high-dose-rate brachytherapy as a monotherapy. Brachytherapy 8(1):45–51. doi:10.1016/j.brachy.2008.09.004

138. Grills IS, Martinez AA, Hollander M et al (2004) High dose rate brachytherapy as prostate cancer monotherapy reduces toxicity compared to low dose rate palladium seeds. J Urol 171(3):1098–1104. doi:10.1097/01.ju.0000113299.34404.22

139. Komiya A, Fujiuchi Y, Ito T et al (2013) Early quality of life outcomes in patients with prostate cancer managed by high-dose-rate brachytherapy as monotherapy. Int J Urol 20(2):185–192. doi:10.1111/j.1442-2042.2012.03125.x

140. Kukiełka AM, Dąbrowski T, Walasek T, Olchawa A, Kudzia R, Dybek D. High-dose-rate brachytherapy as a monotherapy for prostate cancer–Single-institution results of the extreme fractionation regimen. Brachytherapy. 2015;14(3):359–365. doi:10.1016/j.brachy.2015.01.004

141. Mark R, Anderson P, Akins R (2010) Interstitial high-dose-rate brachytherapy as monotherapy for early stage prostate cancer: Median 8-year results in 301 patients. (Abstract). Brachytherapy 9:76

142. Martin T, Baltas D, Kurek R et al (2004) 3-D conformal HDR brachytherapy as monotherapy for localized prostate cancer. A pilot study. Strahlenther Onkol 180(4):225–232. doi:10.1007/s00066-004-1215-4

143. Martinez AA, Demanes J, Vargas C et al (2010) High-dose-rate prostate brachytherapy: an excellent accelerated-hypofractionated treatment for favorable prostate cancer. Am J Clin Oncol 33(5):481–488. doi:10.1097/COC.0b013e3181b9cd2f

144. Prada PJ, Jimenez I, González-Suárez H et al (2012) High-dose-rate interstitial brachytherapy as monotherapy in one fraction and transperineal hyaluronic acid injection into the perirectal fat for the treatment of favorable stage prostate cancer: treatment description and preliminary results. Brachytherapy 11(2):105–110. doi:10.1016/j.brachy.2011.05.003

145. Díez P, Mullassery V, Dankulchai P et al (2014) Dosimetric analysis of urethral strictures following HDR (192)Ir brachytherapy as monotherapy for intermediate- and high-risk prostate cancer. Radiother Oncol 113(3):410–413. doi:10.1016/j.radonc.2014.10.007

146. Tselis N, Tunn UW, Chatzikonstantinou G et al (2013) High dose rate brachytherapy as monotherapy for localised prostate cancer: a hypofractionated two-implant approach in 351 consecutive patients. Radiat Oncol 8:115. doi:10.1186/1748-717X-8-115

147. Ghadjar P, Oesch SL, Rentsch CA et al (2014) Late toxicity and five year outcomes after high-dose-rate brachytherapy as a monotherapy for localized prostate cancer. Radiat Oncol 9:122. doi:10.1186/1748-717X-9-122

148. Vargas C, Ghilezan M, HOLLANDER M et al (2005) A new model using number of needles and androgen deprivation to predict chronic urinary toxicity for high or low dose rate prostate brachytherapy. J Urol 174(3):882–887. doi:10.1097/01.ju.0000169136.55891.21

149. el Din KE, Koch WF, Wildt MJ et al (1996) Reliability of the International Prostate Symptom Score in the assessment of patients with lower urinary tract symptoms and/or benign prostatic hyperplasia. J Urol 155(6):1959–1964

150. Rosen RC, Allen KR, Ni X et al (2011) Minimal clinically important differences in the erectile function domain of the International Index of Erectile Function scale. Eur Urol 60(5):1010–1016. doi:10.1016/j.eururo.2011.07.053

151. Stone NN, Potters L (2007) Davis BJ et al: Customized dose prescription for permanent prostate brachytherapy: insights from a multicenter analysis of dosimetry outcomes. Int J Radiat Oncol Biol Phys 9(5):1472–1477. doi:10.1016/j.ijrobp.2007.05.002

152. Stone NN, Stock RG, Cesaretti JA et al (2010) Local control following permanent prostate brachytherapy: effect of high biologically effective dose on biopsy results and oncologic outcomes. Int J Radiat Oncol Biol Phys 76(2):355–360. doi:10.1016/j.ijrobp.2009.01.078

153. Krauss D, Kestin L, Ye H et al (2011) Lack of benefit for the addition of androgen deprivation therapy to dose-escalated radiotherapy in the treatment of intermediate- and high-risk prostate cancer. Int J Radiat Oncol Biol Phys 80(4):1064–1071. doi:10.1016/j.ijrobp.2010.04.004

154. Freeman DE, King CR (2011) Stereotactic body radiotherapy for low-risk prostate cancer: five-year outcomes. Radiat Oncol 6:3. doi:10.1186/1748-717X-6-3

155. King CR, Brooks JD, Gill H et al (2009) Stereotactic body radiotherapy for localized prostate cancer: interim results of a prospective phase II clinical trial. Int J Radiat Oncol Biol Phys 73(4):1043–1048. doi:10.1016/j.ijrobp.2008.05.059

156. King CR, Brooks JD, Gill H et al (2012) Long-term outcomes from a prospective trial of stereotactic body radiotherapy for low-risk prostate cancer. Int J Radiat Oncol Biol Phys 82(2):877–882. doi:10.1016/j.ijrobp.2010.11.054

157. McBride SM, Wong DS, Dombrowski JJ et al (2012) Hypofractionated stereotactic body radiotherapy in low-risk prostate adenocarcinoma: preliminary results of a multi-institutional phase 1 feasibility trial. Cancer 118(15):3681–3690. doi:10.1002/cncr.26699

158. Teh BS, Ishiyama H, Mathews T et al (2010) Stereotactic body radiation therapy (SBRT) for

genitourinary malignancies. Discov Med 10(52): 255–262

159. Fuller DB, Naitoh J, Mardirossian G (2014) Virtual HDR CyberKnife SBRT for localized prostatic carcinoma: 5-year disease-free survival and toxicity observations. Front Oncol 4:321. doi:10.3389/fonc.2014.00321

160. Spratt DE, Scala LM, Folkert M et al (2013) A comparative dosimetric analysis of virtual stereotactic body radiotherapy to high-dose-rate monotherapy for intermediate-risk prostate cancer. Brachytherapy 12(5):428–433. doi:10.1016/j.brachy.2013.03.003

161. Fuller DB, Naitoh J, Lee C et al (2008) Virtual HDR CyberKnife treatment for localized prostatic carcinoma: dosimetry comparison with HDR brachytherapy and preliminary clinical observations. Int J Radiat Oncol Biol Phys 70(5):1588–1597. doi:10.1016/j.ijrobp.2007.11.067

162. Aluwini S, van Rooij P, Hoogeman M et al (2010) CyberKnife stereotactic radiotherapy as monotherapy for low- to intermediate-stage prostate cancer: early experience, feasibility, and tolerance. J Endourol 24(5):865–869. doi:10.1089/end.2009.0438

163. Bruce JY, Lang JM, McNeel DG et al (2012) Current controversies in the management of biochemical failure in prostate cancer. Clin Adv Hematol Oncol 10(11):716–722

164. Ahmed HU, Pendse D, Illing R et al (2007) Will focal therapy become a standard of care for men with localized prostate cancer? Nat Clin Pract Oncol 4(11):632–642. doi:10.1038/ncponc0959

165. Chen CP, Weinberg V, Shinohara K et al (2013) Salvage HDR brachytherapy for recurrent prostate cancer after previous definitive radiation therapy: 5-year outcomes. Int J Radiat Oncol Biol Phys 86(2):324–329. doi:10.1016/j.ijrobp.2013.01.027

166. Pound CR, Partin AW, Eisenberger MA et al (1999) Natural history of progression after PSA elevation

following radical prostatectomy. JAMA 281(17): 1591–1597

167. Ward JF, Pagliaro LC, Pisters LL (2008) Salvage therapy for radio-recurrent prostate cancer. Curr Probl Cancer 32(6):242–271. doi:10.1016/j.currproblcancer.2008.10.001

168. Lee B, Shinohara K, Weinberg V et al (2007) Feasibility of high-dose-rate brachytherapy salvage for local prostate cancer recurrence after radiotherapy: the University of California-San Francisco experience. Int J Radiat Oncol Biol Phys 67(4):1106–1112. doi:10.1016/j.ijrobp.2006.10.012

169. Oliai C, Yang L, Lee JY (2013) Prospective quality of life and efficacy of high-dose-rate brachytherapy salvage for recurrent prostate cancer. Int J Radiat Oncol Biol Phys 87(2):S396

170. Pellizzon A, Miziara MC. Neviani C, Miziara R (2009) Long-term results of salvage interstitial high-dose brachytherapy for local-only recurrent prostate cancer treated with definitive conventional external beam radiotherapy. ASCO abstract 2009. http://meetinglibrary.asco.org/content/20049-64

171. Scala L, Page PN, Lee JW (2009) Salvage high dose rate brachytherapy for locally recurrent prostate cancer after primary radiotherapy. Int J Radiat Oncol Biol Phys 75(3):S322

172. Tharp M, Hardacre M, Bennett R et al (2008) Prostate high-dose-rate brachytherapy as salvage treatment of local failure after previous external or permanent seed irradiation for prostate cancer. Brachytherapy 7(3):231–236. doi:10.1016/j.brachy.2008.03.003

173. Yamada Y, Kollmeier MA, Pei X et al (2014) A phase II study of salvage high-dose-rate brachytherapy for the treatment of locally recurrent prostate cancer after definitive external beam radiotherapy. Brachytherapy 13(2):111–116. doi:10.1016/j.brachy.2013.11.005

Lower Gastrointestinal Brachytherapy: Rectum

Maria Antonietta Gambacorta, Maura Campitelli,
Rezarta Frakulli, Andrea Galuppi,
Alessio G. Morganti, and Vincenzo Valentini

Abstract

The management of rectal cancer is largely surgical. The treatment can be modulated according to tumor presentation: endoscopic excision and surgery for early tumors, radiotherapy and chemotherapy treatments integrated to definitive surgery, and, in advanced cases, chemotherapy, palliative surgery and/or radiotherapy, or a combination of the above in metastatic tumors.

1 Introduction

Population-based studies showed improved overall outcomes from the 1990s and beyond [1]. However, although the improvement in survival was gained in younger patients, the same result was not reached for the older (>75 years) group.

M.A. Gambacorta, MD • M. Campitelli, MD
V. Valentini, MD (✉)
Gemelli ART (Advanced Radiation Therapy),
Catholic University of the Sacred Heart,
Agostino Gemelli Polyclinic, Rome, Italy
e-mail: vvalentini@rm.unicatt.it

R. Frakulli, MD • A. Galuppi, MD
A.G. Morganti, MD
Radiation Oncology Center,
Department of Experimental,
Diagnostic and Specialty Medicine-DIMES,
University of Bologna, San Orsola-Malpighi
Hospital, Bologna, Italy

This seems to be due to the lesser access to preoperative treatments and to the higher mortality rate at 6 months post-TME for older versus younger patients (14 % vs. 3.3 %) ($p < 0.0001$) [2]. Multimodal treatments, especially including a radical surgery component, may be too demanding for aged, frail patients who more often have associated comorbidities. Many times patients with significant medical illnesses cannot tolerate prolonged anesthesia or morbidity from the surgical approach. This category of patients has been treated, in some series, with conservative surgery or radiotherapy alone, with the intent of either achieving prolonged symptom control or prolonged tumor control, trying to minimize treatment-related side effects [3–5].

Younger or fit patients who undergo radical TME surgery have impaired quality of life due to the inevitable consequences of the surgical procedure: patients with ultra-low rectal cancer who undergo abdominoperineal resection (APR) have to live with the stoma; patients who undergo low anterior resection (LAR) may suffer from defecation

© Springer International Publishing Switzerland 2016
P. Montemaggi et al. (eds.), *Brachytherapy: An International Perspective*, Medical Radiology,
DOI 10.1007/978-3-319-26791-3_20

problems due to the entire removal of the rectum and/or anal sphincteric injury. These symptoms may be more pronounced when radiotherapy is incorporated, likely related to fibrosis of the surrounding tissue of the neo-rectum and the dysfunction of the anal sphincter, when this is included in the treatment field [5, 6].

These side effects, although an accepted trade-off for a cancer cure, may be even more unacceptable for those patients in whom preoperative radiotherapy +/– chemotherapy results in a pathological complete tumor response (ypCR), and thus no residual cancer is found in the surgical specimen after major mutilating surgery leading many patients and physicians to wonder if the surgery was really necessary since definitive data in this circumstance remain elusive.

The achievement of a pCR following neoadjuvant therapy (ypCR), which occurs in approximately 15–20 % of patients, has been shown to reflect better long-term outcomes [7–9]. These findings, together with the intention to improve the quality of life of surviving patients, have stimulated the exploration of more conservative approaches. A number of Phase 2 studies are evaluating the role of conservative treatment in patients who demonstrate substantial clinical response. A completely nonsurgical or minimal surgical approach with "watch and wait" policies after chemoradiotherapy followed in some series by brachytherapy or local excision of the residual tumor is being studied following pathological confirmation of clinical response.

In this setting, decision supportive systems based on analysis of large data bases, through the connection of clinical, radiological, and therapy data, have been created. Nomograms for the prediction of pCR both before surgery and during chemoradiation are now available. These tools may support the multidisciplinary team: (1) to identify the subgroup of patients with an excellent response after chemoradiation who may benefit from conservative treatment and (2) to define, during treatment, categories of patients with different responses, allowing early modulation of preoperative treatment according to response [10, 11].

The definition of prolonged survival in rectal cancer is enlarging to also include metastatic patients.

This circumstance represents a complex category including pluri-metastatic patients needing a systemic approach with the intent to slow the growth of disease and consequently delay the appearance of related symptoms. Oligometastatic disease in some patients now presents an opportunity for salvage cure. In these patients systemic therapy still represents the main treatment to reach multiple tumor sites. However, local therapy directed to the rectum, such as radiotherapy, surgery, or endoscopic strategies, can be considered according to the aim of the treatment. Eradication or control of the primary tumor, in those potentially curable patients or control of tumor-related local symptoms, such as bleeding, pain, constipation, and mucous discharge, is now common, while just a few years ago, this was thought impossible and not much different from pluri-metastatic disease.

Patients with any or all of the above conditions, age unfit, serious comorbidities, and favorable metastatic patients, may benefit from conservative therapies such as local excision, radiotherapy, and brachytherapy, as well as "watch and wait" approaches. In these settings, brachytherapy may play an important role in increasing quality of life by trying to maintain the same outcomes of the standard treatment:

1. Achieving cure or long-term control of the primary tumor, in aged frail and unfit patients, avoiding surgery
2. Increasing, delivered as a boost, the rate of ypCR allowing minor or no surgery, in good responding patients after chemoradiation
3. Achieving symptom palliation related to the primary tumor in pluri-metastatic patients or prolonged tumor control in the oligometastatic patients

2 Rectal Cancer Brachytherapy Techniques

Different types of brachytherapy have been used in rectal cancer and will be briefly summarized in the following paragraphs: contact X-ray brachytherapy, high-dose rate intraluminal rectal brachytherapy, interstitial rectal brachytherapy, and intraoperative radiotherapy (IORT) [12].

2.1   Contact X-Ray Brachytherapy

With this technique, a high dose of low-energy (50 KV) X-ray is delivered to the tumor under direct vision. In France in 1946, Lamarque and Gros were the first to use the handheld Philips RT 50 machine to treat a rectal cancer [13]. In the following decades, Papillon popularized this technique treating more than 300 rectal cancer patients [14]. The treatment can be delivered as an outpatient. An empty rectal ampulla is needed, and therefore a low residue diet for 3–5 days is required, and a mini-rectal enema is given 30 min before the procedure. No general anesthesia is required and generally only local anesthetic gel is used. According to the exact tumor site in the rectum, different treatment positions are recommended. For anterior and lateral tumor localization, a knee-chest position helps to open the rectum and makes it easier to visualize the tumor. For low posterior tumors, the lithotomy position is recommended. Initially, a rigid sigmoidoscope is inserted into the anus and rectum to identify tumor size and location. Based on tumor size, the diameter of the applicator is chosen, inserted, and placed directly to encompass the tumor with a small margin of about 0.1 cm. Different sizes of applicators are available: 3.0, 2.5, and 2.2 cm. One hundred percent of the dose is prescribed at the surface, and the dose falls off to 60 and 55 % at a 0.5 cm depth for 3.0 and 2.2 cm diameter applicators, respectively. The dose rate is close to 20 Gy/min and treatment time does not exceed 1–3 min. Recently, an innovative machine, the Papillon 50TM (Ariane Medical Systems Ltd, Derby, UK), has been designed allowing direct vision during treatment.

2.2   Endoluminal High-Dose-Rate (HDR) Rectal Brachytherapy

This technique was developed in the 1990s by Sun Myint in Clatterbridge [15] and Vuong in Montreal [16]. Both ^{192}Ir- and ^{60}Co-sourced remote afterloader systems are available. Initially in the procedure, radiopaque clips are endoscopically inserted to mark the proximal and distal margins of the tumor. For contact radiotherapy,

general anesthesia is not mandatory and conscious sedation can be substituted if necessary. Patients are placed into the lithotomy position and the rectal applicator is inserted following local anesthetic application. There are two different types of rectal applicators: rectal rigid line (with or without central shielding) or multichannel. A rectal rigid line applicator is a cylindrical tube with an outer diameter of 2.0 cm and a length of 16 cm; it houses a centrally placed stainless steel catheter (0.3 cm in diameter) as the application channel of the iridium source with spacing for shielding. This system allows shielding from 25 to 75 % of the applicator circumference for treatment of tumors with less than complete circumferential mucosal involvement [17]. The alternative system (multichannel) has the advantage that the catheters can be selectively loaded, ensuring more conformal dose delivery and sparing the uninvolved opposite rectal wall. The applicator also contains a balloon, which can be inflated to immobilize the applicator in the desired position within the rectum thus reducing the dose to the normal structures [18]. After applicator positioning, a computerized tomography scan using 0.5 cm slice thickness is performed for planning. Dwell positions are selected to accommodate the outlined clinical target volume (CTV). The CTV is defined as the gross tumor volume (GTV) plus a 0.5 cm margin, and the dose is normalized to the mean of applicator points at a distance from the applicator surface, equidistant between loaded catheters. Sometimes computerized optimization to achieve acceptable coverage (such as V100 ≥90 %) may be necessary.

2.3   Rectal Interstitial Implant

Interstitial implants of the rectum are most often used as a boost after external beam radiation. Initially endorectal ultrasound is useful to identify the thickness of the residual tumor. Patient preparation starts the day before procedure including perineal shaving and cleansing enemas. The procedure is performed under general or spinal anesthesia. Patients are placed in the lithotomy position and a Foley catheter is inserted into the bladder. Using guide needles and a template, needles are sequentially inserted via the perineum approximately 0.3–0.4 cm from the mucosal surface. The distance between needles is 1 cm. A 2.5 cm margin beyond the volume to be covered by isodose is recommended to take account of all the variables (the pull back from patients, the crimped tip, and the tip of sources to the reference isodose using the Paris system). During all treatments a rectal tube is inserted to keep the anal canal open and to push the mucosa opposite the implanted needles away from the defined treated volume. The tube also allows gas and/or fecal evacuation during treatment. A compressive dressing is applied to prevent displacement of the system during irradiation. However, the correct position of the implant has to be monitored daily [19].

3 Rectal Cancer Brachytherapy: Clinical Results

Brachytherapy in the treatment of rectal cancer has been performed since the 1940s and 1950s due to the pioneering contributions of Chaoul [20] and Lamarque and Gros [13] using a nonsurgical approach on small and accessible cancers.

In the 1970s, Papillon et al. [21] published his successful work on endocavitary contact radiotherapy (CXRT) using ^{192}Iridium interstitial brachytherapy in the conservative treatment of 152 rectal cancers, obtaining excellent local control and anal function preservation.

By the end of 1990s, Maingon et al. [22] reported a complete response rate of 93 % with a sphincter preservation rate of 84 % and a normal sphincter function of 98 % in a series of 151 patients affected by T1 to T3 low rectal adenocarcinomas treated by a combination of contact X-ray, interstitial brachytherapy, and external beam radiation therapy (EBRT).

In 1992, the Papillon technique was introduced at Clatterbridge in the UK by Sun Myint, and iridium endoluminal high-dose-rate brachy-

therapy was introduced to Montreal in the 1990s by Vuong.

A number of studies investigated the role of brachytherapy as an alternative preoperative treatment or as a dose escalation procedure, combined with external radiation therapy in elderly or inoperable patients or in a preoperative setting. Their results will be reported here.

3.1 Rectal Cancer Brachytherapy as an Alternative Preoperative Treatment

In an attempt to reduce the toxicity related to radiochemotherapy, 100 patients with resectable rectal adenocarcinoma T2–T4, N0/N1 were treated with a daily dose of 6.5 Gy of endorectal brachytherapy for over 4 consecutive days at McGill University [23]. Immediate tolerance was good in 99 patients who developed no more than grade 2 acute proctitis. Surgery was performed 4–8 weeks after the completion of brachytherapy. Pathologic review demonstrated 29 % of the surgical specimens with a ypCR, comparing favorably with responses achieved with conventional radiochemotherapeutic treatment. At 5 years, the local recurrence rate was 5 %. Surgical complications were not increased with this approach.

Hesselager et al. at Uppsala University in collaboration with Vuong et al. of McGill University [16, 24] recently published the results related to short-term complications following rectal resection in T3–T4 Nx patients preoperatively treated with short-course radiotherapy or high-dose-rate endorectal brachytherapy (HDREBT) or with no preoperative radiotherapy. The brachytherapy technique was the same as described above. They found no major differences in postoperative complications between the groups, with lower rates of reoperation and perioperative bleeding in the high-dose-rate brachytherapy group. Complete tumor regression was obtained in nearly one-quarter of patients in the brachytherapy group with a higher proportion of R0 resection, probably due to a longer interval between radiotherapy and surgery and the higher total dose delivered to the tumor bed by brachytherapy. They concluded that high-dose-rate brachytherapy can be considered a safe alternative to neoadjuvant treatment for patients with resectable rectal cancer, although further studies would be needed to investigate whether a high tumor regression grade will translate into better local control and survival.

Smith et al. [25] at Johns Hopkins University conducted a pilot study on 7 T2 N1 or T3 N0–N1 low rectal adenocarcinoma patients, who were treated with high-dose-rate endorectal brachytherapy. They were compared with historical controls treated with conventional three-dimensional conformal external beam radiotherapy (3DCRT) or intensity-modulated radiotherapy (IMRT). They found results in terms of pCR and toxicity similar to Vuong, with a trend in favor of HDREBT.

In this context, a careful selection of patients is fundamental (i.e., N0–N1 mesorectal only) for brachytherapy success.

3.2 Rectal Cancer Brachytherapy as a Dose Escalation Procedure

Contact X-ray brachytherapy is the only technique whose benefit was proven by a randomized trial, the Lyon R96-02 Phase 3 trial [26]. Between 1996 and 2001, 88 patients with selected distal rectal cancer (T2 or early T3), involving less than 2/3 of the rectal circumference, were randomized between preoperative EBRT (39 Gy in 13 fractions) and the same EBRT with a CXRT boost of 85 Gy in 3 fractions (35, 30 and 20 Gy in sequence). For patients with a complete clinical response 4 weeks after the completion of EBRT, a final boost of 25 Gy could be given to tumor bed using an interstitial iridium-192 brachytherapy implant. The main end point was sphincter preservation. The results, published in 2004, demonstrated that CXRT significantly increased the rate of clinical complete response, pathological response, and sphincter preservation at a mean follow-up of 35 months.

The 10-year follow-up of the Lyon R96-02 trial described a cumulated colostomy rate of 29 % in the EBRT + CXRT group versus 63 % in the EBRT alone group ($p < 0.001$) [27]. The 10-year cumulative colostomy rate according to clinical response was 17 % in patients who had a complete clinical response (15 % of total), 42 % in patients with a clinical response ≥ 50 % (68 % of total), and 77 % in those patients with a clinical response <50 % (17 % of total) ($p = 0.014$). Interestingly, for nine patients with a major/complete clinical response, the therapeutic strategy was to perform an organ-saving approach such as a transanal local excision or other nonoperative treatment, which contributed to the improved rate of sphincter saving observed in the experimental arm. The 10-year rate of local control, disease-free survival, and overall survival were similar between the two arms of the trial, demonstrating that the sphincter preservation did not compromise control of the disease.

The main limits of this study were the small number of total patients and the use of radiotherapy alone without chemotherapy, a context in which dose escalation should be evaluated to improve conservative treatment.

The use of rectal cancer brachytherapy as a boost technique has been evaluated also by Sun Myint in Clatterbridge [15]. They investigated whether the addition of a high-dose rate brachytherapy boost following preoperative chemoradiotherapy could improve surgical outcomes in terms of R0 resection and pCR. They included bulky low non-circumferential or fixed T2 or T3 resectable tumors with threatened circumferential resection margin or multiple suspicious lymph nodes. Thirty-four patients received 45 Gy to the pelvis over 5 weeks concurrently with chemotherapy and a 10 Gy boost at 1.0 cm from the surface of the applicator 6–8 weeks before surgery. Twenty-nine patients went on to operation, and among these, 24 achieved an R0 resection (80 %), while nine (31 %) had a pCR with both rates higher than those reported in literature. No local recurrence was observed after a median follow-up interval of 17 months. As regards to toxicity, there was no increase in grade 3–4 toxicity and no delay in wound healing or increase in anastomotic leakage as compared to historic data. The study demonstrated that increasing the dose of radiation with an HDR brachytherapy boost appears to improve the likelihood of obtaining an R0 resection and pCR rate, but the short follow-up was not sufficient for meaningful survival analysis.

Despite these encouraging early results on the improved tumor response at the time of surgery, the recently published randomized Danish study on long-term results of brachytherapy boost in advanced rectal cancer has not been so enthusiastic [28]. In this study, a cohort of 221 patients T3–T4 N0–N2 M0 was randomized between radiochemotherapies with or without a brachytherapy boost. At a median follow-up of 5.4 years and despite a significant increase in tumor response at the time of surgery (41 % in the brachytherapy boost arm versus 27 % in the standard arm), no differences in 5-year OS (70.6 % vs. 63.6 %, respectively, hazard ratio [HR] = 1.24, p = 0.34) and PFS (63.9 % vs. 52.0 %, respectively, HR = 1.22, p = .32) were observed. Freedom from locoregional failure at 5 years was 93.9 and 85.7 % (HR = 2.60, p = .06) in the standard and in the brachytherapy arms, respectively. Unfortunately the trial did not report data on late toxicity.

The authors concluded that the use of brachytherapy as a boost treatment for locally advanced rectal cancer patients in the preoperative setting cannot be recommended based on the findings of their trial. On the contrary, the role of brachytherapy in other patient groups, such as patients with early rectal cancer treated with definite radiotherapy (as for patients in the Lyon R 96–02) or patients treated with palliative intent, remains open.

Papillion-style contact therapy [29]. This study demonstrated an excellent local control rate of 93 % at 3 years. At a median follow-up of 4.6 years, the overall survival was 71 %, reflecting the advancing age and the poor general condition due to medical comorbidity of the cohort of patients that were treated. The cancer-specific survival was in fact 93 %.

For medically unfit patients with larger tumors (T2/T4), the risk of nodal involvement makes the combination of local radiotherapy (either with contact X-rays or with high-dose-rate brachytherapy) and external beam radiotherapy necessary [30].

In elderly unfit patients, endoluminal brachytherapy in association with external radiotherapy was studied in 41 patients (median age, 82 years) at McGill University [16]. In this study, 40–45 Gy in 4/5 weeks followed by 30 Gy in three fractions of brachytherapy was delivered with and without surgery. Local control at 14 months was 76 % with an incidence of grade 3 rectal bleeding occurring in only seven patients and rectal stenosis occurring in only three patients.

Another interesting use of endocavitary HDR brachytherapy has been evaluated by Chuong et al. in patients who previously received pelvic irradiation at a mean of 11 years prior to their diagnosis of rectal cancer [31]. In this study, ten patients received a total dose of 26 Gy in four consecutive daily 6.5 Gy fractions. Among the six patients who went to surgery in follow-up, two had a pCR and two others a near pCR. Five had negative surgical margins. As for tolerance, there was no grade 3 or higher toxicity and no patients had significant intraoperative or postoperative complications. In this particular population of patients, preoperative endorectal HDR brachytherapy could be considered as an alternative to external irradiation.

3.3 Rectal Cancer Brachytherapy in Medically Unfit Patients and in Re-irradiation

Elderly unfit patients with T1/T2 rectal adenocarcinoma were treated with curative intent by Sun Myint et al. by a combination modality treatment consisting of external radiotherapy and

4 Special Clinical Application: IORT

In cases of suspected positive margins or residual disease, IORT is an alternative to deliver a high dose of local radiation and reduce the risk of local recurrences [32]. Multiple methods of delivery of IORT are available. Either low-energy X-rays (50 kV maximum) or 6–18 MeV electrons have been used in clinical practice [6]. For low-energy X-ray delivery, different diameters of the spherical applicators are available and placed at the tip of a 0.32 cm diameter tube, ranging from 1.5 to 5 cm in 0.5 cm increments. The spherical applicator is placed into the tumor bed by the surgeon and radiation oncologist. Normal structures (small bowel, ureters, etc.) are shielded by small sheets of lead covered by a sterile plastic drape. All present operating room personnel wear leaded aprons and stand behind a shielded screen while IORT is delivered [33]. Additionally, IORT may also be performed using ^{192}I sources although experience is limited [34].

5 Side Effects

Proctitis is the most frequent acute toxicity reported with a grade 3 incidence of approximately 1 % [23]. Late toxicity is mainly represented by bleeding which occurs in 26 % of cases (usually grade 1 and 2) and usually resolves after 6–12 months. No grade 5 toxicity, perforation, or uncontrolled bleeding have been reported following brachytherapy. In patients on anticoagulants medications, bleeding can be troublesome and argon plasma coagulation can be useful in approximately 5 % of cases [35], although this should be used sparingly and when all other options have been exhausted (local steroids and vasoconstrictors). About 10 % of patients develop rectal discomfort, urgency, or tenesmus with steroid enemas being potentially helpful. Fistulas and rectal stenosis occur in less than 1 % and are generally associated with prior surgical intervention.

References

1. Brenner H, Bouvier AM, Foschi R et al (2012) Progress in colorectal cancer survival in Europe from the late 1980s to the early 21st century: the EUROCARE study. Int J Cancer 131(7):1649–1658
2. Rutten H, den Dulk M, Lemmens V et al (2007) Survival of elderly rectal cancer patients not improved: analysis of population based data on the impact of TME surgery. Eur J Cancer 43(15):2295–2300
3. Habr-Gama A, Perez RO, Sabbaqa J et al (2009) Increasing the rates of complete response to neoadjuvant chemoradiotherapy for distal rectal cancer: results of a prospective study using additional chemotherapy during the resting period. Dis Colon Rectum 52(12):1927–1934
4. Papillon J (1990) Present status of radiation therapy in the conservative management of rectal cancer. Radiother Oncol 17(4):275–283
5. Pucciarelli S, De Paoli A, Guerrieri M et al (2013) Local excision after preoperative chemoradiotherapy for rectal cancer: results of a multicentre phase II trial. Dis Colon Rectum 56(12):1349–1356
6. Roeder F, Goetz JM, Habl G et al (2012) Intraoperative Electron Radiation Therapy (IOERT) in the management of locally recurrent rectal cancer. BMC Cancer 12:592–602
7. Capirci C, Valentini V, Cionini L et al (2008) Prognostic value of pathologic complete response after neoadjuvant therapy in locally advanced rectal cancer: long-term analysis of 566 ypCR patients. Int J Radiat Oncol Biol Phys 72(1):99–107
8. Maas M, Nelemans PJ, Valentini V et al (2010) Long term outcome in patients with pathological complete response after chemoradiation for rectal cancer: a pooled analysis of individual patient data. Lancet Oncol 11(9):835–844
9. Martin ST, Heneghan HM, Winter DC (2012) Systematic review and meta-analysis of outcomes following pathological complete response to neoadjuvant chemoradiotherapy for rectal cancer. Br J Surg 99:918–928
10. van Stiphout RGPM, Lammering G, Buijsen J et al (2011) Development and external validation of a predictive model for pathological complete response of rectal cancer patients including sequential PET-CT imaging. Radiother Oncol 98:126–133
11. van Stiphout R, Valentini V, Buijsen J et al (2014) Nomogram predicting response after chemoradiotherapy in rectal cancer using sequential PET CT imaging: a multicentric prospective study with external validation. Radiother Oncol 113:215–222
12. Gerard JP (2012) What is the contribution of brachy therapy in tailoring local therapy? In: Valentini V, Schmoll HJ, Van de Velde CJH (eds) Multidisciplinary management of rectal cancer. Questions and answers. Springer, Berlin/Heidelberg, pp 163–169
13. Lamarque P, Gros C (1946) La radiothérapie de contacte dans les cancers du rectum. J Radiol Electrol 27:333–348
14. Papillon J (1982) Rectal and anal cancer. Conservative treatment by irradiation; an alternative to radical surgery. Springer, Berlin
15. Sun Myint A, Mukhopadhyay T, Ramani VS et al (2010) Can increasing the dose of radiation by HDR brachytherapy boost following pre-operative chemoradiotherapy for advanced rectal cancer improve surgical outcomes? Colorectal Dis 12(Suppl 2):30–36
16. Vuong T, Richard C, Niazi T et al (2010) High dose rata endorectal brachytherapy for curable rectal cancer. Semin Colon Rectal Surg 21:115–119

17. Jakobsen A, Mortensen JP, Bisgaard C et al (2006) Preoperative chemoradiotherapy of locally advanced T3 rectal cancer combined with an endorectal boost. Int J Radiat Oncol Biol Phys 64(2):461–465

18. Devic S, Vuong T, Moftah B (2005) Advantages of inflatable multichannel endorectal applicator in the neo-adjuvant treatment of patients with locally advanced rectal cancer with HDR brachytherapy. J Appl Clin Med Phys 6(2):44 49

19. Grimard L, Stern H, Spaans JH (2009) Brachytherapy and local excision for sphincter preservation in T1 and T2 rectal cancer. Int J Radiat Oncol Biol Phys 74(3):803–809

20. Chaoul H (1950) La roentgenthérapie à courte distance. J Electro Radiol 31:290

21. Papillon J, Montbarbon JF, Gérard JP et al (1989) Interstitial curietherapy in the conservative treatment of anal and rectal cancers. Int J Radiat Oncol Biol Phys 17:1161–1169

22. Maingon P, Guerif S, Darsouni R et al (1998) Conservative management of rectal adenocarcinoma by radiotherapy. Int J Radiat Oncol Biol Phys 40:1077–1085

23. Vuong T, Devic S, Podgorask E (2007) High dose rate endorectal brachytherapy as a neoadjuvant treatment for patients with resectable rectal cancer. Clin Oncol 19:701–705

24. Hesselager C, Vuong T, Pahlman L et al (2013) Short-term outcome after neoadjuvant high dose rate endorectal brachytherapy or short-course external beam radiotherapy in resectable rectal cancer. Colorectal Dis 15(6):662–666

25. Smith JA, Wild AT, Singhi A et al (2012) Clinicopathologic comparison of high-dose-rate endorectal brachytherapy versus conventional chemoradiotherapy in the neoajuvant setting for resectable stage II and III low rectal cancer. Int J Surgical Oncol 2012:1–11

26. Gerard JP, Chapet O, Nemoz C et al (2004) Improved sphincter preservation in low rectal cancer with high- dose preoperative radiotherapy: the Lyon R96-02 randomized trial. J Clin Oncol 22:2404–2409

27. Ortholan C, Romestaing P, Chapet O et al (2012) Correlation in rectal cancer between clinical tumor response after neoadjuvant radiotherapy and sphincter or organ preservation: 10-year results of the Lyon R96-02 randomized trial. Int J Radiation Oncol Biol Phys 83:e165–e171

28. Appelt AL, Vogelius YIR, Pløen ZJ et al (2014) Long-term results of a randomized trial in locally advanced rectal cancer: no benefit from adding a brachytherapy boost. Int J Radiation Oncol Biol Phys 90(1):110–118

29. Sun Myint A, Grieve RJ, McDonald AC et al (2007) Combined modality treatment of early rectal cancer-the UK experience. Clin Oncol 19:674–681

30. Marijnen CA (2007) External beam radiotherapy and high dose rate brachytherapy for medically unfit and elderly patients. Clin Oncol (R Coll Radiol) 19(9):706–710

31. Chuong MD, Fernandez DC, Shridhar R et al (2013) High dose rate endorectal brachytherapy for locally advanced rectal cancer in previously irradiated patients. Brachytherapy 12:457–462

32. Cantero-Muñoz P, Urién MA, Ruano-Ravina A (2011) Efficacy and safety of intraoperative radiotherapy in colorectal cancer: a systematic review. Cancer Lett 306(2):121–133

33. Guo S, Reddy AC, Kolar M et al (2012) Intraoperative radiation therapy with the photon radiosurgery system in locally advanced and recurrent rectal cancer: retrospective review of the Cleveland clinic experience. Radiat Oncol 7:110–117

34. Goes RN, Beart RW Jr, Simons AJ et al (1997) Use of brachytherapy in management of locally recurrent rectal cancer. Dis Colon Rectum 40(10):1177–1179

35. Sun Myint A, Whitmarsh K, Perkins K et al (2013) A preliminary report on toxicity of contact radiotherapy in first 100 patients treated by the new RT50 Papillon machine. Colorectal Dis 15:Abst. P081

Lower Gastrointestinal Brachytherapy: Anus

Stefania Manfrida, Luca Tagliaferri,
Rezarta Frakulli, Maria Antonietta Gambacorta,
Alessio G. Morganti, and Vincenzo Valentini

Abstract

Management of anal canal cancers has special concerns due to the functional and structural relationships of the body, especially as compared to the remarkable radiosensitivity of tumors of this region. We present an outline of the special role of brachytherapy and an analysis of the data to date.

1 Introduction: The Need for Brachytherapy Nowadays

Anal cancer is a rare disease and accounts for only 2 % of digestive tract tumors and 2–4 % of colon, rectal, and anal tumors [1, 2]. The annual incidence is 1 in 100,000, is higher in women, and is increasing [3, 4].

S. Manfrida, MD • L. Tagliaferri, MD
M.A. Gambacorta, MD • V. Valentini (✉)
Gemelli ART (Advanced Radiation Therapy),
Catholic University of the Sacred Heart,
Agostino Gemelli Polyclinic, Rome, Italy
e-mail: vvalentini@rm.unicatt.it

R. Frakulli, MD • A.G. Morganti, MD
Radiation Oncology Center, Experimental,
Diagnostic and Specialty Medicine-DIMES,
Sant'Orsola-Malpighi Hospital, University of
Bologna, Bologna, Italy

1.1 Anatomy and Histology

The anal region is comprised of the anal canal and the anal margin, dividing anal cancers into two categories. However, tumors can involve both the anal canal and the anal margin. The anal canal is the more proximal portion of the anal region and extends from the anorectal junction to the junction with perineal skin (anal verge) as defined by the American Joint Committee on Cancer (AJCC) [5] and the Union Internationale Contre le Cancer (UICC) [6] (Fig. 1). The superior border of the functional anal canal, separating it from the rectum, has been defined as the palpable upper border of the anal sphincter and puborectalis muscles of the anorectal ring. It is approximately 3–5 cm in length, and its inferior border starts at the anal verge, the lowermost edge of the sphincter muscles, corresponding to the introitus of the anal orifice. Useful palpable landmarks are the puborectal sling and the intersphincteric groove. The columnar, or cylindrical, epithelium of the rectum extends to about 1 cm

Fig. 1 Anatomy of the anal region

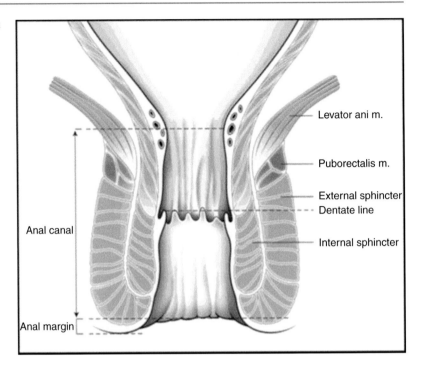

Levator ani m.

Puborectalis m.

External sphincter
Dentate line

Internal sphincter

Anal canal

Anal margin

above the dentate line where the anal transitional zone begins. The *dentate line* is defined as the limits between the columnar epithelium and the stratified squamous epithelium of the anal canal. This junction is not characterized by an abrupt histological change, but rather by a *transition zone* that extends for approximately 0.6–1.2 cm containing epithelial columnar, cuboidal, squamous, and transitional cell subtypes. The stratified squamous epithelium extends just below the dentate line to the *anal verge* defined as the junction of the squamous epithelium of the anal canal with its perianal skin. The pigmented skin within a 5-cm radius around the anal verge is called the *perianal skin* or *anal margin* and is covered by the epidermis. Tumors of the anal margin (below the anal verge and involving the perianal hair-bearing skin) are classified with skin tumors.

Because therapy for anal tumors is determined in large part by location, it is critical that there is universal understanding of anatomic landmarks in this region.

Anatomic definitions of the anal and perianal region have been confusing and controversial. Various definitions of the anal canal exist that are

based on particular physical/anatomic landmarks or histologic characteristics. In some surgical series, the anal canal is defined as the region between the dentate line and the upper margin of the anal sphincter based upon the pathways of lymphatic drainage. Consequently, a tumor arising below the dentate line may be defined as a tumor of the margin [7, 8]. Recently, AJCC and UICC have clarified the definition of the anal canal as the portion that extends from the anorectal ring to the anal verge.

In practice at diagnosis, the precise point of origin is often uncertain, and the distinction between an anal canal and anal margin tumor is often difficult. For this reason, a classification of three distinct regions has been suggested—i.e., intra-anal, perianal (visualized with gentle traction on the buttocks), and skin tumors (beyond a 5-cm radius from the anal verge) [9].

For anal cancer treatment, histological confirmation by biopsy is mandatory.

In the anal canal, the most common histologic type (80 %) is squamous cell carcinoma. Other malignant tumors of the epithelium included cloacogenic, basaloid, and transitional tumors which occur with a lesser prevalence [10]. Uncommon histological presentations of anal carcinomas include adenocarcinoma, undifferentiated cancer, melanoma, neuroendocrine tumors, and small cell carcinomas [11].

Squamous cell carcinoma of the anus is strongly associated with human papillomavirus (HPV) infection which represents the causative agent in 80–85 % of patients (usually from HPV 16 or HPV 18 subtypes in Europe) [12, 13] as is its precursor lesion anal intraepithelial neoplasia (AIN) [14].

Epidermoid carcinoma is a slow growing tumor and usually presents as an intra-anal or perianal mass. Lymph node involvement at diagnosis is observed in about 30 % of cases, while systemic spread is uncommon (5–8 %).

Staging of anal cancer is based upon tumor size and local extension, regional lymph node involvement, and the presence or absence of distant metastases. Magnetic resonance imaging (MRI) and endoanal ultrasound increasingly are utilized to assess tumor depth and sphincter involvement.

Tumors of the anal margin are generally well differentiated and more often occur in men, in contrast to canal tumors which are normally poorly differentiated and more common in women. Because of tumor location and early diagnosis, patients with anal margin tumors tend to have a better prognosis. Very early-stage (T1N0M0) anal margin cancer is similar to treatment for skin cancer by local wide excision. More advanced diseases or lesions that involve the anal verge are managed with combined treatment similar to those for anal canal cancers which will be presented later in this chapter.

1.2 Combined Treatments

External beam radiotherapy with concurrent chemotherapy (RCT) represents the primary standard treatment in squamous anal canal carcinoma. The aim of treatment is to achieve cure with locoregional control and preservation of anal function for the best possible quality of life.

Concomitant use of radiotherapy with chemotherapy was introduced by Nigro et al. in 1974 [15], initially as neoadjuvant therapy preceding radical surgical resection consisting of abdominoperineal resection (APR), thereafter as definitive treatment with surgery reserved for those who failed this regimen [11, 14]. The 5-year overall survival for patients who received nonsurgical radiochemotherapy treatments (50–70 % according to clinical stage) is equivalent to that of patients who received surgical treatment and most are spared the need of colostomy [16].

Six randomized controlled trials conducted in the last three decades assessed the role of concomitant use of external beam radiochemotherapy for patients with epidermoid anal cancer and confirmed the association of radiotherapy with concurrent 5Fu and mitomycin C (MMC) as standard treatment providing better local control and lower colostomy rates [17–23].

RCT offers a complete response rate of approximately 80–90 % in early-stage disease, associated with a high rate of local control and sphincter preservation with locoregional failures of 15 %. However, especially for more advanced patients treated with standard schedules, there is still a 30–40 % rate of locoregional recurrence. In an effort to reduce locoregional recurrence and the colostomy rate coupled with the observation of high level of overall grade 3 and 4 acute toxicity during radiochemotherapy in about 1/3 of the overall treated population (skin, hematological, and gastrointestinal) [18, 20], three randomized trials explored different chemotherapeutic agents and schedules (cisplatin instead of mitomycin C induction or maintenance chemotherapy) [4, 21].

Data from these trials and a recent systematic review [24, 25] continue to support the paradigm of external beam radiotherapy with concurrent 5Fu and MMC developed over 30 years ago as the standard of care for lower colostomy and local failure rates with less acute toxicity.

Disappointingly, the 5-year survival has changed little in the last two decades. In the United States, the overall 5-year survival rate in a patient cohort treated from 1994 to 2000 was 60 % for men and 78 % for women [4].

Radiotherapy techniques, total dose, fraction, planned interruption, and boost dose vary in the randomized clinical trials, and the optimal radiotherapy approach in combination with concurrent chemotherapy has not been directly explored in randomized trials.

From evidence of randomized trials and systematic reviews, international guidelines have been formulated that suggest doses of at least 45–50 Gy without a treatment gap are recommended for T1–2 N0 tumors [26, 27]. Higher doses may be required for more advanced lesions, particularly if a planned treatment gap is used. The importance of delivering a total dose of ≥55–59 Gy to the tumor bed to patients with stage II/III anal canal carcinoma as supported by retrospective studies showed better local control rates at these dose levels even if significantly associated with acute and late toxicity [19, 28, 29].

Uninterrupted treatment (avoiding a gap) is considered radiobiologically to be the most effective treatment. Shorter overall treatment time (OTT) is associated with improved outcome [30], while prolonged OTT over 60 days showed a detrimental impact [20, 31], even for total doses over 54Gy [29]. Therefore, in order to optimize local control rates, individualized treatment breaks as necessary due to acute adverse effects may be preferred over planned treatment interruptions [33].

The introduction of 3D conformal radiotherapy-based treatments allows practitioners to identify normal as well as target soft tissue structures on axial CT images, which has led to improved treatment accuracy during delivery. Moreover, the evolution of conformal treatment strategies such as intensity-modulated radiotherapy (IMRT) while sparing organs at risk may result in a reduction of acute and long-term toxicity in normal tissue and may allow full or even escalated doses to be achieved within a shorter overall treatment time [16, 32, 34]. The potential clinical benefits of the dosimetric advantages of these techniques in the treatment of anal canal cancer patients are under prospective evaluation.

Boost doses to the primary tumor have usually ranged from 9 to 20 Gy, with higher doses applied for observed poor clinical response.

International guidelines support the utility of a boost after RCT [26, 27].

2   Brachytherapy

Brachytherapy (BT) has an important role in the local dose escalation for the treatment of anal cancer because of the physical and biological advantages which offer a highly conformal treatment (steep dose falloff around the source) which is able to deliver a high dose to the primary tumor, sparing surrounding normal tissues such as the contralateral mucosa and sphincter.

Nevertheless, its role has not been evaluated extensively, and at the moment there is no clear evidence in the literature to guide the choice of brachytherapy boost versus external beam boost after initial external beam radiotherapy (EBRT) for anal cancer [35].

The most frequently applied BT methods are low-dose rate (LDR), pulsed dose rate (PDR), or high-dose rate (HDR). These methods are characterized by the different dose rates delivered by the radiation sources (LDR/PDR, 0.5–1 Gy/h; HDR, >12 Gy/h). The isotope iridium-192 (Ir192) is commonly used for remote afterloading procedures.

2.1   Indications

The Groupe Européen de Curiethérapie-European Society for Radiotherapy and Oncology (GEC-ESTRO) guidelines suggest interstitial brachytherapy for delivering the boost to the tumor bed after 45 Gy (conventional EBRT or chemoradiation) for T1–T2 and selected small T3 anal tumors responding to external beam radiotherapy [36]. In patients with anal canal cancer, a brachytherapy boost after radiotherapy or chemoradiotherapy leads to high local control rates with acceptable acute and late toxicity. Brachytherapy *alone* is effective in controlling most small lesions, but causes painful reactions in half of the patients and late necrosis in 10–15 %, and is therefore contraindicated [37, 38].

In order to preserve the sphincter function, there are some limitations for the use of BT in anal cancer. Implantation of more than the half of the circumference and a longitudinal length of more than 5 cm should be avoided. As well, the thickness of the tumor usually should not generally extend to more than 1.0 cm. In daily clinical practice, patients who may benefit from BT have localized tumors and are generally good responders to radiochemotherapy even in case of a locally advanced clinical presentation. A more aggressive approach, which could also integrate surgery, should be considered for poorly responding patients.

Clinical response assessment after RCT is a crucial aspect in the indication of a brachytherapy boost. A time gap between RCT and BT allows recovery of acute normal tissue toxicity and regression of tumor volume; however, the exact time for response evaluation and boost delivery vary among the randomized trials. In this context, important prognostic issues for local control are the time gap between EBRT and BT boost and OTT, with a negative impact on local control when the time gap between EBRT and boost is >37.5 days [32, 39]. In addition, boost radiotherapy after a treatment interruption of 6 weeks could result in increased late adverse effects instead of local control [40].

Regarding the impact of the OTT, data from the CORS-03 trial showed the negative influence on local control for OTT >80 days without influence by the boost technique. But if the OTT is shortened to <80 days, local control is increased significantly using the BT boost instead of an EBRT boost [41].

In summary, a complete response after RCT, even for a locally advanced presentation, should be managed with a lower brachytherapy dose thereby reducing the need for colostomy and limiting irradiated normal tissue volume, thereby decreasing late toxicity as documented in Peiffert and Lestrade papers [42, 43]. Incomplete tumor response after RCT with lesions that require large volume and higher dose cause a more severe toxicity without a real gain in terms of local control; therefore, these situations represent a contraindication to the use of interstitial BT.

2.2 Anal Canal Brachytherapy Techniques

In the past, the positioning of brachytherapy needles was performed by assessing the tumor extent and target volume using clinical findings and not with imaging; moreover, the treatment was primarily done with linear sources. Image-guided brachytherapy (IGBT) and intensity-modulated brachytherapy (IMBT) due to 3D compatible applicators allow a sectional image-based approach with a better assessment of gross tumor volume (GTV) and clinical target volume (CTV) compared to traditional approaches. Nowadays, it is strongly recommended to perform anal brachytherapy with 3D imaging support and with a delivery system that incorporates stepping source technology (IMBT). Also, the European Society for Medical Oncology-European Society of Surgical Oncology-European Society of Radiotherapy and Oncology (ESMO-ESSO-ESTRO) anal cancer clinical practice guidelines (2014) state that double-plane or volume implants may be related to a risk of late necrosis and radiation proctitis; hence, they underline the advantage in the use of computerized 3D image-based treatment planning which allows optimal dose distribution [44].

2.3 Pretreatment Evaluation and Patient Preparation

Before the brachytherapy procedure, it is necessary to evaluate the patient to rule out BT and anesthesia contraindications. BT contraindications are length of the tumor greater than 5 cm, infiltration thickness exceeding 1.0-cm depth, infiltration of the external sphincter, tumor involving more than half the circumference of the anal canal, primary tumor with excessive invasion of the skin, and rectovaginal fistula. Regarding anesthesia, many centers use a general anesthesia, while others prefer a spinal anesthesia because it is safer and causes less systemic effects. Based on clinical findings, imaging is also necessary to define the BT technique as in some selected cases, it is possible to use intracavitary brachytherapy. It is mandatory in cases being considered for intracavitary BT to an accurate prediction of possible dose distribution as the contralateral mucosa could receive a much higher and injurious dose. In such cases, it is preferable to perform an interstitial implant. The preparation of the patient depends on the type of brachytherapy (HDR or LDR/PDR). For HDR implantation, an enema is recommended the evening before and in the early morning of the day of the procedure, a light dinner is suggested. For an LDR/PDR procedure, it is preferable to prescribe laxatives and fast the day before the procedure. The bowel should be kept quiescent thereafter. Before bringing the patient to the theater, preparation of the perianal area with shaving and antiseptic cleansing as well as placing a bladder catheter are required.

2.4 Template Needle Implant Procedure

After anesthesia, the patient is placed in the lithotomy position. The template is positioned and secured to the skin with sutures. The template allows transcutaneous implantation of needles through holes placed at regular, equidistant, and parallel geometric positions which are well defined dosimetrically. Templates are either available commercially or can be fashioned in-house. The needles are positioned under real-time imaging (US or MRI) or according to the indications of the pretreatment plan. When performing a US-guided brachytherapy (Figs. 2, 3, and 4), it is necessary to have a template with a central hole to insert the probe of US devices. Generally, the template is

provided with a central cylinder which is inserted into the anus to stabilize the system and to keep straight the anus and the rectum in order to avoid piercing of the mucosa. Often for performing a US-guided brachytherapy, the cylinder is hollow inside and made of US translucent material. For RM-guided BT, the template must be MRI compatible. In general, the needles are made of stainless steel; however, for MRI-guided BT, they must be plastic or titanium for compatibility.

2.5 CTV Definition

Using brachytherapy as a boost, the CTV is defined by transrectal exploration and imaging exams after EBRT±CT. The most widely used

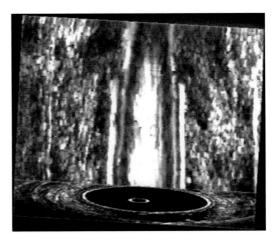
Fig. 3 Ultrasonographic image of needle insertion

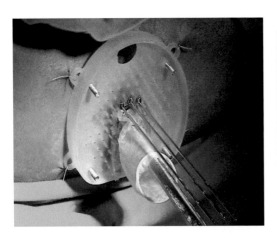
Fig. 2 In-house-made template for US-guided BT in use at the Catholic University of Rome

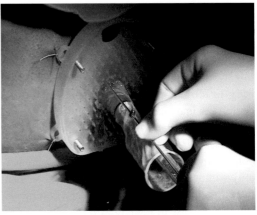
Fig. 4 Needle insertion under ultrasound guidance

imaging method for exact guidance of interstitial radiotherapy in anal cancer brachytherapy is endoanal ultrasound (EAUS) [35] due to excellent target delineation and easiness of application. The EAUS-guided interstitial HDR brachytherapy for anal cancer was introduced in the 1990s and is the first choice in anal canal BT for implant guidance. Doniec [45] in his pilot study demonstrated that EAUS-guided BT for anal cancer is safe in terms of side effects compared to conventional brachytherapy. In addition, the use of this technology in combination with brachytherapy improves local tumor control and minimizes morbidity in patients with anal carcinoma. Moreover, under ultrasound control the needles are implanted directly into the tumor or tumor bed and real-time treatment planning is possible [46]. Regarding other image-guided technique, Christensen et al. in 2008 and Niehoff in 2014 reported the possible use of MRI in the practice of interstitial BT of the anus. The stated limitations were the possibility of having an open MRI machine and the necessity of MRI-compatible templates and needles [42, 47]. A pre-procedure exam is useful to define the target because after the implantation the needles may create artifact. Additionally, MRI is useful if the simulation is performed with only the treatment planning computer (TC) where the lesion is difficult to detect. In these cases, fusion software can be very useful.

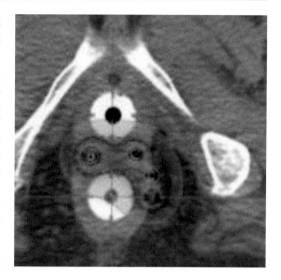

Fig. 5 Example of a treatment plan on TC with dose optimization

2.6 Dosimetry

Following needle implantation, the patient undergoes imaging. Three-dimensional imaging is strongly recommended. It can be 3D US, CT, or MRI. The dose planning process should follow the general rules of the Paris system, with additional manual volume optimization (Fig. 5). The CTV and dose to organs at risk (OARs) should be documented using a dose-volume histogram (DVH). The OARs are the rectum, bladder, and the uninvolved anus. For planning evaluation, it is appropriate to calculate the volume coverage with 200 % of prescribed dose (V200), 150 % (V150), 100 % (V100), and 85 % (V85). Other quality indicators for the treatment plan are D90, D100 (dose delivered to 90 % and 100 % of the CTV, respectively), and the DHI (dose homogeneity index, [V100–V150]/V100). All parameters have to be reported in the BT metrics [48].

The dose nonuniformity ratio (DNR) is calculated as D150/D100 and should not generally exceed 0.32. However, in the analysis published in 2014 by Kapoor et al. [49], the DHI was 0.83 and the DNR was 0.37. In another study published in the same year by Falk et al. [48], these parameters were 0.58 and 0.38, respectively. Major et al. considered that the larger target volume involves longer active length and the increase of active length improves the dose uniformity and the optimal dosimetry. DNR and DHI distant from recommended indications could be justified by a low treatment volume because the implant geometry is applicator dependent [50, 51].

2.7 Anal Cancer Brachytherapy: Clinical Results

In this section, we reviewed the literature on BT boost in anal cancer. In Table 1, a summary of clinical results of multiple studies is reported.

In 1994 Wagner et al. published the results of 96 patients treated with an interstitial ^{192}Ir implant

Table 1 Summary of studies using interstitial brachytherapy boost in anal cancer

Author (year)	Period	No. of pts	EBRT dose (Gy)	CT	Interval between EBRT and boost (days)	Boost	BT technique/dose(Gy)	FU (months)	Outcomes (5 years)
Gerard et al. (1998) [53]	1982–1993	95	Papillion technique (30 Gy direct perineal field+18 Gy sacral field or 3-fields, 39 Gy)	5Fu+CDDP	Median, 56	BT, 85 pts	LDR median dose, 19.1 (range 14–28)	64	OS, 84 %; CSS, 90 %; CFS, 71 %
Weber et al. (2001) [32]	1981–1998	90	40	5Fu+MMC	Median, 37.5	EBRT, 41 pts; BT, 49 pts	LDR median dose, 18	76.2	OS, 76.7 %; LRC, 72.5 %
Hannoun-Levi et al. (2011) [54]	2000–2004	162	Median, 45.1	5Fu+CDDP	Median, 36	EBRT, 76 pts; BT, 86 pts	LDR median dose, 17.4 (range 10–25)	62	OS, 78 %; CRLR, 21 %; CFS (BT), 71 %; CFS (EBRT), 56 %
Oblak et al. (2012) [39]	2003–2010	84	45	5Fu+MMC	Mean, 27	EBRT, 33 pts; BT, 49 pts	PDR BED, 30–40	43	LRC, 71 %; OS, 67 %; CFS, 85 %; DFS, 68 %
Moureau Zabotto et al. (2013) [41]	2000–2005	99	Median, 45.1	5Fu+CDDP	Median, 31	EBRT, 49 pts; BT, 50 pts	LDR median does, 17.2 (range 10–25)	71.5	CRLR, 21 %; CRDR, 19 %; CFS, 63 %; OS, 74.4 %
Lestrade et al. (2014) [43]	1992–2009	209	Median, 45	CDDP+5Fu or 5Fu+MMC	Median, 32	BT, 209 pts	LDR or PDR median dose, 18 (range 10–31.7)	72.8	OS, 80.9 %; LC, 78.6 %; CSS, 85.7 %; CFS, 79.4 %

BT brachytherapy, *CDDP* cisplatin, *CT* chemotherapy, *CRLR* cumulative rate of local recurrence, *CFS* colostomy-free survival, *CSS* cancer-specific survival, *CRDR* cumulative rate of distant recurrence, (including nodal), *DFS* disease-free survival, *5Fu* 5-fluorouracil, *FU* follow-up, *LDR* low-dose rate, *LRC* locoregional control, *LC* local control, *MMC* mitomycin C, *OS* overall survival, *PDR* pulsed dose rate boost. A complete response was recorded 2 months after BT in 104/108 patients (96 %). Five-year overall survival (OS) and specific survival were 64 % ± 6 and 72 % ± 8, respectively. Sphincter preservation was achieved in 85 % of patients [52].

Gerard et al. reported a retrospective analysis of 95 patients treated with external beam radiotherapy (EBRT) followed by BT. During EBRT, all patients received one course of 5Fu and cisplatin. The OS at 5 and 8 years was 84 % and 77 %, respectively, and the cancer-specific survival was 90 % and 86 %, respectively. The colostomy-free survival (CFS) was 71 and 67 %, respectively, in the same time frame [53].

Weber and colleagues analyzed the impact of gap duration on locoregional control in 90 patients treated with 40 Gy EBRT + chemotherapy followed by 20 Gy BT (49 patients) or EBRT (41 patients) [32]. The median gap was 37.5 days. In both univariate and multivariate analyses, a prolonged gap (>37.5 days) was reported as an independent unfavorable prognostic factor for locoregional control (p, 0.02). Also age <65 years was a significant independent factor (p, 0.01). Based on multivariate analysis, the authors stratified the patients in four prognostic groups:

- Group 1 (favorable prognosis): older patients with a shorter gap (<37.5 days)
- Groups 2–3 (intermediate prognosis): older patients with a prolonged gap and younger patients with a short gap
- Group 4 (unfavorable): young patients and prolonged gap

In older patients, 5-year actuarial LRC was 92.3 % and 75.0 % for shorter and longer gaps, respectively. In younger patients, the corresponding values were 73.7 % and 50.0 %, respectively. Locoregional control (LRC) for all patients was 72.5 %.

Widder and coworkers retrospectively analyzed factors influencing local control and survival in patients treated with chemoradiation for anal cancer [31]. In this study, 18 % (23/129) of patients received a BT boost. Median overall treatment time (OTT) was 63 days for the EBRT boost cohort and 55 days for BT boost cohort. In stage T1–2 tumors, a shorter OTT favored local control (p, 0.015). For T3–T4, higher total radiation dose and female gender were associated with improved local control (p, 0.021). Five-year OS and LRC were 57 % and 87 %, respectively.

Oblak and colleagues published the results of 84 patients treated with 45 Gy EBRT with concurrent chemotherapy (5-fluorouracil and mitomycin C), followed by BT or EBRT boost [39]. At 6 and 18 weeks after treatment, complete response was recorded in 65.5 % and 79.8 %, respectively. At multivariate analysis, complete clinical response was identified as an independent prognostic factor for locoregional control (LRC), disease-free survival (DFS), and disease-specific survival (DSS). The 5-year LRC, DFS, DSS, OS, and CFS rates were 71 %, 68 %, 81 %, 67 %, and 85 %, respectively. Skin toxicity was the most frequent G3–G4 acute toxicity, occurring in 58.2 % of patients. The most frequent late G3–G4 toxicities were incontinence and anal stenosis, occurring in 18 % of patients. In the BT boost group, less late side effects were observed compared to the EBRT boost.

A multicenter retrospective French study (CORS-03) compared EBRT versus BT boost after 45 Gy EBRT [54]. In this study, 86 patients received 17.4 Gy (range 10–25 Gy) low-dose-rate BT boost and 76 patients received a mean dose of 18.3 Gy (range 8–25 Gy) EBRT boost, respectively. The mean OTT was 82 days (range, 45–143) for the EBRT group and 67 days (range, 37–128) for the BT group. Five-year cumulative rate of local recurrence (CRLR) was 21 %. At multivariate analysis, BT boost was the only prognostic factor associated with lower CRLR. In the subgroup of patients with OTT <80 days, 5-year CRLR was significantly reduced by delivery of a BT boost (BT 9 % versus EBRT 28 %) ($p=0.03$)). In a multivariate analysis of a subgroup of 99 patients with lymph node involvement, BT boost in N1 patients was the unique prognostic factor for CRLR (4 % for BT versus 31 % for EBRT; p, 0.042). Five-year CRLR and OS were 21.0 % and 74.4 %, respectively.

Recently, Lestrade and colleagues reported a retrospective analysis of 209 patients treated with 45 Gy EBRT + chemotherapy followed by 18 Gy BT boost (low dose rate or pulsed dose rate) [43]. Severe acute and late G3–G4 toxicity occurred in 11.2 % and 6.3 % of patients, respectively. The univariate analysis showed that pelvic treatment volume ($p = 0.046$) and total dose ($p = 0.02$) were associated with a risk of severe acute and late toxicities, respectively. Local control (LC) rates at 5 and 10 years were 78.6 % and 73.9 %, respectively. Overall, BT showed an acceptable toxicity profile and high local control rates.

2.8 Future Perspectives

The combination of RCT and BT allows higher doses to be delivered to the tumor. Improvements in local control and reductions in toxicity therefore become possible by integration of more advanced external beam delivery techniques (such as IMRT) with new BT techniques, such as high-dose-rate BT (HDR-BT) with the aim to reduce local failure and the risk of late radiation proctitis [55].

The evolution of the modern image-based 3D treatment planning for BT and the possibility of intensity modulation in brachytherapy (IMBT) may offer the most conformal treatment available to boost small volumes after radiochemotherapy for a higher possibility of success and better tolerance. The introduction of transrectal ultrasound (TRUS) and magnetic resonance imaging (MRI) make possible image-based implants, resulting in high precision therapy. The use of image-guided brachytherapy (IGBT) allows a better target volume definition and is recommended to guide the implantation procedure [56]. Imaging allows for control of the dose distribution and ensures that the whole of the tumor is covered by the reference isodose.

Prospective studies are needed to assess better the BT role and its clinical meaning in the multidisciplinary and tailored approach to this disease in the era of image guided radiotherapy (IGRT).

References

1. Ryan DP, Compton CC, Mayer RJ (2000) Carcinoma of the anal canal. N Engl J Med 342:792–800
2. Siegel R, Ma J, Zou Z, Jemal A (2014) Cancer statistics, 2014. CA Cancer J Clin 64:9–29
3. Jemal A, Simard EP, Dorell C et al (2013) Annual Report to the Nation on the Status of Cancer, 1975–2009, featuring the burden and trends in human papillomavirus (HPV)-associated cancers and HPV vaccination coverage levels. J Natl Cancer Inst 105: 175–201
4. Ries LAG, Harkins D, Krapcho M et al (2005) SEER cancer statistics review, 1975-2003. National Cancer Institute, Baltimore, pp 1–103
5. Edge SB, Byrd DR, Compton CC et al (2010) AJCC cancer staging manual, 7th edn. Springer, New York, pp 167–169
6. Sobin LH, Wittekind C (eds) (1997) TNM classification of malignant tumors. 5th ed. Wiley-Liss, New York, pp 91–95
7. Brown DK, Oglesby AB, Scott DH et al (1998) Squamous cell carcinoma of the anus: a twenty-five year retrospective. Am Surg 54(6):337–342
8. Greenall MJ, Quan SH, Urmacher C et al (1985) Treatment of epidermoid carcinoma of the anal canal. Surg Gynecol Obstet 161(6):509–517
9. Welton ML, Sharkey FE, Kahlenberg MS (2004) The etiology and epidemiology of anal cancer. Surg Oncol Clin N Am 13(2):263–275
10. Fenger C, Frisch M, Marti AC et al (2000) Tumours of the anal canal. In: Hamilton SR, Aaltonen LA (eds) Pathology and genetics of the digestive system. IARC Press, Lyon, pp 145–155
11. Cummings BJ, Ajani JA, Swallow CJ (2008) Cancer of the anal region. In: DeVita VT Jr, Lawrence TS, Rosenberg SA et al (eds) Cancer: principles & practice of oncology, 8th edn. Lippincott, Williams & Wilkins, Philadelphia
12. Frisch M, Glimelius B, van den Brule AJ et al (1997) Sexually transmitted infection as a cause of anal cancer. N Engl J Med 337:1350–1358
13. Hoots BE, Palefsky JM, Pimenta JM et al (2009) Human papillomavirus type distribution in anal cancer and anal intraepithelial lesions. Int J Cancer 124:2375–2383
14. Watson AJ, Smith BB, Whitehead MR et al (2006) Malignant progression of anal intra-epithelial neoplasia. ANZ J Surg 76:715–717
15. Nigro N, Vaitkevicius V, Considine S (1974) Combined therapy for cancer of the anal canal: a preliminary report. Dis Colon Rectum 17:354–356
16. Myerson RJ, Garofolo MC, Naqa IE et al (2009) Elective clinical target volumes for conformal therapy in anorectal cancer: an RTOG Consensus Panel Contouring Atlas. Int J Radiat Oncol Biol Phys 74(3):824–830
17. Ajani JA, Winter KA, Gunderson LL et al (2008) Fluorouracil, mitomycin, and radiotherapy vs

fluorouracil, cisplatin, and radiotherapy for carcinoma of the anal canal: a randomized trial. JAMA 299:1914–1921

18. Bartelink H, Roelofsen F, Eschwege F et al (1997) Concomitant radiotherapy and chemotherapy is superior to radiotherapy alone in the treatment of locally advanced anal cancer: results of a phase III randomized trial of the European Organization for Research and Treatment of Cancer radiotherapy and gastrointestinal cooperative groups. J Clin Oncol 15: 2040–2049

19. Bosset JF, Pavy JJ, Roelofsen F et al (1997) for the EORTC Radiotherapy Gastrointestinal Cooperative Groups: combined radiotherapy and chemotherapy for anal cancer. Lancet 349:205–206

20. Flam M, John M, Pajak TF et al (2006) The role of mitomycin-C in combination of 5-FU and radiotherapy, and of salvage chemoradiation therapy in the definitive nonsurgical treatment of epidermoid cancer of the anal canal. Results of a phase III randomized RTOG/ECOG intergroup study. J Clin Oncol 14:2527–2539

21. James RD, Glynne-Jones R, Meadows HM et al (2013) Mitomycin or cisplatin chemoradiation with or without maintenance chemotherapy for treatment of squamous-cell carcinoma of the anus (ACT II): a randomised, phase 3, open-label, 2x2 factorial trial. Lancet Oncol 14:516–524

22. Peiffert D, Tournier-Rangeard L, Gerard JP et al (2012) Induction chemotherapy and dose intensification of the radiation boost in locally advanced anal canal carcinoma: final analysis of the randomized UNICANCER ACCORD 03 trial. J Clin Oncol 30(16):1941–1948

23. UKCCCR Anal Cancer Trial Working Party (1996) Epidermoid anal cancer: results from the UKCCCR randomized trial of radiotherapy alone versus radiotherapy, 5-FU and mitomycin-C. Lancet 348:1049–1054

24. Lim F, Glynne-Jones R (2011) Chemotherapy/chemoradiation in anal cancer: a systematic review. Cancer Treat Rev 37:520–532

25. Spithoff K, Cummings B, Jonker D et al (2014) Gastrointestinal Cancer Disease Site Group Chemoradiotherapy for squamous cell cancer of the anal canal: a systematic review. Clin Oncol (R Coll Radiol) 26(8):473–487

26. Myerson RJ, Karnell LH, Menck HR et al (1997) The national cancer data base report on carcinoma of the anus. Cancer 80:805–815

27. National Comprehensive Cancer Network (2015) http://www.nccn.org/professionals/physician_gls/f_guidelines.asp#anal. Accessed 6 Jan 2015

28. Ferrigno R, Nakamura RA, Dos Santos Naovaes PE et al (2005) Radiochemotherapy in the conservative treatment of anal canal carcinoma: retrospective analysis of results and radiation dose effectiveness. Int J Rad Oncol Biol Phys 61:1136–1142

29. Huang K, Haas-Kogan D, Weinberg V et al (2007) Higher radiation dose with shorter treatment duration improves outcome for locally advanced carcinoma of anal canal. World J Gastroenterol 13:895–900

30. Ben-Josef E, Moughan J, Ajani JA et al (2010) Impact of overall treatment time on survival and local control in patients with anal cancer: a pooled data analysis of Radiation Therapy Oncology Group trials 87-04 and 98-11. J Clin Oncol 28:5061–5066

31. Widder J, Kastenberger R, Fercher E et al (2008) Radiation dose associated with local control in advanced anal cancer: retrospective analysis of 129 patients. Radiother Oncol 2008(87):367–375

32. Weber DC, Kurtz JM, Allal AS (2001) The impact of gap duration on local control in anal canal carcinoma treated by split course radiotherapy and concomitant chemotherapy. Int J Radiat Oncol Biol Phys 50(3):675–680

33. Meyer A, Meier zu Eissen J, Karstens JH (2006) Chemo-radiotherapy in patients with anal cancer: impact of length of unplanned treatment interruption on outcome. Acta Oncol 45:728–735

34. Salama JK, Mell LK, Schomas DA et al (2007) Concurrent chemotherapy and intensity-modulated radiation therapy for anal canal cancer patients: a multicentre experience. J Clin Oncol 25:4581–4586

35. Oehler-Janne C, Seifert B, Lutolf UM et al (2007) Clinical outcome after treatment with a brachytherapy boost versus external beam boost for anal carcinoma. Brachytherapy 6:218–222

36. Gerbaulet A, Pötter R, Mazeron JJ et al (2002) The GEC ESTRO handbook of brachytherapy (ISBN 90–804532–6). Bruxelles, pp 505–514. (The Authors and ESTRO)

37. Gérard JP, Chapet O, Samiei F et al (2001) Management of inguinal lymph node in patients with carcinoma of the anal canal. Experience in a series of 270 patients treated in Lyon and review of the literature. Cancer 92:77–84

38. Otmezguine Y, Grimard L, Calitchi E et al (1989) A new combined approach in the conservative treatment of rectal cancer. Int J Radiat Oncol Biol Phys 17:539–545

39. Oblak I, Petric P, Anderluh F et al (2012) Long term outcome after combined modality treatment for anal cancer. Radiol Oncol 46(2):145–152

40. Glynne-Jones R, Sebag-Montefiore D, Adams R et al (2011) "Mind the gap" the impact of variations in the duration of the treatment gap and overall treatment time in the first UK Anal Cancer Trial (ACT 1). Int J Radiat Oncol Biol Phys 81:1488–1494

41. Moreau-Zabotto L, Ortholan C, Hannoun-Levi JM et al (2013) Role of brachytherapy in the boost management of anal carcinoma with node involvement (CORS-03 study). Int J Radiat Oncol Biol Phys 85(3):135–142

42. Peiffert D, Bey P, Pernot M et al (1997) Conservative treatment by irradiation of epidermoid cancers of the anal canal: prognostic factors of tumoral control and complications. Int J Radiat Oncol Biol Phys 37:313–324

43. Lestrade L, De Bari B, Pommier P et al (2014) Role of brachytherapy in the treatment of cancers of the anal canal. Long-term follow-up and multivariate analysis of a large monocentric retrospective series. Strahlenther Onkol 190:546–554

44. Glynne-Jones R, Nilsson PJ, Aschele C et al (2014) ESMO; ESSO; ESTRO. Anal cancer: ESMO-ESSO-ESTRO clinical practice guidelines for diagnosis, treatment and follow-up. Radiother Oncol 111(3): 330–339

45. Doniec JM, Schniewind B, Kovács G et al (2006) Multimodal therapy of anal cancer added by new endosonographic-guided brachytherapy. Surg Endosc 20(4):673–678

46. Löhnert M, Doniec JM, Kovács G et al (1998) New method of radiotherapy for anal cancer with three-dimensional tumor reconstruction based on endoanal ultrasound and ultrasound-guided afterloading therapy. Dis Colon Rectum 41(2):169–176

47. Christensen AF, Nielsen BM, Engelholm SA (2008) Three-dimensional endoluminal ultrasound-guided interstitial brachytherapy in patients with anal cancer. Acta Radiol 49(2):132–137

48. Falk AT, Claren A, Benezery K et al (2014) Interstitial high-dose rate brachytherapy as boost for anal canal cancer. Radiat Oncol 9:240

49. Kapoor R, Khosla D, Shukla AK et al (2014) Dosimetric and clinical outcome in image-based high-dose-rate interstitial brachytherapy for anal cancer. Brachytherapy 13(4):388–393

50. Major T, Polgár C, Somogyi A et al (2000) Evaluation of the dose uniformity for double-plane high dose rate interstitial breast implants with the use of dose reference points and dose non-uniformity ratio. Radiother Oncol 54(3):213–220

51. Major T, Polgár C, Fodor J et al (2002) Conformality and homogeneity of dose distributions in interstitial implants at idealized target volumes: a comparison between the Paris and dose-point optimized systems. Radiother Oncol 62(1):103–111

52. Wagner JP, Mahe MA, Romestaing P et al (1994) Radiation therapy in the conservative treatment of carcinoma of the anal canal. Int J Radiat Oncol Biol Phys 29(1):17–23

53. Gerard JP, Ayza L, Hun D et al (1998) Treatment of anal canal carcinoma with high dose radiation therapy and concomitant fluorouracil-cisplatinum. Long-term results in 95 patients. Radiother Oncol 46:249–256

54. Hannoun-Levi JM, Ortholan C, Resbeut M et al (2011) High-dose split-course radiation therapy for anal cancer: outcome analysis regarding the boost strategy (CORS-03 study). Int J Radiat Oncol Biol Phys 80:712–720

55. Saarilahti K, Arponen P, Vaalavirta L et al (2008) The effect of intensity-modulated radiotherapy and high dose rate brachytherapy on acute and late radiotherapy-related adverse events following chemoradiotherapy of anal cancer. Radiother Oncol 87:383–390

56. Niehoff P, Kovács G (2014) HDR brachytherapy for anal cancer. J Gastrointest Oncol 5(3):218–222

Brachytherapy of the Skin: Cancers and Other Diseases

James Fontanesi, Brian Kopitzki, and Eric Van Limbergen

Abstract

Skin…We tan it, we burn it, we pierce it, we ink it, and we moisturize it. When it is wet, we try to dry it, we shave it, and we inject it, and all these things are done in an effort to enhance the appearance of it. Brachytherapy has been used in the management of skin cancer since the first days of therapeutic intervention shortly after the discovery of radium. We present this chapter as a complete reference not only in the standard of care, but to highlight novel applications of the science.

1 Introduction

Skin is the largest organ of the body, and for most individuals, it encompasses approximately 20 square feet of protective surface which we often take for granted. Our skin protects us from various infections and from the elements by helping to maintain and regulate body temperature. It permits tactile sensation and most importantly has a great capacity for healing. However, there are situations in which the damage that occurs to the skin results in conditions which require medical attention. In some of these conditions, the utilization of radiation has been very effective in helping to alleviate and control both malignant and benign problems.

In this chapter we will discuss the use of brachytherapy in the treatment of various skin conditions. We will discuss when to consider brachytherapy, review published guidelines and clinical results, and discuss various technical aspects that make brachytherapy for skin applications so unique.

2 Anatomy

The skin is comprised of three individual layers (Fig. 1); they are the following:

1. The *epidermis*, which is the outermost layer. It provides a waterproof barrier and is

J. Fontanesi, MD (✉)
Radiation Oncology, Botsford Cancer Center,
Oakland University/William Beaumont School of
Medicine, Farmington Hills, MI, USA
e-mail: jfontanesi@comcast.net

B. Kopitzki, DO
Department of Dermatology, Michigan State College
of Osteopathic Medicine, East Lansing, MI, USA

E. Van Limbergen, MD, PhD
Department of Radiotherapy, University of
Gasthuisberg, Leuven, Belgium

© Springer International Publishing Switzerland 2016
P. Montemaggi et al. (eds.), *Brachytherapy: An International Perspective*, Medical Radiology,
DOI 10.1007/978-3-319-26791-3_22

365

Fig. 1 Skin anatomy

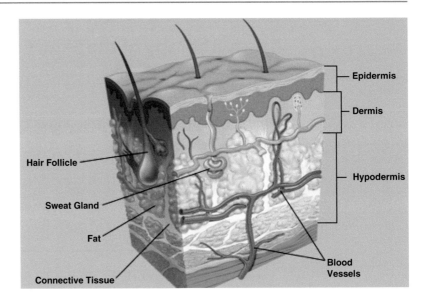

responsible for creating our skin tone. The epidermis is probably the single most abused organ in the human body on a day-to-day basis.

2. The *dermis*, which lies below the epidermis. It contains connective tissue, hair follicles, and sweat glands.

3. The subcutaneous tissue, also known as the *hypodermis*, is made up of fat and connective tissues. It also helps structurally facilitate vascular supply.

The skin's color is created by special cells called *melanocytes* which are located in basal layer of the epidermis. These are critically important as they help protect us from sun damage by the production of melanin which is able to absorb ultraviolet rays. It is known that prolonged exposures to the sun will increase the melanocytic production and in many cases help with the darkening of the skin as a protective mechanism. The skin is essential in the activation of vitamin D which is critical to the integrity of the osseous system. It is also known that the skin is not uniform in its thickness. The thinnest areas of the skin in the body are located around the eyelids, while the thickest resides on the palms and the soles of the feet [1].

2.1 Skin Layer Activities

2.1.1 Epidermis

As noted, the epidermis is the outermost layer of the skin. It is responsible for fluid management and prevention of pathogen introduction and plays a major role in body temperature regulation. It is composed of stratified squamous epithelium, and keratinocytes make up the majority of cells in this layer compromising 95 % of the epidermis, while other selected cells such as the Merkel cells, melanocytes, and Langerhans cells are also present. Beginning with the outermost portion of the epidermis, there are five layers:

Stratum corneum
Stratum lucidum (which is located only in the palms and soles)
Stratum granulosum
Stratum spinosum
Stratum germinativum (which is also known as the stratum basale)

The keratinocytes in the stratum germinativum layer proliferate through mitosis, and these daughter cells move up the various strata toward the surface of the skin changing their shape and composition as they undergo multiple stages of cell differentiation until they eventually become anucleated. As this process occurs, these cells produce keratin proteins and lipids which help in the formation of an extracellular matrix that provides mechanical strength to the skin. Once the cells reach the outer layer, they are eventually shed from the surface in a process which is known as desquamation. The transitional zone between the epidermis and the dermis is defined by a thin sheet of fibers which is known as the "basement membrane." This basement membrane controls the migration of the cells and molecules between these two layers and also contains a variety of cytokines and growth factors which are used as a reserve for controlled release during physiological remodeling or repair [2].

2.1.2 Dermis

This is the second layer of skin that consists of connective tissues and helps provide tensile strength and elasticity through an extracellular matrix composed of collagen microfibrils and elastic fibers embedded in proteoglycans. This layer has also many of the nerve endings that help to provide tactile, thermal, and pain sensation. It also contains hair follicles, sweat glands, sebaceous glands, apocrine glands, and lymphatic and vascular structures. The vascular structures in this layer are important as they help with providing nutrients and also in waste removal from the epidermis. The dermis is often considered to be divided into two regions, and the region closer to the epidermis is known as the "papillary region." The deeper area, which is thicker, is known as the "reticular region."

The papillary region is composed of connective tissue and provides the dermis with the ability to interact with the epidermis strengthening the connection between these two layers of skin.

The reticular region is composed mostly of dense irregular connective tissues with a dense concentration of collagenous elastic and reticular fibers. It is these fibers that give the dermis strength, extensibility, and elasticity. Within this region are blood vessels, sweat and sebaceous glands, and the roots of hair and nails [3].

2.1.3 Hypodermis

The purpose of the hypodermis is to attach the skin to the underlying bone, muscle, and connective tissues as well as maintaining the supply of blood vessels and nerves. It consists of connective tissue and elastin with the main cell types being fibroblasts, macrophages, and adipocytes. It should be noted that the hypodermis contains 50 % of the body fat. This fat serves as padding and insulation for the body [4].

Despite the importance that the skin plays in our overall health, insults occur not only on a natural basis but also deliberately and sometimes on a daily basis. These insults often result in conditions which require intervention for both malignant and benign processes.

In this chapter we will discuss these various conditions and how brachytherapy has been utilized in their management and treatment. We will cover squamous cell carcinoma, basal cell carcinoma, and melanoma as the main oncologic foci. In addition, we will discuss benign processes such as keloid/heterotopic scar formation, hidradenitis suppurativa, and other benign conditions which have been treated with brachytherapy techniques.

---

3 Skin Cancer

A recent review of 75 studies conducted over the past half century looked at geographic variations in trends worldwide in non-melanomic skin cancers, and not surprisingly, the highest rates occurred in areas in which there was prevalent sun exposure [5]. Skin cancers now represent the number one cancer diagnosis, not only in the United States, but worldwide. As the medium age of the population increases and with ever increasing exposure to various environmental factors that allow for the development of these cancers, the numbers of new skin cancers will continue to grow in the future [6].

While there are traditionally identified causative effects related to the development of various malignancies of the skin that do not need to be rediscussed in this chapter, there are other less reported causative events which do need to be noted as often skin cancers related to these factors have a perceived more virulent course. These factors include previous exposure to ionizing radiation [7, 8], patients who are immunocompromised secondary to infectious diseases Ebstein Barr Virus (EBV) or related to immunosuppression in transplant patients [9–11], patients who develop malignancy in scar tissue or chronic inflamed tissue [12], and patients with a known genetic predisposition such as those with xeroderma pigmentosum or those with nevoid basal cell carcinoma (Gorlin syndrome) [13].

The two most diagnosed skin cancers are basal cell carcinoma, which compromises approximately 65 % of all skin malignancy, and squamous cell carcinoma, which accounts for approximately 30 % [5].

Basal cell carcinomas are lesions that arise from the basal cells of the skin and appear with various presentations. Clinically, five different subtypes are discerned: superficial spreading, nodular, morphea-like, pigmented, and ulcus rodens that invades and destroys the local anatomy. If left alone, they can grow to large sizes and become quite disfiguring. However, they rarely metastasize beyond the original site [14]. It is estimated that there are over 2.8 million cases of basal cell carcinoma diagnosed in the United States each year (Fig. 2). Often patients have multiple sites of involvement at diagnosis.

Squamous cell carcinomas, as the name implies, involve abnormal growth of squamous cells which compromise most of the epidermis. They too can present in different ways in terms of their appearance (superficial spreading, exophytic, and ulcerating). While not as prevalent as basal cell carcinomas, it is estimated that over 700,000 squamous carcinomas are diagnosed in the United States annually [15].

What differentiates squamous cell carcinoma clinically from basal cell carcinoma is its higher propensity for the development of lymph node and, eventually, distant metastasis. It is estimated that 2500 individuals yearly will die of squamous cell carcinoma of the skin. Another differentiating factor is that squamous cell carcinomas not only appear in areas exposed to the sun but also can occur in all areas of the body that have squamous cells including the mucus membranes, head and neck, and genital regions (Figs. 3 and 4).

There are certain precancerous growths that can be associated with a development of squamous cell carcinomas. These include actinic keratosis, in which up to 10 %, if left untreated, will advance to squamous cell carcinomas [16] (Fig. 5).

Actinic cheilitis, which most often occurs in the lower lip resulting in a dry, cracked, scaly appearance, is also associated with the development of squamous cell carcinomas [17] (Fig. 6).

Bowen's disease is an entity which is generally considered to be a noninvasive form of

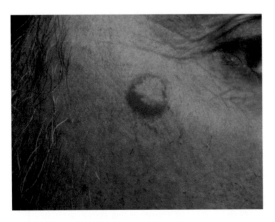

Fig. 2 Solitary lesion/basal cell carcinoma

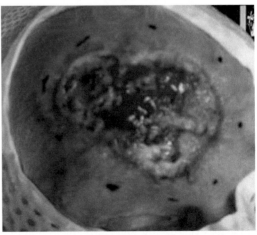

Fig. 3 Supraorbital squamous cell cancer. Figure 3: Squamous cell cancer of the supraorbital scalp

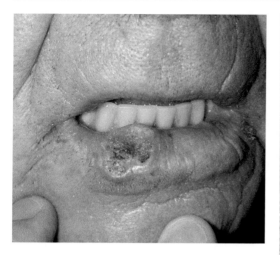

Fig. 4 Squamous cell cancer of mucosal lip

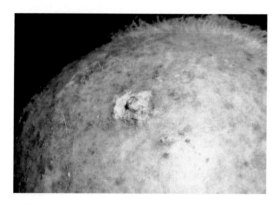

Fig. 5 Actinic keratosis of the scalp

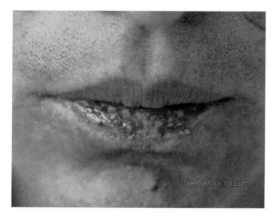

Fig. 6 Actinic cheilitis

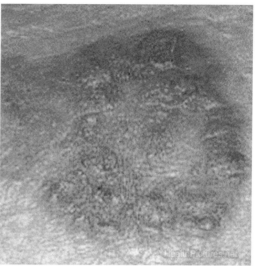

Fig. 7 Bowen's disease

reported that there is even a form of Bowen's disease associated with the human papillomavirus (HPV) [18] (Fig. 7).

While the mainstay of treatment for these lesions remains surgical intervention, there are often cases in which other therapies, including the use of radiotherapy, are required. Radiation therapy is required if the margins are positive after surgical intervention, in patients that are not considered surgical candidates, or in patients who have developed lesions in areas that would result in functional and/or cosmetically displeasing deformities. The latter are usually noted in areas around the eyelid, the nasal labial fold, and the ear. It is these cases in which the use of radiotherapy has been shown to be an effective treatment. We will confine the majority of our comments in this chapter to the basal cell and squamous cell carcinomas.

4   Radiation Therapy Overview

When a patient is referred for radiation therapy for basal or squamous cell carcinoma of the skin, external beam irradiation is most often utilized. It has a strong historical record of long-term local control. Oftentimes because of the ease of application, patients receive only external beam

squamous cell carcinoma, most often presenting as a reddish-brown scaly area that oftentimes is confused for psoriasis or eczema. It has also been irradiation either for unresected lesions or for lesions that have had positive margins.

In recent publications, the clinical/pathological finding of perineural involvement (PNI) has been shown to have a significant influence on local control and potential for metastasis, particularly in squamous cell carcinoma [19, 20]. Thus, this finding must be taken into account especially in sites with adjacent lymphatic drainage, in which case external beam techniques may provide improved dose coverage. Various dose fractionation schemes have been utilized, and the long-term success rates have been quite high. Results of various external beam series for basal cell carcinoma (BCC) and squamous cell carcinoma (SCC) are noted in Table 1.

There is, however, also a rich tradition for the use of brachytherapy for various skin malignancies. Whether using interstitial techniques or surface mold techniques or more recently with the introduction of electronic brachytherapy, the success rates of brachytherapy have been equivalent with those associated with external beam irradiation (Table 2).

The choice of external beam radiotherapy versus brachytherapy often is based on patient presentation, overall condition, and comfort with the treating radiation oncologist's ability to deliver either modality. Oftentimes brachytherapy becomes a more suitable option because of the ability to modulate the dose through the brachytherapy field to various depths because of lesional size, especially in non-resected lesions.

Besides the more traditional diagnosis in which radiation and specifically brachytherapy are used, there are various skin conditions, both malignant and benign, in which brachytherapy applications have been utilized. Malignant melanoma, Merkel cell carcinoma, Kaposi's sarcoma, and cutaneous non-Hodgkin's lymphoma malignancies, although traditionally treated with external beam techniques, have also enjoyed successful "local" results when brachytherapy has been used. The results of several selected reports are listed in Table 3.

The technical aspects of delivery for the "orphan" tumors are similar to that utilized in other skin sites. However, one exception should be noted. At William Beaumont Hospital, a small series of cutaneous NHL patients with extensive scalp involvement were referred for treatment. Because of the extensive skin involvement and curvature of the skull, it was elected to treat with a "bonnet" that was constructed of Aquaplast® with HDR catheters imbedded into it (Figs. 8). It was designed to allow for margins similar that what are used in the traditional external beam literature, but with the advantage of avoiding unnecessary brain irradiation. We treated using a BID schedule of 325–350 cGy/fraction for eight fractions over four treatment days while others have utilized 4 Gy BID × 8 fractions. Our intent was to ensure that not more than 50 % of the treatment volume received greater than 125 % of the prescribed dose. All patients developed alopecia, mostly resolved during follow-up, with no local recurrence at a median of 4 years.

4.1 Target Volume

The clinical target volume we recommend for well-delineated squamous cell or basal cell carcinomas is the palpable visible tumor with a margin of 0.3–0.5 cm for skin cancers and 0.5–0.7 cm for lip cancers. For ill-defined lesions, such as morphea-like basal cell carcinomas, a wider margin is taken (0.7–1.0 cm).

4.2 Commonly Used Techniques

Several techniques are available, and all of them can be carried out under local anesthesia (hypodermic needles, silk wires, and inner nylon tubes) or without anesthesia (mats and molds, Leipzig, Valencia, or electronic brachytherapy). Target depths up to 0.3 cm, less than 3.0 cm diameter, and flat in shape are good candidates for Leipzig or Valencia applicators or electronic brachytherapy. Targets up to 0.5 cm depth, >3.0 cm diameter, and/or with a curved shape can be treated with plastic afterloading catheters spaced 1.0–1.5 cm apart in a mask, mat, or mold. Thicker targets and locations in the lip, inner canthus, or eyelid require an interstitial 5-French plastic afterloading tube implant, usually under general anesthesia.

Table 1 External beam irradiation for BCC/SCC

Author	Year	N	Site	Dose	F/U months	LC	Complications Gr III/IV	Others	Ref
Silva	2000	334	Pinna	35–60 Gy	3.3	79.2 5 years	7.3 % at 5 years Risk with lesion size, fraction size	Failure with low BED, lesion ≥2 cm	[19]
Petrovich	1987	646	Face	30–51 Gy[a]	N/A	≤2 cm 99/98 5/10 years 2–5 cm 92/79 5/10 years >5 cm 60/ 5/8 years	N/A	N/A	[20]
Wilder	1991	115	All	20–73 Gy	40 months	St I–II 95 %/5 years St III/IV 50 %/5 years	3 case STN	Median time to recur 20 months	[21]
Fitzpatrick	1984	498	HN	20–60 Gy in 1–30 Fx[b]	Minimum 36 months	94.7 % 3 years	4.4 % STN 9.6 %	8 % LN Mets 2.6 % ↓ Tumor	[22]
Lin	2012	222	All with path PNI	BCC 55 Gy/20 Fx SCC 55 Gy/25 Fx[c]	62 months BCC 42 months SCC	78 % 5 years SCC 91 % 5 years BCC	N/A	PNI histologically	[23]
Abbatucci	1989	675	Face	3060R/3 Fx	24	96 %	3 %	17 cataracts 20 keratitis 10 enucleations 1 glaucoma 1 vitreous bleed	[24]
Schlienger	1996	850	Eyelid	44–55 Gy	60	97.5	5.7 %		[25]
Locke	2001	531	All	Various based on histology/ site	72	93 for 1° 80 for recur	5.8 %		[26]

[a]For large tumors/cartilage involvement 70 Gy/2 Gy Fx
[b]Most common dose schedule 2000–2250/1 Fx, 3500–4000/5 Fx
[c]Median dose/number fractions
BED Biological equivalent dose

Table 2 Brachytherapy results for BCC/SCC

Author	Year	N	Site	Type Tx	Dose	F/U	LC	Complication	Ref
Guix	2000	136	Face	HRD	60–80 Gy/180cGy/Fx at 0.5 cm	60	99 % for 1° 87 % for recur	0 %	[27]
Crook	1990	468	Nasal	LDR	60 Gy at 85 % IDL	60	97.5 %	2 %	[28]
Mazeron	1989	762[a]	All	IR-192 Ro1-226 Gs-137 Sr-90	NA	24	95 % for 1° 94 % for recur	2 %	[29]
Gauden	2013	236	All	HDR	36 Gy/3 Fx at 0.3–0.4 cm	66	98 %	71 % Gr I 34 % Gr II	[30]
Bhatnagor	2013	171	All	e HDR	40 Gy	10 months	100 %	9.2 % Gr I–II	[31]
Krengli	2014	60	Eyelid	LDR (R-192)	51–70 Gy (mean 65 Gy)	36 months	96.7 %	3 % Gr III	[32]
Rio	2005	97	All[b]		50–65 Gy (55 Gy) 50–60 Gy (52 Gy)	60	91 % 80 %	100 % Desquamation healed by 10 weeks	[33]
Ducassou	2011	132[c]	Facial	LDR	Group A 60–70 Gy Med = Gy Group B 60–65 Gy Mean = 60[d]	72	87 % 0.5 years	28.6 % Gr I 7.5 % Gr III with dose rate >98C GY/h	[34]

IDL isodose line, e electronic

[a]762/1676 treated with brachytherapy

[b]Group 1, no surgery; Group 2, surgery → brachytherapy

[c]Group A, primary treatment; Group B, recurrent treatment

[d]Group A, dose rate 65.2–144 cGy/HR; MED=99.4; Group B, dose rate 74–115 cGy/HR;MED=92.5

Table 3 Other malignant skin conditions treated with brachytherapy

Name	Year	# pts	Tumor type	Dose	Local control	F/U	Complications	Other information	Ref
Hobbs	2011	1	MM	30 Gy EBI + 18 Gy/3Fx	N	N/A	N/A	Initial "good" response in field but eventually fails	[36]
Scepanovic	2013	1	MM	10×4 Gy at 3 mm×2/weeks	Y	N/A	N/A	Developed systemic disease	[37]
Shi	2014	24	MM	Perm I-125	55 % at 2 years	19.6	–	Estimated 2 years LC 83 %	[38]
Chaudhuri	2011	6	MM	1R-192 HDR 30–36 Gy/5-6 Fx	100 %	23	1/6 Gr IV skin	↓ 2/6 from distant disease	[39]
Smithers	2011	3	MM	32 Gy/8 Fx 42 Gy/7 Fx	100 %	21		Fibrosis/telangiectasis	[40]
Garibvan	2013	10 pts/152 lesions	MCC	10–12 Gy 12 Fx at depth 5–10 MM	99 %	34	Gr II 20 %	4/10 ↓ distant disease	[41]
Kasper	2013	16	KS	24 Gy/4 FX 35 Gy/6 Fx	100 %	41	13/16 Gr I 2/16 Gr II	All lesion < 2 cm Tx volume = Lesion + 4 mm Leipzig	[42]
Desimone	2013	10 pts 23 Lesion	NHL	8 Gy/2 Fx at 3 mm	100 %	6.3	N/A	N/A	[43]

Legend *MM* malignant melanoma, *KS* Kaposi sarcoma, *MCC* Merkel cell carcinoma, *NHL* non-Hodgkin's lymphoma

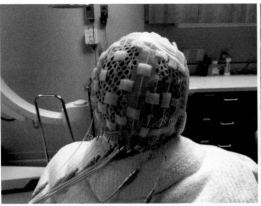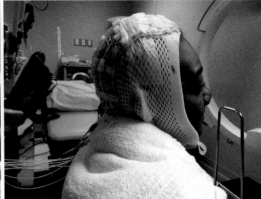

Figs. 8 The "bonnet" technique

Most skin cancers can be treated by a single-plane implant, using parallel catheters, spaced 1.0–1.5 cm from each other. The treated thickness of such implants varies. Consequently the source carriers must be implanted 0.2–0.5 cm beneath the skin surface. Implants which are more superficial may result in late visible telangiectasia along the source positions.

For curved planes, which frequently occur in skin cancers of the face, the reference isodose projects further at the concave than the convex surface. The arrangement of implanted catheters in those cases must take into account this shift in the isodose lines. Thicker lesions may have to be treated by double-plane implants. However, sometimes it is easier to shave the exophytic part of the tumor with electrocoagulation.

4.3 Afterloading Technique

4.3.1 Classic Plastic Tubes "Henschke"
Classic plastic tube implants (0.16–0.19 cm external diameter) can be used for large lesions of the periorbital area, the cheek, and the shoulder region. Because of the large volume that has to be anesthetized, general anesthesia is usually required (Figs. 9 and 10).

There are cases that are clinically challenging, and our initial instinct may be that there is little we can do; however, each case should be individualized and considered. Even the most untoward appearing tumor may sometimes be managed by brachytherapy (Figs. 11, 12, and 13).

5 Dosimetry

Source reconstruction is done using 3-D images as is target delineation GTV and CTV. For skin tumors, usually no PTV margin is added, unless there is an uncertainty of mold, mat, or mask positioning. In the case of interstitial implants, mean central dose (MCD) is determined. The prescribed dose to the minimal target dose usually corresponds to 85 % of MCD (Paris System). With parallel interstitial lines, application of geometrical optimization is advised to reduce the indentation of the prescription isodose. The prescription dose after geometrical optimization is possible on the 90 % of the mean central dose. In an ideal implanted target, this 90 % isodose should cover the target completely. In cases where the CTV is not covered, increasing dwell times and/or prescribing at a lower isodose line can help to improve the dose distribution. However, as recommended by ICRU Report 51, the prescription (minimal target dose as well as the % to MCD) value should always be recorded and reported.

For surface applicators and molds, the dose is prescribed at the appropriate depth: at 0.8 cm for Leipzig, Valencia, or electronic BT, at 0.3–0.5 cm

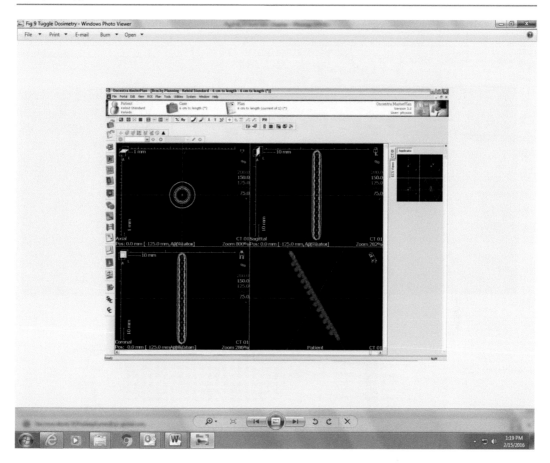

Fig. 9 Five-French plastic tube implant for interstitial HDR BT of a basal cell carcinoma of the right lower eyelid. Eight fractions of 4 Gy were delivered in 4 days

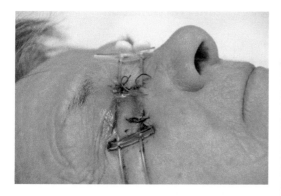

Fig. 10 Five-French plastic tube interstitial implant, spaced 1.8 cm for a Merkel cell tumor of the right lower eyelid with a wide (5 cm) safety margin toward the lymphatics of the cheek. Eight fractions of 4 Gy were given in 4 days

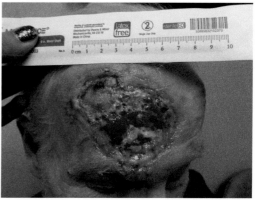

Fig. 11 Large basal cell cancer 4 weeks post Mohs surgery

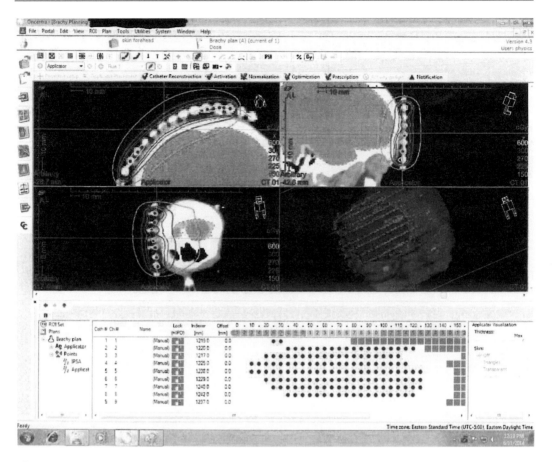

Fig. 12 Scalp brachytherapy plan

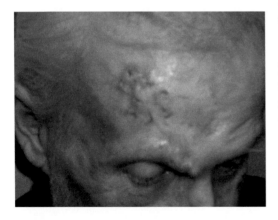

Fig. 13 The same patient 1 year post brachytherapy alone

for molds, mats, or masks. The surface epidermal dose constraint is approximately 10 Gy if five fractions of 7 Gy are given [35].

6 Dose, Dose Rate, and Fractionation

For LDR BT, the GEC-ESTRO prescribed dose is 60 Gy at the 85 % reference isodose, at dose rates between 30 and 90 cGy/h [44]. Usually a dose rate of 45–70 cGy/h is desired. Therefore, the linear activity of iridium sources should be in the range of 5.5–7.7 cGy/h linear air kerma rate at 1 m. Depending on the linear activity and the source spacing and length, it will take 4–6 days to deliver the required dose. Although doses up to 70 Gy can be given in some large tumors, the increase in cosmetic damage is greater than the gain in local control expected from a dose increase above 60 Gy [45].

Other total dose, dose rate, and fractionation schemes have been reported in the literature. Again much depends on whether low dose rate or high dose rate is utilized. For those not using the Paris System, either the Manchester System (uneven source loading for a more homogeneous dose which is equivalent to geometrical optimization in a stepping source PDR or HDR application) or the Patterson-Parker System (even source loading/dose inhomogeneity) is used.

Many centers prescribe the total dose and dose rate to the treatment volume. This usually will be the tumor volume plus a margin. Recommendations for hourly low dose rates generally run 35–60 cGy/h which corresponds to 840–1440 cGy/day. Total dose recommendations will be based on individual patient needs but will usually be 50–60 Gy.

For cases in which HDR BT is utilized, a great deal will depend on size and location. There have been some reports of single fraction treatment using between 700 and 1000 cGy for lesions less than 1 cm that have been resected but harbor positive margins. For more traditional use, either once daily or BID treatments can be utilized. Again treatment prescriptions can be via the Paris System or prescribed to the tumor volume edge plus a margin. For single fractions/day, doses between 5 and 12 Gy per fraction to total doses of 36–60 Gy have been reported with good success (Table 2).

For BID schedules, we recommend 300–400 cGy/fraction to similar total doses as utilized in the single fraction per day recommendation. One important aspect of our treatment policy is to try and minimize dose inhomogeneity across the tumor volume. This is often more realistic to accomplish with HDR brachytherapy due to source optimization. When uniform dose across the tumor volume plus margin cannot be achieved, we try to limit the 150 % isodose volume to less than 25 % of the treatment volume.

Whatever prescription is used in interstitial BT, one should always record the prescription isodose as well as its relation to the MCD. For surface applications, always record and report the depth and resulting prescription isodose (MTD) as well as the maximum surface dose at the epidermal surface.

7 Melanoma of the Eyelid

At one of the author institutions (Van Limbergen), we have treated four eyelids in three patients with excision and postoperative BT using eight fractions of 4 Gy HDR interstitial BT (32 Gy total) using two parallel plastic tubes. With a follow-up interval of 2.5 years, no patient has developed a recurrence.

8 Nonmalignant Skin Applications

8.1 Keloid

The earliest known description of keloids was by Egyptian surgeons around 1700 BC [46]. However, it was not until 1806 that Baron Jean-Louis Alibert identified them as a specific entity [47].

Keloids are histologically characterized by an abundance of an extracellular matrix of connective tissue. The formation of this type of scar is usually composed of a reduced amount of type 3 (early) and an increased amount of type 1 (late) collagen. It has been suggested that

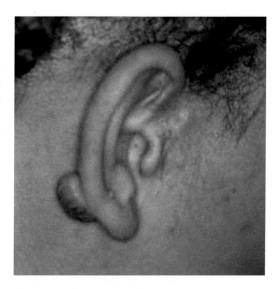

Fig. 14 Traditional keloid of the pinna

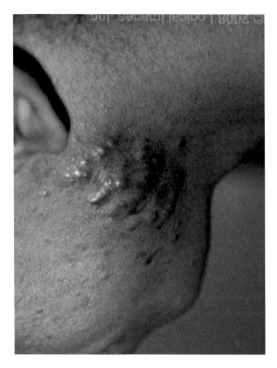

Fig. 15 Hypertrophic scar

there are two possible mechanisms for the deposition of collagen in keloid lesions. The traditional theory is that the keloid results from the localized loss of control of extracellular matrix production of fibroblasts. A second suggested mechanism is that the reduced degradation of newly synthesized procollagen polypeptides may contribute to collagen depositions in keloids [48].

Recently an analysis of 8393 differentially expressed genes in keloids and in normal skin has been reported [49]. In this study, 402 genes (4.79 %) had different expression levels between the keloid and normal skin. Two hundred and fifty of these genes, including the transforming growth factor (TGF)-beta 1 and the NGF (nerve growth factor) gene, were upregulated (2.98 %), and 152 were downregulated (1.81 %). It was noted that there was a higher expression of TGF-Beta 1 and NGF in keloids when compared with normal skin. This was also identified using reverse transcription polymerase chain reaction analysis. Possible genetic mutations of chromosomes 2q23 and 7p11 have been suggested [52]. It is also postulated that in the posttraumatic and chronic inflammatory phases of wound develop-

ment, these mediators may play an important role in the keloid microenvironment and are crucial for keloid fibroblast abnormalities to develop. This has led to suspicion that the upregulation of the pro-inflammatory gene expression in keloid lesions maybe responsible for development [50].

Keloid scars should not be confused with hypertrophic scars which are raised and do not grow beyond the boundaries of the original wound, unlike those of keloids which may progress in a clawlike growth pattern into the normal skin region (Figs. 14 and 15). Keloids also have the capacity to cause symptoms, the most common of which are pain and itching. Complications associated with itching include infection and ulceration of the keloid and surrounding tissues.

Although they usually occur at the site of some injury, keloids can also arise spontaneously. While they are often associated with trauma, interestingly enough, they can be quite different in the same individual. A patient that is prone to developing keloid scars does not necessarily develop keloid with every insult to the skin.

Keloids are a "quiet" skin tissue which is more prevalent than most realize. There is a suggestion of racial disparity with people of Chinese and African background potentially at increased risk of development [51]. It has been reported that overall between 5 and 15 % of all wounds will develop a keloid.

Various treatments have been utilized in the management of keloids. Most commonly surgical intervention is utilized and often is combined with injections of corticosteroids, laser treatment, retinoic acid, silicone gel, and other local therapies in an effort to prevent recurrences of keloid formation.

In general the use of non-radiation-based postoperative therapies has resulted in local control rates of 40–90 % (Table 4).

The use of postoperative radiation therapy, whether using external beam techniques or brachytherapy, has enjoyed a long history of excellent long-term local control. Various articles including meta-analyses have described various doses utilized. However, what seems to be the most important is the initiation of therapy within 24 h of surgical resection. The results of various external beam series are presented in Table 5.

Header: Brachytherapy of the Skin: Cancers and Other Diseases — 379

Table 4 Nonradiation treatment of keloids

Author	Year	Number	Treatment	Results	F/U	Others	Ref
Wang	2014	186	Surgery (22) Steroid injection (34) Surgery and steroid (130)	55 % 56 % 97 %	12 months		[53]
Wu	2009	166	Surgery and 5 FU/steroids	47 % "cured" 53 % "effective"	9 months	Normal auricular shape 93 %	[54]
Davison	2009	102	5 FU/steroid 5 FU/steroid/excision Steroid/excision	81 % lesion reduction 92 % lesion reduction 73 % lesion reduction			[55]
Jin	2013 (Meta-analysis)	919	Laser	71 % for scar prevention 65 % for heterotrophic or 72 % for keloid		585/595-nm pulsed dye laser and 532 nm with best response	[56]
Litrowski	2013	97	Surgery → cryotherapy	71 % major flattening	43	Partial ear amputation three cases hypopigmentation	[57]
Obrien	2013	873	Silicone gel			Meta-analysis	[58]
Mamalis	2013					Meta-analysis	[59]
Soray	2005	15	Bleomycin injection	73 % flattened			[60]
Janssen	1980	28	Retinoic acid	77 % "favorable"		2–6 sessions improved pain and pruritis scores	[61]
Park	2011	1436	Surgery → pressure	89.4 %	18		[62]

Table 5 External beam irradiation results for resected keloids

Author	Year	#	Dose	Local control	F/U	Others	Ref
Ogawa	2007	109	10 Gy surgery → 15 Gy 20 Gy	71 % prior 2002 86 % after 2002	18 months	Electrons	[63]
Wang	2014	139	Surgery 5 Gy × 4 4 Gy × 5 surgery → alone	91 % 67 %		Difference noted chest wall/shoulder/ back vs face (0.009)	[64]
Kol	2005	Meta-analysis	Surgery → post-op X RT	90 % if BED 30 Gy		Meta-analysis	[65]
Ogawa	2013	174 (earlobe)	XRT-5 Gy Surgery + 10 Gy	96 %	18 months	86 % 1 14 % recurrent, no difference in dose	[66]
Flickenger	2011	Meta-analysis	Surgery alone-29 % Surgery→post-op XRT 71 %	90–95 % if 16–19Gy/3Fx/10 days earlobes 21.5–24.8/3 Fx/10 days Other sites		Meta-analysis	[67]
Sulfane	1996	31 (randomized	Steroid surgery Radiation	8/12 (67 %) 14/16 (91.5 %)	12 months		[68]
Kovalic	1989	113	Surgery →12 Gy	73 %	6 years	2 cm, previous Tx males with recurrate; med time to recur 12 months	[69]
Locomotor	2009	194	XRT → 16–40 Gy Surgery→	89 % with ≥20 Gy 57 % <20 Gy	36 months	20 Gy/5 Fx "optimal" dose	[70]

Table 6 Brachytherapy results for keloids

Author	Year	#	Treatment	Dose	Local control	F/U	Others	Ref
Guix	2001	169	Surgery→Bx 22 – Bx	12 Gy/4 Fx HDR	96 % 142/147 = 96.5 18/22 = 82 %	84 months		[71]
Escarmont	1993	570	Surgery→Bx	8–30 Gy/1–2Fx	79 %	6.9 years	91 % recur in 12 months 25 % hyperpigmentation 13 % hyperpigmentation	[72]
Kuribayashi	2011	36	Surgery→Bx (superficial)	15 Gy/3 Fx @ 2 mm 20 Gy/4 Fx @ 2 mm	90 %	18 months	Median fail 12 months Only failures were on chest wall No grade II complications	[73]
Fontanesi	2008	49	Surgery→Bx	1000@3 mm/1Fx	94 %	42	No grade II complication	[74]
Moglei	2000	114	Surgery→1r	20.4 Gy@5 mm	87 %	24		[75]
Vioni	2009	892	Sr 90Y	20 Gy/10 Fx	88 %	61	0.5 cm Fx margin	[76]
DeCicco	2014	96	LDR (46) surgery HDR (50)	16 Gy 12 Gy	70 % 65 %			[77]
Rio	2010	73	LDR	15–40 Gy (20 Gy med)@5 mm	86 %	44.5 months		[78]

While the use of external beam irradiation has shown an excellent long-term prevention of keloid recurrence in the postoperative setting, so has the use of postoperative brachytherapy. Technical aspects will be addressed later in this chapter; however, there are certain advantages that brachytherapy provides. Various scries, using different isotopes, techniques (HDR vs LDR), and fraction schemes (single vs multiple), have noted long-term keloid recurrence prevention rates ranging from 68 to 96 % (Table 6).

The advantages include reduced overall time to complete treatment in many cases and direct visualization and placement of applicators into the wound by the surgeon. Another consideration when planning adjunctive treatment for keloids is the potential for serious side effects. For example, the use of different topical/injected chemotherapeutic agents such as 5-fluorouracil/bleomycin has well-defined dose-dependent side effects. These include skin darkening, susceptibility to enhanced sun/skin reaction, itching, blistering, rash, and potential allergic reaction.

However, these side effects rarely occur with the use of any radiation technique. Of more concern in this modality is the potential for the development of radiation-induced malignancies. Recent reports have identified this risk [79]. Based on a Medline search of years 1901–2009, Ogawa identified only five cases of malignancy associated with postoperative radiation for keloid prevention [80]. The article concluded that the risk was "very low when preformed with adequate doses and under conditions that provide adequate protection of surrounding issues." For this reason BT can be advocated as the radiation treatment of choice since the CTV is very small (0.5 cm around the incision) which reduces the treated volume dramatically as compared to external beam radiotherapy where a larger PTV margin must be taken into account.

8.2 Technical Aspects and Dosing in Keloid Brachytherapy

It is critically important that any patient being considered for postoperative brachytherapy be seen preoperatively. This will allow for evaluation of the lesion and should include measurement of lesions but also allows for photographic images to be obtained. It is also critical to obtain informed consent with discussion of potential side effects including the possible development of radiation-induced malignancies.

The surgical technique is critical in understanding the length of treatment required. Issues related to tension created in the wound postoperatively can play a significant role in treatment planning and catheter placement. If the tissue is undermined in order to be able to provide primary closure, that undermined tissue can come under the same influences as the primary resected keloid scar. This is perhaps the single most important reason for failure to obtain local control and the reason most radiation oncologists prefer to use external beam techniques.

8.3 Technical Considerations

It is critical that the radiation oncologist be in the operating theater at the time of catheter placement. Generally one of the two common techniques is employed. The first is the one preferred by the authors: the "blind end" technique. In this technique, the catheter's distal end is "buried" approximately 1 cm beyond the end of the wound/undermined tissue that has to be treated. The second technique is the "through-and-through" technique. In this technique, there are both entrance and exit sites. If this technique is utilized, the distal exit site should be 1.0 cm from the end of the wound/undermined tissue.

One of the advantages of brachytherapy is the single fraction treatment scheme. In our hands we prescribe a dose of 1000 cGy calculated at 0.7 cm in all directions and treat to the single exit skin site using the blind end technique that we prefer. Other doses such as 20 Gy prescribed to a 0.5 cm margin with LDR BT or two fractions of 7 Gy with a 6 h interval have been used successfully. If using the through-

and-through technique, the dose should be carried to both entrance/exit sites.

8.4 Treatment Timing

In our experience, treatment can most often be delivered in the first 24 h. Often we treat on the day of surgery, similar to external beam techniques. When the patient presents in the postoperative setting, we perform a CT simulation with dummy wires placed in the catheters for accurate assessment. It is beneficial that the radiation oncologist be present in the operating theater, in order to identify any specific peculiarities that may have occurred during catheter placement. Once the planning CT is obtained, treatment planning occurs. With single catheter use, this is relatively straightforward. However, with multicatheter placement, we try to minimize dose inhomogeneity. We attempt to ensure that no more than 25 % of the treatment area receives 125 % of prescription dose. One way in which this is accommodated is by securing the catheters in at least two but often three areas of the wound to ensure only minimal movement occurs, if any. We attempt to space catheters at 1.0 cm if only two catheters are used. If three or more are used, which is extremely rare, we recommend 1.0 cm from the "outside" edge catheters to the next inside catheter and internal catheter spacing of 1.0–1.5 cm.

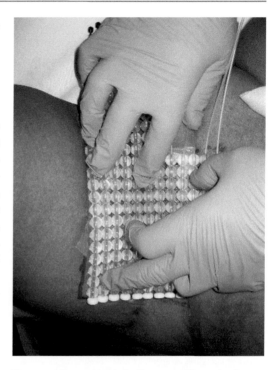

Fig. 17 Above with brachytherapy applicator in place

9 Hidradenitis Suppurativa

Hidradenitis suppurativa is a benign skin condition that is characterized by chronic recurrent infections often localized to axillary, groin, and gluteal regions [81]. It has been considered a "silent" disease, in that there is not much discussion about it in the public domain despite estimates of up to 4 % prevalence in certain populations [82]. Patients often undergo many localized surgical treatments in addition to antibiotic therapy and other therapies. There are data on the effectiveness of external beam irradiation for this entity, and when combined with antibiotic therapy, weight loss in obese patients, and aggressive skin care, treatment often results in successful long-term control [83–86]. Our institution (Fontanesi) has treated over 100 sites with external beam doses similar to those published; however, we have found that about one third of our patients require re-treatment at future time points because of reactivation of these sites.

We have noted that the sites most common to require re-treatment were those in "creased" areas

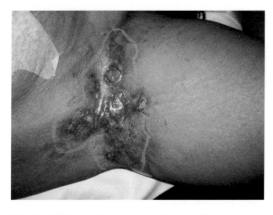

Fig. 16 Hidradenitis suppurativa in the axilla

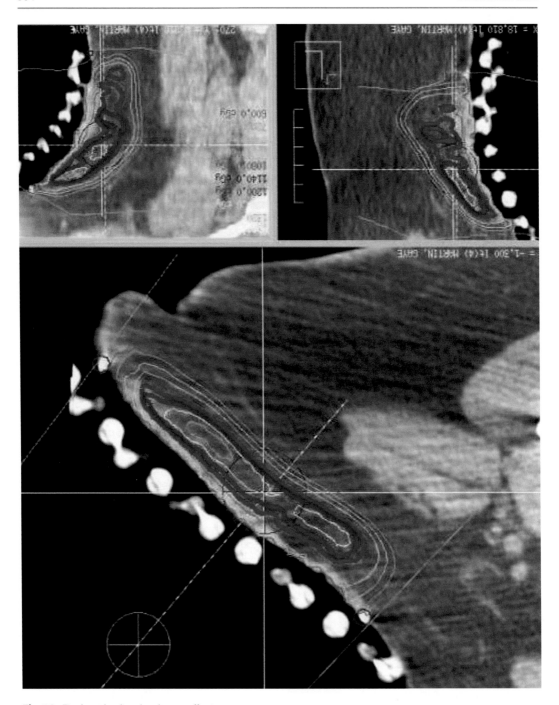

Fig. 18 Dosimetric plan showing excellent coverage

of the body such as the groins and gluteal regions, where the use of electron beams has some uncertainty due to the sloping nature of the skin in these areas. We have also noted on our CT treatment planning scans that these areas often have various depths of involvement, thus making external beam techniques more difficult to deliver homogeneous dose coverage. Thus in a limited number of patients, "surface" mold brachytherapy has been utilized. We attempt to cover all CT-based abnormalities with a 1 cm margin (Figs. 16, 17, and 18) utilizing the same daily and total dose recommendation as with electron beam therapy (150 cGy per day × 8 fractions). This experience is very early but the results and dosimetric improvements will continue to be evaluated.

Conclusions

Brachytherapy has a long history of use in the treatment of skin malignancies and non-skin malignancies such as NHL. Excellent results have also been reported in the prevention of keloid recurrence postoperatively with little second malignancy risk.

Newer brachytherapy application for non-traditional use in entities such as hidradenitis suppurativa has been also utilized with initial success. What is critical to all these sites/applications is the close cooperation between the radiation oncology and the surgical teams. This enhanced communication leads to better definition of tumor volume and allows, in many cases, improved catheter placement especially as it relates to wound closure.

Various dose rate/total dose recommendations have been published with similar results and complication rates. It is clear with increased hourly dose rates (LDR), dose/fraction (HDR), and total dose delivered, there are increased complications without increase benefit of improved local control.

Whether the Paris, Manchester, or Patterson-Parker System (LDR) is used or if HDR dose optimization programs are utilized, dose inhomogeneity is important as it can dramatically change complication rates.

In any skin site, the only limitation to the use of brachytherapy is imagination of the physician.

Acknowledgements The authors wish to thank Susan King for her assistance in the editing and preparation of this chapter.

References

1. Tay SS, Roediger B, Tong PL et al (2013) The skin-resident immune network. Curr Dermatol Rep 28(3):13–22
2. Madison KC (2003) Barrier function of the skin: "la raison d'être" of the epidermis. J Invest Dermatol 121(2):231–41
3. McGrath JA, Eady RA, Pope FM (2004) Rook's textbook of dermatology, 7th ed, vol 3. Blackwell Publishing, Hoboken NJ, pp 1–3
4. Orphanidou C, McCargar L, Birmingham C et al (1994) Accuracy of subcutaneous fat measurement: comparison of skinfold calipers, ultrasound, and computed tomography. J Am Diet Assoc 94(8):855–858
5. Lomas A, Leonardi-Bee J, Bath-Hextall F (2004) A systematic review of worldwide incidence of non-melanoma skin cancer. Br J Dermatol 166:1069–1080
6. Staples Margaret P, Mark E, Burton Robert C (2006) Non-melanoma skin cancer in Australia: the 2002 national survey and trends since 1985. Med J 184(1):6–10
7. Sanat K (2012) Malignant neoplasms following radiotherapy. Int J Environ Res Public Health 9:4744–4759
8. Berrington de Gonzalez A, Curtis RE, Kry SF et al (2011) Proportion of second cancers attributable to radiotherapy treatment in adults: a cohort study in the US SEER cancer registries. Lancet Oncol 12(4):353–60
9. Salavoura K, Aggeliki K, Tsangaris G et al (2008) Development of cancer in patients with primary immunodeficiencies. Anticancer Res 28:1263–1270
10. Safai B, Diaz B, Schwartz J (1992) Malignant neoplasms associated with human immunodeficiency virus infection. CA Cancer J Clin 42(2):74–95
11. Zwald FO, Brown M (2011) Skin cancer in solid organ transplant recipients: advances in therapy and management: part I. Epidemiology of skin cancer in solid organ transplant recipients. J Am Acad Dermatol 65(2):253–61
12. Wallingford SC, Olsen CM, Plasmeijer E et al (2011) Skin cancer arising in scars: a systematic. Review Dermatol Surg 37(9):1239–1244
13. Nikolaou V, Stratigos AJ, Tsao H (2012) Hereditary nonmelanoma skin cancer. Semin Cutan Med Surg 31(4):204–10
14. McCusker M, Basset-Seguin N, Dummer R et al (2014) Metastatic basal cell carcinoma: prognosis dependent on anatomic site and spread of disease. Eur J Cancer 50(4):774–83
15. Cancer Facts & Figures (2014) Estimated numbers of new cancer cases for 2014, excluding basal cell and squamous cell skin cancers and in situ carcinomas except urinary bladder. American Cancer Society. http://www.cancer.org/acs/groups/content/@research/documents/document/acspc-041780.pdf
16. Cantisani C, De Gado F, Ulrich M et al (2013) Actinic keratosis: review of the literature and new patents. Recent Pat Inflamm Allerg Drug Discov 7(2):168–75
17. Dufresne R, Curlin A (1997) Actinic cheilitis. A treatment review. Dermatol Surg 23(1):15–21
18. Neubert T, Lehmann P (2008) Bowen's disease – a review of newer treatment options. Ther Clin Risk Manag 4(5):1085–1095
19. Lin C, Tripcomy L, Keller J et al (2012) Perineural infiltration of cutaneous squamous cell carcinoma and basal cell carcinoma without clinical features. Int J Radiat Oncol Biol Phys 82(1):334–40
20. Panizza B, Solares CA, Redmond M et al (2012) Surgical resection for clinical perineural invasion

from cutaneous squamous cell carcinoma of the head and neck. Head Neck 34(11):1622–7

21. Silva JJ, Tsang RW, Panzarella T et al (2000) Results of radiotherapy for epithelial skin cancer of the pinna: the Princess Margaret Hospital experience, 1982–1993. Int J Radiat Oncol Biol Phys 47(2):451–9

22. Petrovich Z, Kuisk H, Langholz B et al (1987) Treatment results and patterns of failure in 646 patients with carcinoma of the eyelids, pinna, and nose. Am J Surg 154(4):447–50

23. Wilder RB, Kettelson JM, Shimm DS (1991) Basal cell carcinoma treated with radiation therapy. Cancer 68(10):2134–7

24. Fitzpatrick PJ (1984) Skin cancer of the head-treatment by radiotherapy. J Otolaryngol 13(4):261–6

25. Abbatucci JS, Boulier N, Laforge T et al (1989) Radiation therapy of skin carcinomas: results of a hypofractionated irradiation schedule in 675 cases followed more than 2 years. Radiother Oncol 14:113–19

26. Schlienger P, Brunin F, Desjardins L et al (1996) External radiotherapy for carcinoma of the eyelid: report of 850 cases treated. Int J Radiat Oncol Biol Phys 34:277–87

27. Locke J, Karimpour S, Young G et al (2001) Radiotherapy for epithelial skin cancer. Int J Radiat Oncol Biol Phys 51:748–55

28. Guix B, Finestres F, Tello JI et al (2000) Treatment of skin carcinomas of the face by high-dose-rate brachytherapy and custom-made surfaces mold. Int J Radiat Oncol Biol Phys 47:95–102

29. Crook JM, Mazeron JJ, Marinello G et al (1990) Interstitial Iridium 192 for cutaneous carcinoma of the external nose. Int J Radiat Oncol Biol Phys 18:243–48

30. Mazeron JJ, Chassagne D, Crook J et al (1988) Radiation therapy of carcinomas of the skin of nose and nasal vestibule: a report of 1676 cases by the Groupe Europeen de Curiethèrapie. Radiother Oncol 13:165–73

31. Gauden R, Pracy M, Avery AM et al (2013) HDR brachytherapy for superficial non-melanoma skin cancers. J Med Imaging Radiat Oncol 57(2):212–7

32. Bhatnagar A (2013) Non-melanoma skin cancer treated with electronic brachytherapy: results at 1 year. Brachytherapy 12(2):134–40

33. Krengli M, Masini L, Comoli AM et al (2014) Interstitial brachytherapy for eyelid carcinoma: outcome analysis in 60 patients. Strahlenther Onkol 190(3):245–249

34. Rio E, Bardet E, Ferron C et al (2005) Interstitial brachytherapy of periorificial skin carcinomas of the face: a retrospective study of 97 cases. Int J Radiat Oncol Biol Phys 63(3):753–7

35. Ducassou A, David I, Filleron T et al (2011) Retrospective analysis of local control and cosmetic outcome of 147 periorificial carcinomas of the treated with low-dose rate interstitial brachytherapy. Int J Radiat Oncol Biol Phys 81(3):726–31

36. Hobbs C, Harper J (2011) The use of high dose rate brachytherapy palliation after failed palliative exter-nal beam radiotherapy for a cutaneous malignant melanoma of the foot: a case report. J Palliat Med 14(4):521–3

37. Scepanovic D, Paluga M, Rybnikarova M et al (2013) Brachytherapy as a treatment for malignant melanoma of the nasal cavity and nasopharynx; case report. J Contemp Brachytherapy 5(3):157–63

38. Shi F, Zhang X, Wu K et al (2014) Metastatic malignant melanoma: computed tomography-guided 125l seed implantation treatment. Melanoma Res 24(2):137–43

39. Chaudhuri A, De-Groot C, Seel M et al (2011) Treatment of regional cutaneous nodular metastases from melanoma using high-dose rate mould brachytherapy. J Med Imaging Radiat Oncol 55(2):206–12

40. Smithers FA, Moaveni Z, De Groot C (2011) The role of radiotherapy in the palliation of cutaneous melanoma metastases: a case series of 3 patients. J Plast Reconstr Aesthet Surg 64(4):550–3

41. Garibyan L, Cotte SE, Hansen JL et al (2013) Palliative treatment for in-transit cutaneous metastases of Merkel cell carcinoma using surface-mold computer-optimized high-dose-rate brachytherapy. Cancer J 19(4):283–7

42. Kasper ME, Richter S, Warren N et al (2013) Complete response of endemic Kaposi sarcoma lesions with high-dose-rate brachytherapy: treatment method, results, and toxicity using skin surface applicators. Brachytherapy 12(5):495–9

43. DeSimone JA, Guenova E, Carter JB et al (2013) Low-dose high-dose-rate brachytherapy in the treatment of facial lesions of cutaneous T-cell lymphoma. J Am Acad Dermatol 69(1):61–5

44. Van Limbergen E, Mazeron JJ Skin cancer. The GEC ESTRO handbook of brachytherapy. http://estro-education.org/publications/Documents/final%20 introduction.pdf

45. Maes A, Van Limbergen E (2001) LDR – brachytherapy for non melanoma skin cancer of the face: local control rate, functional and cosmetic outcomes in 173 patients. Radiother Oncol 60(suppl 1):S16

46. Berman B, Flores F (1999) Comparison of a gel filled cushion and silicone gel sheeting in the treatment of Hypertrophic scar of keloid scars. Dermatol Surg 25(6):484–6

47. Albert JLM (1817) Quelques resherches surla cheloide. Mem Soc Med d'Emul 744–752

48. Abergel RP, Pizzurro D, Meeker CA et al (1985) Biochemical composition of the connective tissue in keloids and analysis of collagen metabolism in keloid fibroblast cultures. J Invest Dermatol 84(5):384–90

49. Chen W, Fu X, Sun X et al (2003) Analysis of differentially expressed genes in keloids and normal skin with cDNA microarray. J Surg Res 113(2):208–16

50. Dong Z, Mao S, Wen H (2013) Upregulation of proinflammatory genes in skin lesions may be the cause of keloid formation (Review). Biomed Rep 1(6):833–836

51. Alhady SM, Sivanantharajah K (1969) Keloids in various races. A review of 175 cases. Plast Reconstr Surg 44(6):564–6
52. Marneros AG, Norris JE, Watanabe S et al (2004) Genome scans provide evidence for keloid susceptibility loci on chromosomes 2q23 and 7p11. J Invest Dermatol 122(5):1126–32
53. Wang QG, Li XM, Zhang M et al (2014) Effect of two dose fra Chapters 11, 12, 27 and 30 ctionations on postoperative radiotherapy of keloid: an analysis of 107 patients. Beijing Da Xue Xue Bao 46(1):169–72
54. Wu XL, Gao Z, Song N et al (2009) Clinical study of auricular keloid treatment with both surgical excision and intralesional injection of low-dose 5-fluorouracil and corticosteroids. Zhonghua Yi Xue Za Zhi 89(16):1102–5
55. Davison SP, Dayan JH, Clemens MW et al (2009) Efficacy of intralesional 5-fluorouracil and triamcinolone in the treatment of keloids. Aesthet Surg J 29(1):40–6
56. Jin R, Huang X, Li H et al (2013) Laser therapy for prevention and treatment of pathologic excessive scars. Plast Reconstr Surg 132(6):1747–58
57. Litrowski N, Boullie MC, Dehesdin D et al (2014) Treatment of earlobe keloids by surgical excision and cryosurgery. J Eur Acad Dermatol Venereol 28(10):1324–1331
58. O'Brien L, Jones D (2013) Silicone gel sheeting for preventing and treating hypertrophic and keloid scars. Cochrane Database Syst Rev (9):CD003826
59. Mamalis AD, Lev-Tov H, Nguyen DH et al (2014) Laser and light-based treatment of Keloids – a review. J Eur Acad Dermatol Venereol 289(6):689–699
60. Saray Y, Gulec AT (2005) Treatment of keloids and hypertrophic scars with dermojet injections of bleomycin: a preliminary study. Int J Dermatol 44(9):777–84
61. Janssen De Limpens AM (1980) The local treatment of hypertrophic scars and keloids with topical retinoic acid. Br J Dermatol 103(3):319–23
62. Park TH, Seo S, Kim JK et al (2011) Outcomes of surgical excision with pressure therapy using magnets and identification of risk factors for recurrent keloids. Plast Reconstr Surg 128(2):431–9
63. Ogawa R, Tsuguhiro M, Hiko H et al (2007) Postoperative radiation protocol for keloids and hypertrophic scars statistical analysis of 370 sites followed for over 18 months. Department of Plastic and Reconstructive Surgery and Department of Radiation Oncology, Nippon Medical School, 1-1-5 Sendagi Bunkyo-ku, Tokyo
64. Wang F, Yang H, Liao H et al (2014) Treatment of auricular keloids with surgery and intralesional injection of compound betamethasone. Zhonghua Zheng Xing Wai Ke Za Zhi 30(1):7–10
65. Kal HB, Veen RE (2005) Biologically effective doses of postoperative radiotherapy in the prevention of keloids: dose-effect relationship. Strahlenther Onkol Niv 181(11):7017–23
66. Ogawa R, Huang C, Akaishi S et al (2013) Analysis of surgical treatments for earlobe keloids: analysis of 174 lesions in 145 patients. Plast Reconstr Surg 132(5):818e–825e
67. Flickinger JC (2011) A radiobiological analysis of multicenter data for postoperative keloid radiotherapy. Int J Radiat Biol Phys 79(4):1164–70
68. Sclafani A, Gordon L, Chadha M et al (1996) Prevention of earlobe keloid recurrence with postoperative corticosteroid injections versus radiation therapy. Dermatol Surg 22(6):569–574
69. Kovalic JJ, Perez CA (1989) Radiation therapy following keloidectomy: a 20 year experience. Int J Radiat Oncol Biol Phys 17(1):77–80, Radiation Oncology Center, Mallinckrodt Institute of Radiology, St. Louis, MO
70. Sakamoto T, Oya N, Shibuya K et al (2009) Dose-response relationship and dose optimization in radiotherapy of postoperative keloids. Radiother Oncol 91(2):271–6
71. Guix B, Henriquez I, Andres A et al (2001) Treatment of keloids by high-dose-rate brachytherapy: a seven – year study. Int J Radiat Oncol Biol Phys 50(1):167–172
72. Escarmant P, Zimmermann S, Amar A (1992) The treatment of 783 keloid scars by iridium 192 interstitial irradiation after surgical excision. Int J Radiat Oncol Biol Phys 26:245–251
73. Kuribayahi S, Miyashita T, Ozawa Y et al (2011) Post-keloidectomy irradiation using high-dose-rate superficial brachytherapy. J Radiat Res 52:356–368
74. Fontanesi J, Griffin A (2008) Brachytherapy in the treatment of resected keloids. Author presentation to the 2008 World Congress of Brachytherapy, Boston
75. Maalej M, Frikha H, Bouaouina N et al (2000) Intraoperative brachytherapy in the management of keloids: apropos of 114 cases. Cancer Radiother 4(4):274–8
76. Viani GA, Stefano EJ, Afonso SL et al (2009) Postoperative strontium-90 brachytherapy in the prevention of keloids: results and prognostic factors. Int J Radiat Oncol Biol Phys 73(5):15010–6
77. De Cicco L, Vischioni B, Vavassori A et al (2014) Postoperative management of keloids: low-dose-rate and High-dose-rate brachytherapy. Brachytherapy 13(5):508–513
78. Rio E, Bardet E, Peuvrel P et al (2010) Perioperative interstitial brachytherapy for recurrent keloid scars. Cancer Radiother 14(1):65–8
79. Fortson JK, Rosenthal M, Patel V et al (2012) Atypical presentation of mucoepidermoid carcinoma after radiation therapy for the treatment of keloids. Ear Nose Throat J 91(7):286–8
80. Ogawa R, Yoshitatsu S, Yoshida K et al (2009) Is radiation therapy for keloids acceptable? The risk of radiation-induced carcinogenesis. Am Soc Plastic Surg 124:1196. http://www.plasticsurgery.org/Documents/news-resources/statistics/2009-statistics/2009-US-cosmeticreconstructiveplasticsurgeryminimally-invasive-statistics.pdf
81. Attanoos RL, Appleton MAC, Douglas-Jones AG (1995) The pathogenesis of hidradenitis suppurativa; a closer look at apocrine and apoeccrine glands. Br J Dermatol 133:254–258

82. Jemec GB, Heidenheim M, Nielsen NH (1996) The prevalence of hidradenitis suppurativa and its potential precursor lesions. J Am Acad Dermatol 35:191–194
83. Frohlich D, Baaske D, Glatzel M (2000) Strahlentherapie der Hidradenitis axillaris-heute noch aktuell? Strahlenther Onkol 176:286–289
84. Krause GP (1994) Die Rontgenbehandlung der Schweißdrusenabszesse. Strahlentherapie 79:253–256
85. Trombetta M, Werts ED, Parda D (2010) The role of radiotherapy in the treatment of hidradenitis suppurativa; case report and review of the literature. Dermatol Online J 16(2):16–19
86. Pape R, Golles D (1950) Was leisten Rontgenmikrodosen bei der Hydrosadenitis axillaris? Strahlentherapie 81:565–576

Soft Tissue Sarcoma Brachytherapy

James Fontanesi, Michael Mott, Jeffrey Margolis, Gabrielle Monit, and Alain Gerbaulet

Abstract

Soft tissue sarcomas (STS) are a diffuse group of malignancies that arise from connective tissues such as fat, muscle, nerves, and blood vessels. They account for approximately 1 % of all adult malignancies and approximately 10 % of pediatric malignancies. They do not respect age, appearing in all age groups. Here we present brachytherapy as primary therapy or an adjunct to management.

1 Introduction

Although reportedly described in ancient Egyptian text, it appears the first published account of soft tissue sarcomas was from

J. Fontanesi, MD (✉)
Radiation Oncology, Botsford Cancer Center,
Oakland University/William Beaumont School
of Medicine, Farmington Hills, MI, USA
e-mail: jfontanesi@comcast.net

M. Mott, MD
Orthopedic Oncology, Henry Ford Hospital,
Detroit, MI, USA

J. Margolis, MD
Department of Oncology, Oakland University,
William Beaumont Medical School,
Rochester, MI, USA

G. Monit, MS, PA-C
Oakland Medical Group, Michigan Healthcare
Professionals, Oakland, MI, USA

A. Gerbaulet, MD
Department of Radiotherapy, Institut
Gustave-Roussy, Villejuif, France

Morgagni in 1761 in his famous textbook *De Sedibus, et Causis Morborum per Anatomen Indagatis Libri Quinque* [1].

This heterogeneous group of rare tumors arises predominantly from the embryonic mesoderm although some have been noted to arise from the neuroectoderm. It is also estimated that there are approximately 50 subtypes [2].

These malignancies can arise anywhere in the body however with the majority occurring in the limb, limb girdle, retroperitoneal, and intraperitoneal sites, among others.

It is estimated that approximately 12,420 adults will be diagnosed with a soft tissue sarcoma in 2014. Unfortunately, approximately 4740 will die from their disease [3]. There is a slight male predominance within the adult age group. The most common diagnosed histology is malignant fibrous histiocytoma (MFH), followed by liposarcoma and leiomyosarcoma.

With STS we must not only address the primary disease site but we must have knowledge of

© Springer International Publishing Switzerland 2016
P. Montemaggi et al. (eds.), *Brachytherapy: An International Perspective*, Medical Radiology,
DOI 10.1007/978-3-319-26791-3_23

potential lymphatic and distant disease spread. It has been noted that up to 16 % of adult STS patients will have lymph node involvement at diagnosis or at some time during their disease course [4]. The histological type of STS influences lymph node involvement with the highest rates seen in angiosarcoma, embryonal rhabdomyosarcoma (RMS), and epithelioid sarcoma, while neurofibrosarcoma, liposarcoma, and leiomyosarcoma generally have less than a 5 % risk of involvement [5, 6]. Site can also influence lymph node involvement, with the highest rates being identified in lesions of the lower extremity (up to 45 %) and the lowest with truncal presentations (1–15 %) [7].

Distant disease diagnosed at initial presentation can greatly affect treatment decisions. It has been reported that between 25 and 50 % of patients with intermediate- or high-grade lesions measuring more than 5 cm will have distant disease at diagnosis or during their disease course, compared with less than 10 % in those with low-grade lesions less than 5 cm. Most distant spread will involve the lungs, at least initially [8, 9].

2   Pediatric Soft Tissue Sarcoma

As noted STS are not age discriminatory; it is estimated that about 6800 new cases of STS will be diagnosed in children less than 19 years old in 2014 [10] (Table 1).

Rhabdomyosarcoma (RMS), with its three distinct variants, is the most common STS in children less than 14 years old and accounts for approximately 50 % of tumors in this age group. RMS will account for approximately 7 % of all childhood tumors. The remaining STS known as non-rhabdomyosarcoma STS (NRSTS) will account for approximately 3 % of childhood tumors; the most common of which are fibrosar-

Table 1 Age distribution of soft tissue sarcomas (STSs) in children aged 0–19 years (SEER 1975–2008)

	Age <5 years	Age 5–9 years	Age 10–14 years	Age 15–19 years	% of the total number of STS cases <20 years
All soft tissue and other extraosseous sarcomas	1130	810	1144	1573	100
Rhabdomyosarcomas	710	466	364	350	41
Fibrosarcomas, peripheral nerve, and other fibrous neoplasms	151	64	132	192	12
Fibroblastic and myofibroblastic tumors	131	31	57	86	6.5
Nerve sheath tumors	19	32	74	104	5
Other fibromatous neoplasms	1	1	1	2	0.1
Kaposi's sarcoma	*1*	*2*	*0*	*12*	*0.3*
Other specified soft tissue sarcomas	*198*	*220*	*512*	*856*	*38*
Ewing tumor and Askin tumor of soft tissue	22	28	57	81	4
pPNET of soft tissue	21	19	29	42	2.4
Extrarenal rhabdoid tumor	37	3	8	3	1
Liposarcomas	5	6	22	66	2
Fibrohistiocytic tumors[a]	53	69	171	293	12
Leiomyosarcomas	13	19	22	57	2.4
Synovial sarcomas	12	39	133	204	8.3
Blood vessel tumors	15	7	11	33	1.4
Osseous and chondromatous neoplasms of soft tissue	1	5	9	16	0.6
Alveolar soft parts sarcoma	3	7	19	26	1
Miscellaneous soft tissue sarcomas	16	18	31	35	2
Unspecified soft tissue sarcomas	*70*	*58*	*163*	*163*	*9*

pPNET peripheral primitive neuroectodermal tumors, *SEER* Surveillance, Epidemiology, and End Results
[a]Dermatofibrosarcoma accounts for 75 % of these cases

coma, synovial sarcoma, MFH, and malignant peripheral nerve sheath tumors.

Again one must be mindful of lymph nodes/distant metastases in pediatric STS/NRSTS. While unusual at diagnosis, certain non-RMS lesions have a higher propensity for lymph node involvement; these include epithelioid and clear cell sarcomas [11].

Prognostic factors for pediatric non-RMS STS have been difficult to ascertain since few institutions have large enough numbers of these rare cases to enable evaluation. However, St. Jude Children's Research Hospital did publish on a series of 121 patients. In a multivariate analysis, positive surgical margins, intra-abdominal primary site, and omission of radiation therapy predicted for increased risk or local failure, while size ≥5 cm, high-grade designation, and invasiveness predicted increased distant metastases [12].

Another factor that makes pediatric STS diagnosis intriguing is the genetic predisposition of certain patients for the development of soft tissue sarcomas. Included in these populations are the Li-Fraumeni syndrome, in which changes in the p53 tumor suppressor gene can lead to an increased risk of development of non-RMS lesions, bone sarcomas, breast cancer, brain tumors, and acute leukemia [13]. Patients with neurofibromatosis type 1 have approximately 4 % chance of developing a malignant peripheral nerve sheath tumor [14], while patients with familial adenomatous polyposis (FAP) have an increased risk for developing desmoid tumors [15]. In those patients with the Werner syndrome, an increased susceptibility to STS and premature aging is noted [16], and in patients with germline mutations of the retinoblastoma gene, there is an increased risk of development of STS, especially leiomyosarcoma [17].

Certain environmental factors also can play a role in the development of both adult and pediatric STS. Previous therapeutic radiation exposure results in an increased risk of development of "in-field" non-RMS sarcoma, most commonly malignant fibrous histiocytoma (MFH) [18]. AIDS patients with known Epstein-Barr virus infections (EBV) are at increased risk for the development of leiomyosarcoma, in addition to the

known risk of development of Kaposi's sarcoma [19]. Pediatric patients who develop non-RMS sarcoma also have an association with chromosomal alteration. A list of some of the most commonly seen is found in Table 2.

3 Soft Tissue Sarcoma Location Influences

Often the site of origin helps in determining the type of soft tissue sarcoma which is being investigated. Examples include MFH/fibrosarcoma which most often develops in the legs, arms, and trunks, while leiomyosarcoma often presents in the uterus and digestive tract. Synovial sarcomas are usually associated with the linings of joints and tendon sheaths and most often present in the legs (Table 3).

4 Diagnosis

Often the clinical symptoms associated with the diagnosis of STS are nonspecific. They can often present as a painless, slow growing, enlarging mass that is often mistaken for a benign process. Tumors that are readily visible are often diagnosed at an earlier time frame and are often smaller then corresponding soft tissue sarcomas that develop in the retroperitoneal areas because of lack of visibility.

Workup of these lesions includes a detailed history and physical and imaging studies. Imaging is critical in the development of the diagnosis of soft tissue sarcomas in that it not only helps to delineate the extent of tumor, lymph node involvement, and metastatic disease but also can identify any pseudo capsule which may help the surgeon in their quest for total exenteration at the time of surgery.

Plain radiographs are often used to help to detect calcifications and/or rule out primary bone malignancies such as osteogenic sarcoma. Chest X-rays are essential in helping to establish metastatic disease, as the lung is often the preferable site for metastatic deposits. Imaging using computed tomography of the thorax, abdomen, and pelvis is critical along with MRI

Table 2 Frequent chromosomal aberrations seen in non-rhabdomyosarcoma STS

Histology	Chromosomal aberrations	Genes involved
Alveolar soft part sarcoma	t(x;17)(p11.2;q25)	$ASPL/TFE_3$ [29–31]
Angiomatoid fibrous histiocytoma	t(12;16)(q13;p11)(q33;q12), t(12;22)(q13;q12)	FUS/ATF_1, $EWSR_1$ [32], EWS/ATF_1
Clear cell sarcoma	t(12;22)(q13;q12), t(2;22)(q33;q12)	ATF_1/EWS, $EWSR_1/CREB_1$
Congenital (infantile) Fibrosarcoma/mesoblastic nephroma	t(12;15)(p13,q25)	$ETV-NTRK_3$
Dermatofibrosarcoma protuberans	t(17;22)(q22;q13)	$COL_1A_1/PDGFB$
Desmoid fibromatosis	Trisomy 8 or 20, loss of 5q21	$CTNNB_1$ or APC mutations
Desmoplastic small round cell tumors	t(11;22)(p13;q12)	EWS/WT_1 [33]
Epithelioid hemangioendothelioma	t(1;3)(p36;q25) [34]	$WWTR_1/CAMTA_1$
Epithelioid sarcoma	Inactivation $SMARCB_1$	$SMARCB_1$
Extraskeletal myxoid chondrosarcoma	t(9;22)(q22;q12), t(9:17)(q22;q11), t(9;15), (q22;q21), t(3;9)(q11;q22)	$EWSR_1/NR_4A_3$, TAR_2N/NR_4A_3, TCF_{12}/NR_4A_3, TGF/NR_4A_3
Hemangiopericytoma	t(12;19)(q13;q13.3) and t(13;22)(q22;q13.3)	
Inflammatory myofibroblastic tumor	t(1;2)(q23;q23), t(2;19)(q23;q13) 0, t(2;17)(q23;q23), t(2;2)(p23;q13), t(2;11)(p23;p15) [35]	TPM_3/ALK, TPM_4/ALK, $CLTC/ALK$, $RANBP_2/ALK$, $CARS/ALK$
Low-grade fibromyxoid sarcoma	t(7;16)(q33;p11), t(11;16)(p11;p11)	$FUS/CREB_3L_2$, $FUS/CREB_3L_1$
Malignant peripheral nerve sheath tumor	17q11.2, loss or rearrangement 10p, 11q, 17q, 22q	NF_1
Myxoid/round cell liposarcoma	T(12;16)(q13;p11), t(12;22)(q13;q12)	FUS/DD_1T_3, $EWSR/DD_1T_3$
Rhabdoid tumor	Inactivation $SMARCB_1$	$SMARCB_1$
Synovial sarcoma	t(x;18)(p11.2;q11.2)	SYT/SSX
Tenosynovial giant cell tumor	t(1;2)(p13;q35)	CSF_1

Table 3 Major types of soft tissue sarcomas in adults

Tissue of origin	Type of cancer	Usual location in the body
Fibrous tissue	Fibrosarcoma	Arms, legs, trunk
	Malignant fibrous histiocytoma	Legs
	Dermatofibrosarcoma	Trunk
Fat	Liposarcoma	Arms, legs, trunk

Muscle
   Striated muscle
   Smooth muscle
	Rhabdomyosarcoma
	Leiomyosarcoma
		Arms, legs
		Uterus, digestive tract

Blood vessels	Hemangiosarcoma	Arms, legs, trunk
	Kaposi's sarcoma	Legs, trunk
Lymph vessels	Lymphangiosarcoma	Arms
Synovial tissue (linings of joint cavities, tendon sheaths)	Synovial sarcoma	Legs
Peripheral nerves	Malignant peripheral nerve sheath tumor/neurofibrosarcoma	Arms, legs, trunk
Cartilage and bone-forming tissue	Extraskeletal chondrosarcoma	Legs
	Extraskeletal osteosarcoma	Legs, trunk (not involving the bone)

imaging. PET scans have also been used to help and more accurately stage STS (Figs. 1, 2, and 3). However, what is interesting is that a recent meta-analysis has disputed the benefit of use of PET imaging in its current state, especially in low-grade tumors [20].

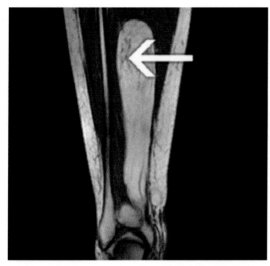

Fig. 1 Well-differentiated liposarcoma. Coronal plane T1 sequence; *arrow* shows stranding within tumor mass

Following identification of what is believed to be a soft tissue sarcoma, diagnosis with histological sampling becomes imperative. Percutaneous core needle biopsy is often utilized, but it is important to have a pathologist who is experienced in examining soft tissue sarcomas to make the diagnosis. If core needle biopsy is unsuccessful in establishing a diagnosis, more extensive procedures may be required. Having an accurate diagnosis becomes critical in that it has been well established that if surgery is to play a role in the treatment of an STS, initial en bloc resection with negative margins becomes critical. There are numerous articles that have indicated that incomplete resection with positive margins has dire effect on the overall local control and survival of these patients [21, 22].

Additionally, establishing not only the primary tumor diagnosis but the size, lymph node involvement, and distant metastatic involvement allows us to use the tumor-node-metastasis (TNM) staging system, developed both by the American Joint Committee on Cancer (AJCC) for soft tissue sarcoma and the International Union Against Cancer Committee (UICC) to correctly "stage" these patients and establish treatment goals (Table 4).

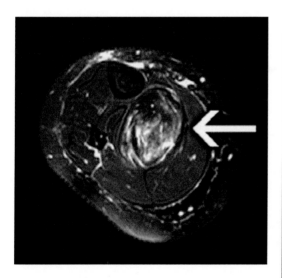

Fig. 2 Axial plane T2 sequence with fat suppression; arrow shows high (bright) signal throughout cross-section of tumor

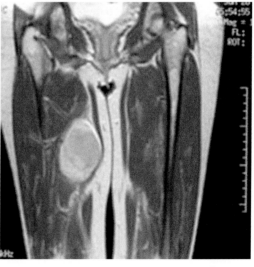

Fig. 3 Large basal cell carcinoma of scalp vertex

Table 4 Descriptions of stages, grades, and the tumor-node-metastasis (TNM) system of the American Joint Committee on Cancer for soft tissue sarcoma and the International Union Against Cancer committee

Grade And TNM	Description	T1a	T1b	T2a	T2b
G1	Well differentiated	Stage			
G2	Moderately differentiated	G1or G2	IA	IB	IIA
G3	Poorly differentiated	G3 or G4	IIB	IIC	III
G4	Undifferentiated	N1			
T1	Tumors 5 cm in largest dimension	M1	IV		
T1a	Superficial to deep fascia				
T1b	Deep to deep fascia (includes retroperitoneal, intrathoracic and most head and neck tumors)				
T2	Tumors >5 cm in largest dimension	5 –YR survival			
T2a	Superficial to deep fascia	Stage	%		
T2b	Deep to deep fascia(includes retroperitoneal, intrathoracic and most head and neck tumors)	I	86		
		II	72		
N1	Regional nodal metastasis	III	52		
M1	Distant metastasis	IV	10-20		

5 Treatment of Adult STS

Once the diagnosis of soft tissue sarcoma has been made, surgical intervention often becomes the center piece of therapy. While amputation was once considered the only surgical approach available for extremity soft tissue sarcomas, a report from Rosenberg et al. showed that the use of limb savage had equivalent local control rates to amputation [23]. Because of this study and others that followed, limb savage became more common. Soon after, other reports began to identify poor prognostic factors for local control; the chief among these was a positive surgical margin. Based on these citations, others followed with reports on adjunctive therapies such as chemotherapy and radiation, either alone or in combination, in efforts to mitigate these factors [23, 24].

However, surgical margin status is not the only prognostic factor that is considered important. Size of the tumor (less than or greater than 5 cm), tumor grade (high versus low), location, and histological subtype are just a few of the factors that must be considered when treatment of soft tissue sarcoma is decided upon. In fact, several of these criteria are included in the AJCC staging system for soft tissue sarcomas [25, 26].

While it is widely accepted that high-grade tumor designation is a significant prognostic factor, marginal status has more recently come under reinvestigation with several authors questioning the influence of the notion of (positive) margins and the eventual ability to establish local control. Both Baldini and Curtis have reported that margin status did not affect local control [27, 28].

As noted, multiple clinical trials have been reported using both pre- and postoperative chemotherapy alone or in combination with radiation. Radiation has also been evaluated in the preoperative setting or in conjunction with (boost) radiation therapy usually based on surgical margin status. Postoperative radiation by itself has also been evaluated. It is interesting to note that regardless of what additional therapy is employed in conjunction with surgical intervention, local control rates appear to be very similar (Table 5).

There have also been recent clinical reports which have looked at how radiation is delivered

Table 5 External/intraoperative radiation in treatment of soft tissue sarcoma

Author	Year	# Patients	Initial TX/factors	Boost type	LC	Complication	Notes
Pan [32]	2014	61	Preop EBI/positive margin	EBI 10 RT Bx	100 % 5 years	N/A	Longer survival with <5 cm low-grade boost
Folkert [31]	2014	319	Surg/pre	EBI	IMRT – 92 % 5 years EBI – 85 % 5 years	Gr III II 5 %	↓ LF with IMRT
Dincbas [33]	2014	60	Preop EBI → surg Y-ctx	EBI for positive margins	81 % 5 years	8 Gr III 3 Gr IV	CTX if >5 cm/high grade
Mullen [34]	2012	48	CTX/preop/≥8 cm	16 Gy for positive margin	83 % control 90 % MAID	(−)	1 PT with myelodysplastic syndrome death
Look- Hong [35]	2013	66	MAID/EBI → surg → ctx ± boost	EBI for close/pos margin	91 % at 46 months 78 % at 5 years	20/66 Wound complications	↓LC/surv with MFH
Cai [30]	2013	164	Various pre-/post-op EBI/ctx	EBI	83 % 5 years	Gr III 6 %	↑LC with dose >60 Gy
Felderhof [36]	2013	118	Surg → post-op EBI (60 Gy)	EBI	91 % at 5 years	Gr III/IV 21 %	↑LF age >50 Stage II histology
Curtis [28]	2011	112	Various	N/A	89 % 3 years	34 %	↑ Complications with chemo/ radiation
Trovik [37]	2001	1613	Various	EBI	83 %	N/A	Doubt LF cause distant mets

EBI external beam irradiation, *CTX* chemotherapy, *LF* local failure, *LC* local control and its influences on the establishment of local control. Some have evaluated the use of intensity-modulated radiation therapy IMRT and compared it to more traditional treatment approaches. These reports have shown that there appears to be improved local control with the use of intensity-modulated radiation therapy. Whether this is due to the technical delivery or the ability to increase the amount of dose delivered is unclear. There have been several clinical reports in which it has been shown that doses greater than 60 Gy helped to improve local control [29–31].

Based on multiple clinical reports and experiences, various national and international organi-

zations have met and issued recommendations/guidelines that would assist physicians in their approach to patients with soft tissue sarcomas. These organizations included the National Comprehensive Cancer Network (USA), American Brachytherapy Society (USA), GEC/ESTRO (Europe), British Sarcoma Group (UK), and ESMO (Europe) [38–42] (Table 6).

Despite having access to these guidelines which are very similar in their recommendations, a recent report had some disturbing conclusions. Bagaria et al. reported that despite NCCN recommendations of no postoperative radiation for stage 1 tumors, 25 % of

Table 6 Radiation recommendation for selected published guidelines

ESMO [38]	2014	Low/high grade; superficial; ≥5 cm Low grade; deep; ≤5 cm	50–50.4 at 1.8–2 Gy Boost to 66 Gy	External beam
ABS [39]	2013	Close/positive margin LR after previous surgery Lesion ≥5 cm Lesion deep to/invading superficial fascia High grade ≤50 year	Table 3 from ABS paper P 186	
British Sarcoma Group [40]	2010	Intermediate/high grade Low grade; >5 cm; positive margins	50 Gy at 2 Gy/Fx	Preoperative
			60–66 Gy	Postoperative
GEC/ESTRO [41]		Low grade; >5 cm; positive margin Intermediate/high grade Local recurrence	60–70 Gy at 40–60 Gy/HR :	LDR
			70–80 Gy/25–35 from brachy tx :	Combined EBI/brachy
NCCN [42]		Preop		16–18 Gy EBI (M)
			50 Gy → surg →	20–26 Gy EBI (G)
				16–18 Gy LDR (M)
				20–26 Gy LDR (G)
				14–16 Gy at 3–4 Gy BID HDR (M)
				18–21 Gy at 3–4 Gy BID HDR (G)
				10–12.5 Gy 10 RT (M)
				15 Gy 10 RT (G)
		Post-op for positive margins		10–16 Gy boost (negative margin)
			50 Gy +	16–18 Gy boost (M)
				20–26 Gy boost (G)
			10 RT 10–16 Gy + 50 Gy	
			LDR – 10–20 Gy (positive margin)	
				OR] → 50 Gy EBI
			HDR – 14–16 Gy (positive margin)	
			LDR – 45 Gy (negative margin)	
			HDR – 36 Gy (negative margin)	

M microscopic margin, *G* gross margin

these patients were eventually treated. More concerning was that *only* 60 % of those in whom a recommendation for postoperative irradiation was appropriate actually received it, proving again that you can lead a horse to water but you cannot make it drink [32].

Implant Technique at Institut Gustave-Roussy (IGR)

Soft tissue sarcomas: Adult
Technique

In the majority of cases, brachytherapy (BT) is performed during the surgical procedure. The plastic tubes are implanted perpendicularly to the surgical incision. The implant follows the Paris system rules, that is, with the after loading tubes equidistant, parallel, and spaced 1–2 cm apart. The CTV is determined according to the preoperative MRI and in consideration of the surgical and pathological findings.

For LDR BT alone, prescription dose is between 60 and 75 Gy delivered in approximately 1 week (35–40 cGy/h). In cases of BT used as a boost, the dose ranges between 25 and 35 Gy at the same dose rate. For HDR BT boost, we follow the recommendations of the ABS with a dose range from 10 to 15 Gy.

Results

Comparison between HDR and LDR BT yields a mean local control of about 80 % with variable complication rates.

Soft tissue sarcoma: Pediatric

Knowing the therapeutic possibilities offered by brachytherapy in STS for adults, the question is: "Is it possible to adapt this modality in children?" Although spectacular progress has been realized in chemotherapy as well in external beam irradiation, brachytherapy can also play a specific role in conservative treatment of STS in pediatric malignancies. Brachytherapy delivers irradiation with a very high dose gradient allowing a diminution of dose to the healthy structures and we know that in a child the growing, normal tissue is very radiosensitive.

At the Institut Gustave-Roussy, more than 50 years ago, the first BT in pediatric malignancies was realized by Chassagne, then by Gerbaulet, and now by Haie-Meder and their colleagues. Many articles and books were published during this past half century, and our experience is essentially based on the use of LDR BT (replaced recently in few patients by PDR BT). In all cases, the Paris system rules were applied for interstitial BT. For endo-cavitary BT, the recommendations of ICRU 38 were applied. More recently, the GEC-ESTRO recommendations are used to specify doses to the tumor, to the critical organs, volumes (GTV, CTV), dose rate, etc.

Four main tumor sites are individualized: trunk and limbs, head and neck, gynecologic, and prostate and bladder

Trunk and limbs

Perioperative BT is used in practically all cases and performed according to tumor surgical resection. In cases of an R2 resection, BT is applied as an anticipated boost of 25–30 Gy before external beam radiotherapy (EBT) (40–45 Gy). In cases where BT is used as monotherapy, LDR BT delivers a complete dose of 50–60 Gy.

Head and neck

In the example of sarcomas of the naso-labial sulcus (a frequent rhabdomyosarcoma [RMS] site), two afterloading systems scan be used, individually or together. Silk threads are used for very superficial lesions, and plastic afterloading tubes for the rest. Usually 3–5 threads/tubes are implanted and spaced at of 1–1.5 cm. The delivered dose with LDR BT is 55–60 Gy, with PDR BT: 40–45 Gy at 50 cGy per pulse, one pulse per hour. For a child younger than 7 years of age, the use of PDR is not recommended.

Gynecologic

For adult patients, the molded applicator devised by Chassagne is usually used, and made specially to order for each girl, which is essential for vaginal-cervix tumors. That allows conformality to tumor topography and to adapt patient by patient the positioning of future radioactive sources. The dose calculation can be complex and may depend on the treatment planning system. For LDR BT, the total dose is 60 Gy with a dose rate of 0.4–0.6 Gy/h.

Prostrate and bladder

The perioperative BT starts as a conservative procedure: tumor resection with partial prostatectomy and/or partial cystectomy in some cases but in all cases urethra preservation. Brachytherapy can be performed for bladder tumor alone by a suprapubic approach; however, the perineal approach is more often used to implant plastic tubes in a loop technique through the open pelvis. A dose of 60 Gy is delivered by LDR BT. In cases of PDR, the same total dose delivered as 40–50 cGy per pulse and one pulse per hour.

Results

Trunk and limbs: In this group of patients the pathology more often is non-RMS, and represents less than 10 % of children receiving BT. The results are worse when compared to those observed when compared to those observed in other tumor sites: 3-year survival rate is 68 %, local failure rate is 31 %; and metastases is 50 %. Still, we must focus on the high level of salvage using BT: 36 %.

Head and neck: For all the groups of children the local control approaches 80 %, but with a high level of sequelae rate of 37 %.

Gynecologic: The 5-year OS rate is 91 %, while the complication rate decreases when the target volume includes only residual disease and not the initial tumor volume.

Prostate and bladder: With a median follow-up of 4 years (10 months–14.5 years), 24 out of 26 boys are alive, 1 patient relapsed locally (out of the BT target volume) and succumbed to disease.

5.1 Complications of Therapy

One of the drawbacks of the use of irradiation in the pre- and postoperative setting is the issue of side effects. Multiple series have reported on significant side effects associated with the delivery of radiation. If one is serious about dose localization and the potential to lessen radiation-related side effects, then brachytherapy becomes the desired way to accomplish this goal. With that in mind, there have been various clinical reports which have utilized different brachytherapy techniques whether using permanent or temporary applications and high-dose or low-dose rates. Regardless of the dosimetric evaluations/prescription system used, the local control rates parallel those that have been reported with external beam series often with reduced grade 3/4 toxicity (Table 7).

There are those that dispute the advantages of brachytherapy when compared to IMRT. A series from Memorial Sloan Kettering in 2011 reported on 134 adults with high-grade STS. Seventy-one received LDR brachytherapy and the remaining patients were treated with IMRT to a median dose of 63 Gy. The 5-year local control was 92 % for the IMRT group and 81 % for the LDR group [51].

Others also dispute the need for any radiation after limb-sparing surgery. Baldini et al. reported on 242 patients with STS of the trunk and extremity [27]. If surgical margin was ≤1.0 cm, the local control was 87 % compared with 100 % local control with margins greater than 1.0 cm. This has been reported by other groups [52, 53].

Table 7 Brachytherapy in treatment of soft tissue sarcoma

Author	Year	Patients	Tx sequence	Local control	Complications	Comments
Ren [43]	2014	110	Surg → I-125p	74 % at 43 months	Wound – 4.5 % Nerve damage – 1.8 %	
Rosenblatt [44]	2014	32	Surg → Bx → ± EBI	87.5 % at 36 months	Gr III/IV wound −16 %	
Petera [45]	2010	45	Surg → Bx → ±EBI	74 % at 5 years	>Gr II – 4.4 %	↑ LC with dose ≥65 Gy
Itami [46]	2010	25	Surg → Bx	78 % 5 years	>Gr II – 11.5 %	50 % positive margin with ↓ LC
San Miguel [47]	2011	60	Surg → Bx → EBI	77 % at 9 years	Gr III – 30 %	↓ DFS with tumor >6 cm, positive margin
Fairweather [48]	2014	46	Surg → I-125p	74 % at 5 years	Gr III/IV – 24 %	
Alektiar [49]	1996	105	Surg → Bx ±EBI	86 % at 2 years	Overall wound – 26–38 %	↑ LC with Bx + EBI for positive margin
Youssef [50]	2002	60	Surg → Bx/Bx and EBI	71 % at 5 years	1 delay wound healing 2 infection	↓ LC with positive margin
Pisters [51]	1996	164	Randomized surg ± Bx	82 % – Bx 69 % – no Tx at 5 years	N/A	Limited advantage for HG lesions
Beltrami [52]	2008	112	Bx/EBI	91 % at 5 years	12 %	12.5 com

LC local control, *EBI* external beam irradiation, *p* permanent, *HG* high grade, *Bx* brachytherapy

6 Treatment of Pediatric STS

While similar treatment interventions are used for pediatric non-rhabdomyosarcoma soft tissue sarcoma, patients with RMS are frequently entered into national clinical trials that are trying to establish the best chemotherapy treatment, often based on histological subtype. The main difference in contemplating the use of radiation in adults and pediatric patients with STS lies in the concern related to potential second malignant neoplasm (SMN) development in addition to the local effects of irradiation such as impaired soft tissue/bone development.

It is well established that the age at which a child receives irradiation can have a profound effect on soft tissue/bone growth especially if treatment is given prior to the age of 7 [54, 55].

While these non-life-threatening side effects of radiation can have a significant effect on the child,

of greater concern is the potential of a radiation- or chemoradiation-induced SMN. These are life threatening. This problem is compounded by the fact that these children may be genetically predisposed to this development [56, 57].

When radiation is employed, there is a clear difference in the doses delivered for those patients who carry a diagnosis of RMS and for all other non-rhabdomyosarcoma (NRS) soft tissue sarcomas. The RMS doses rarely exceed 45 Gy, while treatment of NRS soft tissue sarcomas can include doses of up to 70.2 Gy [58]. There have been reports detailing dose variation based on surgical margin status. In the NRS soft tissue sarcomas series that have been reported, local control rates are similar regardless of dose and parallel most adults series (Table 8).

Because of concerns about local toxicities and the potential for second malignant neoplasm development, the use of brachytherapy has been

Table 8 Pediatric external beam for RMS/NRSTS

Author	Year	Patients	Treatment scheme	Local control	Grade III/IV complication	Comments
Krasin [58]	2010	34 HG NRSTS	Preop: 45–50.4 Post-op: 55–63 Defin 70.2 Brachy 45 Gy	87 %	47 % > Gr II Fibrosis	2 cm margin used 47 % Gr II fibrosis
Rodeberg [59]	2014	Inter risk RMS	Delayed primary resection with various dose schedule	100 – bladder dome 93 % extremity 80 % trunk	N/A	84 % Able to have dose reduction with delay
Cecchetto [60]	2000	25 RMS 27 NRSTS	Various	84–87 %	N/A	Worse LC with CTX alone

Table 9 Pediatric brachytherapy series

Author	Year	# Patients	Treatment scheme	Dose utilized	Med F/U	Local control
Gerbaulet [61]	1985	58	CTX → BX	60–65 Gy/5–7 days (L)	60 months	78 %
Fontanesi [62]	1994	46	Various	LDR	39 months	86 %
Merchant [63]	2000	31	12 BX 19BR + EBI	LDR		100 BX alone 13/14 LC BR/EBI
Pötter [64]	1995	18	BX BX + EBI	HDR/15–43 Gy/ 3–16 FX PDR 13-36 Gy/1 h fraction	14 months	STS 9/12 Ewing 6/6
Martelli [65]	2009	26 (Bladder) RMS	Resect → BX	LDR (60 Gy)	48 months	25/26
Viani [66]	2008	18	HDR HDR + EBI	HDR	79 months	8/8 HDR 9/10 HDR/EBI
Folkert [67]	2014	75	HDR/10 RT 8–12 Gy	HDR	7.8 years	63 % initial 46 % for relapsed case

CTX chemotherapy, *PDR* pulsed dose rate, *Bx* brachytherapy, *EBI* external beam irradiation

investigated. It has a rich history of utilization for more than 30 years and has shown excellent local control rates with acceptable local toxicities and what appears to be a low rate of second malignant neoplasms (Table 9).

7 Technical Aspects of Brachytherapy in the Treatment of STS

With few exceptions, the use of brachytherapy for both adult and pediatric STS is done in an operative theater during the definitive surgical procedure. It is critically important to have coordination with the surgeon and rehabilitation physicians when it comes to limb salvage procedures. This is key in that is allows for better understanding of how the wound will be closed and what strategies to employ in order to get the patient as much future function as possible.

During the surgical procedure, we prefer to have the surgeon outline the gross tumor volume with surgical clips. We request that this be done in at least four positions: proximal, distal, medial, and lateral. If there are special areas that need to be identified, special clip arrangements, such as using double surgical clips, can be utilized. We will request from the pathologist information on the "margins" to determine positivity or negativity. We strive for negative margins where possible. This helps with catheter placement decisions.

Next we pay attention to wound closure. Often tissue has to be undermined in order to affect a primary closure. It is critical for the radiation oncology team to understand how the closure is to take place as it may affect how catheters/seeds are placed.

Once the closure is identified and discussed, we will place the catheters. Generally we will use either a horizontal (perpendicular to wound) or vertical (parallel) catheter placement strategy. In general, the horizontal placement strategy will result in more catheters being placed than in the vertical technique. We always try to place the center or middle catheter first and then proceed to place the remaining catheters at 1–1.5 cm spacing. With each catheter placement, we reassess the wound closure and make adjustments as needed. The catheter will then be secured in either two or three sites with absorbable suture material (we prefer 6-0 chromic suture). In this way we assure that when the closure takes place, the surgeon is aware of the geometry we are trying to achieve. We do not cut any catheter that is extending outside the skin surface until simulation is completed. At that time, if we are using HDR techniques, we make sure 4–5 cm extends from the skin surface. If LDR techniques are being utilized, we like at least 2 cm from the skin surface from the side that is to be loaded.

One of the critical decisions that are made is the implant volume to be treated and the catheter placement technique. The two most common catheter placement techniques are the "buried" technique, where one side of the catheter is blind ended (see Skin chapter) and is buried in one of the margins. This is usually 2–5 cm beyond the clips that have been placed by the surgeons. The second technique employs a through and through technique where both ends of the catheter can be utilized, although blind-ended catheters can also be used effectively.

Our next step is to perform a CT simulation and treatment planning. We try to do this as soon as the surgical team will allow the patient to be brought for evaluation. We also try to ensure that the treatment site is stabilized. This usually occurs 24–48 h after surgery.

Much has been discussed regarding how soon treatment should be initiated. In general we wait for final pathology report to make sure no unusual findings are reported that may alter the brachytherapy decision. If none occur, we start the treatment as the treatment plan is ready and as long as the surgeons are OK with treatment proceeding. Some groups have suggested waiting for up to 7 days before treatment initiation in an effort to reduce wound complications. We believe treatment can be initiated earlier than that, even within 72 h, so long as the surgical team approves. We are concerned that waiting a full 7 days to initiate treatment may allow a "longer" access time for infection to occur even in the face of antibiotic coverage. In addition if one extrapolates from the keloid brachytherapy postoperative data, there is little chance of wound dehiscence when treatment is introduced within 24 h as most of fibroblast depositions for wound closure take place in the first 24–48 h.

Various brachytherapy dose recommendations have been used in both adult and pediatric STS. They are noted in Tables 6, 7, and 9.

Our group most frequently utilizes HDR techniques. The following table outlines our usual recommendation. Note that we try to keep less than 50 % of the treatment volume from receiving 125 % or more of the prescribed dose.

Brachytherapy type	Situation	Dose/FR	# Fx	Schedule
HDR	Monotherapy	325–350	12	BID
		Or		
		600–800	6	QD
	Boost	325–350	6	BID
		Or		
		600–800	3	QD
LDR	Monotherapy	42–50/ HR	N/A	60 Gy total
	Boost	35–45/ HR	N/A	16–24 Gy total

Conclusion

Soft tissue sarcomas present unique challenges to both the patient and treating physician team.

They are unique in that they are age independent, have 50 plus subtypes, and in general their aggressiveness is tied to tumor grade. Soft tissue sarcomas have varied rates of regional (lymphatic)/distant spread, and their presentations are also quite varied. The treatment of soft tissue sarcoma has evolved from amputation first to limb salvage/preservation if possible. In order to improve local control, various adjunct therapies have been introduced. Chemotherapy and radiation have been used in the pre-/postoperative setting with various reported success.

One of the most consistent prognostic factors besides tumor grade has been resection margin positivity but even that has been challenged.

With various opportunities to interdict with radiation, there have been advocates and detractors of both external beam and brachytherapy techniques. However, there is no disputing the greater dose profiling that brachytherapy offers. The main drawback of brachytherapy has been historically related to patient hospitalization requirements for low-dose radiation techniques. However, with high-dose radiation techniques, these issues are mitigated.

Brachytherapy for soft tissue sarcoma requires excellent coordination with the surgical oncology and rehabilitative service participants. This helps the brachytherapist to best understand functional expectations postoperatively and allows for better radiation treatment planning. In general, it is best if patients receive treatment at centers that have dedicated orthopedic/surgical oncology teams that work closely with experienced medical and radiation oncologists and are supported by strong ancillary service teams that recognize the unique challenges which patients with soft tissue sarcoma present.

Acknowledgements The authors wish to thank Susan King for her assistance in the editing and preparation of this chapter.

References

1. Morgagni G. De Sedibus, Et Causis Morborum Per Anatomen Indagatis Libri Quinque. Published 1761 by Ex Typographia Rmondiniana in Venetiis. Written in Latin
2. Gronchi A, Casali PG (2013) Adjuvant therapy for high-risk soft tissue sarcoma in the adult. Curr Treat Options Oncol 14(3):415–424. doi:10.1007/s11864-013-0243-7
3. Cancer Facts & Figures 2014. American Cancer Society
4. Fong Y, Coit DG, Woodruff JM et al (1993) Lymph node metastasis from soft tissue sarcoma in adults. Analysis of data from a prospective database of 1772 sarcoma patients. Ann Surg 217(1):72–77
5. Nelen SD, Vogelaar FJ, Gilissen F et al (2013) Case report, lymph node metastasis after a soft tissue sarcoma of the leg: a case report and a review of the literature. Case Rep Surg 2013:930361. http://dx.doi.org/10.1155/2013/930361
6. Mazeron JJ, Suit HD (1987) Lymph nodes as sites of metastases from sarcomas of soft tissue. Cancer 60(8):1800–1808
7. Daigeler A, Kuhnen C, Moritz R et al (2009) Lymph node metastases in soft tissue sarcomas: a single center analysis of 1,597 patients. Arch Surg 394(2):321–329
8. Billingsley KG, Lewis JJ, Leung DH et al (1999) Multifactorial analysis of the survival of patients with distant metastasis arising from primary extremity sarcoma. Cancer 85(2):389–395
9. Pisters PW, Leung DH, Woodruff J et al (1996) Analysis of prognostic factors in 1,041 patients with localized soft tissue sarcomas of the extremities. J Clin Oncol 14(5):1679–1689
10. Wexler LH, Helman LJ (1994) Pediatric soft tissue sarcomas. CA Cancer J Clin 44(4):211–247
11. Neville HL, Raney RB, Andrassy RJ et al (2000) Multidisciplinary management of pediatric soft-tissue sarcoma. Oncology 14(10):1471–1481; discussion 1482–1486, 1489–1490
12. Spunt S, Catherine S, Poquette A et al (1999) Prognostic factors for children and adolescents with surgically resected nonrhabdomyosarcoma soft tissue sarcoma: an analysis of 121 patients treated at St Jude Children's Research Hospital. J Clin Oncol 17(2):3697–3705
13. Zahm SH, Fraumeni JF (1997) The epidemiology of soft tissue sarcoma. Semin Oncol 24(5):504–514
14. Ferrari A, Bisogno G, Macaluso A (2007) Soft-tissue sarcomas in children and adolescents with neurofibromatosis type 1. Cancer 109(7):1406–1412
15. Campos FG, Martinez C, Novaes M et al (2015) Desmoid tumors: clinical features and outcome of an unpredictable and challenging manifestation of familial adenomatous polyposis. Cancer 14(2):211–219
16. Goto M, Miller RW, Ishikawa Y et al (1996) Excess of rare cancers in Werner syndrome (adult progeria). Cancer Epidemiol Biomarkers Prev 5(4):239–246

17. Kleinerman RA, Schonfeld SJ et al (2012) Sarcomas in hereditary retinoblastoma. Clin Sarcoma Res 2(1):15. doi:10.1186/2045-3329-2-15

18. Cohen RJ, Curtis RE, Inskip PD et al (2005) The risk of developing second cancers among survivors of childhood soft tissue sarcoma. Cancer 103(11):2391–2396

19. McClain KL, Leach CT, Jenson HB et al (1995) Association of Epstein-Barr virus with leiomyosarcomas in children with AIDS. N Engl J Med 332(1):12–18

20. Schwarzbach MH, Dimitrakopoulou-Strauss A, Willeke F et al (2000) Clinical value of [18-F] fluoro-deoxyglucose positron emission tomography imaging in soft tissue sarcomas. Ann Surg 231(3):380–386

21. O'Donnell PW, Griffin AM, Eward WC et al (2014) The effect of the setting of a positive surgical margin in soft tissue sarcoma. Cancer 120(18):2866–2875

22. Zagars GK, Ballio MT, Pisters PW et al (2003) Prognostic factors for patients with localized soft-tissue sarcoma treated with conservation surgery and radiation therapy: an analysis of 1225 patients. Cancer 97(10):2530–2543

23. Rosenberg SA, Tepper J, Glatstein E et al (1982) The treatment of soft-tissue sarcomas of the extremities: prospective randomized evaluations of (1) limb-sparing surgery plus radiation therapy compared with amputation and (2) the role of adjuvant chemotherapy. Ann Surg 196(3):305–315

24. Swallow CJ, Catton CN (2007) Local management of adult soft tissue sarcomas. Semin Oncol 34(3):256–269

25. Levine EA (1999) Prognostic factors in soft tissue sarcoma. Semin Surg Oncol 17(1):23–32

26. Jones NB, Iwenofu H, Scharschmidt T et al (2012) Prognostic factors and staging for soft for soft tissue sarcomas: an update. Surg Oncol Clin N Am 21(2):187–200. doi:10.1016/j.soc.2011.12.003, Epub 2012 Jan 9

27. Baldini EH, Goldberg J, Jenner C et al (1999) Long-term outcomes after function-sparing surgery without radiotherapy for soft tissue sarcoma of the extremities and trunk. Clin Oncol 17(10):3252–3259

28. Curtis KK, Ashman JB, Beauchamp CP et al (2011) Neoadjuvant chemoradiation compared to neoadjuvant radiation alone and surgery alone for Stage II and III soft tissue sarcoma of the extremities. Radiat Oncol 6:91. doi:10.1186/1748-717X-6-91

29. Fein DA, Lee WR, Lanciano RM (1995) Management of extremity soft tissue sarcomas with limb-sparing surgery and postoperative irradiation: Do total dose, overall treatment time, and the surgery-radiotherapy interval impact on local Control? Int J Radiati Oncol Biol Phys 32(4):969–976

30. Cai L, Mirimanoff RO, Mouhsine E et al (2013) Prognostic factors in adult soft tissue sarcoma treated with surgery combined with radiotherapy: a retrospective single-center study on 164 patients. Rare Tumors 5(4):e55. doi:10.4081/rt.2013.e55

31. Folkert MR, Singer S, Brennan MF et al (2014) Comparison of local recurrence with conventional and intensity-modulated radiation therapy for primary soft-tissue sarcomas of the extremity. J Clin Oncol 32(29):3236–3241. doi:10.1200/JCO.2013.53.9452

32. Pan E, Goldberg SI, Chen YL et al (2014) Role of post-operative boost for soft tissue sarcomas with positive margins following pre-operative radiation and surgery. J Surg Oncol 110(7):817–822. doi:10.1002/jso.23741, Epub 2014 Aug 11

33. Dincbas FO, Oksuz DC, Yetmen O et al (2014) Neoadjuvant treatment with preoperative radiotherapy for extremity soft tissue sarcomas; long-term results from a single institution in Turkey. Asian Pac J Cancer Prev 15(4):1775–1781

34. Mullen JT, Kobayashi W, Wang JJ et al (2012) Long-term follow-up of patients treated with neoadjuvant chemotherapy and radiotherapy for large, extremity soft tissue sarcomas. Cancer 118(15):3758–3765. doi:10.1002/cncr.26696

35. Look Hong NJ, Hornicek F, Harmon DC et al (2013) Neoadjuvant chemoradiotherapy for patients with high-risk extremity and truncal sarcomas: a 10 year single institution retrospective study. Eur J Cancer 49(4):875–883. doi:10.1016/j.ejca.2012.10.002

36. Felderhof JM, Creutzberg CL, Putter H et al (2013) Long-term clinical outcome of patients with soft tissue sarcomas treated with limb-sparing surgery and postoperative radiotherapy. Acta Oncol 52(4):745–752. doi:10.3109/0284186X.2012.709947

37. Trovik CS, Scandinavian Sarcoma Group Project (2001) Local recurrence of soft tissue sarcoma. A Scandinavian Sarcoma Group Project. Acta Orthop Scand Suppl 72(300):1–31

38. ESMO/European Sarcoma Network Working Group (2014) ESMO clinical practice guidelines for diagnosis, treatment and follow-up. Soft tissue and visceral sarcomas. Ann Oncol 25(Suppl 3):iii102–iii112. doi:10.1093/annonc/mdu254

39. Holloway C, DeLaney T, Alektiar KM et al (2013) American Brachytherapy Society (ABS) consensus statement for sarcoma brachytherapy. Brachytherapy 12:179–190

40. Grimer R, Judson I, Peake D et al (2010) Guidelines for the management of soft tissue sarcomas: British Sarcoma Group. Sarcoma 2010:506182. doi:10.1155/2010/506182

41. Lartigau E, Gerbaulet A (2002) GEC/ESTRO soft tissue sarcomas of the extremities in adults. ACCO, Leuven, Belgium. GEC-ESTRO Handbook 2002

42. NCCN Guidelines; Version 2 (2014) National comprehensive cancer network, soft tissue sarcoma. http://www.nccn.org/professionals/physician_gls/f_guidelines.asp

43. Ren C, Shi R, Min L et al (2014) Experience of interstitial permanent I 125 brachytherapy for extremity soft tissue sarcomas. Clin Oncol 26(4):230–235. doi:10.1016/j.clon.2014.01.004

44. Rosenblatt E, Meushar N, Bar-Deroma R et al (2003) Interstitial brachytherapy in soft tissue sarcomas: the Rambam experience. Isr Med Assoc J 5(8):547–551

45. Petera J, Soumarova R, Ruzickova J et al (2010) Perioperative hyperfractionated high-dose rate brachytherapy for the treatment of soft tissue sarcomas: a multicentric experience. Ann Surg Oncol 17(1):206–210. doi:10.1245/s10434-00-0684-1

46. Itami J, Sumi M, Beppu Y (2010) High-dose rate brachytherapy alone in postoperative soft tissue sarcomas with close or positive margins. Brachytherapy 9(4):349–353. doi:10.1016/j.brachy.2009.07.012

47. San Miguel I, San Julian M, Cambeiro M et al (2011) Determinants of toxicity, patterns of failure, and outcome among adult patients with soft tissue sarcomas of the extremity and superficial trunk treated with greater that conventional doses of perioperative high-dose-rate brachytherapy and external beam radiotherapy. Int J Radiat Oncol Biol Phys 81(4):e529–e539. doi:10.1016/j.ijrobp.2011.04.063

48. Fairweather M, Wang J, Devlin PM et al (2015) Safety and efficacy of radiation dose delivered via Iodine-125 brachytherapy mesh implantation for deep cavity sarcomas. Ann Surg Oncol 22(5):1455–1463

49. Alektiar KM, Leung DH, Brennan MF et al (1996) The effect of combined external beam radiotherapy and brachytherapy on local control and wound complications in patients with high-grade soft tissue sarcomas of the extremity with positive microscopic margin. Int J Radiat Oncol Biol Phys 36(2):321–324

50. Youssef E, Fontanesi J, Mott M et al (2002) Long-term outcome of combined modality therapy in retroperitoneal and deep-trunk soft-tissue sarcoma: analysis of prognostic factors. Int J Radiat Oncol Biol Phys 54(2):514–519

51. Pisters PW, Harrison LB, Leung DH et al (1996) Long-term results of a prospective randomized trial of adjuvant brachytherapy in soft tissue sarcoma. Clin Oncol 14(3):859–868

52. Beltrami G, Rüdiger HA, Mela MM et al (2008) Limb salvage surgery in combination with brachytherapy and external beam radiation for high-grade soft tissue sarcomas. Eur J Surg Oncol 34(7):811–816

53. Alektiar K, Zelefsky M, Brennan M (2000) Morbidity of adjuvant brachytherapy in soft tissue sarcoma of the extremity and superficial trunk. Int J Radiat Oncol Biol Phys 47(5):1273–1279

54. Dörr W, Kallfels S, Herrmann T (2013) Late bone and soft tissue sequelae of childhood radiotherapy. Relevance of treatment age and radiation dose in 146 children treated 1970 and 1997. Strahlenther Onkol 189(7):529–534. doi:10.1007/s00066-013-0361-y

55. Paulino AC (2004) Late effects of radiotherapy for pediatric extremity sarcomas. Int J Radiat Oncol Biol Phys 60(1):265–274

56. Hennewig U, Kaatsch P, Blettner M et al (2014) Local radiation dose and solid second malignant neoplasms after childhood cancer in Germany: a nested case-control study. Radiat Environ Biophys 53(3):485–493. doi:10.1007/s00411-014-0550-9

57. Guerin S, Guibout C, Shamsaldin A et al (2007) Concomitant chemo-radiotherapy and local dose of radiation as risk factors for second malignant neoplasms after solid cancer in childhood: a case-control study. Int J Cancer 120(1):96–102

58. Krasin MJ, Davidoff AM, Xiong X et al (2010) Preliminary results from a prospective study using limited margin radiotherapy in pediatric and young adult patients with high-grade nonrhabdomyosarcoma soft-tissue sarcoma. Int J Radiat Oncol Biol Phys 76(3):874–878. doi:10.1016/j.ijrobp.2009.02.074

59. Rodeberg RD, Wharam MD, Lyden ER et al (2015) Delayed primary excision with subsequent modification of radiotherapy dose for intermediate-risk rhabdomysarcoma: a report from the Children's Oncology Group Soft Tissue Sarcoma Committee. Int J Cancer 137(1):204–211. 2014 UICC. doi:10.1002/ijc.29351

60. Cecchetto G, Modesto CM, Sotti G et al (2000) Importance of local treatment in pediatric soft tissue sarcomas with microscopic residual after primary surgery: results of the Italian Cooperative Study RMS-88. Med Pediatr Oncol 34:97–101

61. Gerbaulet A, Panis X, Flamant F, Chassagne D (1985) Iridium afterloading curietherapy in the treatment of pediatric malignancies. The Institut Gustave Roussy experience. Cancer 56(6):1274–1279

62. Fontanesi J, Rao BN, Fleming ID et al (1994) Pediatric brachytherapy. The St. Jude Children's Research Hospital experience. Cancer 74(2):733–739

63. Merchant TE, Parsh N, del Valle PL et al (2000) Brachytherapy for pediatric soft-tissue sarcoma. Int J Radiat Oncol Biol Phys 46(2):427–432

64. Pötter R, Knocke TH, Kovacs G et al (1995) Brachytherapy in the combined modality treatment of pediatric malignancies. Principles and preliminary experience with treatment of soft tissue sarcoma (recurrence) and Ewing's sarcoma. Klin Padiatr 207(4):164–173

65. Martelli H, Haie-Meder C, Branchereau S et al (2009) Conservative surgery plus brachytherapy treatment for boys with prostate and/or bladder neck rhabdomyosarcoma: a single team experience. J Pediatr Surg 44(1):190–196. doi:10.1016/j.jpedsurg.2008.10.040

66. Viani GA, Novaes PE, Jacinto AA et al (2008) High-dose-rate brachytherapy for soft tissue sarcoma in children: a single institution experience. Radiat Oncol 3:9. doi:10.1186/1748-717X-3-9

67. Folkert MR, Tong WY, LaQuaglia MP et al (2014) 20-year experience with intraoperative high-dose-rate brachytherapy for pediatric sarcoma: outcomes, toxicity, and practice recommendations. Int Radiat Oncol Biol Phys 90(2):362–368. doi:10.1016/j.ijrobp.2014.06.016

Index

© Springer International Publishing Switzerland 2016
P. Montemaggi et al. (eds.), *Brachytherapy: An International Perspective*, Medical Radiology,
DOI 10.1007/978-3-319-26791-3